Hematologic Cancers and their Treatment

Hematologic Cancers and their Treatment

Edited by Wedge Burton

hayle
medical

New York

Hayle Medical,
750 Third Avenue, 9th Floor,
New York, NY 10017, USA

Visit us on the World Wide Web at:
www.haylemedical.com

ISBN: 978-1-63241-704-6

Cataloging-in-Publication Data

Hematologic cancers and their treatment / edited by Wedge Burton.
    p. cm.
Includes bibliographical references and index.
ISBN 978-1-63241-704-6
1. Hematological oncology. 2. Blood--Cancer--Treatment. 3. Lymphoproliferative disorders.
4. Leukemia. I. Burton, Wedge.
RC280.H47 H46 2019
616.994 18--dc23

Table of Contents

Preface

This book was inspired by the evolution of our times; to answer the curiosity of inquisitive minds. Many developments have occurred across the globe in the recent past which has transformed the progress in the field.

Hematologic cancers are the cancers affecting the blood, lymph, bone marrow and the lymphatic system. These systems are intimately connected with each other through the circulatory and immune system. Thus, a cancer in one element affects the others as well. Malignancies in the hematological system are malignant neoplasms, derived from myeloid and lymphoid cell lines. Chromosomal translocations are a primary reason of hematologic cancer. For the diagnosis of a hematological malignancy, biopsy from a lymph node or a bone marrow biopsy, a blood film and complete blood count may be performed. The treatment of hematologic cancers may be addressed with radiotherapy, chemotherapy, immunotherapy or a bone marrow transplant. If partial or complete remission has been achieved, a follow-up of the patient is undertaken at regular intervals to monitor for secondary malignancies and recurrences. This book is compiled in such a manner, that it will provide in-depth knowledge about hematologic cancers and their treatment. Most of the topics introduced in this book cover new techniques of cancer treatment. It is meant for students who are looking for an elaborate reference text on this domain.

This book was developed from a mere concept to drafts to chapters and finally compiled together as a complete text to benefit the readers across all nations. To ensure the quality of the content we instilled two significant steps in our procedure. The first was to appoint an editorial team that would verify the data and statistics provided in the book and also select the most appropriate and valuable contributions from the plentiful contributions we received from authors worldwide. The next step was to appoint an expert of the topic as the Editor-in-Chief, who would head the project and finally make the necessary amendments and modifications to make the text reader-friendly. I was then commissioned to examine all the material to present the topics in the most comprehensible and productive format.

I would like to take this opportunity to thank all the contributing authors who were supportive enough to contribute their time and knowledge to this project. I also wish to convey my regards to my family who have been extremely supportive during the entire project.

Editor

Prognostic Value of *Isocitrate Dehydrogenase* Mutations in Myelodysplastic Syndromes: A Retrospective Cohort Study and Meta-Analysis

Jie Jin[1,2¶], Chao Hu[1,2¶], Mengxia Yu[1,2¶], Feifei Chen[1,2], Li Ye[1,2], Xiufeng Yin[1,2], Zhengping Zhuang[3], Hongyan Tong[1,2]*

1 Department of Hematology, the First Affiliated Hospital of Zhejiang University, Hangzhou, People's Republic of China, 2 Institute of Hematology, Zhejiang University School of Medicine, Hangzhou, People's Republic of China, 3 Surgical Neurology Branch, National Institute of Neurological Disorders and Stroke, National Institutes of Health, Bethesda, Maryland, United States of America

Abstract

Background: Recent genomic sequencing efforts have identified a number of recurrent mutations in myelodysplastic syndromes (MDS) that may contribute to disease progression and overall survival, including mutations in *isocitrate dehydrogenases 1* and *2* (*IDH1* and *IDH2*).

Methods: Pretreatment bone marrow (BM) samples were acquired from mononuclear cells in 146 adult patients with de novo MDS from January 2006 to June 2013. Polymerase chain reaction (PCR) and direct sequencing were performed on exon 4 of *IDH1/2* genes and mutation status was correlated with overall survival (OS) and leukemia-free survival (LFS). We then performed a meta-analysis combining previously published and current studies to explore the effect of *IDH* mutations on OS and LFS in MDS.

Results: In our study, somatic mutations of either *IDH* gene were discovered in 11 MDS patients (7.53%) and were significantly correlated with poorer OS ($P = 0.007$). *IDH* mutations were specifically associated with a poorer OS in the intermediate-1 risk group by the International Prognostic Scoring System (IPSS) ($P = 0.039$). In addition, we discovered decitabine achieved a better therapeutic effect compared to other treatments in *IDH* mutation-positive patients ($P = 0.023$). We identified six previous studies of *IDH* mutations in MDS. A meta-analysis of these studies included 111 MDS patients *IDH* mutations and 1671 MDS patients with wild-type *IDH1/2*. The hazard ratios (HRs) of OS and LFS for patients with *IDH* mutations were 1.62 (95% CI, 1.27–2.09) and 2.21 (95% CI, 1.48–3.30), respectively.

Conclusion: The results from our study and the meta-analysis provide firm evidence that *IDH* mutations are significantly associated with poorer clinical outcomes in MDS. Identification of *IDH* mutations may be pivotal for better risk stratification in MDS patients and improving IPSS score. Additionally, hypomethylating agents may be an effective treatment option for MDS patients with *IDH* mutations.

Editor: Zhuang Zuo, UT MD Anderson Cancer Center, United States of America

Funding: This study was supported by grants from Zhejiang Province Fund for Distinguished Young Scholars (LR12H08001), the Foundation of Key Innovation Team of Zhejiang Province (2011R50015), National Public Health Grand Research Foundation (201202017), major program of Science Technology Department of Zhejiang Province fund (2013c03043-2) and the National Natural Science Foundation of China (No.30870914, No.81270582). The funders had no role in study design, data collection and analysis, decision to publish, or preparation of the manuscript.

Competing Interests: The authors have declared that no competing interests exist.

* Email: zjuhongyantong@163.com

¶ These authors are co-first authors.

Introduction

Myelodysplastic syndromes (MDS) comprise a heterogeneous group of hematological disorders defined by blood cytopenias due to ineffective hematopoiesis and an increased risk of developing acute myeloid leukemia (AML) [1,2]. Despite recent advances in therapeutic methods, treatments for MDS are currently tailored to individual patient needs, making the precise forecast of the prognosis an important component of treating patients [3]. Current prognostic scoring systems for patients with MDS are mainly based on karyotypic abnormalities and certain clinical features that are used to stratify risk. Although existing systems such as the IPSS [4], Revised-IPSS [5] and WHO-classification-based Prognostic Scoring System (WPSS) [6] help to estimate patient outcomes and guide treatment decisions, there remains significant variability in prognosis. Hence, novel molecular markers may offer more precise cancer phenotypes and more accurate estimation of prognosis for MDS patients.

Until now, the pathogenesis of MDS has not been clearly identified, but it is generally acknowledged that genetic mutations and dysfunction of gene contribute to the development and progression of this preleukemic disease [7,8]. Genetic mutations are not currently used in estimating prognosis in MDS but are likely key determinants of overall survival and clinical phenotypes [9]. Therefore, contributing gene mutations may supplement current prognostic systems to improve the prediction of prognosis for MDS patients.

IDH 1/2 are key metabolic enzymes that convert isocitrate to α-ketoglutarate (α-KG or 2-oxoglutarate, 2-OG), which is an essential cofactor for α-KG dependent dioxygenases [10,11]. These enzymes are associated with diverse cellular processes such as adapting to histone deacetylation, hypoxia, and DNA demethylation [12]. Therefore, *IDH* mutations may be causally linked to the clinical impacts of patients with MDS. We identified 146 patients with primary MDS and analysed *IDH* mutation status with OS and LFS. We then performed a meta-analysis combining our data with those of the published literature to furnish a more accurate estimation of the relationship between *IDH* mutations and MDS.

Methods

Patients

One hundred and forty-six adult patients with de novo MDS diagnosed according to World Health Organization (WHO) 2001 criteria [13] were recruited at the department of hematology, the First Affiliated Hospital of Zhejiang University. MDS patients were stratified by cytogenetic risk according to IPSS protocols [4]. All of the subjects were well-informed about the study and provided written informed consent to participate this study. This study was approved by the Institutional Review boards of the First Affiliated Hospital of Zhejiang University. Follow-up data were obtained by telephoning and reviewing patients' medical records. 7 of 146 patients (4.79%) were lost to follow-up. Treatments were performed for patients including chemotherapy regimens (the GAA regimen (granulocyte-colony stimulating factor (G-CSF) 200 µg/m^2 per day on days 1–14, aclacinomycin 10 mg per day on days 1–14; cytarabine 10 mg/m^2, days 1–14; n = 2); the GHA regimen (G-CSF 200 µg/m^2 per day on days 1–14, homoharringtonine 1 mg/m^2 per day on days 1–14, cytarabine 10 mg/m^2 per day on days 1–14; n = 6); the DA or IA regimen (daunorubicin 40–45 mg/m^2 per day on days 1–3 or idarubicin 8–12 mg/m^2 per day on days 1–3, cytarabine 100 mg/m^2 per day on days 1–7; n = 8); decitabine (20 mg/m^2/day, days 1–5 or 15 mg/m^2, q8 h, days 1–3; n = 44)) and supportive care (antibiotics, androgen, all-*trans* retinoic acid, blood product transfusion and iron chelation therapy; n = 86).

Mutational Analyses for the IDH1 and IDH2 Genes

Pretreatment BM specimens were enriched for mononuclear cells using Ficoll density gradient centrifugation. Genomic DNA was extracted from cryopreserved mononuclear cells using the DNA Kit (Sangon, Shanghai, China) according to the manufacturer's instructions. Approximately 100 ng of DNA was used for each PCR reaction. The primer pairs were the same as those designed by Patnaik et al [14]. The PCR amplification conditions were as follows: 95°C for 5 minutes; followed by 40 cycles of 95°C for 30 seconds, 60°C for 30 seconds, and 72°C for 30 seconds; and finally, 72°C for 5 minutes. PCR products were directly sequenced on both strands using an ABI 3730 automatic sequencer by Sangon.

Statistical Analysis

OS end-points were defined as the time from diagnosis of MDS to death due to any cause or to the time of last follow-up. LFS end-points were defined as the time from MDS diagnosis to either AML progression or death or failure or alive without disease progression at the date of most recent follow-up. Length of survival comparisons were analyzed using the Kaplan-Meier method. For categorical parameters, overall group differences were compared with the χ^2 or Fisher exact test. For continuous variables, overall group differences were evaluated with the Mann-Whitney U test. A Cox proportional hazards model was performed to evaluate the effect of endpoint on OS and LFS for multivariate analysis. Statistical analysis was performed with SPSS 16.0 software package (SPSS, Chicago, USA). All tests were 2-tailed, and a *P*-value of less than 0.05 was considered statistically significant.

Meta-analysis of *IDH1/2* Mutations in MDS

To further assess the relationship between *IDH1/2* mutations and MDS risk, we conducted a meta-analysis combining our study data with published studies on *IDH* mutations in MDS [3,14,15,16,17,18]. Two independent reviewers (CH and MXY) performed a systematic literature search using ISI Web of Science, PubMed and the Cochrane Library for relevant papers published before December 2013 by the search term "(MDS OR myelodysplastic syndrome OR preleukemia OR myelodysplasia) AND (*IDH1* OR *IDH2*)." Reviews and references of related articles were checked for missing information. Eligible papers met all the following criteria: (1) assessed the association between *IDH1/2* mutations and outcomes in MDS; (2) detailed survival information of patients with *IDH1* or *IDH2* mutations; (3) reported the study in English. Animal studies, letters to the editor without original data, reviews and case reports were excluded. In the event of multiple publications from overlapping study populations or the same study, only the one with the largest sample size was selected (Figure 1).

The following data were extracted from each article: first author's name, year of publication, country of origin, participant gender, participant age, sample size, MDS subtype, criteria for classification of MDS, karyotypes and IPSS classification. If the required data for the meta-analysis were not available in the published study, we contacted the corresponding authors for missing data.

A general variance-based method and a mathematical HR approximation method [19] in this meta-analysis were simultaneously used to estimate the summary HRs and their 95% CIs for the combined large sample set. Assessing heterogeneity and choosing fixed-effect or random-effect were performed as described previously [20]. Sensitivity analysis was conducted by sequential omission of individual studies and evaluated influence of each study on the stability of the results. Cumulative analysis was performed by assortment of publication time. Publication bias was assessed by funnel plot and Egger's test [21,22]. All statistical analyses were carried out in STATA 11.0 statistical software (Stata Corporation, College Station, Texas), and a *P*-value less than 0.05 was considered significant.

Results

Patient Characteristics

The current study included 146 patients (85 men and 61 women). The median age was 55 years (range 18–85). According to the WHO criteria, 7 (4.79%) patients were classified as refractory anemia (RA), 3 (2.05%) as RA with ringed sideroblasts (RARS), 50 (34.25%) as refractory cytopenia with multilineage dysplasia (RCMD), 44 (30.14%) as RA with excess blasts type 1 (RAEB1) and 42 (28.77%) as RAEB2 [23]. Cytogenetic results were available for 141 patients. The data demonstrated a low risk in 99 patients, an intermediate risk in 26 patients and a high risk in

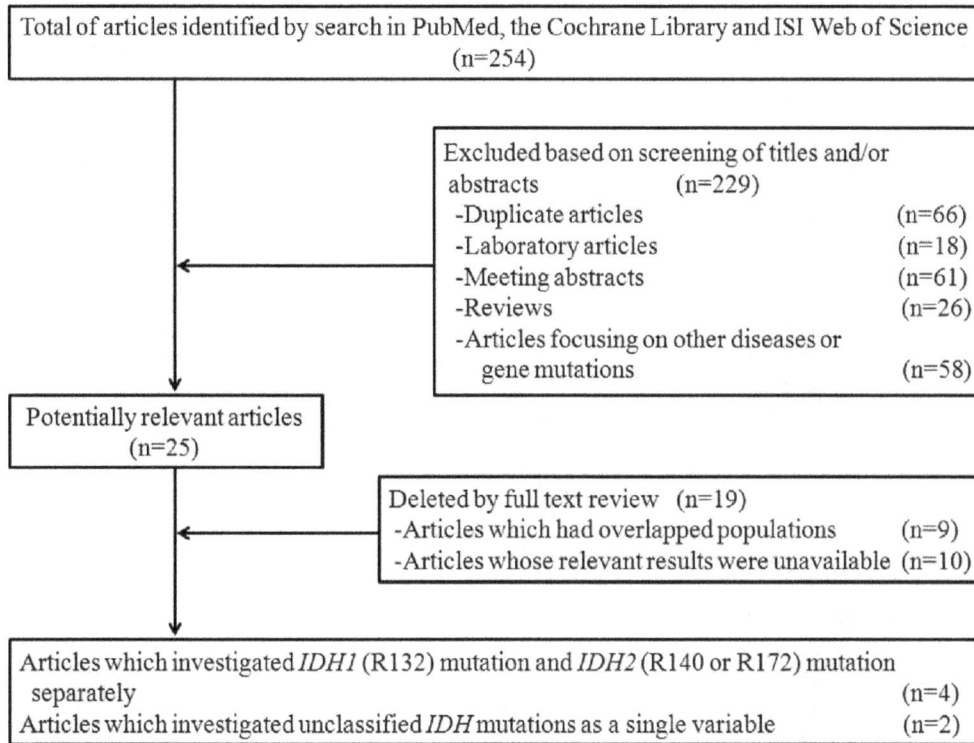

Figure 1. Flow diagram of study selection.

16 patients. IPSS risk distributions were: low risk in 7 patients (4.97%), intermediate-1 risk in 76 patients (53.90%), intermediate-2 risk in 46 patients (32.62%) and high risk in 12 patients (8.51%).

IDH1/2 Mutations in MDS and Association with Clinical Outcomes

IDH1/2 mutations were identified in eleven (7.53%) MDS patients, six (4.11%) had mutations in IDH1 and five (3.42%) had mutations in IDH2 (Table 1). Among MDS patients with IDH1/2 mutations, two (18.18%) were classified as RAEB1, seven (63.64%) as RAEB2 and two (18.18%) as RCMD. Seven MDS patients (64.64%) with IDH mutations had a normal karyotype. Of the four patients with IDH1/2 mutations and abnormal karyotypes, three (75%) carried a −7/7q-. All MDS patients with IDH1 mutations carried an IDH1 R132C mutation, whereas all patients with IDH2 mutations carried an IDH2 R140Q mutation. IDH1/2 mutants carried significantly more bone marrow (BM) blasts than MDS patients with wild-type IDH1/2 (P = 0.022); no significant differences were observed in age, sex, white blood cell (WBC) count, hemoglobin, platelet count, WHO subtype, cytogenetics or IPSS.

The median survival time was 512 days (range 100–924 days) in the IDH1/2 mutant group and 956 days (range, 632–1280 days) in the wild-type IDH1/2 group. Survival analysis demonstrated MDS patients harboring IDH1/2 mutations had significantly shorter OS compared to patients with wild-type IDH1/2 (P = 0.007) (Figure 2A). Further, we found IDH1 mutations negatively affected OS in MDS (P = 0.030) rather than IDH2 mutations (P = 0.067) (Figure 2C, E). The presence of IDH1/2 mutations did not influence the LFS (P = 0.078, 0.195 and 0.201, respectively) (Figure 2B, D, F). Interestingly, our data showed the presence of IDH1/2 mutations was an adverse predictor of OS in the intermediate-1 risk group of IPSS (P = 0.039) (Figure 3A), but not in the intermediate-2 risk (P = 0.410) (Figure 3B) or high risk

(P = 0.685) (Figure 3C) group. Our results also indicated that decitabine achieved a better therapeutic effect in IDH1/2 mutation-positive patients compared to other treatments (including: GHA regimen, n = 3; GAA regimen, n = 2; supportive care, n = 2) (P = 0.023) (Figure 3D).

Multivariable analysis including IDH mutations, age, WBC count, hemoglobin, platelet count, BM blast count, cytogenetic changes and IPSS class showed HRs of IDH1/2 mutations for OS and LFS were 1.83 (95%CI 0.86–3.92) (P = 0.118) and 1.18 (95%CI 0.56–2.50) (P = 0.662), respectively. In addition, HRs of mutant IDH1 for OS and LFS were 1.62 (95%CI 0.55–4.81) (P = 0.383) and 1.07 (95%CI 0.37–3.09) (P = 0.903), and HRs of mutant IDH2 for OS and LFS were 1.93 (95%CI 0.70–5.35) (P = 0.206) and 1.23 (95%CI 0.44–3.40) (P = 0.692), respectively.

Meta-analysis Results

As shown in Figure 1, six studies and our data covering a total of 1782 subjects (111 with IDH1/2 mutations, 1671 with wild-type IDH) were included in the meta-analysis. Two of them were from United States [3,14], one from Germany [15] and three from Asia [16,17,18] (Table 2). Two of these studies found a correlation between IDH1/2 mutations and adverse prognosis in MDS [14,15]. For all studies in this meta-analysis, MDS were diagnosed by the WHO [13] or FAB (French-American-British) criteria [24].

The summary HRs for OS were 1.62 (95% CI, 1.27–2.09) for IDH1/2 mutations (Figure 4A), and 2.21 (95% CI, 1.45–3.38) for IDH1 mutations (Figure 4C), indicating that the presence of IDH1 mutations was a negative prognostic factor for OS, whereas a marginal association was discovered for IDH2 mutations 1.38 (95% CI, 0.95–2.02) (Figure 4E). Figure 4B and 4D showed the results of meta analysis for LFS, the summary HRs of LFS were 2.21 (95% CI, 1.48–3.30) for IDH1/2 mutations and 2.65 (95% CI, 1.53–4.59) for IDH1 mutations. There was moderate

Table 1. Characteristics of patients with MDS.

	IDH1 mutation (n = 6)	IDH2 mutation (n = 5)	Wild-type (n = 135)	P
Sex				0.360
Male	4	4	77	
Female	2	1	58	
Median age, years (range)	69(46–74)	61(36–78)	55(18–85)	0.122
Median WBC, ×10⁹/L (range)	4.1(2.2–15.6)	3(1.3–5.7)	2.8(0.4–26.4)	0.221
Median hemoglobin, g/L (range)	94(60–102)	74(60–82)	80(39–169)	0.850
Median platelets, ×10⁹/L (range)	56(20–86)	89(27–484)	70(4–542)	0.891
Median blasts, %(range)	11.8(5–18)	13(2–19.5)	6(0.5–18.5)	0.022
WHO subtype				0.121
RA	0	0	7	
RARS	0	0	3	
RCMD	0	2	48	
RAEB1	2	0	42	
RAEB2	4	3	35	
Karyotype classification				0.087
Low risk	4	4	91	
Intermediate risk	0	0	26	
High risk	2	1	13	
IPSS				0.364
Low risk	0	0	7	
Intermediate 1	2	2	72	
Intermediate 2	2	3	41	
High risk	2	0	10	

Abbreviations: MDS, myelodysplastic syndromes; WHO, World Health Organization; RA, refractory anemia; RARS, RA with ringed sideroblasts; RCMD, refractory cytopenia with multilineage dysplasia; RAEB-1, RA with excess blasts type 1; WBC, white blood cell count; IPSS, International Prognostic Scoring System.

heterogeneity among studies ($I^2<75\%$), but no publication bias was found. Since significant heterogeneity across studies was detected, we executed sensitivity analyses and the results demonstrated the robust stability of the current results.

Cumulative analysis of the relationship between *IDH* mutations and MDS was performed via the assortment of studies by publication time. Inclinations toward significant association were evident over time. Moreover, the 95% CI became increasingly narrow with accumulation of more data, indicating the exactness of estimates was progressively boosted by the addition of more subjects (Figure 4F).

Discussion

Due to the heterogeneity that still exists in the current prognostic scoring systems of MDS, the inclusion of novel molecular markers in these systems may enhance prognostic information. Although single gene mutations are not currently included in prognostic scoring systems, they may be vital to clinical phenotypes and overall survival in MDS. Actually, a great number of single gene mutations including *EZH2*, *SF3B1*, *TET2*, *ASXL1* and *TP53* have been associated with the development of MDS [25,26]. The illumination of new gene mutations may therefore improve the prevention, diagnosis, prognosis and treatment of MDS.

IDH is a key cytosolic enzyme in the Krebs cycle. It catalyzes the decarboxylation of isocitrate to α-KG, leading to the production of nicotinamide adenine dinucleotide phosphate (NADP) [27,28]. *IDH* mutations were first reported in a metastatic colon cancer in 2006 [29], and then since 2010 recurring *IDH* mutations were successively found in MDS (3.42%~12.27%) [3,14,17,30,31,32]. *IDH* mutations impair the normal enzymes' function, which may be associated with poor prognosis in MDS. However, prior studies have not provided a definitive link between *IDH* mutations and MDS. Meta-analysis is a useful statistical method for integrating results from independent studies for a specified outcome. Combining the relevant studies increases statistical power and thus makes it possible to detect effects that may be missed by individual studies. Therefore, we summarized here the current data available regarding this potential relationship and revealed several valuable points.

Firstly we discovered a significant relationship between *IDH1/2* mutations status and MDS prognosis in the Chinese population, *IDH* mutations predicted more adverse OS for patients with MDS ($P=0.007$). Furthermore, a meta-analysis combining the current and six previously published studies on *IDH1/2* mutations and MDS indicated *IDH1/2* mutations negatively affected OS (HR, 1.62; 95% CI, 1.27–2.09) and LFS 2.21 (95% CI, 1.48–3.30). Cumulative analysis further confirmed the significant correlation, demonstrating the effect of the variant became progressively significant with each accumulation of more data over time. In

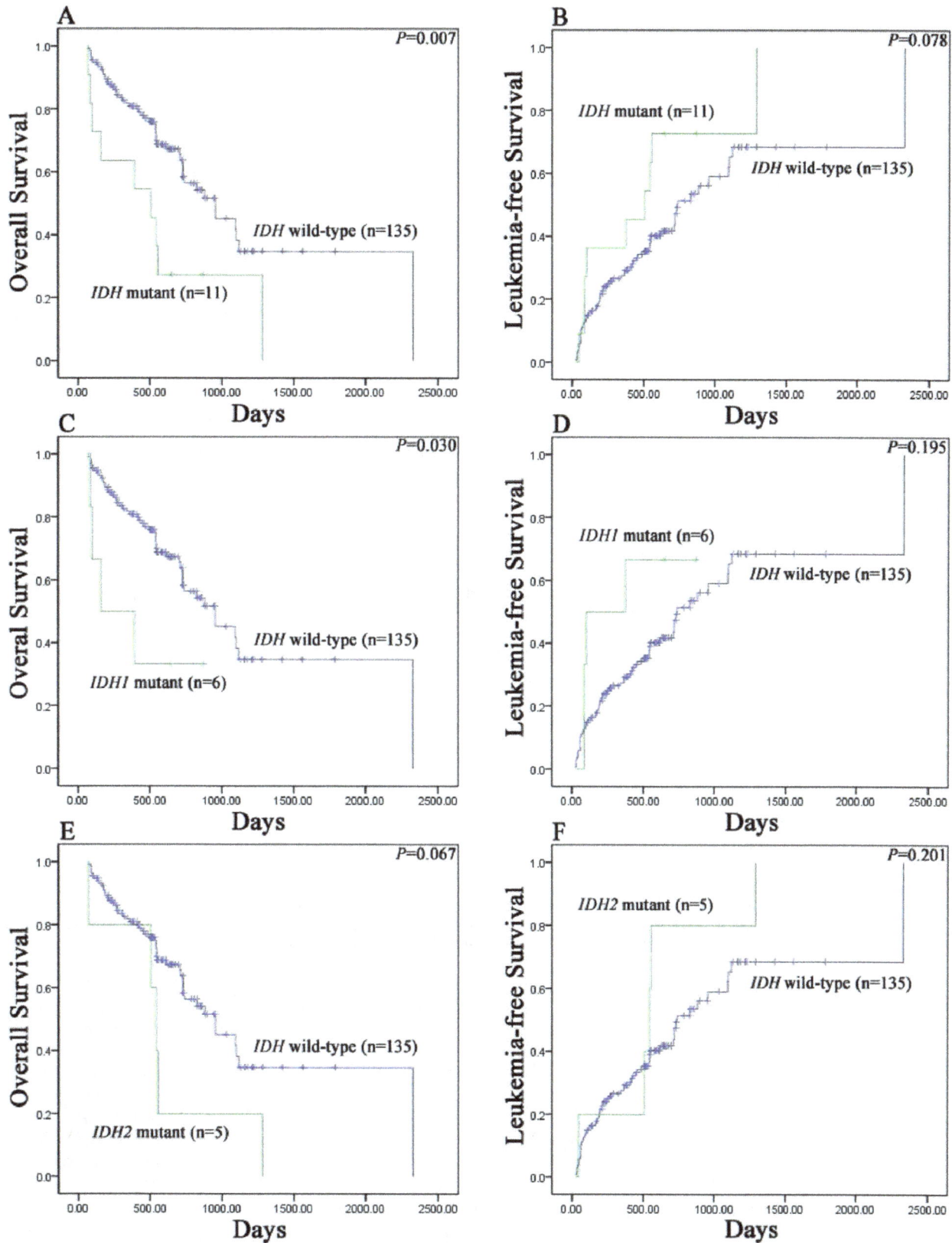

Figure 2. Kaplan–Meier survival curves for survival of MDS patients. (A) Overall survival data for MDS patients stratified by *IDH1/2* mutational status. (B) Leukemia-free survival data for MDS patients stratified by *IDH1/2* mutational status. (C) Overall survival data for MDS patients stratified by *IDH1* mutational status. (D) Leukemia-free survival data for MDS patients stratified by *IDH1* mutational status. (E) Overall survival data for MDS patients stratified by *IDH2* mutational status. (F) Leukemia-free survival data for MDS patients stratified by *IDH2* mutational status.

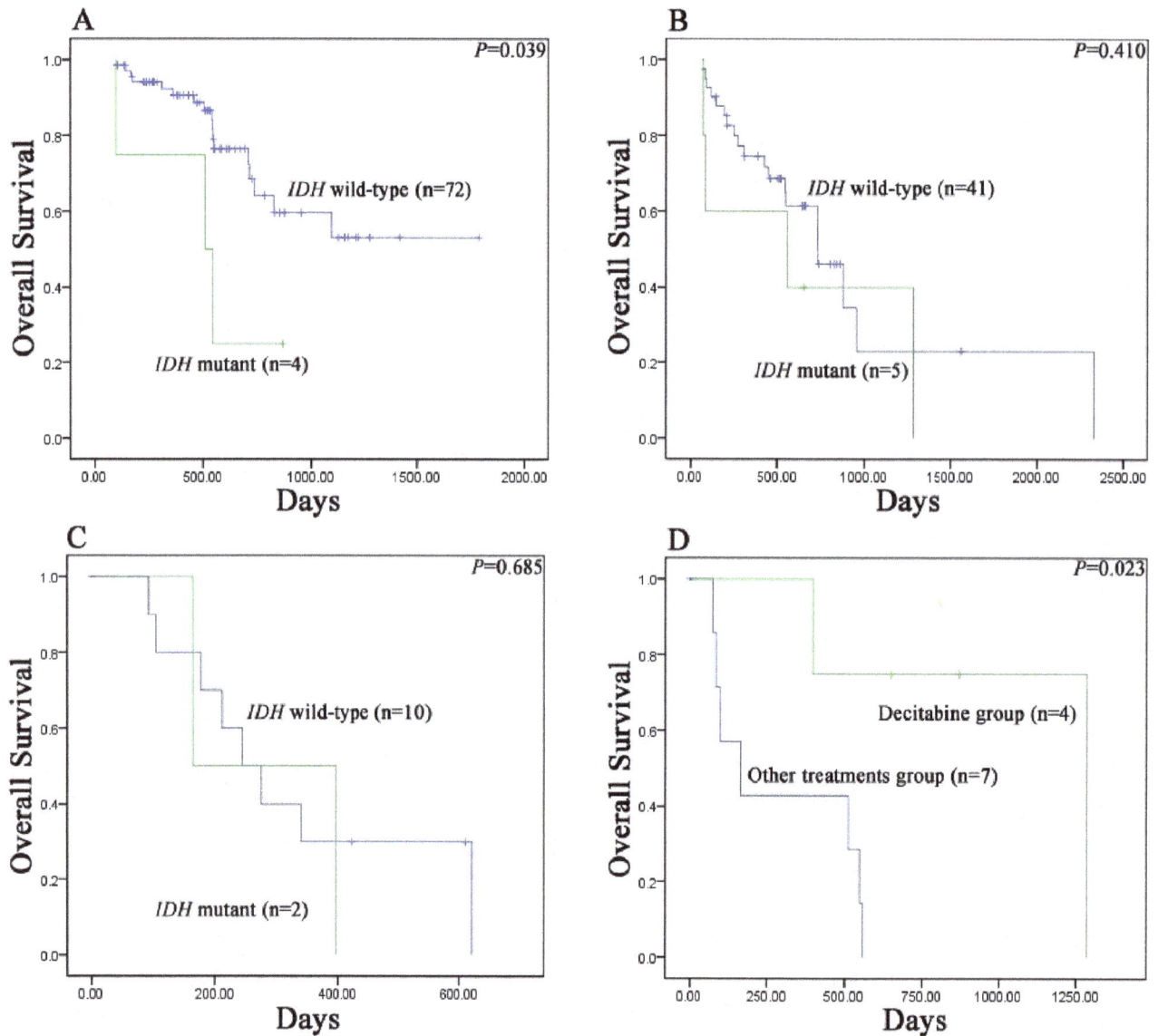

Figure 3. Kaplan–Meier survival curves for overall survival of MDS patients. (A) Overall survival of MDS patients in the intermediate-1 risk group of IPSS. (B) Overall survival of MDS patients in the intermediate-2 risk group of IPSS. (C) Overall survival of MDS patients in the high risk group of IPSS. (D) Kaplan–Meier survival of *IDH* mutant patients with decitabine chemotherapy compared with other treatments.

addition, when we conducted subgroup analyses, our data illustrated that *IDH1* but not *IDH2* mutations negatively affected OS 2.21 (95% CI, 1.45–3.38) and LFS 2.65 (95% CI, 1.53–4.59) in patients with MDS. Secondly, the presence of *IDH1/2* mutations might subdivide the intermediate-1 IPSS risk group as this was associated with a shorter OS in this group ($P = 0.039$). Finally, we found *IDH1/2* mutation-positive patients with MDS who were treated with decitibine had a significantly longer OS ($P = 0.023$) suggesting hypomethylating agents might be an effective treatment option for these patients.

There are several mechanisms by which *IDH1/2* mutations can worsen the prognosis of patients with MDS. (1) *IDH* mutations occur at low frequency (3.42%–12.27%) in MDS, but *IDH1/2* mutations are more frequent in both de novo AML (7.5%–31%) and AML arising from MDS (7.5%) [15,33,34,35,36,37], indicating a role for *IDH* mutations in leukemic transformation of MDS. (2) At the cytogenetic level, Caramazza et al. [38] showed a likely

association between *IDH1/2* mutations and trisomy 8 in MDS, and our results demonstrated 75% (3/4) of *IDH1/2* mutants with abnormal karyotypes carried a −7/7q- karyotype. In MDS, +8 and −7/7q- karyotypes were categorized in the intermediate-risk and high-risk cytogenetic group, respectively, suggesting they were linked to poor outcome in MDS. (3) The mutant IDH proteins displayed a gain of function as they could convert the α-KG that was generated by wild-type IDH proteins into 2-hydroxyglutarate (2-HG). Recent studies [39,40] reported that 2-HG was closely related to therapeutic response and relapse in AML. Since MDS and AML share many similar characteristics [41], it is possible that 2-HG is an oncogenic factor in MDS. (4) DNA hypermethylation played a vital role in MDS pathogenesis [42]. Dang et al [43] reported that mutant IDH1/2 proteins produced 2-HG which competitively inhibited α-KG-dependent enzymes, such as the DNA demethylating protein TET2 (Ten-eleven translocation 2) resulting in DNA hypermethylation. Indeed, Figueroa et al. [44]

Table 2. Main characteristics of studies involving in the meta-analysis.

study	Country	number	age (range)	Sex female	Sex male	MDS subtype RA/RARS	RCMD	RAEB/RAEB-t	Others	MDS classification	IPSS karyotype Good/Intermediate/ Poor/Unknown	IPSS Low+Int1/Int2+ High/Unknown	Number of IDH mutation (IDH1/IDH2)
Thol (2010) [15]	Germany	193	NR(36–92)	119	74	38/20	30	53/0	52	WHO	109/20/23/41	96/51/46	7(7/0)
Bejar (2011) [3]	United States	439	70(NR)	133	306	197/47	0	160/34	1	FAB	310/55/67/7	295/133/11	15(6/9)
Lin (2012) [16]	China	82	NR (20–85)	35	47	8	35	34/0	5	WHO	62/11/7/2	59/21/2	5(2/3)
Patnaik (2012) [14]	United States	277	71 (21–91)	78	199	0/56	130	77/0	14	WHO	NR	190/87/0	34(8/26)
Lin (2013) [17]	China and Japan	168	NR(60–75)	55	113	NR	38	119/0	NR	WHO	NR	73/77/18	17(7/10)
Lin (2013) [18]	China	477	66(18–98)	158	319	207	0	161/56	53	FAB	274/87/85/1	256/190/1	22(3/19)

Abbreviations: MDS, myelodysplastic syndromes; WHO, World Health Organization; FAB, French American British classification; RA, refractory anemia; RARS, RA with ringed sideroblasts; RCMD, refractory cytopenia with multilineage dysplasia; RAEB, RA with excess blasts; RAEB-t, RAEB in transformation; IPSS, International Prognostic Scoring System; IDH, isocitrate dehydrogenase.

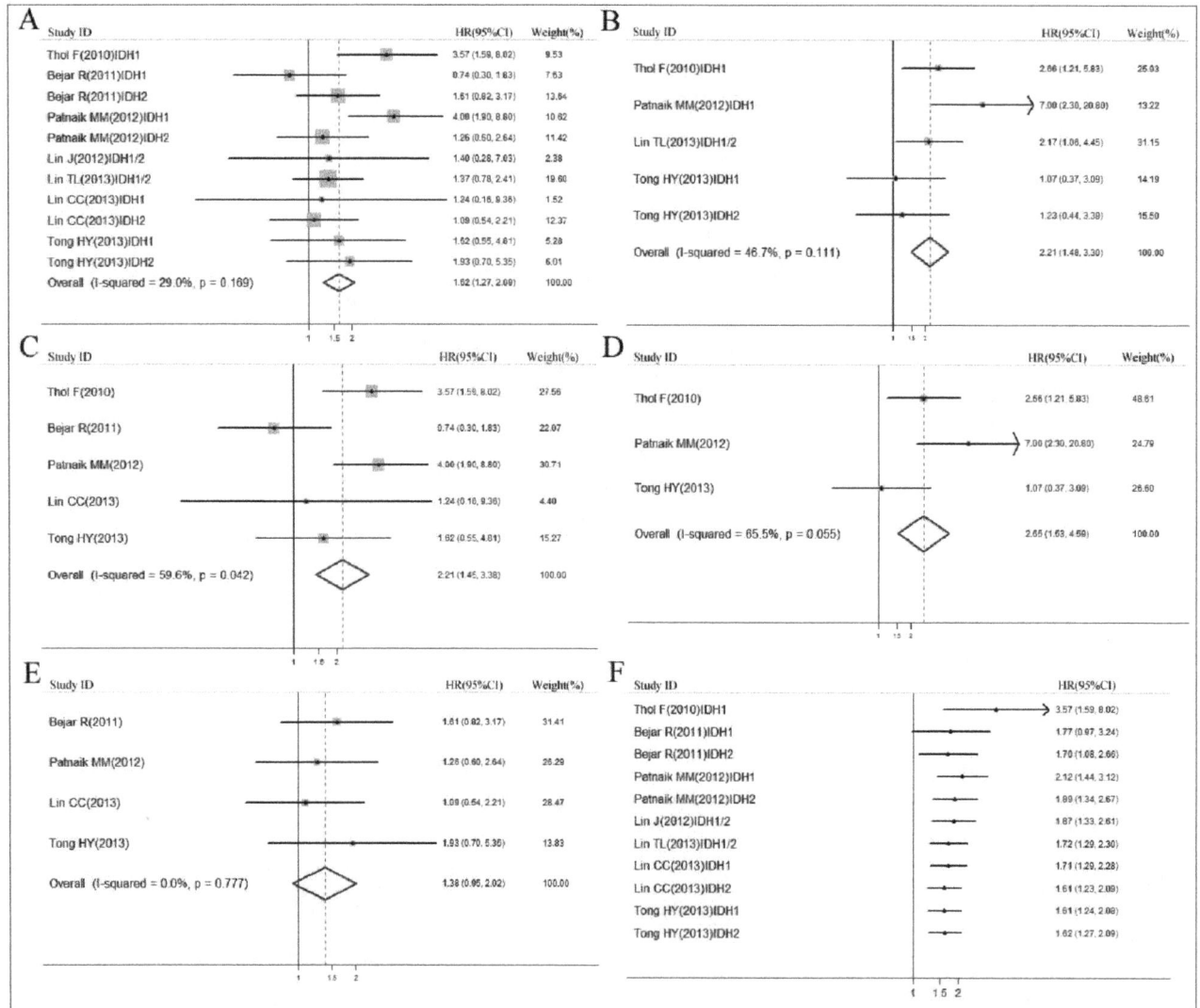

Figure 4. Forest plots describing the association between *IDH* mutations and MDS. (A) Forest plots of HR and 95% CI for *IDH1/2* mutations in MDS comparing with *IDH* wild-type by OS endpoints. (B) Forest plots of HR and 95% CI for *IDH1/2* mutations in MDS comparing with IDH wild-type by LFS endpoints. (C) Forest plots of HR and 95% CI for *IDH1* mutations in MDS comparing with *IDH*1 wild-type by OS endpoints. (D) Forest plots of HR and 95% CI for *IDH*1 mutations in MDS comparing with *IDH*1 wild-type by LFS endpoints. (E) Forest plots of HR and 95% CI for *IDH*2 mutations in MDS comparing with *IDH*2 wild-type by OS endpoints. (F) Forest plots of cumulative meta-analysis of *IDH* mutations in association with MDS for OS by published year.

found that AML patients with *IDH1/2* mutations shared a similar methylation profile to those with *TET2* mutations, and both mutations led to a block in myeloid differentiation and leukemogenesis. This might also be a potential reason for affecting outcomes in MDS. (5) Accumulation of 2-HG might lead to DNA damage by generating reactive oxygen species (ROS) [45] and inhibit EGLN (Egg-laying defective Nine) with subsequent stabilization of hypoxia-inducible factor 1α (HIF-1α) [46]. DNA damage and HIF-1α stabilization have been reported to be closely linked to MDS pathogenesis [47,48]. There are thus several mechanisms by which *IDH1/2* mutations may contribute to MDS pathophysiology but further research is needed to elucidate their exact contributions to the disease.

While the findings of this study are largely consistent with previous studies on *IDH1/2* mutations in MDS, several limitations should be addressed. First, analyses were based on observational rather than experimental studies. Cohort studies are prone to several types of bias including selection bias and loss-to-follow-up [49]. Second, we did not uncover unpublished studies and chose to collect only published articles in English, which could bring publication bias, despite there being no significant evidence of publication bias observed in Egger's test. Third, our study did not assess the potential effects of gene-gene interactions known to influence outcome in MDS such as *TET2* mutation-associated hypermethylation [44]. Similarly, we did not account for other known genetic contributions to leukemic transformation in MDS such as *ASXL1* loss-of-function [50]. This could lead to possible confounding in our study results. However, since *IDH1/2* mutations and *TET2* mutations were previously found to be mutually exclusive in patients with AML [44], it is not likely this particular interaction significantly contributed to our results.

In conclusion, we screened exon 4 of the *IDH1/2* gene in a large cohort of Chinese patients with MDS. Consistent with previous observations, we found that *IDH* mutations were present in some patients with MDS. *IDH1* mutations rather than *IDH2* mutations were significantly associated with shorter OS and LFS in patients with MDS. Further studies with larger sample sizes and functional assays of mutant IDH proteins are essential to decipher the role of *IDH* mutations in the development of MDS. Given that *IDH* mutations may adversely affect outcome in MDS are relatively easy to assess at diagnosis, examining *IDH* mutations in MDS may enhance the current prognostic scoring systems and guide patient-specific treatment in MDS. Finally, the identification of *IDH* mutations in the development and progression of MDS offers the promise of ameliorating the disease using targeted therapeutics against this biochemical pathway.

Supporting Information

Checklist S1　PRISMA checklist.

Acknowledgments

We sincerely thank the sample donors and clinical investigators who participated in this study. We sincerely thank Swallows Cody from NIH for the job in polishing our paper. We are deeply indebted to Pro. Bejar R and Pro. Ebert BL from Harvard Medical School and Brigham and Women's Hospital for supplying us original data.

Author Contributions

Conceived and designed the experiments: JJ HT ZZ. Performed the experiments: CH MY LY. Analyzed the data: CH FC XY. Contributed reagents/materials/analysis tools: CH. Wrote the paper: CH HT.

References

1. Corey SJ, Minden MD, Barber DL, Kantarjian H, Wang JC, et al. (2007) Myelodysplastic syndromes: the complexity of stem-cell diseases. Nat Rev Cancer 7: 118–129.
2. Nimer SD (2008) Myelodysplastic syndromes. Blood 111: 4841–4851.
3. Bejar R, Stevenson K, Abdel-Wahab O, Galili N, Nilsson B, et al. (2011) Clinical effect of point mutations in myelodysplastic syndromes. N Engl J Med 364: 2496–2506.
4. Greenberg P, Cox C, LeBeau MM, Fenaux P, Morel P, et al. (1997) International scoring system for evaluating prognosis in myelodysplastic syndromes. Blood 89: 2079–2088.
5. Greenberg PL, Tuechler H, Schanz J, Sanz G, Garcia-Manero G, et al. (2012) Revised international prognostic scoring system for myelodysplastic syndromes. Blood 120: 2454–2465.
6. Malcovati L, Germing U, Kuendgen A, Della Porta MG, Pascutto C, et al. (2007) Time-dependent prognostic scoring system for predicting survival and leukemic evolution in myelodysplastic syndromes. J Clin Oncol 25: 3503–3510.
7. Bejar R, Levine R, Ebert BL (2011) Unraveling the molecular pathophysiology of myelodysplastic syndromes. J Clin Oncol 29: 504–515.
8. Shih AH, Levine RL (2011) Molecular biology of myelodysplastic syndromes. Semin Oncol 38: 613–620.
9. Garcia-Manero G, Shan J, Faderl S, Cortes J, Ravandi F, et al. (2008) A prognostic score for patients with lower risk myelodysplastic syndrome. Leukemia 22: 538–543.
10. Reitman ZJ, Yan H (2010) Isocitrate dehydrogenase 1 and 2 mutations in cancer: alterations at a crossroads of cellular metabolism. J Natl Cancer Inst 102: 932–941.
11. Chung YR, Schatoff E, Abdel-Wahab O (2012) Epigenetic alterations in hematopoietic malignancies. Int J Hematol 96: 413–427.
12. Kaelin WG Jr (2011) Cancer and altered metabolism: potential importance of hypoxia-inducible factor and 2-oxoglutarate-dependent dioxygenases. Cold Spring Harb Symp Quant Biol 76: 335–345.
13. Vardiman JW, Harris NL, Brunning RD (2002) The World Health Organization (WHO) classification of the myeloid neoplasms. Blood 100: 2292–2302.
14. Patnaik MM, Hanson CA, Hodnefield JM, Lasho TL, Finke CM, et al. (2012) Differential prognostic effect of IDH1 versus IDH2 mutations in myelodysplastic syndromes: a Mayo Clinic study of 277 patients. Leukemia 26: 101–105.
15. Thol F, Weissinger EM, Krauter J, Wagner K, Damm F, et al. (2010) IDH1 mutations in patients with myelodysplastic syndromes are associated with an unfavorable prognosis. Haematologica 95: 1668–1674.
16. Lin J, Yao DM, Qian J, Chen Q, Qian W, et al. (2012) IDH1 and IDH2 mutation analysis in Chinese patients with acute myeloid leukemia and myelodysplastic syndrome. Ann Hematol 91: 519–525.
17. Lin TL, Nagata Y, Kao HW, Sanada M, Okuno Y, et al. (2013) Clonal leukemic evolution in myelodysplastic syndromes with TET2 and IDH1/2 mutations. Haematologica.
18. Lin CC, Hou HA, Chou WC, Kuo YY, Liu CY, et al. (2013) IDH mutations are closely associated with mutations of DNMT3A, ASXL1 and SRSF2 in patients with myelodysplastic syndromes and are stable during disease evolution. Am J Hematol.
19. Tierney JF, Stewart LA, Ghersi D, Burdett S, Sydes MR (2007) Practical methods for incorporating summary time-to-event data into meta-analysis. Trials 8: 16.
20. Tong H, Hu C, Yin X, Yu M, Yang J, et al. (2013) A Meta-Analysis of the Relationship Between Cigarette Smoking and Incidence of Myelodysplastic Syndromes. PLoS One 8: e67537.
21. Begg CB, Mazumdar M (1994) Operating characteristics of a rank correlation test for publication bias. Biometrics 50: 1088–1101.
22. Egger M, Davey Smith G, Schneider M, Minder C (1997) Bias in meta-analysis detected by a simple, graphical test. BMJ 315: 629–634.
23. Bennett JM (2000) World Health Organization classification of the acute leukemias and myelodysplastic syndrome. Int J Hematol 72: 131–133.
24. Bennett JM, Catovsky D, Daniel MT, Flandrin G, Galton DA, et al. (1982) Proposals for the classification of the myelodysplastic syndromes. Br J Haematol 51: 189–199.
25. Tothova Z, Steensma DP, Ebert BL (2013) New strategies in myelodysplastic syndromes: application of molecular diagnostics to clinical practice. Clin Cancer Res 19: 1637–1643.
26. Muto T, Sashida G, Oshima M, Wendt GR, Mochizuki-Kashio M, et al. (2013) Concurrent loss of Ezh2 and Tet2 cooperates in the pathogenesis of myelodysplastic disorders. J Exp Med 210: 2627–2639.
27. Krell D, Assoku M, Galloway M, Mulholland P, Tomlinson I, et al. (2011) Screen for IDH1, IDH2, IDH3, D2HGDH and L2HGDH mutations in glioblastoma. PLoS One 6: e19868.
28. Jin G, Reitman ZJ, Spasojevic I, Batinic-Haberle I, Yang J, et al. (2011) 2-hydroxyglutarate production, but not dominant negative function, is conferred by glioma-derived NADP-dependent isocitrate dehydrogenase mutations. PLoS One 6: e16812.
29. Sjoblom T, Jones S, Wood LD, Parsons DW, Lin J, et al. (2006) The consensus coding sequences of human breast and colorectal cancers. Science 314: 268–274.
30. Yoshida K, Sanada M, Kato M, Kawahata R, Matsubara A, et al. (2011) A nonsense mutation of IDH1 in myelodysplastic syndromes and related disorders. Leukemia 25: 184–186.
31. Rocquain J, Carbuccia N, Trouplin V, Raynaud S, Murati A, et al. (2010) Combined mutations of ASXL1, CBL, FLT3, IDH1, IDH2, JAK2, KRAS, NPM1, NRAS, RUNX1, TET2 and WT1 genes in myelodysplastic syndromes and acute myeloid leukemias. BMC Cancer 10: 401.
32. Kosmider O, Gelsi-Boyer V, Slama L, Dreyfus F, Beyne-Rauzy O, et al. (2010) Mutations of IDH1 and IDH2 genes in early and accelerated phases of myelodysplastic syndromes and MDS/myeloproliferative neoplasms. Leukemia 24: 1094–1096.
33. Abbas S, Lugthart S, Kavelaars FG, Schelen A, Koenders JE, et al. (2010) Acquired mutations in the genes encoding IDH1 and IDH2 both are recurrent aberrations in acute myeloid leukemia: prevalence and prognostic value. Blood 116: 2122–2126.
34. Pardanani A, Lasho TL, Finke CM, Mai M, McClure RF, et al. (2010) IDH1 and IDH2 mutation analysis in chronic- and blast-phase myeloproliferative neoplasms. Leukemia 24: 1146–1151.
35. Tefferi A, Jimma T, Sulai NH, Lasho TL, Finke CM, et al. (2012) IDH mutations in primary myelofibrosis predict leukemic transformation and shortened survival: clinical evidence for leukemogenic collaboration with JAK2V617F. Leukemia 26: 475–480.
36. Chou WC, Lei WC, Ko BS, Hou HA, Chen CY, et al. (2011) The prognostic impact and stability of Isocitrate dehydrogenase 2 mutation in adult patients with acute myeloid leukemia. Leukemia 25: 246–253.
37. Chou WC, Hou HA, Chen CY, Tang JL, Yao M, et al. (2010) Distinct clinical and biologic characteristics in adult acute myeloid leukemia bearing the isocitrate dehydrogenase 1 mutation. Blood 115: 2749–2754.
38. Caramazza D, Lasho TL, Finke CM, Gangat N, Dingli D, et al. (2010) IDH mutations and trisomy 8 in myelodysplastic syndromes and acute myeloid leukemia. Leukemia 24: 2120–2122.
39. Fathi AT, Sadrzadeh H, Borger DR, Ballen KK, Amrein PC, et al. (2012) Prospective serial evaluation of 2-hydroxyglutarate, during treatment of newly diagnosed acute myeloid leukemia, to assess disease activity and therapeutic response. Blood 120: 4649–4652.
40. Dinardo CD, Propert KJ, Loren AW, Paietta E, Sun Z, et al. (2013) Serum 2-hydroxyglutarate levels predict isocitrate dehydrogenase mutations and clinical outcome in acute myeloid leukemia. Blood 121: 4917–4924.
41. Steensma DP (2006) Are myelodysplastic syndromes "cancer"? Unexpected adverse consequences of linguistic ambiguity. Leuk Res 30: 1227–1233.

42. Khan H, Vale C, Bhagat T, Verma A (2013) Role of DNA methylation in the pathogenesis and treatment of myelodysplastic syndromes. Semin Hematol 50: 16–37.

43. Dang L, White DW, Gross S, Bennett BD, Bittinger MA, et al. (2009) Cancer-associated IDH1 mutations produce 2-hydroxyglutarate. Nature 462: 739–744.

44. Figueroa ME, Abdel-Wahab O, Lu C, Ward PS, Patel J, et al. (2010) Leukemic IDH1 and IDH2 mutations result in a hypermethylation phenotype, disrupt TET2 function, and impair hematopoietic differentiation. Cancer Cell 18: 553–567.

45. Ward PS, Patel J, Wise DR, Abdel-Wahab O, Bennett BD, et al. (2010) The common feature of leukemia-associated IDH1 and IDH2 mutations is a neomorphic enzyme activity converting alpha-ketoglutarate to 2-hydroxyglutarate. Cancer Cell 17: 225–234.

46. Zhao S, Lin Y, Xu W, Jiang W, Zha Z, et al. (2009) Glioma-derived mutations in IDH1 dominantly inhibit IDH1 catalytic activity and induce HIF-1alpha. Science 324: 261–265.

47. Tong H, Hu C, Zhuang Z, Wang L, Jin J (2012) Hypoxia-inducible factor-1alpha expression indicates poor prognosis in myelodysplastic syndromes. Leuk Lymphoma 53: 2412–2418.

48. Head DR, Jacobberger JW, Mosse C, Jagasia M, Dupont W, et al. (2011) Innovative analyses support a role for DNA damage and an aberrant cell cycle in myelodysplastic syndrome pathogenesis. Bone Marrow Res 2011: 950934.

49. Grimes DA, Schulz KF (2002) Cohort studies: marching towards outcomes. Lancet 359: 341–345.

50. Abdel-Wahab O, Adli M, LaFave LM, Gao J, Hricik T, et al. (2012) ASXL1 mutations promote myeloid transformation through loss of PRC2-mediated gene repression. Cancer Cell 22: 180–193.

2

Toll-Like Receptor (TLR)-1/2 Triggering of Multiple Myeloma Cells Modulates Their Adhesion to Bone Marrow Stromal Cells and Enhances Bortezomib-Induced Apoptosis

Jahangir Abdi[1], Tuna Mutis[2], Johan Garssen[1], Frank A. Redegeld[1]*

1 Division of Pharmacology, Utrecht Institute for Pharmaceutical Sciences, Faculty of Science, Utrecht University, Utrecht, the Netherlands, 2 Department of Clinical Chemistry & Hematology, University Medical Center Utrecht, Utrecht, the Netherlands

Abstract

In multiple myeloma (MM), the malignant plasma cells usually localize to the bone marrow where they develop drug resistance due to adhesion to stromal cells and various environmental signals. Hence, modulation of this interaction is expected to influence drug sensitivity of MM cells. Toll-like receptor (TLR) ligands have displayed heterogeneous effects on B-cell malignancies and also on MM cells in a few recent studies, but effects on adhesion and drug sensitivity of myeloma cells in the context of bone marrow stromal cells (BMSCs) have never been investigated. In the present study, we explored the modulatory effects of TLR1/2 ligand (Pam3CSK4) on adhesion of human myeloma cells to BMSCs. It is shown that TLR1/2 triggering has opposite effects in different HMCLs on their adhesion to BMSCs. Fravel, L363, UM-6, UM-9 and U266 showed increased adhesion to BMSC in parallel with an increased surface expression of integrin molecules $\alpha4$ and $\alpha V\beta3$. OPM-1, OPM-2 and NCI-H929 showed a dose-dependent decrease in adhesion upon TLR activation following a downregulation of $\beta7$ integrin expression. Importantly, TLR1/2 triggering increased cytotoxic and apoptotic effects of bortezomib in myeloma cells independent of the effect on stromal cell adhesion. Moreover, the apoptosis-enhancing effect of Pam3CSK4 paralleled induction of cleaved caspase-3 protein in FACS analysis suggesting a caspase-dependent mechanism. Our findings uncover a novel role of TLR activation in MM cells in the context of bone marrow microenvironment. Stimulation of TLR1/2 bypasses the protective shield of BMSCs and may be an interesting strategy to enhance drug sensitivity of multiple myeloma cells.

Editor: Andrei L. Gartel, University of Illinois at Chicago, United States of America

Funding: This research has been funded by the Utrecht University. The funders had no role in study design, data collection and analysis, decision to publish, or preparation of the manuscript.

Competing Interests: The authors have declared that no competing interests exist.

* E-mail: f.a.m.redegeld@uu.nl

Introduction

Adhesion of multiple myeloma (MM) cells to bone marrow stromal cells (BMSCs), mediated mostly by the integrin family of adhesion molecules, renders the tumor cells resistant against drugs and apoptotic stimuli, and contributes to other complications of the disease including osteolytic lesions and angiogenesis[1,2,3]. Several cytokines derived from both bone marrow stromal cells and MM cells have been indicated to maintain this interaction [4,5,6]. Toll-like receptors (TLRs) are a family of pathogen recognition receptors expressed mainly by the innate immune cells, but also by a variety of human cancer cells including those of B cell malignancies especially MM [7,8,9,10,11,12]. TLR activation by microbial or endogenous ligands has been implicated in linking inflammation to cancer, with the transcription factor NFκB activation as the main establishing event [13,14,15,16,17,18]. However, activation of NFκB in human myeloma cell lines (HMCLs) and primary MM cells has been explained partly by detection of some mutations in NFκB-controlled/related genes (mostly in alternative pathway) [19,20], and are probably independent of TLR signaling which is normally through the canonical pathway [21,22].

Possible contribution of TLRs to inflammation-related malignancy is indicated mostly by induction of pro-inflammatory cytokines in tumor environment [23], upregulation of cell adhesion molecules on cancer cells and their adhesion or migration following TLR triggering [12,24,25,26]. Recent studies in cells of B lymphoid malignancies including MM also demonstrated that TLR triggering would result in both positive and negative outcomes, including induction of growth and proliferation, drug resistance, immune evasion and cell death. Nonetheless, the modulatory effect of TLR activation in MM cells on their adhesion to bone marrow microenvironment components including BMSCs has not been explored to date. Hence, regarding the fact that TLRs of MM cells may be activated in the inflammatory environment of bone marrow, possibly by microbial/endogenous ligands, we hypothesized that TLR triggering on MM cells might modulate their adhesion to BMSCs and subsequently modulate MM cells survival and drug resistance. In a recent study, we demonstrated that TLR1/2 activation either increased or decreased adhesion of human myeloma cells to fibronectin and modulated cytotoxicity of bortezomib in HMCLs [27]. In this study, we extend these previous observations and show using an *in vitro* adhesion system that TLR-1/2 triggering on MM cells by Pam3CSK4 modulated their interaction with BMSCs involving adhesion molecules of β1 integrin family. Furthermore, Pam3CSK4 treatment of HMCLs increased their apoptotic response to bortezomib in the context of BMSCs, which suggests that TLR1/2 triggering may be of therapeutic use to decrease cellular resistance to the cytotoxic action of chemotherapeutic agents.

Materials and Methods

Reagents and Antibodies

TLR-1/2 specific ligand, Pam3CSK4, was obtained from Invivogen (San Diego, CA, USA). Rat anti-human beta 7 integrin (clone FIB504, for both FACS and blocking), mouse anti-human αVβ3 integrin (CD51/CD61, clone 23C6, for both FACS and blocking), mouse anti-human VCAM-1 (CD106)-PE (clone STA), mouse anti-human CD49e (α5 integrin, clone P1D6)-PE, mouse anti-human CD49d (α4 integrin, clone 9F10)-PE, anti-mouse IgG-FITC, and mouse IgG2b, κ isotype control were all from eBioscience. Monoclonal rabbit anti-human MyD88 (clone D80F5) and anti-human cleaved caspase-3 (clone D3E9) were obtained from Cell Signaling Technology (Danvers, MA, USA). Mouse anti-human CD49d (clone HP2/1, for blocking) was from ABD Serotec (MorphoSys, Oxford, U.K). Alexa Fluor 488 rabbit anti-rat IgG (H+L) was purchased from Invitrogen. Anti-beta actin and horseradish peroxidase-conjugated goat anti-rabbit IgG were also from Santa Cruz Biotechnology, CA, USA. Bortezomib was obtained from LC Laboratories (Woburn, MA, USA) and dissolved in DMSO to make 100 mM stock. DMSO concentrations in all drug exposure tests never exceeded 0.05%. PMS (Phenazine methosulfate) and XTT were also supplied by Sigma-Aldrich.

Cell Lines and Cell Culture

The HMCLs, Fravel, L363, OPM1, OPM2, U266, and NCI-H929, were obtained from American Type Culture Collection (Manassas, VA, USA). UM-6 and UM-9 had been established by the Department of Clinical Chemistry & Hematology, University Medical Center Utrecht, Utrecht, the Netherlands [28,29]. UM6 is IL-6 dependent and others are IL-6 independent. All the cell lines were maintained in RPMI-1640 culture medium containing 2-mM L-glutamine supplemented with 5 or 10% fetal bovine serum and intermittently with antibiotics, in a 37°C incubator with 5% CO_2. To UM6 cell line was added 5 ng/mL of recombinant human IL-6 (from eBioscience, San Diego, CA, USA). To NCI-H929 cell line medium were also added 1 mM sodium pyruvate and 50 μM 2-mercaptoethanol. Normal human bone marrow stromal cell line, HS-5, was obtained from American Type Culture Collection. This cell line was maintained in DMEM medium supplemented with 10% FBS and intermittently with antibiotics.

For isolating primary stromal cells, frozen vials of patient bone marrow samples were thawed, suspended in fresh warm DMEM medium and applied to Ficoll Hypaque density gradient centrifugation to possibly remove cellular debris and dead cells. The remaining fractions were suspended in DMEM medium and kept in a T-75 culture flask for a few hours in a 37°C incubator. Then the floating cells were gently aspirated and the adhered fraction was maintained in DMEM supplemented with 10% FBS, 100 IU/ml penicillin and 100 μg/ml streptomycin. The medium was refreshed twice per week to yield a confluent layer in 3–4 weeks. Confluent wells were passaged after detachment with trypsin-EDTA. The stromal cells at passage 1–3 were seeded in 12-well plates for survival experiments. Bone marrow samples were surplus

material from bone marrow isolated for diagnostic procedures. All patients approved use of surplus material for scientific purposes by written informed consent. Use of surplus material has been discussed with and approved by the review board of the University Medical Center Utrecht. Due to the nature of the samples i.e. surplus sample remaining after diagnostic procedures, no formal approval number was needed and provided by the Ethics Committee.

Cell Stimulation

To stimulate HMCLs, Pam3CSK4 was used in 1.0, 2.0 and 5.0 μg/ml concentrations. Before any treatment, cells were washed once with PBS, suspended in warm RPMI medium supplemented with 5% FBS. Incubation time in a 37°C incubator with 5% CO_2 was 24 hours.

Flow Cytometry

In FACS experiments, indirect or indirect staining was performed. Briefly, 10^5 cells from indicated conditions were washed and suspended in FACS staining buffer (PBS+0.5% BSA+ 0.01% sodium azide). Cells were incubated with primary antibodies (β7 and αVβ3) followed by relevant fluorescent conjugated secondary antibodies. Direct staining method was also used for anti-VCAM-1 (CD106), anti-CD49d (α4) and anti-CD49e (α5) with fluorochrome-conjugated antibodies. Finally, the samples were washed, suspended in FACS buffer and analyzed with a FACSCantoII flow cytometer (BD Biosciences). Gated live cell populations were analyzed using Cell Quest or FACS Diva software.

Fluorometric Adhesion Assay

Two to three days before adhesion experiments, 3×10^4 cells of the bone marrow stromal cell line, HS-5, or MM primary BMSC were seeded on 96-well plates. Immediately before adhesion, the plates were washed twice with warm PBS. For adhesion analysis, 10^6 HMCLs (treated or untreated) were harvested, washed twice in PBS buffer and suspended in 1 ml of room temperature RPMI medium without any additive. Cell suspensions were labeled with Calcein-AM (1 μM) for 30 minutes at room temperature with gentle mixing after 15 min. To stop labeling, samples were treated with ice cold RPMI and spun twice at 4°C. One milliliter of RPMI plus 2% FBS at room temperature was added to all samples and 10^5 cells were seeded on stromal cell coated 96-well plates and incubated at 37°C for 2 hours. At the end of incubation time, total and background fluorescence were measured with a plate reader (Mithras LB 940, Berthold Technologies, Germany). For measuring fluorescence of adhered cells, non-adhered cells were removed with three gentle washes with warm RPMI, 100 μL RPMI was added to each well and the fluorescence was measured. In some experiments to determine the adhesion molecules involved, anti-β7 (5 μg/ml), anti-αVβ3 and anti-α4 (10 μg/ml) antibodies were added to appropriate number of cells for 15 min at 4°C, the cells were then washed once with cold RPMI to remove free antibody molecules and then added to coated plates. For background readings, fluorescence of the wells containing cells adhered only to BSA was considered. The following formula was used to calculate percentage of adhesion: (Fluorescence reading of adhered cells-background reading)×100/(Total fluorescence reading-spontaneous reading).

Cell Survival: Drug Cytotoxicity Assay

Drug sensitivity measurements were performed using modification of an *acute exposure* approach as described previously [30].

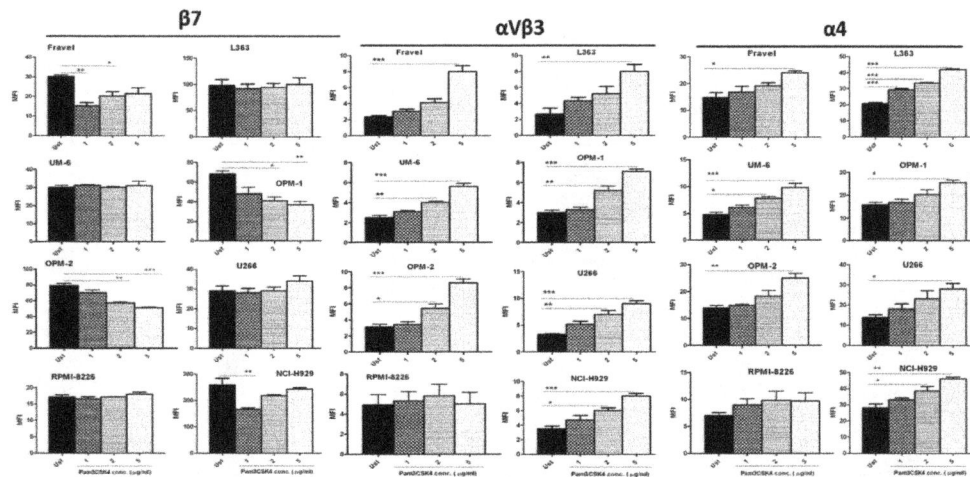

Figure 1. TLR-1/2 activation effects on expression of β7, αVβ3 and α4 integrins in HMCLs. HMCLs were stimulated with Pam3CSK4 for 24 hours and then applied to FACS analysis for expression of integrin molecules as explained in materials and methods. Pam3CSK4 downregulated β7 expression in Fravel, OPM-1, OPM-2, and NCI-H929 in a dose-dependent manner. No change in β7 expression was observed in any other cell line. Pam3CSK4 up-regulated αVβ3 and α4 expression dose-dependently in all HMCLs except RPMI-8226. The results are the statistical analyses of data in 3 separate experiments expressed as mean ± SEM, *P<0.05, **P<0.01, ***P<0.001. (Ust: Unstimulated).

HMCLs were first stimulated with 2 μg/ml (OPM-1, OPM-2, and NCI-H929) or 5 μg/ml (L363 and U266) Pam3CSK4 for 24 hours. Cells were washed twice with PBS and 5×10^4 cells were treated with indicated concentrations of bortezomib in RPMI+ 5%FBS in separate 96-well round bottom plates for one hour at a 37°C incubator, with gentle shaking after 30 minutes. Cells were then washed with warm RPMI, resuspended in drug-free RPMI+ FBS and transferred completely to the 96-well flat bottom plates pre-coated with HS-5. These plates were further incubated for 2–3 days. At the last 4 hours of incubation, 25 μl from XTT reagent which already contained PMS was added and incubation continued. Finally, the absorbance of each well was measured using a plate reader. The percent survival of cells was calculated by using non-linear regression. In each plate run, wells for solvent control (medium+cells+DMSO, for assay validity and also as 100% viability), blank (medium+DMSO), and growth control (medium+cells, for quality control) were also included. The readings of the blank wells were subtracted from those of all test samples.

Cell Survival: Annexin-V/PI and Cleaved Caspase-3 Apoptosis Assay

Five hundred thousand cells from each HMCL were incubated in the presence or absence of Pam3CSK4 for 24 hours, washed and treated with 5 μM bortezomib in RPMI+FBS for one hour (*acute exposure*). Conditions without drug treatment were also included. Cells were then washed, resuspended in drug-free RPMI containing FBS and added to 12-well plates pre-coated with 1×10^5 cells from HS-5cell line or patient BMSCs for 2 hours. Then unattached cells were removed and fresh medium containing protein was added and plates were incubated for 24–48 hours. In parallel, cells were also put in uncoated wells and treated as mentioned. Finally, cells were removed with cold 5 mM EDTA in PBS, washed and suspended in FACS buffer (cold PBS containing 1% BSA and 0.01% sodium azide). Samples were first stained with anti-CD138-APC for 45 minutes on ice, washed once with above FACS buffer and once with binding buffer (eBioscience). The cell pellets were then suspended in 200 μl binding buffer containing 5 μl FITC-conjugated annexin-V and incubated for 10 minutes at

room temperature. After washing with binding buffer, 5 μl propidium iodide in 200 μl of this buffer was added to each well and samples were applied to FACS analysis in a BD FACS Canto II machine. The gate of CD138 positive cells was selected, and the percent-specific apoptosis was calculated using the following formula [27]: (Test-control)×100/(100-control). Test refers to the treatment with Pam3CSK4, bortezomib or Pam3CSK4+ bortezomib, and control is the cells without any stimulation (baseline).For cleaved caspase-3 analysis, cells were first stained with andi-CD138 as above, fixed with a permeabilization/fixation buffer (eBioscience) for 30 minutes on ice, and then stained with anti-human cleaved caspase-3 for one hour at 4°C. At the next step, FITC-conjugated secondary antibody (anti-rabbit IgG) was added for 30 minutes on ice. After washing, samples were applied to FACS analysis as above.

Statistical Analysis

We used unpaired t-test or ANOVA (one way) in GraphPad prism 5 software for statistical analysis, and the values with a p< 0.05 were considered as significant.

Results

TLR-1/2 Triggering in HMCLs Modulates Surface Expression of Different Adhesion Molecules

We first determined the effect of Pam3CSK4 on surface expression of integrin molecules β7, αVβ3, CD49d (α4) and CD49e (α5). Incubation with Pam3CSK4 resulted in down-regulation of β7 integrin on Fravel, OPM-1, OPM-2 and NCI-H929 cell lines in a dose-dependent manner (Fig. 1), with a pattern in OPM-1, OPM-2 and NCI-H929 cell lines closely matching their adhesion behavior (see Fig. 2). No change in β7 expression (or only minimal increase with the 5 μg/ml concentration) was observed in other cell lines. All cell lines displayed a dose dependent increase in the expression of α4 and αVβ3 integrins, except RPMI-8226 which showed only small non-significant changes (Fig. 1). The α5 integrin was not detected on any of the cell lines except RPMI-8226 in which α5 expression was not affected by Pam3CSK4 treatment (data not shown).

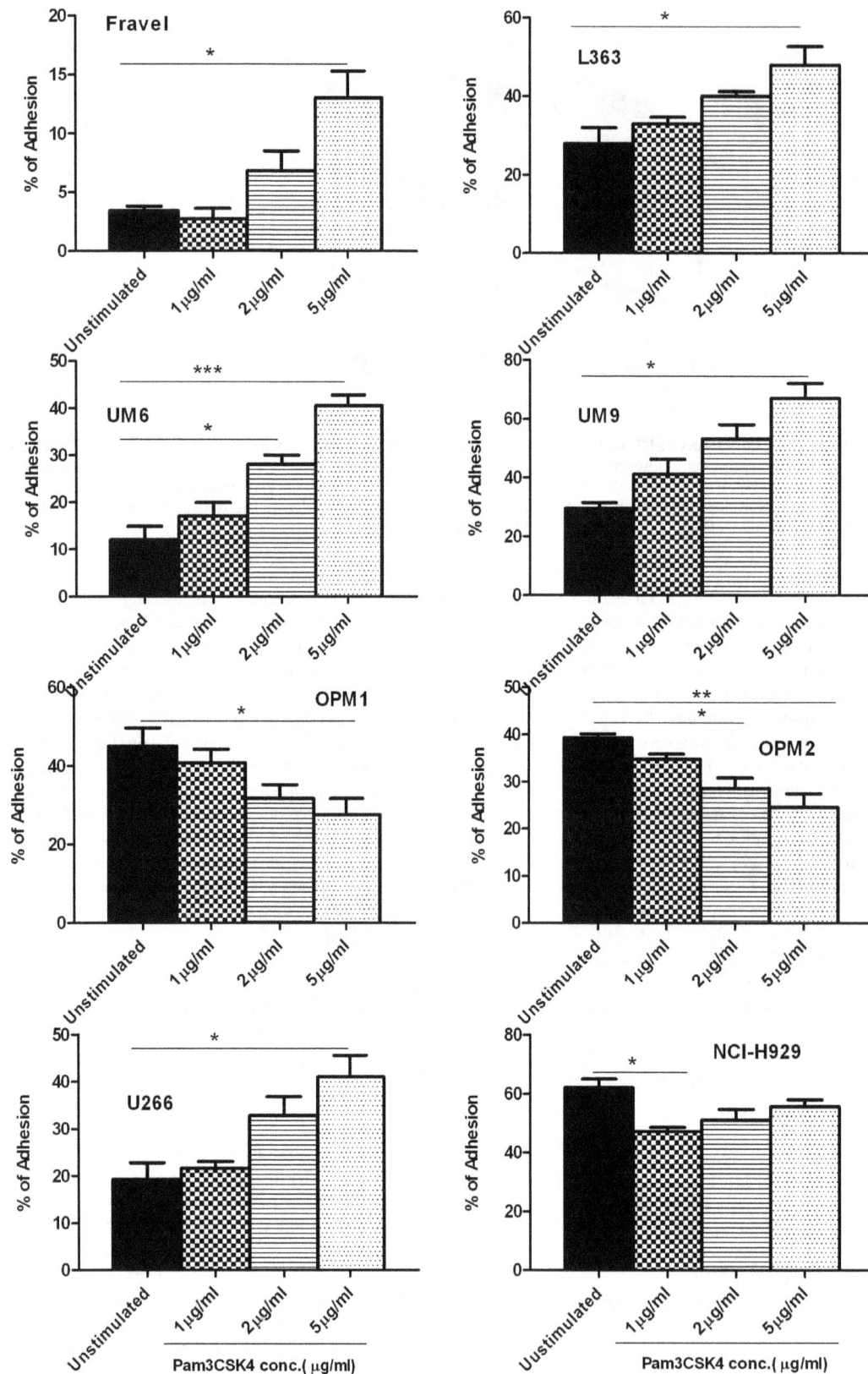

Figure 2. The effect of Pam3CSK on adhesion of HMCLs to BMSCs. HMCLs were stimulated with Pam3CSK4 for 24 hours and then exposed to HS5-coated wells for adhesion assay as explained in materials and methods. Pam3CSK4 decreased adhesion of OPM-1, OPM-2, and NCI-H929 cell lines to HS-5 in a dose-dependent manner. On the contrary, adhesion of L363, UM-6, UM-9 and U266 cell lines increased dose-dependently. The results are the statistical analyses of data in at least 3 separate experiments expressed as mean $\pm$ standard error of mean, *$P < 0.05$, **$P < 0.01$, ***$P < 0.001$.

A)-Blocking the induced
adhesion using anti-β7 antibody

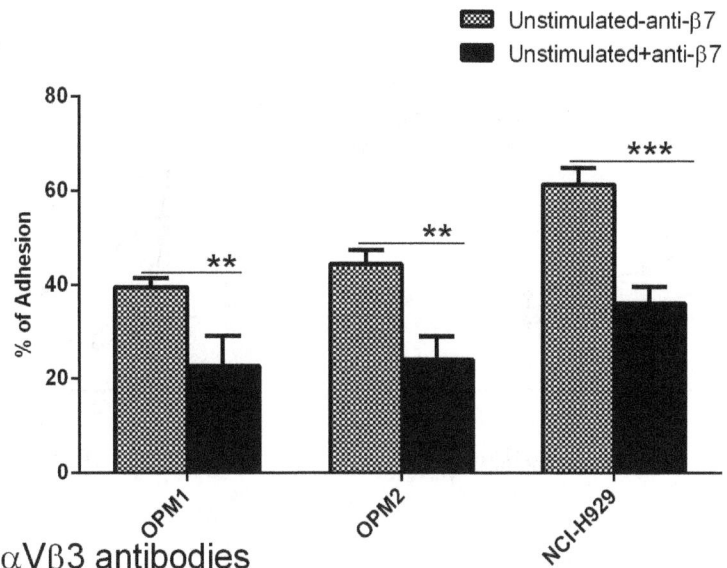

B)-Blocking the induced
adhesion using anti-α4 and anti-αVβ3 antibodies

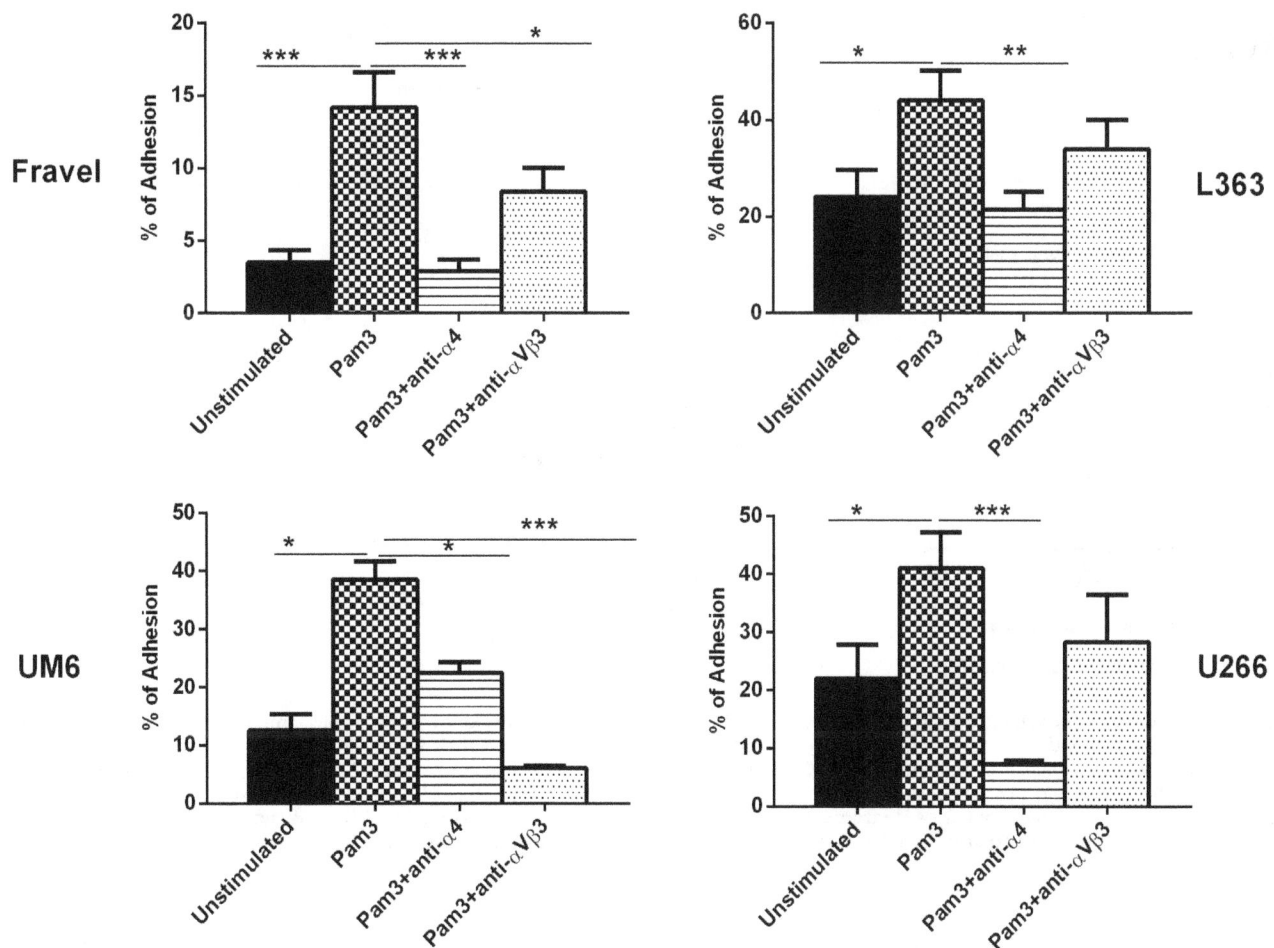

Figure 3. Blocking experiments with anti-β7, anti-α4 and anti-αVβ3 antibodies for adhesion to HS-5 stromal cells. Panel A, Blocking with anti-β7. HMCLs were stimulated with Pam3CSK4 for 24 hours and then treated with anti-β7 antibody before adhesion to HS5-coated wells. Panel B, Blocking experiments with anti-α4 and anti-αVβ3 antibodies for adhesion to HS-5. HMCLs were stimulated with Pam3CSK4 for 24 hours and then treated with anti-α4 and anti-αVβ3 antibodies before adhesion to HS5-coated wells. The results are the statistical analyses of data in 3 separate experiments rexpressed as mean ± SEM, *P<0.05, **P<0.01, ***P<0.001.

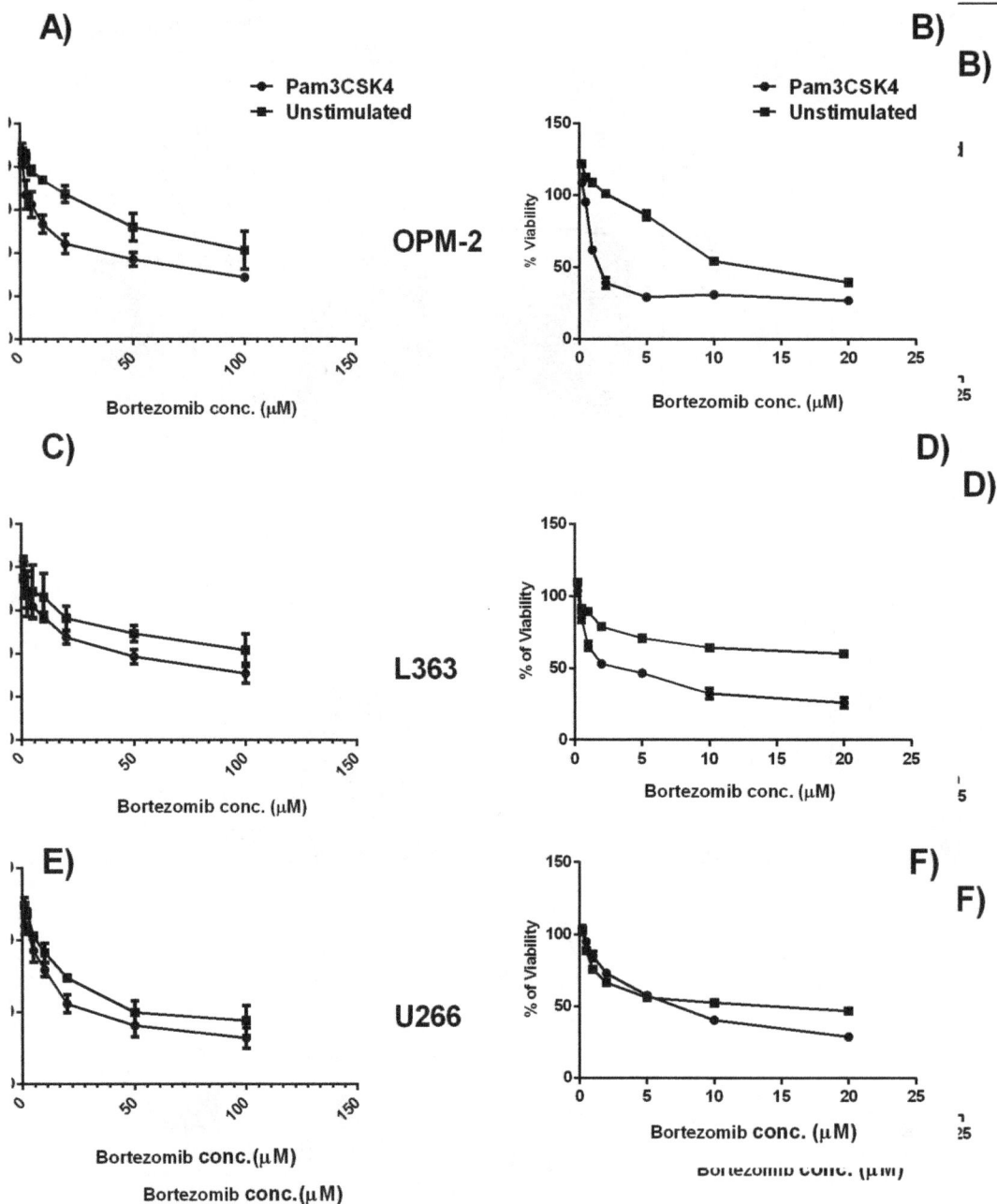

Figure 4. Pam3CSK4 increased sensitivity of HMCLs to bortezomib in the context of BMSCs. Myeloma cells were stimulated with Pam3CSK4 for 24 hours, and exposed to increasing drug concentrations in an acute manner. Panels A, C, E: HMCL adhered to BMSCs. Panels B, D, F: HMCLs in stroma-free conditions. OPM-2 (A, B), L363 (C, D) and U266 (E, F) HMCLs. Pam3CSK4 stimulated cells displayed a higher sensitivity to bortezomib in the presence or absence of stroma, however, the level of sensitivity was lower for HMCLs in BMSCs context than cells in the stroma-free condition. IC50s (µM of the drug): OPM-2: **stroma**, Pam3 (7.5 µM), unst (38.5 µM); **stroma-free**, Pam3 (1.9 µM), unst (15.6 µM); L363: **stroma**, Pam3 (12.8 µM), unst (41.1 µM); **stroma-free**, Pam3 (5.0 µM), unst (14.9 µM); U266: **stroma,** Pam3 (13.5 µM), unst (14.9 µM); **stroma-free,** Pam3 (5.6 µM), unst (11.2 µM).

TLR-1 Triggering in HMCLs has Different Modulatory Effects on their Adhesion to BMSCs

We next investigated the effect of TLR1/2 ligand Pam3CSK4 on the interaction of MM cells with BMSCs, regarding the critical importance of this interaction in MM biology and pathogenesis. TLR1/2 activation modulated adhesion of HMCLs to BMSCs, yet with a heterogeneous pattern (Fig. 2). Fravel, L363, UM-6,

UM-9 and U266 showed a dose-dependent increase in adhesion. Interestingly, Fravel and UM-6 showed quite low baseline adhesions (3.4% and 12%, respectively) which were highly increased with 5 µg/ml Pam3CSK4 (13% and 40%, respectively). OPM-1 and OPM-2 showed a dose-dependent decrease in adhesion. NCI-H929 showed maximal reduction of adhesion already at 1 µg/ml Pam3CSK4. The response of RPMI 8226 to

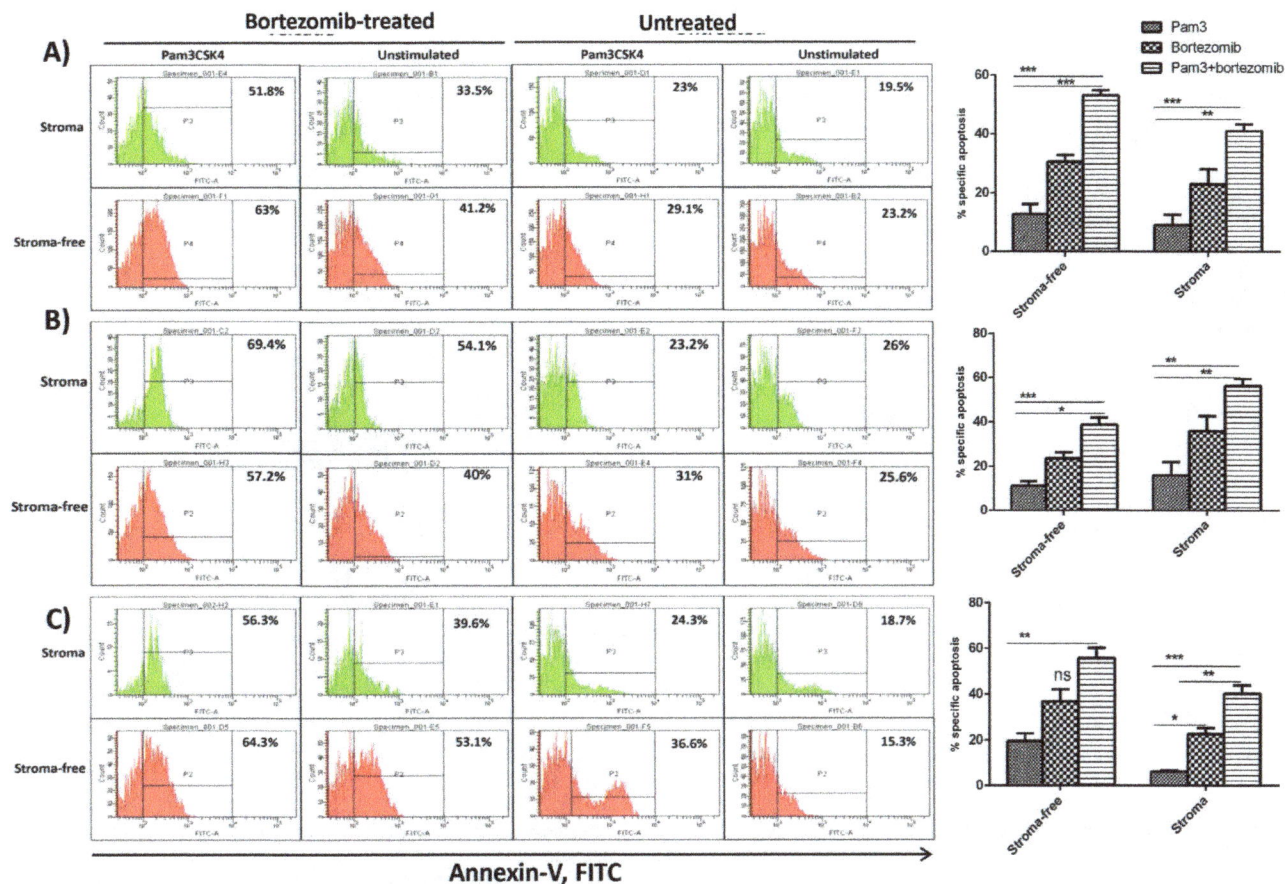

Figure 5. The apoptosis enhancing effect of Pam3CSK4 on HMCLs in the context of HS-5 stromal cells. Apoptosis in L363 (panel **A**), OPM-2 (panel **B**) and U266 (panel **C**) was determined by flow cytometric analysis of annexin-V binding. Percentage of apoptotic cells was calculated by selecting the gated CD138 positive cells. Left panels are one representative out of three separate experiments for each cell line and the right panels are statistical analyses of all experiments. HMCLs were stimulated for 24 hours with Pam3CSK4, adhered to HS-5 cells and then exposed to drug treatment as explained in materials and methods. The results are the statistical analyses of data in 3 separate experiments expressed as mean ± SEM, *P<0.05, **P<0.01, ***P<0.001.

TLR1/2 stimulation was inconsistent with respect to adhesion and therefore not further analyzed (data not shown).

Modulation of HMCLs Adhesion to BMSCs following TLR-1 Activation Possibly Involves Different Integrin Molecules

Based on the above findings, it seemed conceivable that β7 integrin could mediate down-regulatory and αVβ3 and α4 integrins up-regulatory effects of Pam3CSK4 on adhesion of HMCLs to BMSCs. To investigate this, we used anti-β7 antibody to block baseline adhesion to BMSCs in OPM-1, OPM-2, and NCI-H929. The anti-β7 antibody decreased baseline adhesion in these lines as much as 17%, 20%, and 25%, respectively (Fig. 3, panel A), indicating that β7 was involved in the adhesion of these HMCLs.

To investigate the involvement of αVβ3 and α4 integrins in adhesion, anti-αVβ3 and anti-α4 antibodies were used to inhibit adhesion of Fravel, L363, UM-6 and U266 cells at baseline or upon Pam3CSK4 stimulation (Fig. 3, panel B). The experiments indicated that Pam3CSK4-induced upregulation of adhesion was mediated by α4 and/or αVβ3 integrins. Adhesion of Fravel, L363 and U266 cell lines was shown to be mainly α4-mediated, as anti-α4 fully blocked the up-regulated level plus a large part of the baseline adhesion.

Blockade of αVβ3 integrin reduced Pam3CSK4-induced adhesion in Fravel, L363 and U266 cells but not as significantly as α4 blockade. This suggested that α4 integrin subunit was one of the main adhesion molecules engaged by above cell lines in adhesion to BMSCs. Adhesion of UM-6 was regulated by both α4 and αVβ3 integrins. These data confirmed the contribution of β7, α4, αVβ3 integrins to adhesion of HMCLs to stromal cells and suggested that there might be a heterogeneous response to TLR1/2 stimulation on their functional expression in HMCLs.

TLR1 Activation in HMCLs Enhances Cytotoxic Effects of Bortezomib in the Context of Bone Marrow Stromal Cells

Drug resistance of HMCLs can be greatly influenced by adhesion. In the next experiments, we investigated if the changed adhesion due to TLR1/2 stimulation would influence the drug sensitivity of HMCLs. L363 and U266 which showed upregulated and OPM-2 which showed downregulated adhesion following Pam3CSK4 treatment were selected for further investigation. As expected, IC50 of the HMCLs for bortezomib was higher when they adhered to stroma cells (Fig. 4). However, Pam3CSK4 treatment increased drug sensitivity of all HMCLs to bortezomib in the presence or absence of stromal cells suggesting that the Pam3CSK4-induced increases in bortezomib cytotoxicity were adhesion-independent.

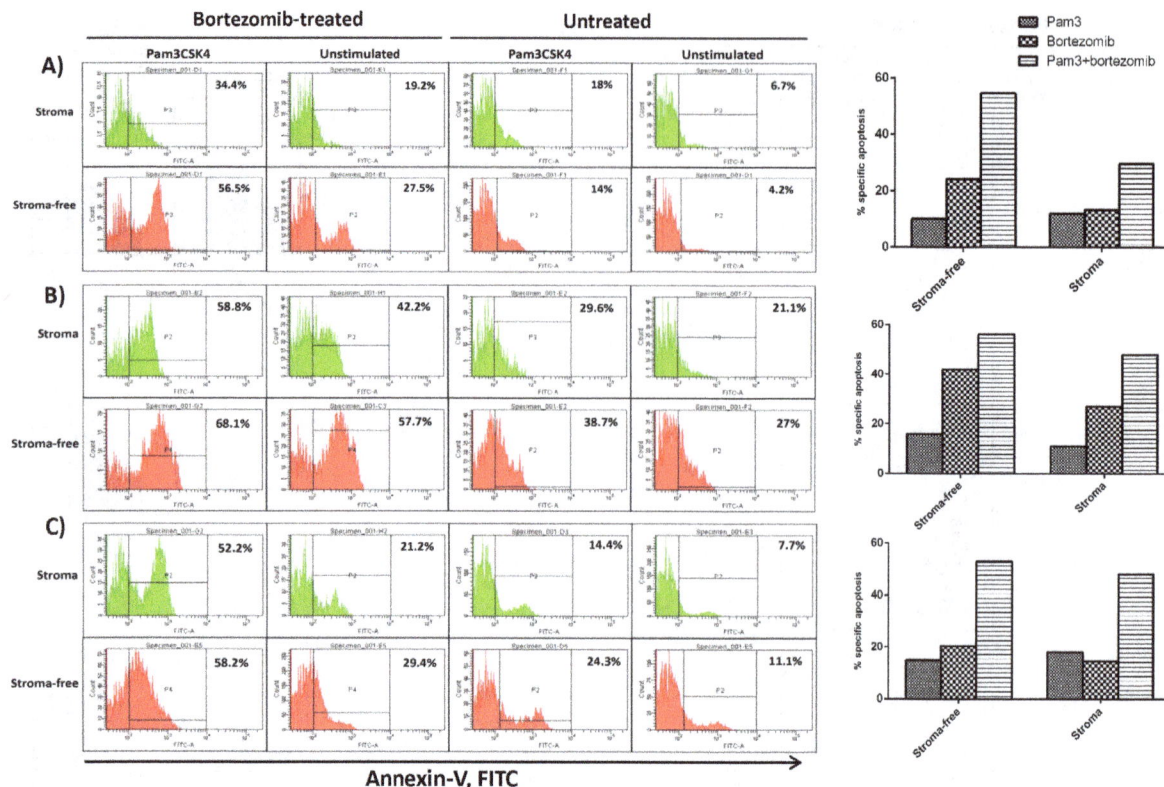

Figure 6. The apoptosis enhancing effect of Pam3CSK4 on HMCLs in the context of myeloma patient bone marrow stromal cells. L363 (panel **A**), OPM-2 (panel **B**) and U266 (panel **C**) were stimulated for 24 hours with Pam3CSK4, adhered to human bone marrow isolated stromal cells and then exposed to drug treatment as explained in materials and methods. Data are representative for the analysis of two MM primary BMSC samples.

TLR1 Activation in HMCLs Enhances the Apoptotic Response to Bortezomib in the Context of Bone Marrow Stromal Cells

Next, we explored if increased cytotoxicity to bortezomib in HMCLs after treatment with Pam3CSK4 was due to an increase in apoptosis. HMCLs were first stimulated with Pam3CSK4 for 24 hours, washed and exposed to acute bortezomib treatment and seeded onto HS-5 cells (Fig. 5) or patient BMSCs (Fig. 6), as described in materials and methods. In gated CD138$^+$ cells, the percentage of annexin-V positive cells was determined to calculate specific apoptosis. As depicted in figure 5, Pam3CSK4 treatment increased the level of bortezomib-induced apoptosis in all cell lines in the presence or absence of HS-5 cells, which further confirmed the adhesion-independent effect of TLR1/2 stimulation on HMCLs viability. Of note, Pam3CSK4 itself also left a partial apoptotic effect which was more pronounced in U266 cell line. Interestingly, varying levels of cell adhesion-mediated drug resistance (CAM-DR) were detected in the context of patient primary BMSCs for all cell lines, which was reversed by the Pam3CSK4+bortezomib treatment (Fig. 6). These findings demonstrate that Pam3CSK4 increases the apoptotic effect of bortezomib in the context of BMSCs.

Apoptosis Enhancing Effects of Pam3CSK4 on HMCLs in BMSCs Context may be Caspase Dependent

Only limited details are known on the effect of TLR activation on apoptotic signaling pathways. We further investigated if Pam3CSK4 could mediate increased apoptosis via caspase-3 activation. HMCLs were first Pam3CSK4-stimulated and drug-treated as detailed in materials and methods. Using FACS analysis the percent apoptotic cells was determined after gating CD138-positive cells (Fig. 7). As expected bortezomib increased cleaved caspase-3 in all conditions for all cell lines indicating it activated caspase-3 pathway [31]. Treatment with Pam3CSK4 alone augmented the cleaved caspase-3 level to different extents in the 3 HMCLs and combination of Pam3CSK4 with bortezomib increased the level of cleaved caspase-3 mostly in an additive manner. Above findings suggest that Pam3CSK4 may contribute to apoptosis through the activation of caspase-3.

Discussion

In the present study, we found that TLR1/2 triggering results in a heterogeneous functional response of HMCLs in terms of integrin surface expression and adhesion to BMSCs. OPM-1, OPM-2 and NCI-H929 myeloma cell lines showed a decrease in adhesion to BMSCs after TLR-1/2 activation, which was accompanied with a down-regulation in surface expression of β7 integrin. Furthermore, blocking experiments confirmed a significant contribution of β7 integrin in their adhesion, although this may not exclude the involvement of other integrins such as α4 and αVβ3 in their basal adhesion. Additionally, OPM-1, OPM-2 and NCI-H929 displayed significant increases in surface expression of α4 and αVβ3 following TLR-1/2 activation, but this upregulation appeared to have no functional effects in the adhesion to BMSCs. The integrin α4β7 has also been involved in adhesion of MM peripheral B cells to FN and BMSC [32]. Of note, the anti-β7 antibody used for blocking experiments is well known to detect only β7 epitopes regardless of its heterodimer partners [33], and

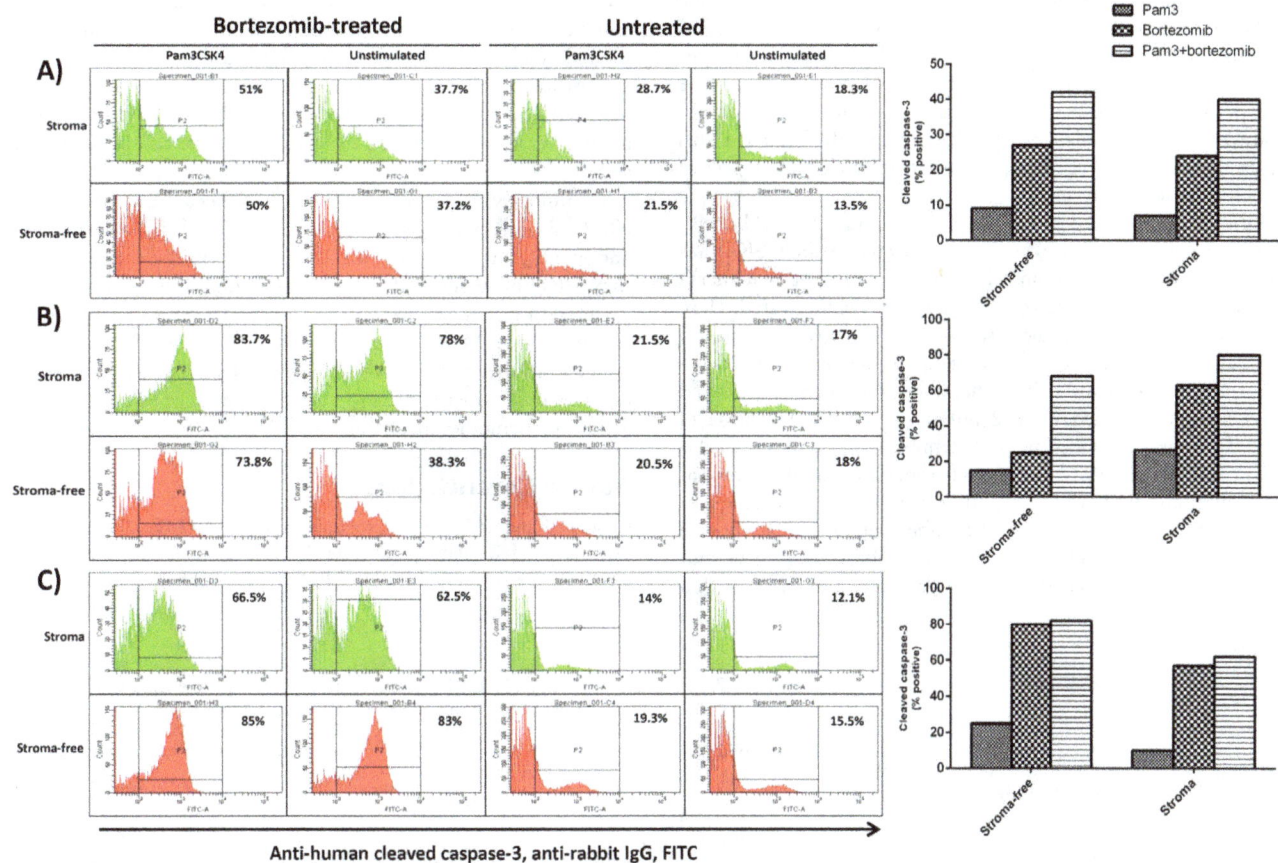

Figure 7. Pam3CSK4 induces apoptosis enhancing effects in bortezomib-treated HMCLs partly through caspase-3 activation. L363 (panel **A**), OPM-2 (panel **B**) and U266 (panel **C**) were stimulated for 24 hours with Pam3CSK4, adhered to primary human bone marrow isolated stromal cells and then exposed to drug treatment and cleaved caspase-3 FACS analysis, as explained in materials and methods. Pam3CSK4 alone weakly induced cleaved caspase-3 expression (compared to baseline) and its combination with bortezomib induced a higher level of cleaved caspase-3 protein in L363 and OPM-2 cell lines. Data are representative for the analysis of two MM primary BMSC samples.

thus affirms the involvement of this integrin in adhesion to BMSCs. Fravel, L363, UM-6, UM-9 and U266 HMCLs showed an increase in adhesion to BMSCs upon TLR1/2 activation. This up-regulated adhesion was demonstrated to be α4 and/or αVβ3 mediated and these two integrins are also involved in part of the baseline adhesion. It is well established that these two integrins can mediate binding of MM cells to FN and BMSCs [34,35], and αVβ3 has been shown to be involved in invasiveness of MM cells [35], Moreover, overexpression of αVβ3 in cervical cancer has been associated with poor prognosis [36]. On the other hand, in normal human PBMCs, TLR1/2 activation increased surface expression of α4 and β7 integrins in T cells, B cells and monocytes (unpublished observation), which rather supports a common mechanism by TLR1/2 activation for α4 modulation, but also indicates a specific mechanism (possibly unique to MM cells) for β7 modulation. Preliminary experiments in siRNA-treated HMCL to knockdown MyD88 indicated the involvement of MyD88 in the TLR1/2-induced modulatory effects on expression of integrins (data not shown). Taken together, these findings imply that TLR1/2 triggering can differentially modulate α4-, αVβ3- and β7 surface expression on MM cells and α4-, αVβ3- and β7-mediated adhesion to stromal cells.

Adhesion of MM cells to BMSCs is well known to render myeloma cells resistant against cytotoxic and apoptotic signals [37,38,39,40,41]. Furthermore, adhesion-induced drug resistance

is suggested to be associated with increased adhesion to fibronectin and with up-regulation of α4, thus cells with a higher expression of this integrin molecule display a drug-resistant phenotype [30]. In this study it is shown that Pam3CSK4 treatment upregulates expression of α4 in all HMCLs. However, some cell lines showed increased adhesion to BMSCs, while others showed decreased adhesion. The effect TLR1/2 activation in HMCLs on viability and drug sensitivity was further shown in three cell lines L363, OPM-2 and U266. Interestingly, Pam3CSK4 increased sensitivity (lower IC50) to bortezomib in the presence or absence of BMSCs, which was accompanied with increased apoptosis. Pam3CSK4 alone stimulated a low apoptotic effect in all HMCLs in the presence or absence of HS-5 or primary BMSCs, while combination with bortezomib induced a higher level of apoptosis. It should be noted that CAM-DR detected in some cell lines was completely eliminated by combined treatment of Pam3CSK4+ bortezomib. These findings suggest that the effect of TLR1/2 stimulation on adhesion to BMSCs does not control their drug resistance or sensitivity. Thus, upregulation of adhesion to BMSCs which was shown to be mostly α4 integrin-mediated did not reduce drug-induced cell death. Likewise, downregulation of adhesion to BMSCs which was shown to be β7 integrin-mediated did not increase drug-induced cell death. A recent study demonstrated that knocking down the β7 integrin gene in MM cells decreased their adhesion to FN and BMSCs and reversed

CAM-DR [33]. Additionally, blocking α4 integrin with specific antibodies increased their drug sensitivity in MM cells [30,42], and bortezomib reversed CAM-DR in MM cells through downregulation of α4 integrin [43]. These studies support involvement of α4 and β7 integrins in controlling drug sensitivity of MM cells. However, in this study, Pam3CSK4 apparently bypassed this involvement and increased drug sensitivity of HMCLs irrespective of their adhesion pattern.

Bortezomib stimulates caspase-3 activation in MM cells, triggering apoptosis [31]. The TLR1/2 ligand (Pam3CSK4) has been shown to induce apoptosis in monocytes [44], but whether it activates caspase-3 in MM cells has not been demonstrated. Here we show that Pam3CSK4 increases the level of activated caspase-3 in HMCLs in the presence or absence of BMSCs. Combining bortezomib with Pam3CSK4 increased the level of cleaved caspase-3 in L363 and OPM-2 but not in U266. The level of cleaved caspase-3 induced by bortezomib alone paralleled CAM-DR in L363 and OPM-2 cell lines (stroma compared to stroma-free conditions) but not in U266. Although the role of caspase-3 in the induction apoptosis is well-established, other studies showed that other isoforms such as caspase-2 contributes to bortezomib-induced apoptosis in HMCL [45]. Our study also suggests that

Pam3CSK4 may engage other mechanisms than caspase-3 to enhance bortezomib-induced apoptosis in HMCLs, and that inhibition of caspase signaling may only partly explain CAM-DR at least in some HMCLs. Further studies using specific inhibitors or expression-knockdown approaches should delineate the role of different caspase isoforms in TLR1/2-stimulated apoptosis in MM cells.

In summary, this study is the first to delineate the modulatory effects of TLR1/2 triggering on adhesion of HMCLs to BMSCs and identify the integrin molecules involved in this interaction. It shows that following TLR1/2 activation on HMCLs, expression of β7 integrin is downregulated, and that Pam3CSK4 increases drug sensitivity of HMCLs in the context of BMSCs. On this basis, although further research is essential, our findings suggest TLR1/2 as a potential target in MM to decrease resistance to the cytotoxic action of chemotherapeutic agents.

Author Contributions

Conceived and designed the experiments: JA TM JG FR. Performed the experiments: JA. Analyzed the data: JA TM FR. Contributed reagents/materials/analysis tools: JA TM. Wrote the paper: JA FR.

References

1. Anderson KC, Carrasco RD (2011) Pathogenesis of myeloma. Annu Rev Pathol 6: 249–274.

2. Hideshima T, Mitsiades C, Tonon G, Richardson PG, Anderson KC (2007) Understanding multiple myeloma pathogenesis in the bone marrow to identify new therapeutic targets. Nat Rev Cancer 7: 585–598.

3. Mitsiades CS, McMillin DW, Klippel S, Hideshima T, Chauhan D, et al. (2007) The role of the bone marrow microenvironment in the pathophysiology of myeloma and its significance in the development of more effective therapies. Hematol Oncol Clin North Am 21: 1007–1034.

4. Bloem AC, Lamme T, de Smet M, Kok H, Vooijs W, et al. (1998) Long-term bone marrow cultured stromal cells regulate myeloma tumour growth in vitro: studies with primary tumour cells and LTBMC-dependent cell lines. Br J Haematol 100: 166–175.

5. Tai YT, Li XF, Breitkreutz I, Song W, Neri P, et al. (2006) Role of B-cell-activating factor in adhesion and growth of human multiple myeloma cells in the bone marrow microenvironment. Cancer Res 66: 6675–6682.

6. Gupta D, Treon SP, Shima Y, Hideshima T, Podar K, et al. (2001) Adherence of multiple myeloma cells to bone marrow stromal cells upregulates vascular endothelial growth factor secretion: therapeutic applications. Leukemia 15: 1950–1961.

7. Abdi J, Engels F, Garssen J, Redegeld F (2011) The role of toll-like receptor mediated signalling in the pathogenesis of multiple myeloma. Crit Rev Oncol Hematol 80: 225–240.

8. Chiron D, Bekeredjian-Ding I, Pellat-Deceunynck C, Bataille R, Jego G (2008) Toll-like receptors: lessons to learn from normal and malignant human B cells. Blood 112: 2205–2213.

9. Chiron D, Pellat-Deceunynck C, Amiot M, Bataille R, Jego G (2009) TLR3 ligand induces NF-{kappa}B activation and various fates of multiple myeloma cells depending on IFN-{alpha} production. J Immunol 182: 4471–4478.

10. Bohnhorst J, Rasmussen T, Moen SH, Fløttum M, Knudsen L, et al. (2006) Toll-like receptors mediate proliferation and survival of multiple myeloma cells. Leukemia 20: 1138–1144.

11. Xu Y, Zhao Y, Huang H, Chen G, Wu X, et al. (2010) Expression and function of toll-like receptors in multiple myeloma patients: toll-like receptor ligands promote multiple myeloma cell growth and survival via activation of nuclear factor-kappaB. Br J Haematol 150: 543–553.

12. Abdi J, Mutis T, Garssen J, Redegeld F (2013) Characterization of the Toll-like Receptor Expression Profile in Human Multiple Myeloma Cells. PLoS One 8: e60671.

13. Chen R, Alvero AB, Silasi DA, Mor G (2007) Inflammation, cancer and chemoresistance: taking advantage of the toll-like receptor signaling pathway. Am J Reprod Immunol 57: 93–107.

14. Rakoff-Nahoum S, Medzhitov R (2009) Toll-like receptors and cancer. Nat Rev Cancer 9: 57–63.

15. Chen R, Alvero AB, Silasi DA, Steffensen KD, Mor G (2008) Cancers take their Toll-the function and regulation of Toll-like receptors in cancer cells. Oncogene 27: 225–233.

16. Chen K, Huang J, Gong W, Iribarren P, Dunlop NM, et al. (2007) Toll-like receptors in inflammation, infection and cancer. Int Immunopharmacol 7: 1271–1285.

17. Pikarsky E, Porat RM, Stein I, Abramovitch R, Amit S, et al. (2004) NF-kappaB functions as a tumour promoter in inflammation-associated cancer. Nature 431: 461–466.

18. Maeda S, Omata M (2008) Inflammation and cancer: role of nuclear factor-kappaB activation. Cancer Sci 99: 836–842.

19. Klein B (2010) Positioning NK-kappaB in multiple myeloma. Blood 115: 3422–3424.

20. Demchenko YN, Glebov OK, Zingone A, Keats JJ, Bergsagel PL, et al. (2010) Classical and/or alternative NF-kappaB pathway activation in multiple myeloma. Blood 115: 3541–3552.

21. Kawai T, Akira S (2010) The role of pattern-recognition receptors in innate immunity: update on Toll-like receptors. Nat Immunol 11: 373–384.

22. Kawai T, Akira S (2007) Signaling to NF-kappaB by Toll-like receptors. Trends Mol Med 13: 460–469.

23. Zhang Y, Xu CB, Cardell LO (2009) Long-term exposure to IL-1beta enhances Toll-IL-1 receptor-mediated inflammatory signaling in murine airway hyperresponsiveness. Eur Cytokine Netw 20: 148–156.

24. Hung C-H, Wu D, Lin F-Y, Yuan R-Y, Hu CJ (2010) Toll-like Receptor 4 and Vascular Cell Adhesion Molecule 1 in Monocyte-Endothelium Adhesion Induced by Lipopolysaccharide. J Exp Clin Med 2: 297–301.

25. Omagari D, Mikami Y, Suguro H, Sunagawa K, Asano M, et al. (2009) Poly I:C-induced expression of intercellular adhesion molecule-1 in intestinal epithelial cells. Clin Exp Immunol 156: 294–302.

26. Hennessy EJ, Sheedy FJ, Santamaria D, Barbacid M, O'Neill LA (2011) Toll-like receptor-4 (TLR4) down-regulates microRNA-107, increasing macrophage adhesion via cyclin-dependent kinase 6. J Biol Chem 286: 25531–25539.

27. Abdi J, Mutis T, Garssen J, Redegeld F (2013) Stimulation of Toll-like receptor-1/2 combined with Velcade increases cytotoxicity to human multiple myeloma cells. Blood Cancer J 3: e119.

28. van de Donk NW, Kamphuis MM, Lokhorst HM, Bloem AC (2002) The cholesterol lowering drug lovastatin induces cell death in myeloma plasma cells. Leukemia 16: 1362–1371.

29. van der Veer MS, de Weers M, van Kessel B, Bakker JM, Wittebol S, et al. (2011) Towards effective immunotherapy of myeloma: enhanced elimination of myeloma cells by combination of lenalidomide with the human CD38 monoclonal antibody daratumumab. Haematologica 96: 284–290.

30. Damiano JS, Cress AE, Hazlehurst LA, Shtil AA, Dalton WS (1999) Cell adhesion mediated drug resistance (CAM-DR): role of integrins and resistance to apoptosis in human myeloma cell lines. Blood 93: 1658–1667.

31. Saha MN, Jiang H, Jayakar J, Reece D, Branch DR, et al. (2010) MDM2 antagonist nutlin plus proteasome inhibitor velcade combination displays a synergistic anti-myeloma activity. Cancer Biol Ther 9: 936–944.

32. Masellis-Smith A, Belch AR, Mant MJ, Pilarski LM (1997) Adhesion of multiple myeloma peripheral blood B cells to bone marrow fibroblasts: a requirement for CD44 and alpha4beta7. Cancer Res 57: 930–936.

33. Neri P, Ren L, Azab AK, Brentnall M, Gratton K, et al. (2011) Integrin beta7-mediated regulation of multiple myeloma cell adhesion, migration, and invasion. Blood 117: 6202–6213.

34. Sanz-Rodriguez F, Ruiz-Velasco N, Pascual-Salcedo D, Teixido J (1999) Characterization of VLA-4-dependent myeloma cell adhesion to fibronectin and VCAM-1. Br J Haematol 107: 825–834.

35. Ria R, Vacca A, Ribatti D, Di Raimondo F, Merchionne F, et al. (2002) Alpha(v)beta(3) integrin engagement enhances cell invasiveness in human multiple myeloma. Haematologica 87: 836–845.

36. Werner J, Decarlo CA, Escott N, Zehbe I, Ulanova M (2012) Expression of integrins and Toll-like receptors in cervical cancer: effect of infectious agents. Innate Immun 18: 55–69.

37. Nefedova Y, Landowski TH, Dalton WS (2003) Bone marrow stromal-derived soluble factors and direct cell contact contribute to de novo drug resistance of myeloma cells by distinct mechanisms. Leukemia 17: 1175–1182.

38. Wang X, Li C, Ju S, Wang Y, Wang H, et al. (2011) Myeloma cell adhesion to bone marrow stromal cells confers drug resistance by microRNA-21 up-regulation. Leuk Lymphoma 52: 1991–1998.

39. Markovina S, Callander NS, O'Connor SL, Xu G, Shi Y, et al. (2010) Bone marrow stromal cells from multiple myeloma patients uniquely induce bortezomib resistant NF-kappaB activity in myeloma cells. Mol Cancer 9: 176.

40. Nefedova Y, Cheng P, Alsina M, Dalton WS, Gabrilovich DI (2004) Involvement of Notch-1 signaling in bone marrow stroma-mediated de novo drug resistance of myeloma and other malignant lymphoid cell lines. Blood 103: 3503–3510.

41. Perez LE, Parquet N, Shain K, Nimmanapalli R, Alsina M, et al. (2008) Bone marrow stroma confers resistance to Apo2 ligand/TRAIL in multiple myeloma in part by regulating c-FLIP. J Immunol 180: 1545–1555.

42. Damiano JS, Dalton WS (2000) Integrin-mediated drug resistance in multiple myeloma. Leuk Lymphoma 38: 71–81.

43. Noborio-Hatano K, Kikuchi J, Takatoku M, Shimizu R, Wada T, et al. (2009) Bortezomib overcomes cell-adhesion-mediated drug resistance through down-regulation of VLA-4 expression in multiple myeloma. Oncogene 28: 231–242.

44. Aliprantis AO, Yang RB, Mark MR, Suggett S, Devaux B, et al. (1999) Cell activation and apoptosis by bacterial lipoproteins through toll-like receptor-2. Science 285: 736–739.

45. Gu H, Chen X, Gao G, Dong H (2008) Caspase-2 functions upstream of mitochondria in endoplasmic reticulum stress-induced apoptosis by bortezomib in human myeloma cells. Mol Cancer Ther 7(8): 2298–2307.

3

Overexpression of Wilms Tumor 1 Gene as a Negative Prognostic Indicator in Acute Myeloid Leukemia

Xiaodong Lyu[1,3]*[9], Yaping Xin[2][9], Ruihua Mi[1], Jing Ding[1], Xianwei Wang[1], Jieying Hu[1], Ruihua Fan[1], Xudong Wei[1], Yongping Song[1], Richard Y. Zhao[3]*

1 Henan Institute of Hematology, Affiliated Tumor Hospital of Zhengzhou University, Zhengzhou, Henan, China, 2 Department of Endocrinology and Metabolic Diseases, the Second Affiliated Hospital of Zhengzhou University, Zhengzhou, Henan, China, 3 Division of Molecular Pathology, Department of Pathology, University of Maryland School of Medicine, Baltimore, Maryland, United States of America

Abstract

Chromosomal aberrations are useful in assessing treatment options and clinical outcomes of acute myeloid leukemia (AML) patients. However, 40~50% of the AML patients showed no chromosomal abnormalities, *i.e.*, with normal cytogenetics aka the CN-AML patients. Testing of molecular aberrations such as *FLT3* or *NPM1* can help to define clinical outcomes in the CN-AML patients but with various successes. Goal of this study was to test the possibility of Wilms' tumor 1 (*WT1*) gene overexpression as an additional molecular biomarker. A total of 103 CN-AML patients, among which 28% had overexpressed *WT1*, were studied over a period of 38 months. Patient's response to induction chemotherapy as measured by the complete remission (CR) rate, disease-free survival (DFS) and overall survival (OS) were measured. Our data suggested that *WT1* overexpression correlated negatively with the CR rate, DFS and OS. Consistent with previous reports, CN-AML patients can be divided into three different risk subgroups based on the status of known molecular abnormalities, *i.e.*, the favorable (*NPM1*^{mt}/no *FLT3*^{ITD}), the unfavorable (*FLT3*^{ITD}) and the intermediate risk subgroups. The *WT1* overexpression significantly reduced the CR, DFS and OS in both the favorable and unfavorable groups. As the results, patients with normal *WT1* gene expression in the favorable risk group showed the best clinical outcomes and all survived with complete remission and disease-free survival over the 37 month study period; in contrast, patients with *WT1* overexpression in the unfavorable risk group displayed the worst clinical outcomes. *WT1* overexpression by itself is an independent and negative indicator for predicting CR rate, DFS and OS of the CN-AML patients; moreover, it increases the statistical power of predicting the same clinical outcomes when it is combined with the *NPM1*^{mt} or the *FLT3*^{ITD} genotypes that are the good or poor prognostic markers of CN-AML.

Editor: Yuntao Wu, George Mason University, United States of America

Funding: This work was supported by the Social Public Service Foundation of Henan Technology Department [072103810503] to Xiaodong Lyu who was a visiting physician scientist in the RZ's laboratory at the University of Maryland School of Medicine when this manuscript was written. The authors would like to thank Ge Li for helpful discussions and revision. The funders had no role in study design, data collection and analysis, decision to publish, or preparation of the manuscript.

* E-mail: xiaodonglv2007@sina.com (XL); RZhao@som.uamryland.edu (RZ)

[9] These authors contributed equally to this work.

Introduction

Acute myeloid leukemia (AML) is defined as hematopoietic stem cell malignancy characterized by clonal expansion of myeloid blasts. It is typically divided into three different risk groups, *i.e*, the favorable, the intermediate and the unfavorable group based on the types of chromosomal aberrations. About half (40~50%) of the AML patients have normal karyotype or normal cytogenetics that typically belong to the intermediate risk group in terms of patient's survival [1,2]. However, inconsistencies were found among this group of patients in their responses to chemotherapy and prognosis that sometimes makes it difficult to make the right decision for therapeutic treatment and/or assessment of the possible treatment outcome of the patients.

Adding examination of molecular aberrations is thought to be helpful in addressing the differences as described above. Few molecular markers have been used to predict treatment response

and prognosis in cytogenetically normal acute myeloid leukemia (CN-AML), such as the nucleoplasmin (*NPM1*) gene and the fms-like tyrosine kinase 3 (*FLT3*) gene. A typical *NPM1* gene mutation includes small insertions (4~11 bp) in the coding region of exon 12. The *FLT3* gene mutations usually include a D835 point mutation in the tyrosine kinase domain (TKD) of the exon 20 or internal tandem duplications (ITD) in the exon of 14 or 15. Detection of these *NPM1* and *FLT3* gene mutations has been used to evaluate clinically biological behavior of leukemia cell in the CN-AML patients [2,3].

The Wilms' tumor 1 (*WT1*) gene, which is located on the chromosome 11p13, encodes a zinc-finger transcriptional factor that has emerged as an important regulator of normal and malignant hematopoiesis. *WT1* is also one of the molecules that are known to control cellular apoptosis [4]. Resistance of leukemia blasts to apoptosis may cause poor clinical outcomes. Therefore, regulation of apoptotic or anti-apoptotic pathways has high clinical relevance with regard to the remission therapy and the overall survival of the AML patients. Interestingly, high *WT1* gene expression was consistently found in peripheral blood (PB) or bone marrow (BM) in the AML patients in comparison with normal controls [5]. However, the significance of *WT1* overexpression in therapeutic response and prognosis are still elusive in CN-AML [6–8]. Goal of this study was to examine possible correlation of *WT1* gene expression with therapeutic response and prognosis in the CN-AML patients. In addition, we also examined the possible interactions of *WT1* gene overexpression with the *NPM1* or *FLT3* gene status, which are known molecular markers associated with the survival and treatment outcomes of AML patients.

Materials and Methods

Patient Population

A total of 103 CN-AML patients consisting of 58 males and 45 females with a median age of 42 years (range, 17–82 years) were recruited for the *WT1* overexpression study. All patients were newly diagnosed patients with CN-AML at the Henan Cancer Hospital from the time period of September of 2009 to October, 2012, *i.e.*, a total of 38 months. The diagnosis of AML was made according to the FAB classification. The M3 patients were not included in this study because of the success in chemotherapy based on all-trans-retinoic acid and arsenic trioxide. The standard RHG banding techniques were employed in the karyotyping of leukemia. One milliliter of bone marrow was collected in the EDTA vacutainer from all 103 patients before treatment. This clinical study was approved by the Committee of International and Scientific Research at the Affiliated Tumor Hospital of Zhengzhou University. Written informed consents were obtained from all patients for this study. If a minor was enrolled in this study, a letter of authorization will be first obtained from minor's guardian along with a signed informed consent by the guardian.

The *WT1* overexpression was defined in this study as ≥ 250 copies/10^4 *ABL* as previously recommended [9]. When the *WT1* gene was not detected by real-time PCR or the copy number was under the lower limit of detection (3×10^2 copies/mL), we denoted this *WT1* gene copy number as "non-detectable" or "ND". Based on this criterion, the *WT1* gene overexpression was detected in 29 of 103 patients (28%) with a median value of 720 copies/10^4 *ABL* (ranged from ND to 8.2×10^6 copies/mL).

Among these patients, 29% (30/103) of them carried 3 different *NPM1*^{mt} mutant genotypes. The most common *NPM1*^{mt} mutation was the type A (80%, 24/30), which had a "TCTG" insertion in exon 12. In addition, 4 of 30 patients (13%) had the type B mutation ("CATG" insertion), and 2 of 30 patients (7%) had the type 13 mutation ("TAAG" insertion) [10]. Seven of the 30 *NPM1*^{mt} carrying patients (23%) also showed high *WT1* gene expression.

The *FLT3* mutation was detected in 27% of the total patient cohort (28/103), which included the *FLT3*^{TKD} and *FLT3*^{ITD} mutations, respectively. In which 10 out of the 28 patients (36%) carried the *FLT3*^{TKD} mutation including the D835H (80%, 8/10), D835V (10%, 1/10) and D835Y (10%, 1/10) point mutations, respectively. The *FLT3*^{ITD}, which is generally associated with unfavorable outcome [2,3], was identified in 18 of the 28 patients (64%) that carried the internal tandem duplication in exon 14 (61%, 11/18), intron 14 (6%, 1/18) and exon 15 (33%, 6/18). As shown in **Table 1**, 30% (3/10) of the *FLT3*^{TKD}–carrying patients and 44% (8/18) of the *FLT3*^{ITD}–carrying patients also showed *WT1* gene overexpression.

Treatment

All patients received one or two courses of induction chemotherapy with DA (daunorubicin 45 mg/m$^2 \times 3$ days; cytarabine 100–200 mg/m^2 every 12 hours×7 days) or HA (harringtonine 4–6 mg/m$^2 \times 7$ days; cytarabine 100–200 mg/m^2 every 12 hours ×7 days). If patients get complete remission, they would receive consolidation chemotherapy with high-dose cytarabine (3 g/m^2 every 12 hours on days 1, 3, 5 and 7 for a total of 24 g/m^2). Otherwise they would continue to receive other induction chemotherapies. Whether patient will receive hematopoietic stem cell transplantation (HSCT) will depend on comprehensive clinic situation.

DNA and RNA Extraction

Genomic DNA was extracted by using the Genomic DNA Extraction Kit (Tiangen, Beijing, China). Total RNA was isolated using the Trizol reagent (Invitrogen, Carlsbad, USA). All protocols were conducted according to manufacturer's instructions. The quality and concentration of DNA and RNA were analyzed with a Biophotometer (Eppendorf AG, Hamburg, Germany).

Quantification of *WT1* Gene Expression

Real-time reverse-transcriptase polymerase chain reactions (RT-PCR) using patient-derived RNA were carried out on the 7300 real-time PCR system (Applied Biosystems, Foster City, CA, USA). Commercially available *WT1* mRNA quantification kit (Yuanqi, Shanghai, China) was used to detect *WT1* gene expression. A housekeeping gene *ABL* was used as an internal control for calibration of possible variations caused by the variable efficiencies of RNA extraction, RT-PCR and operation. The relative levels of the *WT1* expression to the *ABL* control of the clinical samples were calculated by simultaneous reaction with series standards of known concentrations ($3 \times 10^{3-6}$ copies/ml). To calculate copy number of a specific sample, we first established a standard curve by using a series of known commercial standards from 3×10^3 to 3×10^6 copies/mL. The linear dynamic range of this method was from 3×10^2 copies/mL to 3×10^7 copies/mL. If a samples copy number was above the top limit, the sample will be re-measured with dilutions.

The data were analyzed using the Sequence Detection Software Version 1.2 (Applied Biosystems). For analysis of samples, detectable *WT1* copy numbers were expressed as copies per 10^4 *ABL* copies according to manufacturer's instruction. The cutoff for normal *WT1* expression was defined as 250 copies/10^4 *ABL* as previously used in BM [10].

Detection of *NPM1* and *FLT3* Gene Mutations

For detection of the *NPM1* and *FLT3* mutations, we carried out PCR gene amplification by using the 9700 PCR amplification system (Applied Biosystems). Exon 12 of the *NPM1* gene and exon 14, 15 and 20 of the *FLT3* gene were amplified using respective primer pairs, *NPM1* ex12-F (5′-TTAACTCTCTGGTGGTA-GAATGAA-3′), *NPM1* ex12-R (5′- TGTT ACAGAAATGAAA-TAAGACGG-3′), *FLT3* ex14-F (5′-TTCCCTTT CATCCAA-GAC-3′), *FLT3* ex14-R (5′-AAACATTTGGCACATTCC-3′), *FLT3* ex15-F (5′-GCAATTTAGGTATGAAAGCCAGC-3′), *FLT3* ex15-R (5′-CTTTCAGCATTTTG ACGGCAACC-3′), *FLT3* ex20-F (5′-CCAGGAACGTGCTTGTCA-3′) and *FLT3* ex20-R (5′-TCAAAAA TGCACCACAGTGAG-3′). PCR reaction was performed in a total volume of 25 μL containing 100 ng of DNA, 10 μM of each primer and 12.5 μL 2×PCR buffer (containing MgCl$_2$, dNTP mix and Taq polymerase) (Tiangen). PCR reactions were carried out as follows: denaturation at 95°C

Table 1. Correlation of WT1 overexpression with clinical data, FAB subtypes, and molecular abnormalities in CN-AML patients.

Variant	Total (N = 103)	WT1^{OP} (N = 29, 28%)	P
Median age, years (range)	42 (17~82)	44 (29~74)	.809
Age in groups, years			.549
≤60	91	27 (30)	
>60	12	2 (17)	
Sex			.238
Male	58	19 (33)	
Female	45	10 (22)	
WBC count, 10^9/L			.906
20 or below	40	11 (28)	
Above 20	63	18 (29)	
FAB subtype			
M0	4	2 (50)	.672
M1	16	3 (19)	.543
M2	41	13 (32)	.515
M4	16	4 (25)	.998
M5	26	7 (27)	.872
Molecular abnormalities			
NPM1^{mt}	30	7 (23)	.485
FLT3^{TKD}	10	3 (30)	1
FLT3^{ITD}	18	8 (44)	.091
Risk molecular subgroups*			
Favorable			
NPM1^{mt}/no FLT3^{ITD}	23	4 (17)	.193
Unfavorable			
FLT3^{ITD}	18	8 (44)	.091
Intermediate			
Others excluding NPM1^{mt}/no FLT3^{ITD} and FLT3^{ITD}	62	17 (27)	.838

WT1^{OP}, WT1 overexpression; FAB, French-American-British; CN-AML, cytogenetically normal acute myeloid leukemia; WBC, white blood cell.
*stratification based on molecular abnormalities [2].

for 5 minutes, annealing at 55°C for 1 min. and extension at 72°C for 1 min. for 40 cycles. Amplification products were detected by 1% agarose gel electrophoresis. If the PCR product size was correct, amplification products were subsequently confirmed by nucleotide sequencing using the ABI PRISM 3100 genetic analyzer (Applied Biosystems) after purification. The sequencing results were then compared with the reference and wild type sequences of (*NPM1*: GenBank, NG-016018.1) or *FLT3* (Gen-Bank, NG-007066.1). Gene mutations were confirmed by nucleotide sequencing with coverage of double-strand DNA by using the forward and reverse primers.

Definitions and Statistical Analysis

Complete remission was characterized by morphologically normal marrow with <5% blasts, neutrophil count >1×10^9/L, platelet count >100×10^9/L and normal physical for more than 1 month. The CR rate was evaluated after received one or two courses of induction chemotherapy. Relapse was defined as the reappearance of blasts in the blood or the finding of more than 5% blasts in the bone marrow or any other evidence of leukemia recurrence. The DFS in patients who achieved CR was estimated from the date of CR to relapse or death. The OS was defined as the time from diagnosis to death by any causes [11].

For descriptive statistics, we calculated median, range and percentage of the cases. Proportion was compared using the Chi-Square test. Survival probability was estimated using the Kaplan–Meier curves and the difference between groups was analyzed by the log-rank test. Multivariate analysis was performed applying the COX regression model. For all statistical analyses, the *p* value that was 2-tailed with less than 0.05 was considered to be statistically significant. Statistical analyses were performed by using the statistical software package SPSS Version 19.0 (SPSS Science).

Results

Correlation of *WT1* Overexpression with Clinical Parameters

A total of 103 CN-AML patients, consisting of 58 males and 45 females with a median age of 42 years (range, 17–82 years) were recruited to this study. The *WT1* overexpression was defined as ≥ 250 copies/10^4 *ABL*. Objective of this part of the study was to examine the possible correlation of the *WT1* gene overexpression with various common clinical features or molecular abnormalities.

Specifically, the *WT1* gene overexpression was detected in 29 of 103 patients (28%) with a median value of 720 copies/10^4 *ABL* (range: ND to 8.2×10^6). Comparisons of *WT1* gene overexpression with various clinical parameters and their possible statistical significance are summarized in **Table 1**. Initial comparisons of the *WT1* gene overexpression with common clinical parameters such as age, sex, WBC counts and the FAB subtypes showed no significant differences between the patient groups with or without *WT1* gene overexpression. In order to examine the possible role of *WT1* gene overexpression in assessing treatment response, prognosis and survival of AML patients with normal cytogenetics, All CN-AML patients were divided into three different risk subgroups based on their known molecular abnormalities such as the *FLT3* and *NPM1* gene mutation statuses. As recommended previously [2,3], the favorable outcome subgroup (n = 23) are those CN-AML patients who have the *NPM1* gene mutation (*NPM1*^{mt}) but do not have the internal tandem duplication in the *FLT3* gene (*FLT3*^{ITD}). The unfavorable outcome subgroup (n = 18) are those patients with the FLT3^{ITD} gene mutations. The remaining patients (n = 62), who do not have the *NPM1*^{mt}/no *FLT3*^{ITD} nor the *FLT3*^{ITD} genotypes were defined as the intermediate risk subgroup [2,3]. No statistical significant differences were found in all of these risk groups. Together, these data suggest that the *WT1* overexpression is not associated with any particular risk group or a clinical parameter.

Role of *WT1* Overexpression in Response to Induction Chemotherapy

To examine the potential role of *WT1* overexpression in predicting treatment outcome of the CN-AML patients, we first evaluated the impact of the *WT1* overexpression on patient's response to induction chemotherapy. Complete remission (CR) rates were used and calculated for this evaluation. As shown in **Figure 1A**, the CR rate was significantly influenced by the level of *WT1* gene expression [$p = .003$]. While about 76% (56/74) of the CN-AML patients in the normal *WT1* gene control group had complete remission after treatment, close to half of those patients 45% (13/29) with *WT1* overexpression had complete remission.

Since the *WT1* overexpression clearly showed its impact on patient's response to induction chemotherapy, we next tested the possible role of *WT1* overexpression in measuring CR rates among the 3 different risk groups as defined by the *FLT3* and *NPM1* mutation status. Consistent with the previous classification [2,3], the CR rates in our patient cohort were positively correlated with the three defined risk molecular subgroups (**Figure 1B**), i.e., the CR rates were found to be 91% (21/23), 69% (43/62) and 28% (5/18) in the favorable (*NPM1*^{mt}/no *FLT3*^{ITD}), intermediate and unfavorable (*FLT3*^{ITD}) groups, respectively.

The *WT1* gene expression status was then added to the data analyses and compared for their CR rates among the 3 different risk groups. As shown in **Figure 1C**, it is evident that *WT1* gene expression status had no effect on CR rate in the intermediate risk group. However, statistically significant differences were revealed between patient groups with or without high *WT1* gene expression in the favorable (*NPM1*^{mt}/no *FLT3*^{ITD}) and the unfavorable (*FLT3*^{ITD}) risk groups. For example, in the favorable (*NPM1*^{mt}/no *FLT3*^{ITD}) patient group, complete remission was seen in all 19 patients when the *WT1* gene was expressed at the normal level. However, only half of those patients (2 out of 4) showed complete remission when *WT1* gene was overexpressed ($p = .024$). Remarkably, in the unfavorable (*FLT3*^{ITD}) risk group, none of the patient with *WT1* overexpression showed complete remission whereas about half of this group of patient (5 out of 10) with normal *WT1* expression had complete remission ($p = .036$).

Altogether, the CR rate analyses suggested that *WT1* overexpression alone has no clear role in predicting CR in the intermediate risk group. It however could potentially play a

functional role in predicting CR of the CN-AML patients either in the favorable (*NPM1*^{mt}/no *FLT3*^{ITD}) or the unfavorable (*FLT3*^{ITD}) groups. Specifically, when *WT1* overexpression is added to the predefined risk groups, it may increase the risk or abridge the favorable outcome of the CN-AML patients by interactions with the favorable group or with the unfavorable group, respectively.

Role of *WT1* Overexpression in Predicting Disease-free and Overall Survivals

Since *WT1* overexpression appeared to play a functional role in predicting complete remission of the CN-AML patients especially when it is combined with the favorable *NPM1*^{mt}/no *FLT3*^{ITD} or the unfavorable *FLT3*^{ITD} genotypes, we next examined the potential impact of *WT1* overexpression on the disease-free survival (DFS) and the overall survival (OS) of the studied CN-AML patient cohort. The CN-AML patients were followed in a time period of 1–38 months with a median value of 18 months for DFS or 13 months for OS, respectively. The Kaplan-Meier overall survival analysis was used to calculate the DFS and OS. The potential difference between each testing groups was analyzed by the log-rank test. The final results are summarized in **Figure 2**.

Comparison of the DFS and OS between the *WT1* overexpression group with the *WT1* control group showed that *WT1* overexpression has significantly reduced patient's DFS (**Figure 2A**; log rank = 5.847, $p = .016$) and the OS (**Figure 2B**; log rank = 8.616, $p = .003$). As comparison references for the effect of *WT1* overexpression, the impact of other single gene mutational effect such as the *FLT3*^{ITD}, *NPM1*^{mt} or *FLT3*^{TKD} mutations on DFS and OS was also evaluated. Consistent with the prior report [2], the *FLT3*^{ITD} genotype played a strong role in predicting DFS and OS (log rank = 20.641, $p = 0$ for DFS and log rank = 19.157, $p = 0$ for OS). In contrast, little or no significant influence was detected in patients with the *NPM1*^{mt} genotype (log rank = 2.146, $p = .143$ for DFS and log rank = 2.325, $p = .127$ for OS); or with the *FLT3*^{TKD} genotype (log rank = 0.712, $p = .399$ for DFS and log rank = 0.176, $p = .675$ for OS).

Disease-free survival and the overall survival were also calculated against the three different risk subgroups. Consistent with previous classifications, significant differences in DFS and OS were indeed found among the three risk subgroups. Specifically, patients in the favorable risk group (*NPM1*^{mt}/no *FLT3*^{ITD}) showed excellent DFS and OS; while the high risk or the unfavorable risk (*FLT3*^{ITD}) group displayed very poor outcomes of the DFS and OS (**Figure 2C and 2D**) with the intermediate groups lied in between.

When combining the *WT1* overexpression with the three different risk groups, a very similar contributing patterns of the *WT1* overexpression, as we saw in calculation of the CR rates, were observed with regard to its interaction with the three different risk subgroups. Specifically, the *WT1* overexpression did not seem to affect the DFS and OS in the intermediate subgroup (**Figure 2G and 2H**; log rank = 0.270, $p = .603$ for DFS, log rank = 0.089, $p = .765$ for OS). The average survivals of this group of patients with normal WT1 (*WT1*^{ctr}; n = 45) or high WT1 (*WT1*^{op}; n = 17) expression were 25.4±1.9 and 24.8±2.1 mo ($p = .603$) for DFS, and 30.6±1.8 and 29.9±2.5 mo ($p = .765$) for OS, respectively. However, the *WT1* overexpression significantly reduced the DFS and OS in the favorable risk (*NPM1*^{mt}/no *FLT3*^{ITD}) patient group (**Figure 2E and 2F**, log rank = 4, $p = .046$ for DFS, log rank = 5, $p = .025$ for OS). The average survivals of this group of patients with normal WT1 (*WT1*^{ctr}; n = 19) lived well beyond the study period, however, 7 out the 8 (88%) patients in the high WT1 (*WT1*^{op}; n = 8) group had DFS of less than 16.0 mo ($p = .046$) or OS of about 21.0 mo ($p = .025$), respectively. The other patient

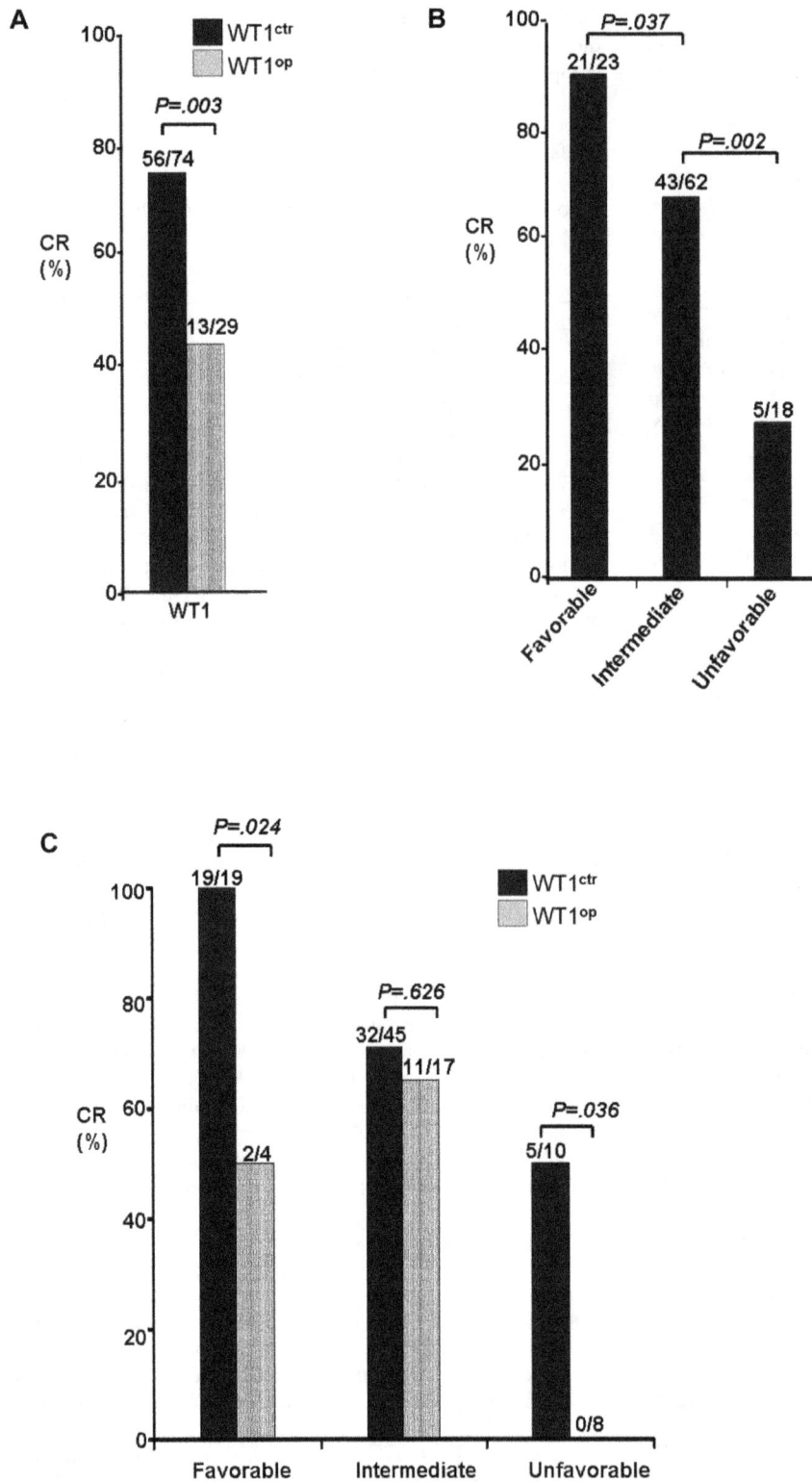

Figure 1. Complete remission (CR) rate analysis based on the *WT1* expression status and other molecular abnormalities in the CN-AML patients. (**A**) Comparison of the CR rates between the CN-AML patients with normal (*WT1*[ctr]) or high (*WT1*[op]) *WT1* gene expression. (**B**) Comparison of the CR rates among three different risk subgroups that were stratified based on molecular abnormalities, *i.e.*, the favorable risk group included CN-AML patients that are carrying the *NPM1*[mt]/no *FLT3*[ITD] genotypes; the unfavorable risk group with the *FLT3*[ITD] genotypes; and the intermediate group are those patients other than the two other risk groups, *i.e.*, lack of the *NPM1*[mt]/no *FLT3*[ITD] and *FLT3*[ITD] genotypes [8]. (**C**) Possible role of *WT1* overexpression in determining the CR rates among the three risk subgroups. Abbreviations: *WT1*[ctr], normal *WT1* expression; *WT1*[op], *WT1* overexpression.

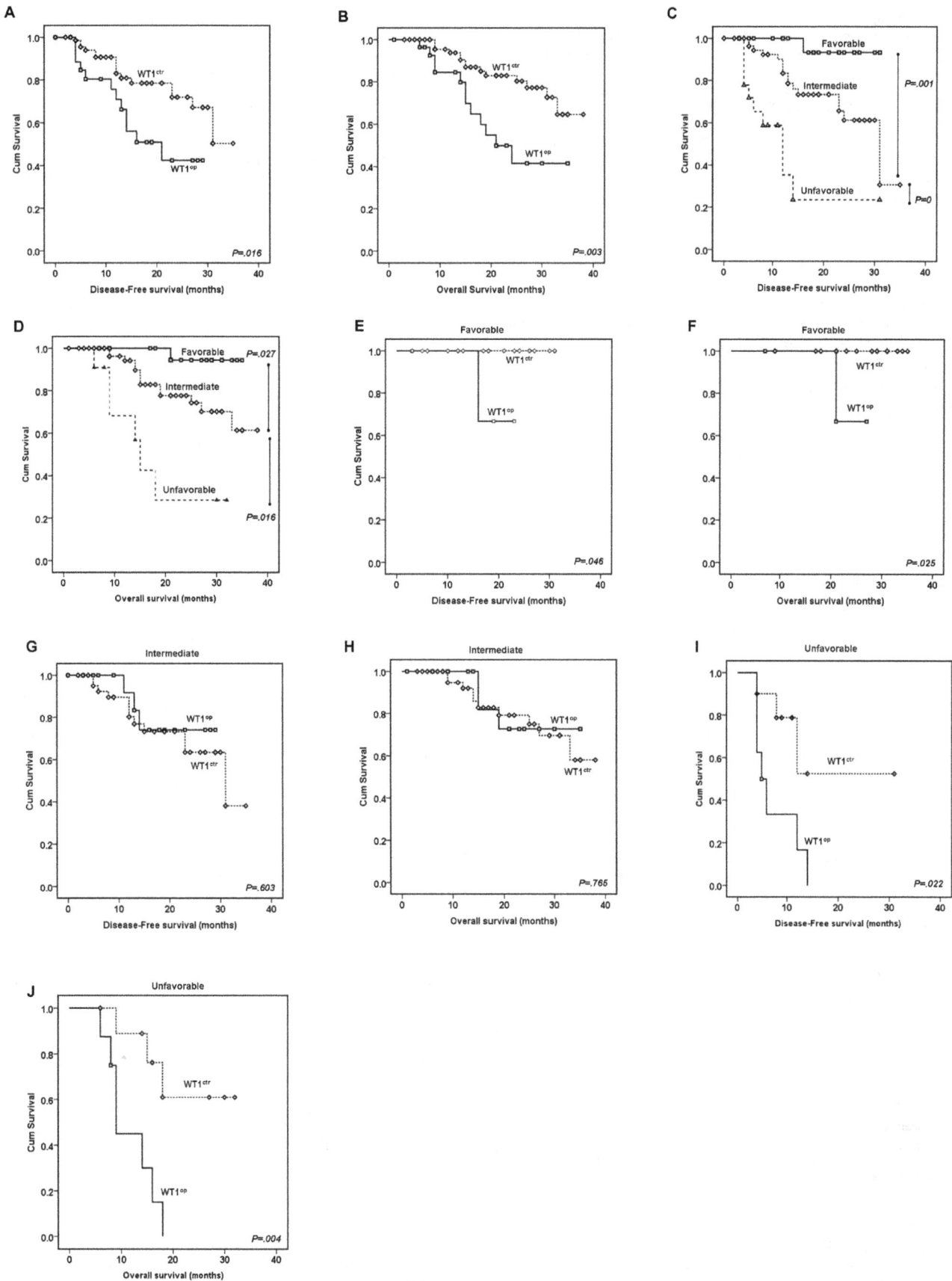

Figure 2. Determination of the diease-free survival (DFS) and overall survival (OS) in the CN-AML patients based on the *WT1* **expression status and other molecular abnormalities.** (**A–B**) Comparison of the DFS (**A**) and OS (**B**) between the CN-AML patients with normal

($WT1^{ctr}$) or high ($WT1^{op}$) WT1 gene expression. The mean DFS and OS of patients with $WT1^{op}$ (n = 29) or $WT1^{ctr}$ (n = 74) were 18.9±2.1 vs. 27.8±1.4 mo (p = .016); and 23.6±2.3 vs. 32.5±1.3 mo (p = .003), respectively. (**C–D**) Comparison of the DFS (**C**) and OS (**D**) among three different risk subgroups that were stratified based on molecular abnormalities, i.e., the favorable risk group included CN-AML patients that are carrying the $NPM1^{mt}$/no $FLT3^{ITD}$ genotypes; the unfavorable risk group with the $FLT3^{ITD}$ genotypes; and the intermediate group are those patients other than the two other groups, i.e., lack of the $NPM1^{mt}$/no $FLT3^{ITD}$ and $FLT3^{ITD}$ genotypes [6]. The average DFS of the patients with favorable (n = 23), intermediate (n = 62) or unfavorable genotype (n = 18) were 30.0±1.0, 26.6±1.6 and 13.9±3.0 mo, respectively. The average OS of the patients with favorable (n = 23), intermediate (n = 62) or unfavorable genotype (n = 18) were 34.2±0.85, 31.4±1.5 and 19.0±2.5 mo, respectively. (**E–J**) Possible role of WT1 overexpression in determining the DFS (**E, G and I**) and OS (**F, H, and J**) among the favorable (**E–F**; $NPM1^{mt}$/no $FLT3^{ITD}$), the intermediate (**G–H**) and the unfavorable (**I–J**; $FLT3^{ITD}$) molecular and risk subgroups. Note that patients with $WT1^{op}$ in the favorable (n = 4) or unfavorable (n = 8) had inferior DFS and OS than their control $WT1^{ctr}$ groups (favorable, n = 19; unfavorable, n = 10). No significant differences of DFS and OS were observed between normal and high WT1 gene expression in the intermediate group. Abbreviations: $WT1^{ctr}$, normal WT1 expression; $WT1^{op}$, WT1 overexpression.

was only followed up to 10 months; thus no specific DFS or OS could be assigned at the completion of this study. Most significantly, the *WT1* overexpression appeared to abruptly shorten patent's survival of the unfavorable risk group patients in both categories (**Figure 2I and 2J**; log rank = 5.246; *p = .022* for DFS, log rank = 8.481; *p = .004* for OS).

Based on these results, we suggest that *WT1* overexpression by itself could play an important but negative role in predicting DFS and OS of the CN-AML patients; moreover, the *WT1* overexpression, when combined with the *NPM1*^mt or the *FLT3*^ITD genotypes, will serve as a poor prognostic marker in reducing DFS and OS in the favorable risk (*NPM1*^mt/no *FLT3*^ITD) patient group or worsening the patient outcomes in the unfavorable risk (*FLT3*^ITD) group.

Multivariate Analysis of the *WT1* Overexpression and its Role in Prognosis of CN-AML

Here we were interested in further testing whether *WT1* overexpression is an independent prognostic factor in predicting DFS or OS the CN-AML patients. Multivariate analysis was carried out by using the cause-specific Cox regression model to analyze the relationship among age (age ≤60 years *vs.* >60 years), the *WT1* overexpression, other single gene mutations and the three molecular risk subgroups. As shown in **Table 2** that age, *FLT3*^ITD and *NPM1*^mt/no *FLT3*^ITD are all independent prognostic markers as previously reported [2,3]. Significantly and indeed,

the *WT1* overexpression also appeared to be an independent prognostic marker for DFS and OS (*p = .028*).

Discussion

Chromosomal aberrations have traditionally been used to assess treatment response, prognosis and survival of the AML patients. Subsequent studies showed, however, that about 85% of the CN-AML patients carried one or more molecular mutations [12]. Indeed, characterization of gene mutations such as *FLT3* or *NPM1* further helped to define the clinical outcomes of AML patients especially when these patients present with normal cytogenetics. Therefore, identification of new molecular biomarker and testing its association with the existing biomarkers are of particular importance for better characterization and risk stratification of CN-AML patients and thus for better patient care.

WT1 overexpression has been shown to play a role in hematologic malignancy [5]. However, molecular mechanism of WT1 overexpression in CN-AML remains to be elusive. There are a number of downstream effectors of the *WT1* genes [13]. For example, the heparin-binding growth factor midkine (*MK*) gene is a prognostic biomarker for various cancers [14,15]. The insulin-like growth factor I receptor (IGF-I-R) is another known downstream effector [16]. More importantly, many of those downstream effectors are indeed involved in cellular growth or survival. Early study by using antisense oligonucleotides has showed that WT1 is required not only for proliferation but also for

Table 2. Multivariate analysis (Cox regression) for clinical and molecular variables of DFS and OS in CN-AML patients.

Variant	DFS		OS	
	Hazard ratio (95% CI)	P	Hazard ratio (95% CI)	P
Age#	0.32 (0.12~0.87)	.025*	0.37 (0.13~1.07)	.037*
WT1^op	2.17 (0.96~4.92)	.034*	2.50 (1.10~5.68)	.028*
NPM1^mt	1.68 (0.41~6.82)	.470	0.92 (0.25~3.40)	0.9
FLT3^TKD	2.71 (0.89~8.33)	.082	2.01 (0.55~7.28)	.289
FLT3^ITD	3.35 (1.26~8.92)	.016*	3.91 (1.42~10.72)	.008*
Risk molecular subgroups				
Favorable				
NPM1^mt/no FLT3^ITD	0.07 (0.01~0.88)	.039*	0.16 (0.07~1.01)	.041*
Unfavorable				
FLT3^ITD	3.35 (1.26~8.92)	.016*	3.91 (1.42~10.72)	.008*
Intermediate				
Others excluding NPM1^mt/no FLT3^ITD and FLT3^ITD	1.15 (0.25~5.39)	.86	1.27 (0.34~6.16)	.81

CN-AML, cytogenetically normal acute myeloid leukemia; DFS, disease-free survival; OS, overall survival; CI, confidence interval; WT1^op, WT1 overexpression.
#age ≤60 years vs. >60 years.
*P values <.05.

inhibiting apoptosis in tumor cell cultures [17]. Therefore, *WT1* overexpression could potentially be used as a tumor-specific target for cancer treatment. Intriguing, an early trial by using peptide vaccines against WT1 in leukemia patients did show promising results [18].

In this study, we examined the possible role of *WT1* gene overexpression in CN-AML patient's responses to induction chemotherapy and in predicting the treatment outcome such as the disease-free survival or overall survival. We further evaluated the possible contribution of *WT1* overexpression to the identification of risk groups that are typically stratified by genotypes such as the *NPM1* or *FLT3* mutation status, which are known molecular markers associated with the survival and treatment outcomes of the AML patients.

From this study, we found that *WT1* overexpression by itself conversely correlated with the CR rate, DFS and OS (**Figure 1 and 2**). Furthermore, *WT1* overexpression also contributes, as a negative prognostic marker, to the prognosis and therapeutic response of the CN-AML patients in the favorable ($NPM1^{mt}$/no $FLT3^{ITD}$) and the unfavorable ($FLT3^{ITD}$) molecular subgroups (**Figure 1 and 2**). Specifically, based on the observations of this CN-AML patient cohort, patients with the *WT1* overexpression/$FLT3^{ITD}$ genotypes showed the worst CR rate, OS and DFS ($WT1^{op}$ in **Figure 2I and 2J**). Conversely, patients with normal *WT1* expression and the $NPM1^{mt}$/no $FLT3^{ITD}$ genotypes displayed the best outcome ($WT1^{ctr}$ in **Figure 2E and 2F**). Altogether, our data suggest that the *WT1* gene overexpression is an independent and negative prognostic factor in predicting patient's response to induction chemotherapy and treatment outcomes. In addition, when combined with the $NPM1^{mt}$ or the $FLT3^{ITD}$ genotypes, the *WT1* overexpression also contribute negatively to patient's response to induction chemotherapy and treatment outcomes. Please note that any clear therapeutic effect of complete remission described here is almost certainly contributed by multifactorial factors such as age, patient's physical status, peripheral white blood counts among other molecular factors, *e.g.*, $NPM1^{mt}$, $FLT3^{ITD}$, *etc*. What we have showed here suggesting *WT1* gene overexpression is at least one of the molecular factors that could play a negative prognostic role in predicting complete remission.

WT1 plays an important role in pathogenesis of AML, but its specific function remains elusive or controversial [5]. In some of the earlier studies, the *WT1* overexpression at diagnosis was shown to be as an adverse predictor for CR rate, DFS and OS in AML patient. In contrast, other studies suggested that *WT1* overexpression was not associated with disease outcome [19,20]. Moreover, previous CN-AML studies on the *WT1* overexpression was mainly used as a molecular marker to detect minimal residual disease. Little was known about the prognostic significance of the *WT1* overexpression in CN-AML. Intriguingly, Frederik Damm and co-

workers did suggest earlier that *WT1* overexpression could potentially be used as one of the several biomarkers to formulate some kind of integrative prognostic risk score for the stratification of CN-AML [21]. Indeed, our data showed here that the *WT1* overexpression can not only be used as a negative prognostic marker for CN-AML but also, for the first time to the best of our knowledge, contributes to the identification of the CN-AML risk subgroups that are normally stratified by the *NPM1* and *FLT3* mutation status.

It was noticed that the percentage of the *WT1* overexpression showed in our study cohort was somewhat lower than the previous reports (28% *vs.* 48%–73%) [7,8]. One obvious difference between our study and the other reports was the use of the reference gene in determining the level of *WT1* gene expression. For example, the housekeeping gene *ABL* was used in our study as an internal control for the calculation of the *WT1* gene expression. The cutoff for normal *WT1* expression was defined as 250 copies/10^4 *ABL* as previously recommended [9]. In contrast, different cutoff value of the *ABL* gene or other housekeep gene such as *GAPDH* gene was used in the other studies [7,20]. It is also possible that other molecular aberrations, *e.g.*, MiR-15a/16-1, which is as a tumor suppressor that down-regulates *WT1* expression in the process of leukemia cell proliferation [22], could be another contributing factor to the observed differences in the *WT1* overexpression. In spite of the observed differences in the percentages of the *WT1* gene expression, this difference should not affect the fact that *WT1*, when it is overexpressed, contributes negatively to the pathogenesis of CN-AML.

Combining with all of our data, our results strongly suggest that *WT1* overexpression is an independent and negative prognostic biomarker that could potentially be used to evaluate response to induction chemotherapy and prognosis of AML patients with normal cytogenetics. In addition, the use of *WT1* overexpression as an additional biomarker seems to enhance the statistical power in the identification of risk subgroups that are normally stratified solely based on the *NPM1* or the *FLT3* mutational status. Therefore, adding profiling of *WT1* gene expression level in the future decision-making of patient's response to induction chemotherapy or prognosis of the CN-AML patients could potentially provide better or more effective care of this group of patients.

Acknowledgments

The authors would like to thank Ge Li for helpful discussions and revision.

Author Contributions

Wrote the paper: XL RZ. Designed the study and analyzed the data: XL YX. Carried out sequencing experiments: RM JD RF. Performed real-time PCR experiments: X. Wang X. Wei. Contributed to analysis of cytogenetics: JH YS.

References

1. Mrozek K, Marcucci G, Paschka P, Whitman SP, Bloomfield CD (2007) Clinical relevance of mutations and gene-expression changes in adult acute myeloid leukemia with normal cytogenetics: are we ready for a prognostically prioritized molecular classification? Blood 109: 431–448.

2. Lyu XD, Zhao RY, Chen Q (2013) Personalized Approach to Diagnosis and Treatment of Acute Myeloid Leukemia. J Clin Exp Patho 3: 143–145.

3. Dohner H, Estey EH, Amadori S, Appelbaum FR, Büchner T, et al. (2010) Diagnosis and management of acute myeloid leukemia in adults: Recommendations from an international expert panel, on behalf of the European LeukemiaNet. Blood 115: 453–474.

4. Yang L, Han Y, Suarez Saiz F, Minden MD (2007) A tumor suppressor and oncogene: the *WT1* story. Leukemia 21: 868–876.

5. Bergmann L, Maurer U, Weidmann E (1997) Wilms tumor gene expression in acute myeloid leukemias. Leuk Lymphoma 25: 435–443.

6. Garg M, Moore H, Tobal K, Liu Yin JA (2003) Prognostic significance of quantitative analysis of *WT1* gene transcripts by competitive reverse transcription polymerase chain reaction in acute leukaemia. Br J Haematol 123: 49–59.

7. Miglino M, Colombo N, Pica G, Grasso R, Clavio M, et al. (2011) *WT1* overexpression at diagnosis may predict favorable outcome in patients with de novo non-M3 acute myeloid leukemia. Leuk Lymphoma 52: 1961–1969.

8. Barragán E, Cervera J, Bolufer P, Ballester S, Martín G, et al. (2004) Prognostic implications of Wilms' tumor gene (*WT1*) expression in patients with de novo acute myeloid leukemia. Haematologica 89: 926–933.

9. Cilloni D, Renneville A, Hermitte F, Hills RK, Daly S, et al. (2009) Real-Time Quantitative Polymerase Chain Reaction Detection of Minimal Residual Disease by Standardized WT1 Assay to Enhance Risk Stratification in Acute Myeloid Leukemia: A European LeukemiaNet Study. J Clin Oncol 27: 5195–5201.

10. Rau R, Brown P (2009) Nucleophosmin (NPM1) mutations in adult and childhood acute myeloid leukaemia: towards definition of a new leukaemia entity. Hematological Oncology 27: 171–181.

11. Cheson BD, Bennett JM, Kopecky KJ, Büchner T, Willman CL, et al. (2003) Revised recommendations of the International Working Group for Diagnosis, Standardization of Response Criteria, Treatment Outcomes, and Reporting Standards for Therapeutic Trials in Acute Myeloid Leukemia. J Clin Oncol 21: 4642–4649.

12. Marcucci G, Haferlach T, Dohner H (2011) Molecular genetics of adult acute myeloid leukemia: Prognostic and therapeutic implications. J Clin Oncol 29: 475–486.

13. Adachi Y, Matsubara S, Pedraza C, Ozawa M, Tsutsui J, et al. (1996) Midkine as a novel target gene for the Wilms' tumor suppressor gene (WT1). Oncogene 13: 2197–2203.

14. Jono H, Ando Y (2010) Midkine: a novel prognostic biomarker for cancer. Cancers (Basel) 2: 624–641.

15. Ma Z, Li H, Wang B, Shen Q, Cui E, et al. (2013) Midkine mRNA level in peripheral blood mononuclear cells is a novel biomarker for primary non-small cell lung cancer: a prospective study. J Cancer Res Clin Oncol 139: 557–562.

16. Werner H, Roberts CT Jr, Rauscher FJ 3rd, LeRoith D (1996) Regulation of insulin-like growth factor I receptor gene expression by the Wilms' tumor suppressor WT1. J Mol Neurosci 7: 111–123.

17. Tuna M, Chavez-Reyes A, Tari AM (2005) HER2/neu increases the expression of Wilms' tumor 1 (WT1) protein to stimulate S-phase proliferation and inhibit apoptosis in breast cancer cells. Oncogene 24: 1648–1652.

18. Oka Y, Tsuboi A, Taguchi T, Osaki T, Kyo T, et al. (2004) Induction of WT1 (Wilms' tumor gene)-specific cytotoxic T lymphocytes by WT1 peptide vaccine and the resultant cancer regression. Proc Natl Acad Sci USA 101: 13885–13890.

19. Spassov BV, Stoimenov AS, Balatzenko GN, Genova ML, Peichev DB, et al. (2011) Wilms' tumor protein and *FLT3*-internal tandem duplication expression in patients with de novo acute myeloid leukemia. Hematology 16: 37–42.

20. Miyawaki S, Hatsumi N, Tamaki T, Naoe T, Ozawa K, et al. (2010) Prognostic potential of detection of *WT1* mRNA level in peripheral blood in adult acute myeloid leukemia. Leuk Lymphoma 51: 1855–1861.

21. Damm F, Heuser M, Morgan M, Wagner K, Görlich K, et al. (2011) Integrative prognostic risk score in acute myeloid leukemia with normal karyotype. Blood 117: 4561–4568.

22. Gao SM, Xing CY, Chen CQ, Lin SS, Dong PH, et al. (2011) MiR-15a and miR-16-1 inhibit the proliferation of leukemic cells by down-regulating *WT1* protein level. J Exp Clin Cancer Res 30: 110.

4

The Osteoblastogenesis Potential of Adipose Mesenchymal Stem Cells in Myeloma Patients Who Had Received Intensive Therapy

Hsiu-Hsia Lin[1], Shiaw-Min Hwang[2], Shang-Ju Wu[1], Lee-Feng Hsu[2], Yi-Hua Liao[3], Yi-Shuan Sheen[3], Wen-Hui Chuang[1], Shang-Yi Huang[1]*

1 Department of Internal Medicine, National Taiwan University Hospital, Taipei, Taiwan, 2 Bioresource Collection and Research Center, Food Industry Research and Development Institute, Hsinchu, Taiwan, 3 Department of Dermatology, National Taiwan University Hospital, Taipei, Taiwan

Abstract

Multiple myeloma (MM) is characterized by advanced osteolytic lesions resulting from the activation of osteoclasts (OCs) and inhibition of osteoblasts (OBs). OBs are derived from mesenchymal stem cells (MSCs) from the bone marrow (BM), however the pool and function of BMMSCs in MM patients (MM-BMMSCs) are reduced by myeloma cells (MCs) and cytokines secreted from MCs and related anti-MM treatment. Such reduction in MM-BMMSCs currently cannot be restored by any means. Recently, genetic aberrations of MM-BMMSCs have been noted, which further impaired their differentiation toward OBs. We hypothesize that the MSCs derived from adipose tissue (ADMSCs) can be used as alternative MSC sources to enhance the pool and function of OBs. Therefore, the purpose of this study was to compare the osteogenesis ability of paired ADMSCs and BMMSCs in MM patients who had completed intensive therapy. Fifteen MM patients who had received bortezomib-based induction and autologous transplantation were enrolled. At the third month after the transplant, the paired ADMSCs and BMMSCs were obtained and cultured. Compared with the BMMSCs, the ADMSCs exhibited a significantly higher expansion capacity (100% vs 13%, respectively; $P = .001$) and shorter doubling time (28 hours vs 115 hours, respectively; $P = .019$). After inducing osteogenic differentiation, although the ALP activity did not differ between the ADMSCs and BMMSCs (0.78 U/μg vs 0.74±0.14 U/μg, respectively; $P = .834$), the ADMSCs still exhibited higher calcium mineralization, which was determined using Alizarin red S (1029 nmole vs 341 nmole, respectively; $P = .001$) and von Kossa staining (2.6 E+05 μm^2 vs 5 E+04 μm^2, respectively; $P = .042$), than the BMMSCs did. Our results suggested that ADMSCs are a feasible MSC source for enhancing the pool and function of OBs in MM patients who have received intensive therapy.

Editor: Pablo Menendez, Josep Carreras Leukaemia Research Institute, University of Barcelona, Spain

Funding: This study was supported by grants from the National Science Council (NSC97-2314-B-002-036-MY3; NSC101-2314-B-002-086; NSC102-2628-B-002-052-MY3) and National Taiwan University Hospital (NTUH 94A19-1, 99-S0131, 100-S1659, 101-S1801, 102-S2161) and Department of Health (DOH100-TD-C-111-001), Taiwan, Republic of China. The funders had no role in study design, data collection and analysis, decision to publish, or preparation of the manuscript.

Competing Interests: The authors have declared that no competing interests exist.

* E-mail: syhuang55@ntuh.gov.tw

Introduction

Multiple myeloma (MM), a malignant B-cell disorder, is characterized by the accumulation of neoplastic plasma cells within bone marrow (BM) and punched-out (lytic) bone lesions [1]. Advanced lytic bone lesions and related pathologic fractures affect nearly 50% of MM patients throughout their disease courses, and are critical clinical concerns that result in 20% higher mortality compared with MM patients without fractures [2]. MM-related bone destruction (MMBD) is caused by increased activity of osteoclasts (OCs) which, however, causes bone loss with concomitant loss of bone repair and growth from the suppression of osteoblasts (OBs) [2]. Myeloma cells (MCs) secrete several cytokines, including the receptor activator of NF-κB ligand (RANKL), interleukin-3 (IL-3), IL-6, and activin A to activate osteoclasts (OCs), and secrete dickkopf-1 (DKK1) and soluble frizzled related proteins (SFRPs) to inhibit the differentiation and maturation of osteoblasts (OBs) [2–7].

Current therapeutic options for MMBD include bisphosphonates, radiotherapy, and surgery, which may reduce bone pain,

the development of new osteolytic lesions, and prevent skeletal-related events (SREs), including pathologic fractures [2]. But only the bisphosphonates are able to inhibit OCs substantially, the effect of radiotherapy and surgery, however, is mainly based on an antitumor and symptomatic effect without an evident role in the modification of the function of OCs. These treatments for MMBD, no matter bisphosphonates or radiation and surgery, do not enhance either the pool or function of OBs; in other words, they do not improve osteoblastogenesis in MM patients [2,4]. It is the reason why in most clinical scenarios, MMBD seldom heal despite adequate treatment, even when the disease is in remission [2,8]. In physiological conditions, OBs are derived from mesenchymal stem cells (MSCs) that reside in the BM [9]. However, human MSCs also reside in various tissues other than the BM and are able to differentiate into multiple tissue lineages, including cartilage and bone [10–13]. Numerous studies on using MSC-related therapy in the regeneration of musculoskeletal and neural tissues and the recovery of endothelial function have been conducted [14,15]. In MMBD, MSCs derived from the BM

(BMMSCs) have been used to heal bone lesions [16]. However, recent studies have shown that BMMSCs from MM patients (MM-BMMSCs) have several aberrant gene expressions and chromosomal abnormalities compared with those from healthy donors [17–19].The origin of these genetic aberrations in MM-BMMSCs is unclear, but the genetic aberrations seemed to persist in the MM-BMMSCs even though the clinical remission of MM was achieved through adequate treatment [19]. Certain aberrant regulatory genes, such as the bone morphogenetic protein (BMP) family have been associated with osteogenic differentiation [17,19,20]. However, according to our thorough review of relevant literature, efforts to repair lytic bone lesions in MM patients by using MM-BMMSCs have not yet succeeded [2,6]. Therefore, we hypothesize that an alternative MSC other than BMMSCs in MM patients can be used as an effective cellular source for repairing osteolytic bone lesions in the future. Adipose-tissue-derived MSCs (ADMSCs) are candidates for repairing osteolytic bone lesions because they reside outside the BM, where the microenvironment might not have been altered by the MCs, and exhibit osteogenic potential [21,22]. Compared with BMMSCs, ADMSCs have similar self-renewal ability [21] and can differentiate into other mesodermal lineages [21,23]. Furthermore, a recent study showed that osteogenesis ability of ADMSCs is less affected by repeated cell passages and donor age than that from BMMSCs [24], indicating that ADMSCs are an ideal alternative MSC source for osteoblastogenesis in MM patients.

The purposes of this study were to compare the osteogenesis potential of paired BMMSCs and ADMSCs obtained from MM patients who completed a bortezomib-based induction regimen followed by high-dose chemotherapy with autologous stem cell transplantation (HDT/AuSCT), a standard treatment for MM patients [1], and to determine whether ADMSCs are a suitable MSC source that can differentiate into adequate and functional OBs in MM patients.

Materials and Methods

MM Patients

From July 2012 to August 2013, 15 MM patients who had received a bortezomib-based induction regimen followed by HDT/AuSCT (200 mg/m^2 of melphalan) were enrolled. The dosage and schedule of the treatment were similar to those reported previously [25]. In brief, bortezomib (1.3 mg/m^2) was administered on Days 1, 4, 8, and 11 in a 21-day cycle, thalidomide (200 mg) was administered daily, and dexamethasone (80 mg) was administered weekly. Seven patients received additional cyclophosphamide (100 mg daily) for the first 4 days in each cycle. One of patient had received doxorubicin (9 mg/m^2 i.v.f. for consecutive 4 days) instead of thalidomide due to personal intolerance.

Paired bone marrow samples and subcutaneous adipose tissues and controls

Paired BM samples and subcutaneous adipose tissues were obtained from eachMM patient at the regular BM examination approximately 3 months after Day 0 of the HDT/AuSCT. Subcutaneous adipose tissues (sizes 0.3–0.5 mm^3) under the BM puncture site were obtained by performing surgical exploration. During the same period of time, bone marrow samples obtained from 5 non-MM patients, including stage I lung cancer (1), perivascular lympocytic dermatitis (1), and stage I/II lymphoma (3) with a median age of 69 years (range: 39–84 y), were used as a non-MM control; while subcutaneous adipose tissues biopsied from another 4 healthy donors with a median age of 38 years

(range 27–73 y) were also obtained. This study was approved by National Taiwan University Hospital Research Ethics Committee (NTUHREC: 201106013RC), and written informed consent was obtained from each study subject in accordance with the Declaration of Helsinki.

Isolation of bone marrow mesenchymal stem cells and adipose tissue-derived mesenchymal stem cells and the cell culture

BM mononuclear cells (BMMNCs) were obtained by conducting equal-volume Ficoll centrifugation (2000 rpm, 40 minutes) (GE Healthcare, UK). The BMMNCs were then seeded in a flask at a cell density of 2×10^6/cm^2. The basic growth medium consisted of α-MEM (GIBCO, CA, USA)+20% FBS (Corning, NY, USA)+4 ng/mL of bFGF (Millipore, MA, USA)+1xPS (GIBCO, CA, USA). The paired subcutaneous adipose tissues were dissected into small pieces and digested with collagenase IV (SERVA Electrophoresis GmbH, Heidelberg, Germany) and hyaluronidase (Sigma-Aldrich, MO, USA), and were cultured in the basic growth medium (α-MEM+20% FBS+4 ng/mL bFGF+ 1xPS) at 37°C for 50 minutes with intermittent shaking. The resulting suspensions were filtered using a 70-μm strainer (BD Bioscience, NJ, USA) to remove debris and then centrifuged at 2000 rpm for 10 minutes. The supernatants were discarded, and the cell pellets were resuspended in the basic growth medium and cultured at density of 1.3×10^5/cm^2 in a tissue flask (37°C, 5% CO$_2$). The basic growth medium was changed every 3 days and the cells were maintained at subconfluent levels (Passage 0, P0). The attached cells (BMMSCs and ADMSCs) were then harvested using trypsin-EDTA (GIBCO, CA, USA), and were subcultured at a density of $2–3 \times 10^3$ cells/cm^2 under the same conditions used in the primary culture (Passage 1, P1).

Flow cytometry

Flow cytometry was performed by employing a FACSVerse flow cytometer (BD Biosciences, NJ, USA) and using a panel of monoclonal antibodies to identify MSCs, namely CD105-PE, CD73-PE, CD44-PE, and CD90-PE (BD Biosciences, NJ, USA) and hematopoietic cells, namely CD14-FITC, CD19-FITC (BD Biosciences, NJ, USA), CD45-FITC/CD34-PE (Thermo Fisher Scientific, MA, USA) [26,27], CD138-FITC and HLA-DR (BD Biosciences, NJ, USA) [28], as well as isotype-matched controls (BD Biosciences, NJ, USA).

Proliferation assay

The proliferation potential of the cultured MSCs from the second passage (P2) to the fourth passage (P4) was evaluated according to the cumulative population doubling level (CPDL) as described previously [29], which was calculated as ln(Nf/Ni)/ln2, where Ni, Nf, and ln are initial seeded cell numbers, final cell numbers on the day of the subculture, and the natural log, respectively. The doubling time (hours) was then obtained by dividing 24 hours by the calculated CPDL.

Expansion capacity of the cultured mesenchymal stem cells

As described previously [29], when the doubling time of the cultured MSCs was greater than 100 hours for a specific passage, the culture was considered to fail. The probability of expansion capacity of the cultured MSCs was estimated by the Kaplan-Meier survival curve, considering that the failure of proceeding culture at the specific passage was an event.

Senescence associated beta-galactosidase staining

Ten thousand MSCs cells were plated in a 24 well plate for 24 h before the staining procedure. The detection of cellular senescence was performed by using the Senescence Detection Kit (Chemicon, USA & Canada) according to the manufacturer's instructions. Briefly, the cells washed with PBS at least 3 times and then fixed by fixation buffer at room temperature for 15 min. Rinsed and washed cells by PBS at least 3 times then stained by beta-galactosidase staining solution and incubated at 37°C overnight in a dry incubator (no CO_2). Under a light microscopic examination, the blue granules developed within the cytoplasms were considered positive for the beta-galactosidase staining, suggesting senescence of the observed cells.

Osteogenic differentiation

The osteogenic differentiation of the cultured MSCs from the second passage (P2) to the fourth passage (P4) was analyzed. The cells were seeded at 5×10^4 cells/well in a 6-well plate ($5 \times 10^3/$ cm^2) and maintained in the basic growth medium until the cells reached 80% confluence. To induce osteogenic differentiation, the culture medium was changed to an osteogenic medium [α-MEM (GIBCO, CA, USA)+10% FBS (Corning, NY, USA)+1xPS (GIBCO, CA, USA)+10 nM dexamethasone (Dex, Sigma-Aldrich, MO, USA), 50 µg/mL of ascorbic acid (Sigma-Aldrich, MO, USA) and 10 mM β-glycerophosphate (Calbiochem, CA, USA)].

Alkaline phosphatase activity

Alkaline phosphatase (ALP) activity of MSCs from passage 2 to 4 each was measured on the Day 4 by using the SensoLyte pNPP alkaline phosphatase assay kit (ANASPEC, Fremont, CA, USA). Briefly, the cells were lysed using an assay buffer with Triton X-100 and then centrifuged at $2500 \times g$ for 10 min at 4°C. The standard curve of ALP was generated using a serial dose of ALP (0–10 ng/well) and incubated with an ALP substrate solution (pNPP) at room temperature for 1 hour in each experiment. The detection range of ALP was 0 to 10 U. The cell lysates were incubated with an ALP substrate solution (pNPP) at room temperature for 1 hour, the reaction was stopped using a stop solution, and the absorbance was read at 405 nm (Perkin Elmer, CA, USA). The ALP activity (U) of cell lysates was calculated according to the ALP standard curve. The obtained ALP activity was then normalized according to the total protein (µg) in the loaded cell lysates and presented as U/µg. The total protein of cell lysates was determined using the Pierce™ BCA protein assay (Thermo Fisher Scientific, IL, USA).

Alizarin red S staining

The cell matrix layer was washed with PBS, fixed with 70% cold ethanol, and stained with a 2% Alizarin red S (ARS) solution with a pH of 4.3 (Sigma-Aldrich, MO, USA) for 15 minutes. The amount of matrix mineralization was determined by dissolving the cell-bound ARS in 10% (w/v) cetylpyridinium chloride (CPC, Sigma-Aldrich, MO, USA) and 10 mM sodium phosphate, pH 7.0, and the standard curve of ARS was generated using a serial dose of ARS (0–100 nmole) in a 10% CPC solution. The absorbance was read at 562 nm (Perkin Elmer, CA, USA). The quantitative measurement of ARS absorbance in MSCs was calculated according to the generated standard curve for ARS

Bone nodule formation and von Kossa staining quantification

Corning Osteo Assay Surface multiple-well plates (Corning, NY, USA) were used to directly assess the osteoblastic activity in

vitro as described previously [30,31]. In brief, the MSCs were seeded at 2×10^4/well ($1 \times 10^4/cm^2$) in a Corning Osteo Surface plate (Corning, NY, USA) with the osteogenic medium. The osteogenic medium was refreshed every 3 days. The formed bone nodules were determined on Day 18 after osteogenic differentiation commenced and were measured using von Kossa staining. Briefly, cells were washed with PBS 3 times and fixed with 4% paraformaldehyde in PBS for 45 minutes at room temperature. After washing with deionized water, the cells were stained with 5% silver nitrate (Sigma-Aldrich, MO, USA) for another 45 minutes at room temperature under a bright light. To stop the silver nitrate reaction, the cells were washed with water and treated with a 5% solution of sodium thiosulfate (Sigma-Aldrich, MO, USA). Following another water wash and air drying, the nodules were visualized as dark staining patches under a light microscope. The area of von Kossa-positive nodules was determined using the public Image J software (developed by NIH, rsb.info.nih.gov/ij/) and the total areas (μm^2) of the von Kossa-positive nodules were calculated.

Statistics

Chi-square or Fisher's exact tests were used for between-group comparisons of the discrete variables. A Student paired t test or one-way ANOVA was used for between-group comparisons of the means. Kaplan-Meier survival curve was constructed to estimate the probability of expansion capacity, as a time to event defined by failure of proceeding further cultures of MSCs cultures, and the differences between groups were compared using the log-rank test. All directional P values were 2-tailed, and a value of .05 or less was considered significant for all tests. All analyses were performed using SPSS 18.0 software (Chicago, IL, USA).

Results

MM Patients

Seven men and 8 women with a median age of 57.5 years (range: 46–67 y) participated in this study. The clinical salient characteristics, treatment content, and response of these patients are summarized in Table 1. The overall response rate, terms of partial response or better, was 100% after the HDC/AuSCT, and the median induction duration was 8 months (range, 3–17 mo).

Characteristics of bone marrow mesenchymal stem cells and adipose tissue-derived mesenchymal stem cells

All of the attached mononuclear cells harvested from subcutaneous adipose tissues and paired BM were immunopositive for CD44, CD73, CD90, and CD105 (Figure 1a), but were immunonegative for CD14, CD19, CD34, CD45, CD138 and HLA-DR (Figure 1b), which are compatible with the surface marker expression of MSCs.

Adipose tissue-derived mesenchymal stem cells exhibited a higher expansion capacity and shorter doubling time than paired bone marrow mesenchymal stem cells did

The expansion capacity of MM-ADMSCs and MM-BMMSCs from P2 to P6 were evaluated and are shown in Figure 2. The expansion capacities of cultured MM-ADMSCs were maintained at 100% from P2 to P6. By contrast, the expansion capacities of paired BMMSCs decreased gradually with the propagation of passages, and dropped to only 13% at P6. The difference in expansion capacities between the MM-ADMSCs and paired BMMSCs was statistically significant ($P = .001$). Notably, except

Table 1. The salient clinical characteristics at diagnosis and treatment response of the 15 MM patients.

Pt	Sex/age (yr)	Stage (DSS/ISS)	M-protein	PC in BM (%)	CA	Osteolytic lesion	Pathologic fracture	ZA	Induction regimen	Induction duration** (m)	Best Response* after HDT/AuSCT
1	F/51	II/I	IgD/kappa	80	no	yes	yes	yes	V+T+C+D	5	PR
2	M/51	IIIb/III	IgD/lambda	90	no	yes	yes	yes	V+T+D	10	CR
3	F/55	II/I	kappa	40	no	no	yes	yes	V+T+C+D	11	CR
4	M/38	I/I	IgA/lambda	5	no	no	yes	yes	V+T+D	8	CR
5	M/57	IIIb/III	IgG/kappa	92	no	yes	yes	yes	V+T+D	8	PR
6	F/60	II/I	IgG/kappa	60	no	no	no	yes	V+T+C+D	13	PR
7	F/58	II/I	IgG/kappa	30	no	yes	no	yes	V+T+C+D	9	CR
8	M/54	IIIa/II	IgG/lambda	30	no	no	no	yes	V+A+D	8	VGPR
9	F/53	II/I	IgG/lambda	50	no	no	no	no	V+T+D	8	VGPR
10	M/45	I/I	IgA/kappa	10	no	yes	yes	no	V+T+D	6	PR
11	F/47	IIIa/III	IgG/kappa	90	no	yes	no	no	V+T+D	3	VGPR
12	F/49	IIIa/II	IgG/kappa	90	yes	yes	yes	yes	V+T+D	5	CR
13	M/63	I/I	IgG/lambda	20	no	yes	no	yes	V+T+C+D	5	CR
14	F/59	IIIa/II	IgG/lambda	30	no	yes	yes	yes	V+T+C+D	17	VGPR
15	M/65	IIIa/II	IgG/kappa	96	yes	yes	yes	yes	V+T+C+D	5	VGPR

* : According to the IMWG criteria, and the evaluation was taken at the 3rd month from the HDT/AuSCT;

** : Defined from commencement of induction treatment to HDT/AuSCT.

Abbreviations: A, doxorubicin; BM, bone marrow; C, cyclophosphamide; CA, cytogenetic abnormalities; CR, complete response; D, dexamethasone; DSS, Durie-Salmon Stage; F, female; HDT/AuSCT, high dose chemotherapy followed by autologous stem cell transplantation; ISS, International Staging System; M, male; M-protein, myeloma immunoprotein; m, month; PC, plasma cell; PR, partial response; Pt, patient; T, thalidomide; V, bortezomib; VGPR, very good partial response; yr, years; ZA, zoledronic acid.

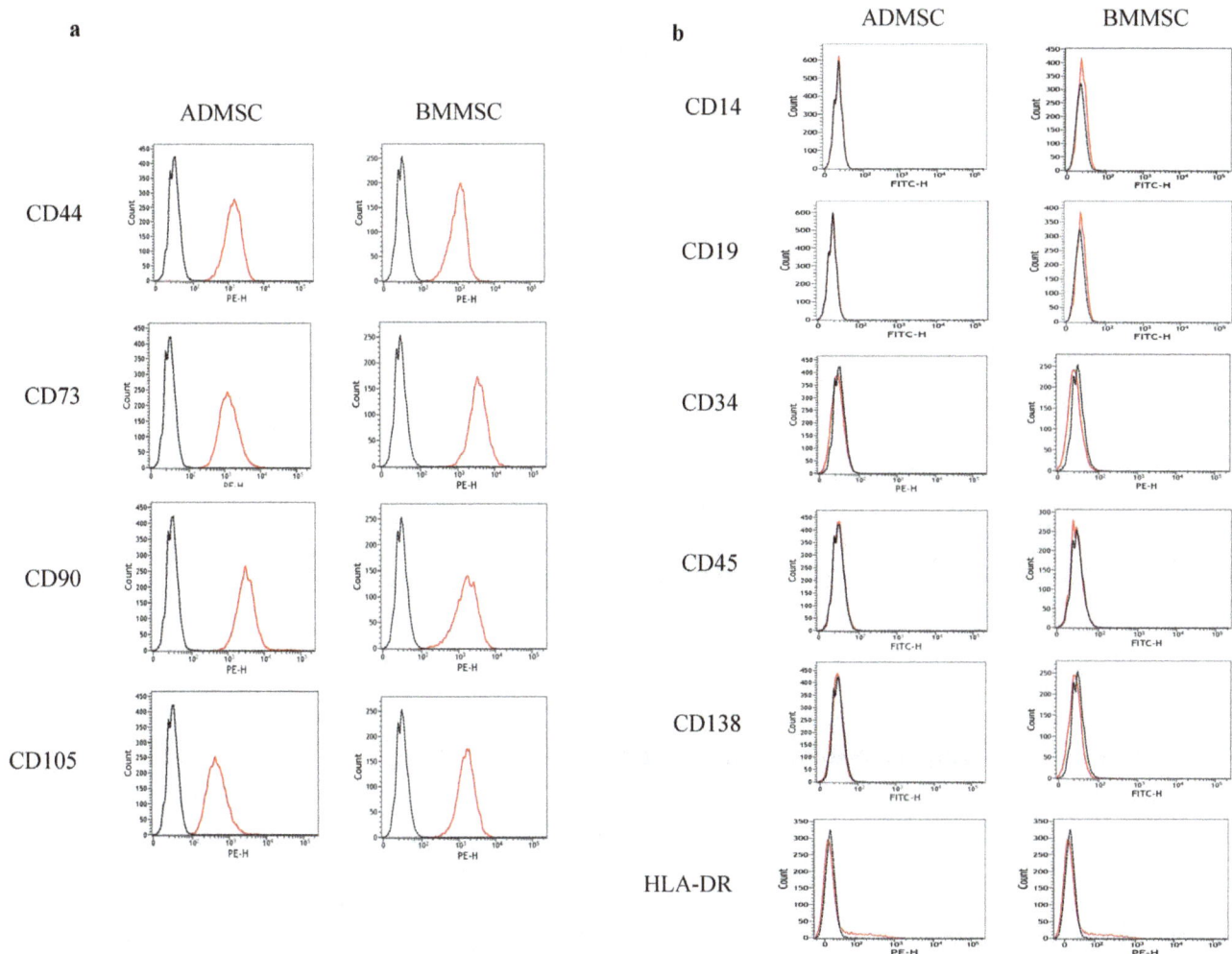

Figure 1. Surface marker analysis of ADMSCs and paired BMMSCs. All the ADMSCs and BMMSCs were immune-positive for the MSCs cell surface markers: CD44, CD73, CD90 and CD105 (a) but immune-negative for the hematopoietic cell surface markers: CD14, CD19, CD34, CD45, CD138 and HLA-DR (b). The results are presented as FACS histograms (isotype control stain = black dot line histogram; surface marker stain = orange solid line histogram).

for the induction duration, which was significantly longer in the failure patients (P2 failure; n = 6) than in the other patients (11.8 mo vs 6.2 mo, respectively; $P = .001$), no other clinical characteristics, including the total white blood cells (WBC), hemoglobin and platelet levels at sampling of BM and adipose tissue, as well as ALP, lactate dehydrogenase (LDH), beta-2-microglobulin (B2MG), whether response to HDC/AuSCT, presence of bone disease, and the type of induction chemotherapy, were associated with BMMSCs from failed cultures. The mean doubling times for MM-ADMSCs and paired BMMSCs were 27.7±1.6 hours and 114.9±31.5 hours, respectively, and the difference was statistically significant ($P = .019$).

Senescence associated beta-galactosidase staining

Typical positive beta-galactosidase stainings were found in most of the cultured MM-BMMSCs (Figure 3a and 3c), but which were not seen in any of the paired ADMSCs (Figure 3b and 3d).

Alkaline phosphatase activity

ALP activity of MSCs from passage 2 to 4 each measured on the Day 4 after the osteogenic induction was 0.78±0.19 U/µg for

MM-ADMSCs and 0.74±0.14 U/µg for the paired BMMSCs, and the differences between the MM-ADMSCs and MM-BMMSCs were not statistically significant ($P = .834$). There was no statistically significant difference for the ALP activity on ADMSCs between healthy donors and MM patients (0.94±0.28 U/µg and 0.74±0.14 U/µg, respectively; $P = .193$), neither on BMMSCs between non-MM control and MM patients (0.77±0.23 U/µg and 0.78±0.19 U/µg, respectively; $P = .975$).

Alizarin red S staining

The cultured MSCs exhibited spindle-shaped and fibroblast-like morphologies before osteogenic differentiation. No differences in the gross morphology were observed between MM-ADMSCs (Figures 4g & 4j) and paired BMMSCs (Figures 4a & 4d). Red granules appeared in positive ARS staining for calcium deposits for both the MM-ADMSCs (Figures 4e & 4k) and paired BMMSCs (Figures 4b & 4h).

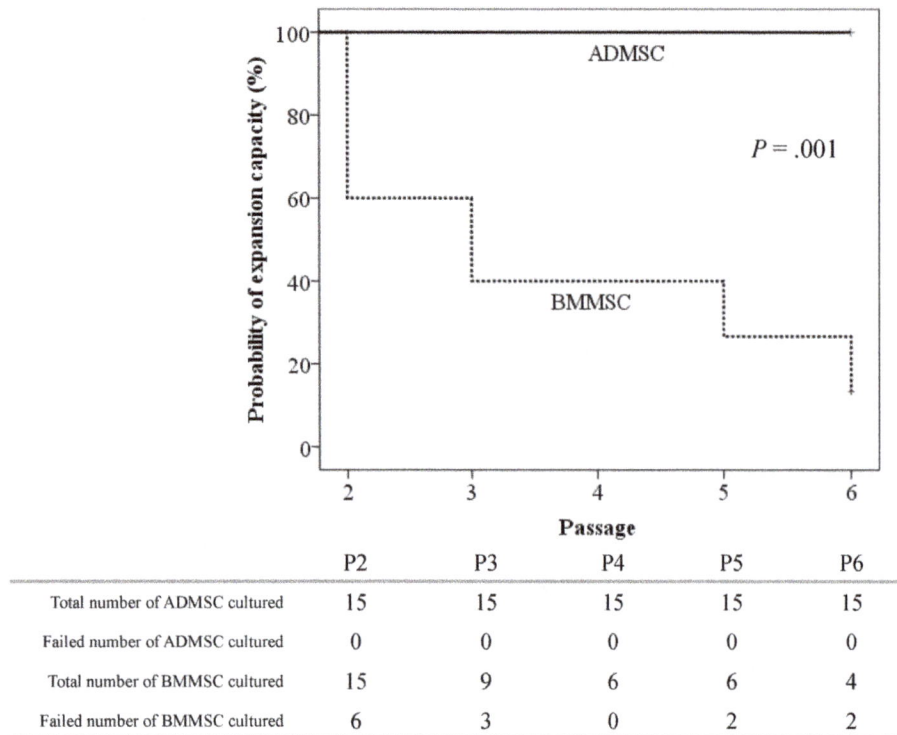

Figure 2. The expansion capacity of MM-ADMSCs and paired BMMSCs.

	P2	P3	P4	P5	P6
Total number of ADMSC cultured	15	15	15	15	15
Failed number of ADMSC cultured	0	0	0	0	0
Total number of BMMSC cultured	15	9	6	6	4
Failed number of BMMSC cultured	6	3	0	2	2

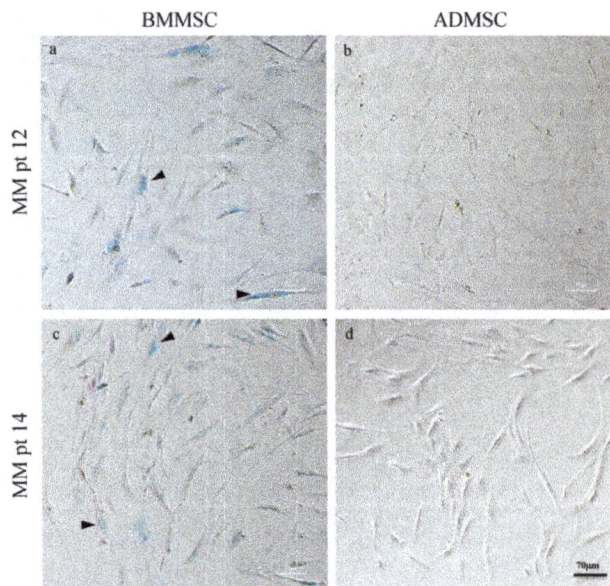

Figure 3. Senescence associated beta-galactosidase staining of cultured ADMSCs and BMMSCs from two representative MM patients. Positive senescence associated beta-galactosidase stainings shown by the blue granules within cytoplasms (arrowhead) were seen in most BMMSCs (a, c), but which were not seen in any of the paired ADMSCs (b, d).

Bone nodule formation and von Kossa stain quantification

Bone nodules were identified using von Kossa staining and were shown in brown-black granules for both the MM-ADMSCs (Figures 4f & 4l) and paired BMMSCs (Figures 4c & 4i). The total von Kossa-positive area on MM-ADMSCs (2.6×10^5 μm^2) was greater than that on paired BMMSCs (5×10^4 μm^2), and the difference was statistically significant ($P = .042$).

Quantification of mineralization

The calcium deposition levels quantified using ARS were 1029 ± 131 nmole for ADMSCs and 341 ± 132 nmole for BMMSCs. The difference was statistically significant ($P = .001$). There was also significant difference on the calcium deposition between BMMSCs from myeloma patients and non-MM control (341 ± 132 nmole vs 1049 ± 202 nmole, respectively; $P = .010$), but on contrast, no significant difference between ADMSCs from healthy donors and MM patients (1388 ± 57 nmole and 1029 ± 131 nmole, respectively; $P = .134$) (Figure 5).

Discussion

Based on our thorough review of relevant literature, this is the first study to evaluate osteoblastogenesis from various MSCs sources, namely paired ADMSCs and BMMSCs, in MM patients who had completed novel-agent-based induction and standard intensive HDT. Our study supports the hypothesis that ADMSCs are a more favorable MSC source for osteoblastogenesis than BMMSCs, because of their higher expansion capacity, shorter doubling time in cell cultures, greater calcium deposition ability and greater osteoblastic activity. In line with our findings, several studies have provided evidence that ADMSCs exhibit advantages over BMMSCs in neural differentiation and myogenesis [32,33].

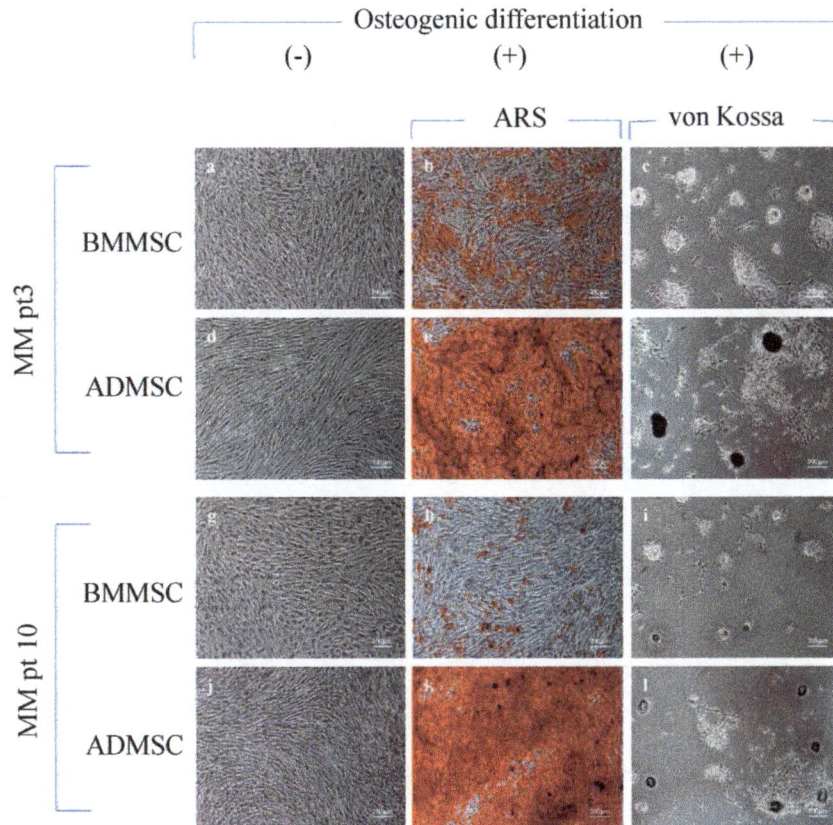

Figure 4. Morphologies, Alizarin Red S and von Kossa staining of cultured ADMSCs and BMMSCs from two representative MM patients. Both ADMSCs (d, j) and BMMSCs (a, g) had typical morphology for MSCs, like spindle shapes, fibroblast-like morphology and aligned in whirl formations. Positive ARS staining for calcium deposits appeared red granules for ADMSCs (e, k) and paired BMMSCs (b, h). Bone nodules were identified by the von Kossa staining and were shown in brown-black granules for ADMSCs (f, l) and paired BMMSCs (c, i).

The sampling of the MSCs was chosen at post- intensive therapy based on the assumption that the impaired osteoblastogenesis in MM patients resulted from the MCs as well as anti-MM therapy [18,34,35]. Therefore, we determined whether BM-targeted therapy in MM affects ADMSCs. Compared to the ADMSCs obtained from healthy donors (n = 4), the osteoblastogenesis potential of the posttherapy MM-ADMSCs did not differ significantly suggesting that MM-ADMSCs might not be affected by MCs and anti-MM treatment. By contrast, the osteogenic differentiation, esp. the calcium deposition, of post-therapy MM-BMMSCs was significantly impaired compared with non-MM control (n = 5; Figure 5). Furthermore, similar to others [35], sign of senescence (ex. positive beta-galactosidase staining) was seen in our MM-BMMSCs, but which was not seen in paired ADMSCs (Figure 3). The underlying mechanism for these observed differences between MM-ADMSCs and MM-BMMSCs is not yet clear; the difference might be due to intrinsic differences between MM-ADMSCs and MM-BMMSCs caused by patients' ages, MCs, and the BM-targeted therapy [35]. To partly support this explanation, the MM-BMMSC cultures that failed at P2 were associated with a longer duration of clinical induction treatment than MM-BMMSCs cultures that propagated beyond P2. Unfortunately, our data was not sufficient to realize how much impact from the anti-MM treatment on the dysfunction of BMMSC, since there was lack of sequential follow-up of the clinical samples at different time points, namely, at diagnosis, after induction, and post HDC/AuSCT; therefore, further studies are required. The BMMSCs and the ADMSCs can be cryopreserved

before commencing anti-MM treatment; however, cryopreservation requires a large storage facility and huge expense to accommodate BMMSCs or ADMSCs for long periods [36]. In addition, certain genetic aberrations have been observed in MM-BMMSCs that are likely to impair the osteogenic differentiation pathways, such as the Wnt and Notch signaling pathways [37,38]. These changes have been reported to persist in BMMSCs from MM patients after extended culture and passage in vitro, indicating that these MM-BMMSCs might be permanently modified [17,18,34,39]. These genetic aberrations might limit the use of BMMSCs in MM patients. Therefore, confirming that ADMSCs can differentiate into functional OBs in MM patients who have received intensive treatment and exhibited the optimal response is clinically relevant. Because MSC treatment for various degenerative diseases requires a large quantity of autologous MSCs, good-manufacturing-practices (GMP)-compliant large-scale ex vivo expansion is essential for future therapeutic purposes [40]; therefore, a favorable MSC source exhibits high viability and potency in an in vitro expansion. The number of BMMSCs in the BM is approximately 1 in 25,000 to 100,000 nucleated cells; however, the average number of ADMSCs in processed lipoaspirate is approximately 2 in 100 nucleated cells [41]. Overall, ADMSCs might be a more suitable MSC source than BMMSCs for clinical use in the future.

Our data also showed that the early osteogenic differentiation capacity determined according to the ALP activity did not differ significantly between the 2 paired MSCs, and this finding was also seen between the BMMSCs from MM patients and the non-MM

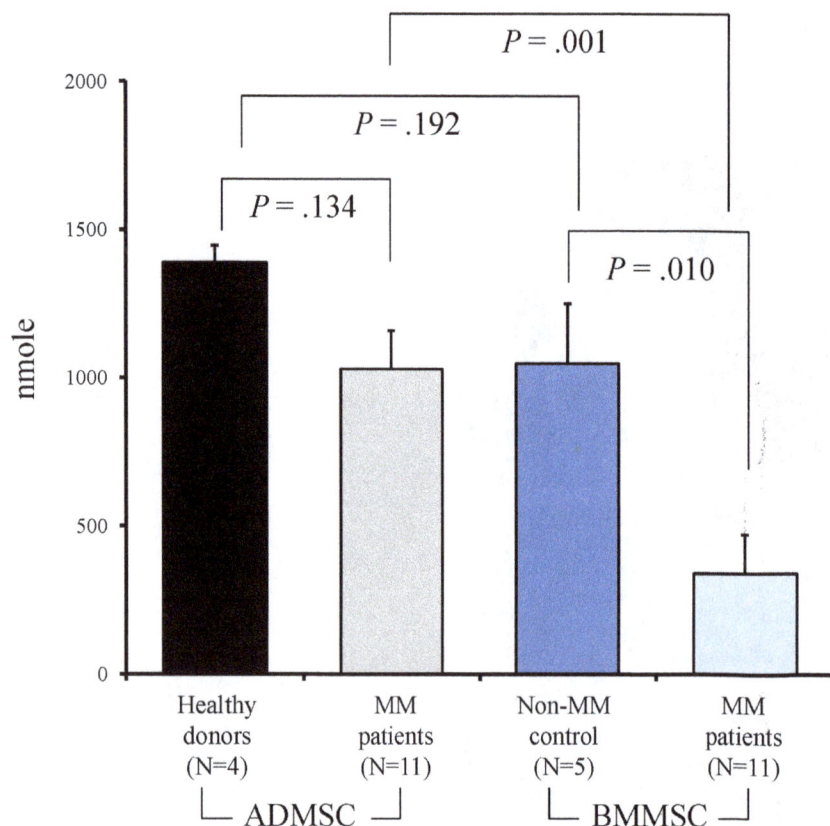

Figure 5. The calcium deposition levels of cultured ADMSCs and BMMSCs from healthy donors, non-MM control and MM patients.

control, suggesting that MCs and/or the related anti-MM therapy primarily affect the late mineralization stage of the osteogenic differentiation of MSCs. Further detailed study, such as molecular profiling of the various stages of differentiation from MSCs to OBs, is required to validate this observation.

This study had several limitations. First, the cohort was small; therefore, the observations must be validated in studies enrolling more patients. However, the paired ADMSCs and BMMSCs obtained from a nearly homogenous patient population who had received uniform treatment procedures provided a great opportunity to minimize the bias caused by the various clinical features of patients, and our data consistently showed that the ADMSCs are a more favorable MSC source than BMMSCs for future cell therapy for MMBD. Second, this study enrolled only relatively young MM patients who could tolerate the HDT/AuSCT. Therefore, we must confirm whether the ADMSCs from elderly MM patients, who are likely to have more prevalent osteopenia and MMBD, are a favorable source for MSC cell therapy. A recent report has indicated that ADMSCs are less affected by patient age than BMMSCs are [24]. Third, the greater calcium deposition ability and osteoblastic activity of ADMSCs compared with BMMSCs did not necessarily indicate that ADMSCs have

greater ability to repair MMBD. In the 2-dimensional culture, we observed that, after osteogenic induction, the MSCs differentiated into OBs and formed osteoid and calcification, but whether these calcified osteoids can heal bone destruction or improve bone strength is unclear. The recent development of 3-dimensional cultures using biological scaffold material, which allows the growth of MSCs within a stereotypical structure [42], will provide the opportunity to assess the ability of building real bony structures by using these 2 MSCs in MM patients.

In conclusion, our findings confirm that osteoblastogenesis can be induced in ADMSCs of MM patients who have received intensive treatment, and that the ADMSCs are a feasible and more favorable MSC source than BMMSCs for future cell therapy for MMBD.

Author Contributions

Conceived and designed the experiments: HHL SMH SYH. Performed the experiments: HHL LFH WHC. Analyzed the data: HHL SYH. Contributed reagents/materials/analysis tools: HSM LFH YHL YSS SYH. Wrote the paper: HHL SJW SYH.

References

1. Palumbo A, Anderson K (2011) Multiple myeloma. N Engl J Med 364: 1046–1060.

2. Raje N, Roodman GD (2011) Advances in the biology and treatment of bone disease in multiple myeloma. Clin Cancer Res 17: 1278–1286.

3. Vallet S, Pozzi S, Patel K, Vaghela N, Fulciniti MT, et al. (2011) A novel role for CCL3 (MIP-1alpha) in myeloma-induced bone disease via osteocalcin downregulation and inhibition of osteoblast function. Leukemia 25: 1174–1181.

4. Christoulas D, Terpos E, Dimopoulos MA (2009) Pathogenesis and management of myeloma bone disease. Expert Rev Hematol 2: 385–398.

5. Tian E, Zhan F, Walker R, Rasmussen E, Ma Y, et al. (2003) The role of the Wnt-signaling antagonist DKK1 in the development of osteolytic lesions in multiple myeloma. N Engl J Med 349: 2483–2494.

6. Papadopoulou EC, Batzios SP, Dimitriadou M, Perifanis V, Garipidou V (2010) Multiple myeloma and bone disease: pathogenesis and current therapeutic approaches. Hippokratia 14: 76–81.

7. Cao Y, Luetkens T, Kobold S, Hildebrandt Y, Gordic M, et al. (2010) The cytokine/chemokine pattern in the bone marrow environment of multiple myeloma patients. Exp Hematol 38: 860–867.

8. Roodman GD (2008) Skeletal imaging and management of bone disease. Hematology Am Soc Hematol Educ Program: 313–319.

9. Charbord P, Livne E, Gross G, Haupl T, Neves NM, et al. (2011) Human bone marrow mesenchymal stem cells: a systematic reappraisal via the genostem experience. Stem Cell Rev 7: 32–42.

10. Sarugaser R, Hanoun L, Keating A, Stanford WL, Davies JE (2009) Human mesenchymal stem cells self-renew and differentiate according to a deterministic hierarchy. PLoS One 4: e6498.

11. Lee OK, Kuo TK, Chen WM, Lee KD, Hsieh SL, et al. (2004) Isolation of multipotent mesenchymal stem cells from umbilical cord blood. Blood 103: 1669–1675.

12. Jiang Y, Jahagirdar BN, Reinhardt RL, Schwartz RE, Keene CD, et al. (2002) Pluripotency of mesenchymal stem cells derived from adult marrow. Nature 418: 41–49.

13. Pittenger MF, Mackay AM, Beck SC, Jaiswal RK, Douglas R, et al. (1999) Multilineage potential of adult human mesenchymal stem cells. Science 284: 143–147.

14. Konno M, Hamabe A, Hasegawa S, Ogawa H, Fukusumi T, et al. (2013) Adipose-derived mesenchymal stem cells and regenerative medicine. Dev Growth Differ 55: 309–318.

15. Moroni L, Fornasari PM (2013) Human mesenchymal stem cells: a bank perspective on the isolation, characterization and potential of alternative sources for the regeneration of musculoskeletal tissues. J Cell Physiol 228: 680–687.

16. Li X, Ling W, Khan S, Yaccoby S (2012) Therapeutic effects of intrabone and systemic mesenchymal stem cell cytotherapy on myeloma bone disease and tumor growth. J Bone Miner Res 27: 1635–1648.

17. Garayoa M, Garcia JL, Santamaria C, Garcia-Gomez A, Blanco JF, et al. (2009) Mesenchymal stem cells from multiple myeloma patients display distinct genomic profile as compared with those from normal donors. Leukemia 23: 1515–1527.

18. Corre J, Mahtouk K, Attal M, Gadelorge M, Huynh A, et al. (2007) Bone marrow mesenchymal stem cells are abnormal in multiple myeloma. Leukemia 21: 1079–1088.

19. Reagan MR, Ghobrial IM (2012) Multiple myeloma mesenchymal stem cells: characterization, origin, and tumor-promoting effects. Clin Cancer Res 18: 342–349.

20. Giuliani N, Mangoni M, Rizzoli V (2009) Osteogenic differentiation of mesenchymal stem cells in multiple myeloma: identification of potential therapeutic targets. Exp Hematol 37: 879–886.

21. Zuk PA, Zhu M, Mizuno H, Huang J, Futrell JW, et al. (2001) Multilineage cells from human adipose tissue: implications for cell-based therapies. Tissue Eng 7: 211–228.

22. Zhang ZY, Teoh SH, Chong MS, Schantz JT, Fisk NM, et al. (2009) Superior osteogenic capacity for bone tissue engineering of fetal compared with perinatal and adult mesenchymal stem cells. Stem Cells 27: 126–137.

23. Zuk PA, Zhu M, Ashjian P, De Ugarte DA, Huang JI, et al. (2002) Human adipose tissue is a source of multipotent stem cells. Mol Biol Cell 13: 4279–4295.

24. Chen HT, Lee MJ, Chen CH, Chuang SC, Chang LF, et al. (2012) Proliferation and differentiation potential of human adipose-derived mesenchymal stem cells isolated from elderly patients with osteoporotic fractures. J Cell Mol Med 16: 582–593.

25. Cavo M, Tacchetti P, Patriarca F, Petrucci MT, Pantani L, et al. (2010) Bortezomib with thalidomide plus dexamethasone compared with thalidomide plus dexamethasone as induction therapy before, and consolidation therapy

after, double autologous stem-cell transplantation in newly diagnosed multiple myeloma: a randomised phase 3 study. Lancet 376: 2075–2085.

26. Nery AA, Nascimento IC, Glaser T, Bassaneze V, Krieger JE, et al. (2013) Human mesenchymal stem cells: from immunophenotyping by flow cytometry to clinical applications. Cytometry A 83: 48–61.

27. Cournil-Henrionnet C, Huselstein C, Wang Y, Galois L, Mainard D, et al. (2008) Phenotypic analysis of cell surface markers and gene expression of human mesenchymal stem cells and chondrocytes during monolayer expansion. Biorheology 45: 513–526.

28. Cocco C, Giuliani N, Di Carlo E, Ognio E, Storti P, et al. (2010) Interleukin-27 acts as multifunctional antitumor agent in multiple myeloma. Clin Cancer Res 16: 4188–4197.

29. Lin TM, Tsai JL, Lin SD, Lai CS, Chang CC (2005) Accelerated growth and prolonged lifespan of adipose tissue-derived human mesenchymal stem cells in a medium using reduced calcium and antioxidants. Stem Cells Dev 14: 92–102.

30. Wang YH, Liu Y, Maye P, Rowe DW (2006) Examination of mineralized nodule formation in living osteoblastic cultures using fluorescent dyes. Biotechnol Prog 22: 1697–1701.

31. Mayr-Wohlfart U, Fiedler J, Gunther KP, Puhl W, Kessler S (2001) Proliferation and differentiation rates of a human osteoblast-like cell line (SaOS-2) in contact with different bone substitute materials. J Biomed Mater Res 57: 132–139.

32. Choi YS, Vincent LG, Lee AR, Dobke MK, Engler AJ (2012) Mechanical derivation of functional myotubes from adipose-derived stem cells. Biomaterials 33: 2482–2491.

33. Zhang HT, Liu ZL, Yao XQ, Yang ZJ, Xu RX (2012) Neural differentiation ability of mesenchymal stromal cells from bone marrow and adipose tissue: a comparative study. Cytotherapy 14: 1203–1214.

34. Garderet L, Mazurier C, Chapel A, Ernou I, Boutin L, et al. (2007) Mesenchymal stem cell abnormalities in patients with multiple myeloma. Leuk Lymphoma 48: 2032–2041.

35. Andre T, Meuleman N, Stamatopoulos B, De Bruyn C, Pieters K, et al. (2013) Evidences of early senescence in multiple myeloma bone marrow mesenchymal stromal cells. PLoS One 8: e59756.

36. Ginis I, Grinblat B, Shirvan MH (2012) Evaluation of bone marrow-derived mesenchymal stem cells after cryopreservation and hypothermic storage in clinically safe medium. Tissue Eng Part C Methods 18: 453–463.

37. Xu S, Evans H, Buckle C, De Veirman K, Hu J, et al. (2012) Impaired osteogenic differentiation of mesenchymal stem cells derived from multiple myeloma patients is associated with a blockade in the deactivation of the Notch signaling pathway. Leukemia 26: 2546–2549.

38. Qiang YW, Chen Y, Stephens O, Brown N, Chen B, et al. (2008) Myeloma-derived Dickkopf-1 disrupts Wnt-regulated osteoprotegerin and RANKL production by osteoblasts: a potential mechanism underlying osteolytic bone lesions in multiple myeloma. Blood 112: 196–207.

39. Pevsner-Fischer M, Levin S, Hammer-Topaz T, Cohen Y, Mor F, et al. (2012) Stable changes in mesenchymal stromal cells from multiple myeloma patients revealed through their responses to Toll-like receptor ligands and epidermal growth factor. Stem Cell Rev 8: 343–354.

40. Sotiropoulou PA, Perez SA, Salagianni M, Baxevanis CN, Papamichail M (2006) Characterization of the optimal culture conditions for clinical scale production of human mesenchymal stem cells. Stem Cells 24: 462–471.

41. Strem BM, Hicok KC, Zhu M, Wulur I, Alfonso Z, et al. (2005) Multipotential differentiation of adipose tissue-derived stem cells. Keio J Med 54: 132–141.

42. Naito H, Dohi Y, Zimmermann WH, Tojo T, Takasawa S, et al. (2011) The effect of mesenchymal stem cell osteoblastic differentiation on the mechanical properties of engineered bone-like tissue. Tissue Eng Part A 17: 2321–2329.

5

Association between the Polymorphism rs3217927 of CCND2 and the Risk of Childhood Acute Lymphoblastic Leukemia in a Chinese Population

Heng Zhang[1◐], Yan Zhou[1◐], Yaoyao Rui[1◐], Yaping Wang[1], Jie Li[2], Liuchen Rong[1], Meilin Wang[3], Na Tong[3], Zhengdong Zhang[3], Jing Chen[4]*, Yongjun Fang[1]*

1 Department of Hematology and Oncology, Nanjing Children's Hospital Affiliated to Nanjing Medical University, Nanjing, China, 2 Department of Hematology and Oncology, Soochow Children's Hospital Affiliated to Soochow University, Suzhou, China, 3 Department of Molecular and Genetic Toxicology, Cancer Center of Nanjing Medical University, Nanjing, China, 4 Department of Hematology and Oncology, Shanghai Children's Medical Center Affiliated to Shanghai, Jiao Tong University, Shanghai, China

Abstract

CyclinD proteins, the ultimate recipients of mitogenic and oncogenic signals, play a crucial role in cell-cycle regulation. CyclinD2, one of the cyclinD family, is overexpressed in T-acute lymphoblastic leukemia (ALL) and B-cell chronic lymphocytic leukemia and involved in the pathogenesis of leukemias. Recent reports indicated that *CCND2* polymorphisms are associated with human cancer risk, thusly we hypothesized that *CCND2* gene polymorphisms may contribute to childhood ALL susceptibility. We selected the polymorphism rs3217927 located in the 3′UTR region of *CCND2* to assess its associations with childhood ALL risk in a case-control study. A significant difference was found in the genotype distributions of rs3217927 polymorphism between cases and controls (P = 0.019) and homozygous GG genotype may be an increased risk factor for childhood ALL (adjusted OR = 1.84, 95% CI = 1.14 —2.99). Furthermore, this increased risk was more pronounced with GG genotype among high-risk ALL (adjusted OR = 1.95, 95% CI = 1.04–3.67), low-risk ALL (adjusted OR = 2.09, 95% CI = 1.13–3.87), B-phenotype ALL patients (adjusted OR = 1.78, 95% CI = 1.08–2.95) and T-phenotype ALL patients (adjusted OR = 2.87, 95% CI = 1.16–7.13). Our results provide evidence that *CCND2* polymorphism rs3217927 may be involved in the etiology of childhood ALL, and the GG genotype of rs3217927 may modulate the genetic susceptibility to childhood ALL in the Chinese population. Further functional studies and investigations in larger populations should be conducted to validate our findings.

Editor: Linda Bendall, Westmead Millennium Institute, University of Sydney, Australia

Funding: This research was partly supported by the National Natural Science Foundation of China (81070436, 81202268), Natural Science Foundation of Jiangsu Province (BK2011775), and a Key Project supported by the Medical Science and Technology Development Foundation, Nanjing Department of Health. The funders had no role in study design, data collection and analysis, decision to publish, or preparation of the manuscript.

Competing Interests: The authors have declared that no competing interests exist.

* E-mail: dryjfang@gmail.com (YF); chenjingscmc@hotmail.com (JC)

◐ These authors contributed equally to this work.

Introduction

Pediatric cancer is now the second most common cause of death by disease in children in developed countries [1]. Acute lymphoblastic leukemia (ALL), the most common childhood malignancy, accounts for 26.8% of all pediatric cancers among children less than 15 years of age, with approximately 38 new cases per million children diagnosed with ALL each year in the developed world [2]. The peak incidence of childhood ALL occurs at age 2 to 5 years, suggesting that ALL may initiate in utero or during the infant period [2,3]. In recent decades, cure rate for childhood ALL have increased from 10% to nearly 85% due to optimized diagnosis, risk stratification, and chemotherapy protocols [4]. Nevertheless, childhood ALL remains a leading cause of cancer death in children. Understanding the potential etiologies of childhood ALL to reduce the incidence of pediatric ALL remains crucial.

It is widely accepted that the interaction between genes and the environment contributes to the pathogenesis of ALL in children. Potential molecular mechanisms implicated include sequential alterations in tumor-suppress genes, proto-oncogenes, and micro-RNA genes of hematopoietic stem cells or their committed progenitors [5]. Multiple recent studies indicate that genetic polymorphisms play an influential role in childhood ALL susceptibility, treatment response, and prognosis [6].

D-type cyclins, the ultimate recipients of mitogenic and oncogenic signals, have been recently recognized as potentially suitable molecular targets for chemotherapy due to their specific over-expression in malignancies [7–9]. The D-type cyclins (cyclinsD1, cyclinsD2, cyclinsD3) are separately encoded by *CCND1*, *CCND2* and *CCND3*. *CCND2* is one of the direct transcriptional targets of Hedgehog signaling and PI3K-AKT signaling pathways [10,11]. Abnormal activation of these two pathways leads to disorders of cell proliferation, metabolism, growth and survival, and has been proven implicated in hematologic malignancies [8,9,12]. Progression of the cell cycle is modulated via the sequential and well-ordered activation of several components. CyclinD2, one of the key components, plays an important role in regulating the G1/S transitions in cell cycle [13]. The abnormal expression of cyclinD2 may influence the repair of DNA damage and initiate of tumorigenesis, including leukemogenesis [14]. Multiple studies of inherited variation in cell cycle genes suggest that genotypes in this pathway may be associated with increased risk of breast cancer, prostate cancer, lung cancer, bladder cancer and oral cancer [15–21]. Recently, a genome-wide association study (GWAS) showed the *CCND2* inherited genetic variations are associated with the risk of colorectal cancer in Europeans and Asians [22,23]. However, few studies have detected the effects of *CCND2* gene polymorphisms on the risk of childhood ALL.

To detect the potential impact of *CCND2* polymorphisms on the risk of developing childhood ALL in a Chinese population, we selected a tagging single nucleotide polymorphism (tSNP) rs3217927 from the data for Chinese in the HapMap database (http://hapmap.ncbi.nlm.nih.gov/), which locates in the 3′ untranslated region (UTR) of *CCND2*. We then genotyped this SNP in 753 patients with childhood ALL and 1088 normal controls in this case control study.

Materials and Methods

Study subjects

The research protocol was approved by the Medical Ethics Committee of Nanjing Children's Hospital affiliated to Nanjing Medical University. Written informed consent was obtained from the parents or legal guardians of all study subjects. From January 2007 to January 2013, 857 subjects with newly diagnosed childhood ALL and 1151 cancer-free controls were recruited from the Nanjing Children's Hospital Affiliated Nanjing Medical University, Shanghai Children's Medical Center Affiliated to Shanghai Jiao Tong University and Soochow University Affiliated Children's Hospital. Parents or legal guardians of the all subjects were interviewed in person to collect demographic data and exposure information, including age, gender, parental alcohol use and tobacco-smoking and painting status of the home. Then the numbers of subjects were reduced into 753 cases and 1088 controls because of the missing of demographic data. The 753 cases included 291 females and 462 males, with a median age of 5 years. Subjects aged from 1 to 18 years and were genetically unrelated to ethnic Han Chinese. All subjects underwent bone marrow aspiration and the diagnosis of ALL was confirmed by morphology, immunohistochemistry, cytogenetics, and molecular biology. Risk stratification of the cases was determined uniformly according to the Suggestion of Diagnosis and Treatment of ALL in Childhood, published by the Society of Pediatrics, Chinese Medical Association in 2006. The control subjects had no history of malignant neoplasm or thrombotic disease and were age and gender matched to the cases.

Genotyping

Genomic DNA was extracted by standard protocols (Qiagen) from isolated peripheral blood lymphocytes. The *CCND2* rs3217927 was genotyped with 384-well ABI 7900HT Real-Time PCR System (Applied Biosystems, Foster City, CA) using TaqMan SNP Genotyping assay. The reaction contained 5 ng genomic DNA, TaqMan Master Mix, forward and reverse primers and probes for the wild type and the mutant allele in a total volume of 5 ul. The primer sequences were 5′-CTGCGCAGGCAAGCAC-TAT-3′ and 5′-CCTGCCAATTCAGTGTGATTGA-3′, and the probes were 5′-FAM-CTCTGCTGAGCGGTA-MGB-3′ and 5′-HEX-CCTCTGCTAAGCGG-MGB-3′, which were devised and manufactured by Nanjing Steed Biotechnology (Nanjing, China). The location of the CCND2 primer sequence is shown in Figure S1. The PCR thermal cycling amplification was performed under the following conditions: 95°C for 10 min followed by 45 cycles of 95°C for 15 s and 60°C for 1 min. The genotype analysis was done blinded and 10% of control samples were randomly repeated for the typing reliability, proven complete concordant.

Expression levels of *CCND2* mRNA

We extracted total RNA from bone marrow in 57 ALL patients from total 753 cases randomly. The total RNA was reverse transcribed into complementary DNA using ReverTra Ace qPCR RT kit (Toyobo, Tsuruga, Japan), and the complementary DNA was used for subsequent real-time PCR analysis (ABI 7300). Glyceraldehyde 3-phosphate dehydrogenase (GAPDH) was used as an internal quantitative control for each sample and each assay was done in triplicate. The primers used for amplification were 5′-TCATTGCTCTGTGTGCCACC-3′and 5′-CAGCTCAGTCA-GGGCATCAC-3′ for *CCND2*, and 5′-GCACCGTCAAGGCT-GAGAAC-3′ and 5′-GGATCTCGCTCCTGGAAGATG-3′ for GAPDH. The PCR thermal cycling protocol consisted of 50°C for 2 min, then 95°C for 10 min followed by 45 cycles of 95°C for 15 s and 60°C for 1 min.

Statistical analysis

Hardy–Weinberg equilibrium of the genotype distribution for each SNP among the control group was examined by a goodness-of-fit χ^2 test. Chi-square (χ^2) test was used to evaluate the distribution differences of selected demographic characteristics as well as each allele and genotypes of rs3217927 between the cases and controls. Unconditional univariate and multivariate logistic regression analyses were performed to obtain crude and adjusted odds ratios (ORs) for estimating risk of childhood ALL and their 95% confidence intervals (CIs) with adjustment for diagnosis age, gender, parental alcohol use, tobacco-smoking and housing painting status. Independent-sample t-test was used for analyzing the results of *CCND2* mRNA expression. Two-sided P values were selected and P<0.05 was considered statistically significant. All the statistical analyses were performed using Statistics Analysis System software (version 9.1; SAS Institute, Cary, NC).

Results

Characteristics of the study subjects

The frequency distributions of all subjects including selected demographic variables are summarized in Table 1. The median age of the recruited subjects was used as the age stratification standard. There was no significant difference in the distribution of age (P = 0.20) and sex (P = 0.89) and smoke (P = 0.08) between the cases and controls. However, compared with the control subjects, the cases had more parental drinkers and home painting exposure during the pregnancy of mother or after the birth (34.5% versus 21.0%, P<0.001; 35.9% versus 26.2%, P<0.001, respectively). Of the 753 ALL patients, 95 (12.6%) were T-ALL, 655 (87.0%) were B-ALL; the others (0.4%) were T-B cell biphenotypic acute lymphoblastic leukemia. Furthermore, 297 (39.4%) patients were in the low-risk, 163 (21.7%) patients were in the medium-risk and the remaining 293 (38.9%) were in the high-risk. All the variables above were further adjusted in the multivariate logistic regression analysis.

Table 1. Frequency distribution of selected variables between cases of childhood ALL and cancer-free controls.

Variables	Cases (n = 753)		Controls (n = 1088)		
	n	%	n	%	P^a
Age (years)					
≤5	404	53.65	551	50.64	0.204
>5	349	46.35	537	49.36	
Gender					
Male	462	61.35	671	61.67	0.890
Female	291	38.65	417	38.33	
Parental smoking status					
Never	314	41.70	498	45.77	0.084
Ever	439	58.30	590	54.23	
Parental drinking status					
Never	493	65.47	860	79.04	<.0001
Ever	260	34.53	228	20.96	
House-painting status					
Never	483	64.14	803	73.81	<.0001
Ever	270	35.86	285	26.19	
Immunophenotype					
B-ALL	655	86.98	-	-	-
T-ALL	95	12.62	-	-	-
Other[b]	3	0.40	-	-	-
Treatment branch					
Low risk	297	39.44	-	-	-
Medium risk	163	21.65	-	-	-
High risk	293	38.91	-	-	-

ALL, acute lymphoblastic leukemia; B-ALL, B-phenotype ALL; T-ALL, T-phenotype ALL; –, data not essential.
[a]Two-sided chi-square test for either genotype distribution or allele frequencies between cases and controls.
[b]Represents T-B cell biphenotypic acute lymphoblastic leukemia and other immunophenotypes.

Association between CCND2 polymorphism and ALL risk

The observed genotype distributions and allele frequencies for *CCND2* rs3217927 polymorphism in cases and controls and their associations with childhood ALL risk are presented in Table 2. The genotype frequencies of rs3217927 polymorphism among the controls were in agreement with Hardy–Weinberg equilibrium (p = 0.461). As shown in Table 2, the frequencies of AA, AG and GG genotypes were 61.5%, 32.9%, and 5.6%, among the cases, and 65.4%, 31.6%, and 3.0%, among the controls, respectively. There was a statistically significant difference in the genotype distributions of the *CCND2* rs3217927 polymorphism between the cases and controls (P = 0.011).

Multivariate logistic regression analysis revealed that the homozygous GG genotype of rs3217927 was associated with an increased risk of childhood ALL compared with the homozygous AA genotype (adjusted OR = 1.84, 95% CI = 1.14 —2.99), while the heterozygous AG was not (adjusted OR = 1.14, 95% CI = 0.93–1.39). We also observed an elevated risk in the recessive model of *CCND2* rs3217927 polymorphisms (adjusted OR = 1.76, 95% CI = 1.10–2.85), but not in the dominant model (adjusted OR = 1.20, 95% CI = 0.99–1.46).

The stratified analysis of the associations between rs3217927 polymorphism and clinical features of ALL

The further stratification analysis was developed to evaluate the risk of *CCND2* rs3217927 polymorphism and some clinical variables of ALL. As shown in Table 3, the increased risk was more pronounced with GG genotype among high-risk ALL (adjusted OR = 1.95, 95% CI = 1.04–3.67), low-risk ALL (adjusted OR = 2.09, 95% CI = 1.13–3.87), B-lineage ALL (B-ALL) patients (adjusted OR = 1.78, 95% CI = 1.08–2.95) and T-lineage ALL(T-ALL) patients (adjusted OR = 2.87, 95% CI = 1.16–7.13). In contrast, with the recessive model, the increased risk was found only in low-risk ALL (adjusted OR = 2.05, 95% CI = 1.12–3.76), B-phenotype ALL patients (adjusted OR = 1.71, 95% CI = 1.03–2.82) and T-phenotype ALL patients (adjusted OR = 2.53, 95% CI = 1.04–6.19). No significant associations were observed between the genotypes and risk of medium-risk ALL.

Association between CCND2 rs3217927 polymorphism and the expression levels of CCND2 mRNA

57 ALL patients with three genotypes of CCND2 (37 patients with AA genotype, 16 patients with AG genotype and 4 patients with GG genotype, respectively) were performed here. As shown in Figure 1 and Figure 2, no obvious difference was found here that A to G mutation changed the expression level of CCND2 mRNA. The expression levels of the AG carriers (P = 0.204) and the GG carriers (P = 0.999) has no significant difference with those of AA carriers. We than conduct a recessive model, no statistical significance has been found, either (P = 0.987).

Discussion

This ongoing study explored the association of *CCND2* rs3217927 polymorphism in 753 newly diagnosed childhood ALL patients and 1088 cancer-free controls. We found that the G allele of *CCND2* polymorphism rs3217927 has a significant association with childhood ALL in a Chinese population and may be a risk factor for the development of the disease. In the stratified analysis, strong evidence were found to prove a pronounced association between homozygous GG and high-risk ALL, low-risk ALL, T-phenotype and B-phenotype ALL sub-groups, thus putting the homozygous GG a potential risk factor for ALL. As shown in Table 1, the epidemiologic data indicates that the cases had more parental alcohol consumption and house painting exposure during the pregnancy or after the birth than the controls, indicating a possible association between parental alcohol use and paint exposure with childhood ALL. Compared with adults, children may be at higher risk of environmental toxicants due to exposure differences, physiologic immaturity, higher cell growth and proliferation [24,25], although there were no observably significant statistical interactions between environmental exposure factors and the polymorphism, which is shown in Table S1.

The human *CCND2* gene, located on chromosome 12p13.32 and spanning 31.6 kb, is a necessary member of the cyclinD gene family which promotes cell growth and proliferation [26]. Once induced by extracellular mitogenic environment, D cyclins will bind and activate the relative cyclin-dependent kinases CDK4 and CDK6 to form the Cyclin/CDK complexes. These complexes promote the cell cycle crossing the restriction-point and subsequently entering the phase of DNA synthesis [26]. In normal mammalian cells, the so-called check-point controls are the G1-to-S and G2-to-M transitions. The progress of cell cycle can stop and delay at these restriction-points to permit cell repairing of damaged DNA and prevent various types of mutations [27].

Table 2. Logistic regression analysis of association between the rs3217927 polymorphisms and the risk of childhood ALL.

Genotypes	Cases (n = 753)		Controls (n = 1088)		Crude OR (95% CI)	Adjusted OR (95% CI)[b]	P[a]
rs3217927	n	%	n	%			
A>G							
AA	463	61.5	712	65.4	1.00 (reference)	1.00 (reference)	0.019
AG	248	32.9	344	31.6	1.11 (0.91 1.36)	1.14 (0.93 1.39)	0.222
GG	42	5.6	32	3.0	2.02 (1.26 3.24)	1.84 (1.14 2.99)	0.013
AG/GG	290	38.5	405	34.6	1.19 (0.98 1.44)	1.20 (0.99 1.46)	0.070
AA/AG	711	94.4	1056	97.0	1.00 (reference)	1.00 (reference)	0.021
GG	42	5.6	32	3.0	1.95 (1.22 3.12)	1.76 (1.10 2.85)	
G allele		0.22		0.19			0.599

[a]Two-sided chi-square test for either genotype distribution or allele frequencies between cases and controls.
[b]Adjusted for age, gender, parental drinking status, parental smoking status, and house painting status.

Over-expression of cyclinD shortens the duration of the G1-phase [14], thereby impeding the repair of damaged DNA, and may result in the development of cancer. The over-expression of cyclin D2 has been observed in many tumors including acute leukemia, and may contribute to unlimited cell division, prevention of programmed death and chemoresistance[28]. Compared with unaffected people, cyclin D2 exhibited over-expression in B-cell chronic lymphocytic leukemia cases and preferentially expressed in human T-lymphotropic virus type I (HTLV-I) infected T cell lines [28,29]. Karrman K and Clappier E *et al.* discovered deregulation of cyclinsD2 by translocational activation in T-cell acute lymphoblastic leukemia [30,31]. Xinliang Mao *et al* demonstrated cyclinsD2 was a therapeutic target of myeloma and leukemia in mouse models and believed decreased D-cyclins may be a biomarker of an anticancer effect [32]. Recent related work declared *CCND2* inherited genetic variations linked with the risk of colorectal cancer and ovarian cancer [22,33]. However, Sheng H *et al.* reported no significant association had been found between *CCND2* rs3217927 and non-small cell lung cancer in a Chinese

population [34]. No reports have found the relationship between genetic variations in *CCND2* and childhood ALL.

In this study, the relevance of tagSNP rs3217927 of *CCND2* and childhood ALL risk was investigated. We found that the homozygous GG genotype of the *CCND2* rs3217927 correlated with a significantly increased risk of childhood ALL. This increased risk was most pronounced in high-risk ALL, low-risk ALL, B-phenotype and T-phenotype ALL patients, but not medium risk group, which may due to the lower number of samples in medium risk group reducing statistical power. A combination between AA genotype and AG genotype is performed as reference to conduct a recessive model, and the homozygous GG genotype still showed a significantly increased risk of childhood ALL among low-risk, B-phenotype and T-phenotype ALL patients, which indicated the importance of the association between homozygous GG and the risk of childhood ALL. Furthermore, the high risk of more parental alcohol consumption and house painting exposure, as well as genetic susceptibilities in rs3217927GG genotype in the subgroup, were

Table 3. Association of rs3217927 (CCND2) polymorphism with clinical risk and immunophenotype of childhood ALL.

Genotype	Controls		Clinical risk						OR (95% CI)[a]			Immunophenotype[b]				OR (95% CI)[a]	
	n = 1088		High n = 293		Medium n = 163		Low n = 297		High	Medium	Low	B-ALL (n = 655)		T-ALL (n = 95)		B-ALL	T-ALL
	n	%	n	%	n	%	n	%				n	%	n	%		
AA	712	65.4	175	59.7	99	60.7	189	63.6	1.00 (reference)	1.00 (reference)	1.00 (reference)	406	62.0	54	56.8	1.00 (reference)	1.00 (reference)
AG	344	31.6	102	34.8	56	34.4	90	30.3	1.21 (0.92 1.61)	1.23 (0.86 1.76)	1.07 (0.80 1.42)	214	32.7	34	35.8	1.14 (0.92 1.41)	1.33 (0.84 2.10)
GG	32	3.0	16	5.5	8	4.9	18	6.1	1.95 (1.04 3.67)	1.58 (0.70 3.58)	2.09 (1.13 3.87)	35	5.3	7	7.4	1.78 (1.08 2.95)	2.87 (1.16 7.13)
AG/GG	405	34.6	118	40.3	64	39.3	108	36.4	1.28 (0.96 1.67)	1.26 (0.90 1.78)	1.16 (0.88 1.53)	249	38.0	41	43.2	1.20 (0.97 1.47)	1.45 (0.94 2.24)
AA/AG	1056	97.0	277	94.5	155	95.1	279	93.9	1.00 (reference)	1.00 (reference)	1.00 (reference)	620	94.7	88	92.6	1.00 (reference)	1.00 (reference)
GG	32	3.0	16	5.5	8	4.9	18	6.1	1.78 (0.95 3.34)	1.49 (0.66 3.35)	2.05 (1.12 3.76)	35	5.3	7	7.4	1.71 (1.03 2.82)	2.53 (1.04 6.19)

[a]ORs and 95% CIs were calculated by logistic regression analysis.
[b]There were three ALL patients diagnosed with B+T-ALL and they were all AA genotype.

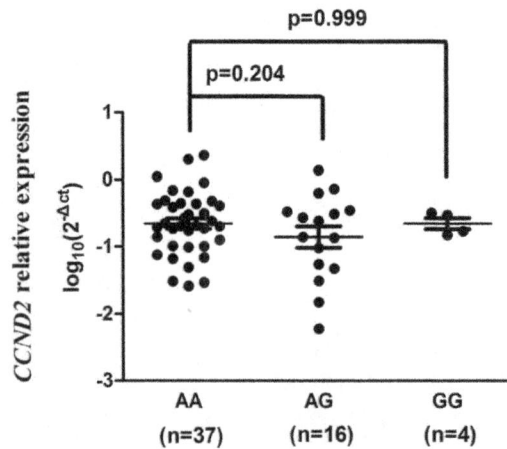

Figure 1. Association between the rs3217927 polymorphism and relative CCND2 mRNA expression. The frequency distributions of the AA, AG and GG genotypes were 37, 16 and 4, respectively. The fold change was normalized against GAPDH. P = 0.204 for AG compared with AA and P = 0.999 for AG compared with AA.

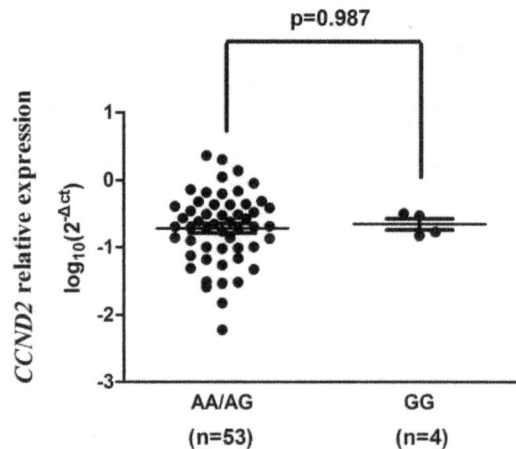

Figure 2. Association between the recessive model of rs3217927 polymorphism and relative CCND2 mRNA expression. The frequency distributions of the AA/AG and GG genotypes were 53 and 4, respectively. P = 0.987 for GG compared with AA/AG.

observed in our study. The result above indicated ALL formation might be subjected to a variety of environmental expose and genetic factors. However, according to recent GWAS, the association between *CCND2* polymorphisms and childhood ALL risk was not observed, as a possible result of ethnic differences [35–38].

It has been reported that the binding affinity between miRNA and its target mRNA may be changed by the SNPs located in miRNA target sites. The difference of those SNPs may lead to degradation of the mRNA and inhibition of the mRNA translation into proteins [39]. For further functional studies of this association between rs3217927 (located in the 3′-UTR region) and ALL, we forecasted the allele-specific targeting miRNAs interacted with complementary sequence motifs of *CCND2* rs3217927 [40]. Based on our bioinformatics analysis using miRanda and TargetScan Database (http://www.bioguo.org/miRNASNP/index.php), has-miR-922 and has-miR-4291 specifically binding the sequence surrounding the variant site came to our sights. Besides, we noticed that the Gibbs free energy was -19.30 kcal/mol for the rs3217927 A allele, and 0 kcal/mol for the G allele. These bioinformatics forecasts indicated that this SNP may change the conformation of the secondary structure of *CCND2* itself and may affect the binding affinity between *CCND2* mRNA and the miRNAs (has-miR-922 or has-miR-4291 or both), which may finally alter the expression of cyclinD2. But no obvious difference was found here indicates A to G mutation changed the expression level of CCND2 mRNA. The reason for this result may be that we only have 57 ALL patients with three genotypes of CCND2 to conduct PCR assay (37 genotype AA, 16 genotype AG and 4 genotype GG, respectively). There are not sufficient GG type samples to provide high certainty. A larger size of subjects is needed to repeat this part of experiment in the following research. Based on discussion above, it is proper to suspect that rs3217927 may influence miRNA biogenesis and function, and may contribute to susceptibility for childhood ALL. Of course, this is just one hypothesis of many unknown pathogenesis. Further functional evaluations in *vitro* and *vivo* with a larger size of samples are needed to confirm our conjecture.

Some limitations of this study should be addressed. Firstly, this study is hospital-based case-control designed, which may give rise to selection bias of subjects related with some particular genotypes. To minimize potential confounding bias, we adopt rigorous exclusion criteria about epidemiological design in recruitment of control subject which is frequency matched to cases by age, sex and ethnicity. The genotype frequencies of rs3217927 polymorphism among the controls in our study were consistent with the information provided by the HapMap Project. Secondly, when designing this experiment, we did notice that an independent validation cohort is necessary but our data was just over the minimum value of statistical power (709 cases and 709 controls), which was performed by Epicacl 2000 based on 1:1 ratio of cases to controls, expected OR 1.35, proportion controls exposed 40.0%, thresholds set on 0.05 and 80% of the calculated degree of certainty. In order to have the most trustworthy relevance, we devoted all our samples into relevance verification. Although we hold the opinion that the current data in this manuscript is enough to analyze the risk of ALL, it will be ideal to carry on a two-stage model. And we are still gathering data. Besides, it is essential to validate our results in a larger size of subjects, which we believe should be at least 4044 subjects in total containing 2022 cases and 2022 controls. This assessment was performed using Epicacl 2000 based on 1:1 ratio of cases to controls, expected OR 1.2, proportion controls exposed 35.0%, thresholds set on 0.05 and 80% of the calculated degree of certainty. Thirdly, the detailed epidemiologic data provided here is not adequate to evaluate gene-environment interaction. In order to provide more detailed interpretation of association between environmental toxic exposure and ALL, it would become an essential pre-work to acquire abundant epidemiologic exposure data and clinical information. Last but not least, our research about the gene susceptibility connected with childhood ALL is only limited on the statistics and epidemiology level and the further functional studies are warranted to validate our findings and reveal the underlying molecular mechanisms.

In conclusion, for the first time we found evidence that rs3217927 polymorphism in the cell cycle gene *CCND2* may be relevant to susceptibility of Childhood ALL in a Chinese population. Further validation in a larger sample size with diverse ethnic populations and functional evaluations in *vitro* and *vivo* are warranted.

Supporting Information

Figure S1 The nucleotide localization of the CCND2 rs3217927 primer sequences.

Table S1 Interaction analyses of CCND2 rs3217927 and parental drinking and house-painting.

References

1. Siegel R, Naishadham D, Jemal A (2013) Cancer statistics, 2013. CA Cancer J Clin 63: 11–30.
2. Kaatsch P (2010) Epidemiology of childhood cancer. Cancer Treat Rev 36: 277–285.
3. Terracini B (2011) Epidemiology of childhood cancer. Environ Health 10 Suppl 1: S8.
4. Armstrong SA, Look AT (2005) Molecular genetics of acute lymphoblastic leukemia. J Clin Oncol 23: 6306–6315.
5. Pui CH (2009) Acute lymphoblastic leukemia: introduction. Semin Hematol 46: 1–2.
6. Mrozek K, Harper DP, Aplan PD (2009) Cytogenetics and molecular genetics of acute lymphoblastic leukemia. Hematol Oncol Clin North Am 23: 991–1010, v.
7. Sicinska E, Aifantis I, Le Cam L, Swat W, Borowski C, et al. (2003) Requirement for cyclin D3 in lymphocyte development and T cell leukemias. Cancer Cell 4: 451–461.
8. Buchakjian MR, Kornbluth S (2010) The engine driving the ship: metabolic steering of cell proliferation and death. Nat Rev Mol Cell Biol 11: 715–727.
9. Siebert R, Willers CP, Opalka B (1996) Role of the cyclin-dependent kinase 4 and 6 inhibitor gene family p15, p16, p18 and p19 in leukemia and lymphoma. Leuk Lymphoma 23: 505–520.
10. Katoh Y, Katoh M (2005) Hedgehog signaling pathway and gastric cancer. Cancer Biol Ther 4: 1050–1054.
11. Katoh Y, Katoh M (2009) Integrative genomic analyses on GLI1: positive regulation of GLI1 by Hedgehog-GLI, TGFbeta-Smads, and RTK-PI3K-AKT signals, and negative regulation of GLI1 by Notch-CSL-HES/HEY, and GPCR-Gs-PKA signals. Int J Oncol 35: 187–192.
12. Han Y, Xia G, Tsang BK (2013) Regulation of cyclin D2 expression and degradation by follicle-stimulating hormone during rat granulosa cell proliferation in vitro. Biol Reprod 88: 57.
13. Chiles TC (2004) Regulation and function of cyclin D2 in B lymphocyte subsets. J Immunol 173: 2901–2907.
14. Ohtsubo M, Roberts JM (1993) Cyclin-dependent regulation of G1 in mammalian fibroblasts. Science 259: 1908–1912.
15. Pharoah PD, Tyrer J, Dunning AM, Easton DF, Ponder BA (2007) Association between common variation in 120 candidate genes and breast cancer risk. PLoS Genet 3: e42.
16. Driver KE, Song H, Lesueur F, Ahmed S, Barbosa-Morais NL, et al. (2008) Association of single-nucleotide polymorphisms in the cell cycle genes with breast cancer in the British population. Carcinogenesis 29: 333–341.
17. Chang BL, Zheng SL, Isaacs SD, Wiley KE, Turner A, et al. (2004) A polymorphism in the CDKN1B gene is associated with increased risk of hereditary prostate cancer. Cancer Res 64: 1997–1999.
18. Hosgood HD 3rd, Menashe I, Shen M, Yeager M, Yuenger J, et al. (2008) Pathway-based evaluation of 380 candidate genes and lung cancer susceptibility suggests the importance of the cell cycle pathway. Carcinogenesis 29: 1938–1943.
19. Ye Y, Yang H, Grossman HB, Dinney C, Wu X, et al. (2008) Genetic variants in cell cycle control pathway confer susceptibility to bladder cancer. Cancer 112: 2467–2474.
20. Wu X, Gu J, Grossman HB, Amos CI, Etzel C, et al. (2006) Bladder cancer predisposition: a multigenic approach to DNA-repair and cell-cycle-control genes. Am J Hum Genet 78: 464–479.
21. Huang M, Spitz MR, Gu J, Lee JJ, Lin J, et al. (2006) Cyclin D1 gene polymorphism as a risk factor for oral premalignant lesions. Carcinogenesis 27: 2034–2037.
22. Jia WH, Zhang B, Matsuo K, Shin A, Xiang YB, et al. (2013) Genome-wide association analyses in East Asians identify new susceptibility loci for colorectal cancer. Nat Genet 45: 191–196.
23. Peters U, Jiao S, Schumacher FR, Hutter CM, Aragaki AK, et al. (2013) Identification of Genetic Susceptibility Loci for Colorectal Tumors in a Genome-Wide Meta-analysis. Gastroenterology 144: 799–807 e724.
24. Whyatt RM, Perera FP (1995) Application of biologic markers to studies of environmental risks in children and the developing fetus. Environ Health Perspect 103 Suppl 6: 105–110.
25. Perera FP (1997) Environment and cancer: who are susceptible? Science 278: 1068–1073.
26. Ely S, Di Liberto M, Niesvizky R, Baughn LB, Cho HJ, et al. (2005) Mutually exclusive cyclin-dependent kinase 4/cyclin D1 and cyclin-dependent kinase 6/cyclin D2 pairing inactivates retinoblastoma protein and promotes cell cycle dysregulation in multiple myeloma. Cancer Res 65: 11345–11353.
27. Sherr CJ (2000) The Pezcoller lecture: cancer cell cycles revisited. Cancer Res 60: 3689–3695.
28. Delmer A, Ajchenbaum-Cymbalista F, Tang R, Ramond S, Faussat AM, et al. (1995) Overexpression of cyclin D2 in chronic B-cell malignancies. Blood 85: 2870–2876.
29. Akagi T, Ono H, Shimotohno K (1996) Expression of cell-cycle regulatory genes in HTLV-I infected T-cell lines: possible involvement of Tax1 in the altered expression of cyclin D2, p18Ink4 and p21Waf1/Cip1/Sdi1. Oncogene 12: 1645–1652.
30. Clappier E, Cuccuini W, Cayuela JM, Vecchione D, Baruchel A, et al. (2006) Cyclin D2 dysregulation by chromosomal translocations to TCR loci in T-cell acute lymphoblastic leukemias. Leukemia 20: 82–86.
31. Karrman K, Andersson A, Bjorgvinsdottir H, Strombeck B, Lassen C, et al. (2006) Deregulation of cyclin D2 by juxtaposition with T-cell receptor alpha/delta locus in t(12;14)(p13;q11)-positive childhood T-cell acute lymphoblastic leukemia. Eur J Haematol 77: 27–34.
32. Mao X, Liang SB, Hurren R, Gronda M, Chow S, et al. (2008) Cyproheptadine displays preclinical activity in myeloma and leukemia. Blood 112: 760–769.
33. Song H, Hogdall E, Ramus SJ, Dicioccio RA, Hogdall C, et al. (2008) Effects of common germ-line genetic variation in cell cycle genes on ovarian cancer survival. Clin Cancer Res 14: 1090–1095.
34. Ma H, Chen J, Pan S, Dai J, Jin G, et al. (2011) Potentially functional polymorphisms in cell cycle genes and the survival of non-small cell lung cancer in a Chinese population. Lung Cancer 73: 32–37.
35. Yang JJ, Cheng C, Yang W, Pei D, Cao X, et al. (2009) Genome-wide interrogation of germline genetic variation associated with treatment response in childhood acute lymphoblastic leukemia. JAMA 301: 393–403.
36. Trevino LR, Yang W, French D, Hunger SP, Carroll WL, et al. (2009) Germline genomic variants associated with childhood acute lymphoblastic leukemia. Nat Genet 41: 1001–1005.
37. Papaemmanuil E, Hosking FJ, Vijayakrishnan J, Price A, Olver B, et al. (2009) Loci on 7p12.2, 10q21.2 and 14q11.2 are associated with risk of childhood acute lymphoblastic leukemia. Nat Genet 41: 1006–1010.
38. Orsi L, Rudant J, Bonaventure A, Goujon-Bellec S, Corda E, et al. (2012) Genetic polymorphisms and childhood acute lymphoblastic leukemia: GWAS of the ESCALE study (SFCE). Leukemia 26: 2561–2564.
39. Medina PP, Slack FJ (2008) microRNAs and cancer: an overview. Cell Cycle 7: 2485–2492.
40. Cai Y, Yu X, Hu S, Yu J (2009) A brief review on the mechanisms of miRNA regulation. Genomics Proteomics Bioinformatics 7: 147–154.

Acknowledgments

We thank Colleen H. McDonough, M.D. from Pediatric Hematology/Oncology Children's Medical Center, Georgia Regents University for her valuable comments of this manuscript.

Author Contributions

Conceived and designed the experiments: YF JC. Performed the experiments: HZ YZ. Analyzed the data: HZ YR. Contributed reagents/materials/analysis tools: YW JL LR MW NT ZZ. Wrote the paper: HZ YF JC.

6

Differences in Meiotic Recombination Rates in Childhood Acute Lymphoblastic Leukemia at an MHC Class II Hotspot Close to Disease Associated Haplotypes

Pamela Thompson[1]*, Kevin Urayama[2,3], Jie Zheng[4,5], Peng Yang[6], Matt Ford[7], Patricia Buffler[2], Anand Chokkalingam[2], Tracy Lightfoot[8], Malcolm Taylor[9]

1 Paediatric & Familial Cancer Research Group, Institute of Cancer Sciences, University of Manchester, St Mary's Hospital, Manchester, United Kingdom, 2 School of Public Health, University of California, Berkeley, Berkeley, California, United States of America, 3 Department of Human Genetics and Disease Diversity, Tokyo Medical and Dental University, Tokyo, Japan, 4 School of Computer Engineering, Nanyang Technological University, Singapore, 5 Genome Institute of Singapore, A*STAR (Agency for Science, Technology, and Research), Biopolis, Singapore, 6 Data Analytics Department, Institute for Infocomm Research, A*STAR, Singapore, 7 Research Computing Services, Faculty of Medical and Human Sciences, University of Manchester, Manchester, United Kingdom, 8 University of York, Heslington, York, United Kingdom, 9 Independent Researcher, Handforth, Cheshire, United Kingdom

Abstract

Childhood Acute Lymphoblastic Leukemia (ALL) is a malignant lymphoid disease of which B-cell precursor- (BCP) and T-cell-(T) ALL are subtypes. The role of alleles encoded by major histocompatibility loci (MHC) have been examined in a number of previous studies and results indicating weak, multi-allele associations between the HLA-DPB1 locus and BCP-ALL suggested a role for immunosusceptibility and possibly infection. Two independent SNP association studies of ALL identified loci approximately 37 kb from one another and flanking a strong meiotic recombination hotspot (DNA3), adjacent to HLA-DOA and centromeric of HLA-DPB1. To determine the relationship between this observation and HLA-DPB1 associations, we constructed high density SNP haplotypes of the 316 kb region from HLA-DMB to COL11A2 in childhood ALL and controls using a UK GWAS data subset and the software PHASE. Of four haplotype blocks identified, predicted haplotypes in Block 1 (centromeric of DNA3) differed significantly between BCP-ALL and controls (P = 0.002) and in Block 4 (including HLA-DPB1) between T-ALL and controls (P = 0.049). Of specific common (>5%) haplotypes in Block 1, two were less frequent in BCP-ALL, and in Block 4 a single haplotype was more frequent in T-ALL, compared to controls. Unexpectedly, we also observed apparent differences in ancestral meiotic recombination rates at DNA3, with BCP-ALL showing increased and T-ALL decreased levels compared to controls. In silico analysis using LDsplit sotware indicated that recombination rates at DNA3 are influenced by flanking loci, including SNPs identified in childhood ALL association studies. The observed differences in rates of meiotic recombination at this hotspot, and potentially others, may be a characteristic of childhood leukemia and contribute to disease susceptibility, alternatively they may reflect interactions between ALL-associated haplotypes in this region.

Editor: Paul J. Galardy, Mayo Clinic, United States of America

Funding: PT is supported by funds from Children With Cancer, UK (http://www.childrenwithcancer.org.uk/). The funders had no role in study design, data collection and analysis, decision to publish, or preparation of the manuscript.

Competing Interests: The authors have declared that no competing interests exist.

* Email: pamela.thompson@manchester.ac.uk

Introduction

Acute lymphoblastic leukemia (ALL) is the most common malignant disease in children under 16 years of age in socio-economically developed countries including the UK [1]. Of the two lymphoid lineages, B-cell ALL comprises 85%, and T-cell ALL approximately 15% of cases; common or B-cell precursor ALL (BCP-ALL) is the most frequent ALL subtype overall. Whilst childhood ALL is predominantly a sporadic disease, a small fraction of cases arise in association with certain rare heritable or congenital genome instability disorders. Genome wide association studies (GWAS) of sporadic ALL have, however, identified single nucleotide polymorphisms (SNPs) in linkage disequilibrium (LD) with 4 genes (IKZF1, ARID5B, CEBPE, CDKN2A) [2,3,4] having roles in B-Cell development [5,6,7,8]. A recent GWAS meta-analysis also identified two further SNPs tagging the genes PIP4K2A and GATA3 as associated with specific BCP-ALL subtypes [9].

Although epidemiological studies have provided indirect support for an infectious etiology of BCP-ALL (reviewed in [10]), no causative agent has yet been identified. Clues provided by evidence that susceptibility to mouse retroviral ALL is linked to the MHC [11], and that certain human leukocyte antigen (HLA) alleles are associated with susceptibility to specific infections (reviewed in [12]), have encouraged the search for HLA allele associations with childhood ALL as a proxy for infection [13,14,15,16,17]. Previous studies of the HLA-DPB1 locus which identified multiple, though weak, allele associations with ALL suggested a role for common antigenic peptide binding pockets in susceptibility. Interactions were identified between the DP1 supertype and proxies for delayed immune exposure in early life, providing further support for HLA-DP function in susceptibility to childhood BCP-ALL [14].

In contrast to these findings, recent GWAS analyses failed to detect SNPs strongly linked to HLA in childhood ALL. However, a modest (non-significant) association with the SNP rs3135034, approximately 97 kb centromeric of *HLA-DPB1*, was reported in a UK GWAS [18]. Furthermore, an independent SNP analysis of the extended MHC (xMHC) in a California ALL study revealed a significant association with rs9296068, located approximately 60 kb centromeric of *HLA-DPB1* [19]. The SNPs identified in these two studies are in close proximity to each other (~37 kb apart) and flank the *HLA-DOA* locus.

In light of these findings, we considered the possibility that previous associations with *HLA-DPB1* alleles might be explained by linkage disequilibrium (LD) with a locus (or loci) in the vicinity of *HLA-DOA*. Our reasoning is based on evidence that the *HLA-DPB1* to *HLA-DOA* interval lies in a region of small haplotype blocks interspersed with pockets of LD breakdown, signifying hotspots of meiotic recombination [20]. The two BCP-ALL associated SNPs occur close to three recombination hotspots, of which *DNA3* is the most intense, leading us to hypothesize that LD breakdown between a putative ALL locus and *HLA-DPB1* could explain the weak allele associations and SNP results. Haplotype associations, LD breakdown and ancestral recombination rates in populations can be detected using estimation-based statistics [21]. Here, we applied these methods to the study of a 316 Kb region from *HLA-DMB* to *COL11A2* encompassing *HLA-DPB1* and *HLA-DOA* and the ALL associated SNPs.

Results

Haplotype frequencies in the *HLA-DMB* to *COL11A2* region in childhood ALL

In view of our results suggesting weak associations between certain *HLA-DPB1* alleles and childhood BCP-ALL [14,16,22], recent evidence [18] that an MHC SNP most strongly associated with childhood ALL (rs3135034) is approximately 97 kb telomeric of *HLA-DPB1*, and a significant association of ALL cases in the Northern California Childhood Leukemia Study (NCCLS) with rs9296068, located approximately 60 kb telomeric from *HLA-DPB1*, we considered that these SNPs might be in LD with BCP-ALL-associated *HLA-DPB1* alleles.

We first examined the association of rs3135034 and rs9296068 with a subset of the ALL cases included in the UK GWAS [18] that identified rs3135034 in the context of childhood ALL. We compared the frequencies of 92 SNPs covering a ~316 kb region of chromosome 6 (GRCh37, Chr6:32924583–33240505), in BCP-ALL and T-ALL cases and controls (N = 447, 44, and 2699, respectively). This region includes the *HLA-DOA* and *HLA-DPB1* loci, as well as rs3135034 and rs9296068. We confirmed the weak association between rs3135034 and BCP-ALL (uncorrected P = 5.4×10^{-3}), but found no evidence of association of this SNP with T-ALL (P = 0.6), or an association of rs9296068 with either ALL subtype (P>0.3)(Figure 1; Table S1).

Using PHASE v2.1.1 [21,23,24,25], we next determined the LD structure of the 316 kb region to identify haplotype blocks. Four haplotype blocks, separated by three recombination hotspots (predicted recombination rate ≥10x the background rate across the region, ρ [25], in at least one sample group) were defined: Block 1, 37.8 kb, with seven SNPs rs209474 - rs206767 (including rs3135034); Block 2, 4.4 kb, with three SNPs, rs172274 - rs3128931; Block 3, 40.1 kb, with 17 SNPs, rs86567 - rs7774158 (including rs9296068); and Block 4, 159.7 kb with 54 SNPs, rs3077 - rs213212 (including *HLA-DPB1*)(Table S1).

Case-control comparisons of overall association of variation within each haplotype block between case groups and controls (1000 permutations) revealed significant differences for BCP-ALL in Block 1 (P = 0.002) and T-ALL in Block 4 (P = 0.049), but no global difference in haplotype frequencies between either case group and controls for haplotype blocks 2 or 3 (P>0.097) (Table 1). Therefore, we compared specific haplotype frequencies in cases and controls using only haplotypes with frequencies >5% in at least one group (BCP-ALL, T-ALL, or controls) in haplotype Blocks 1 and 4. In Block 1, seven control and six case haplotypes had frequencies >5%; two haplotypes (1-C and 1-E) were significantly less frequent in BCP-ALL than controls (7.04% vs. 9.91% and 7.42% vs. 9.72%, respectively; uncorrected P<0.01; Table 2). Haplotype 1-C (P = 0.003) was the only common haplotype >5% to contain the minor allele of rs3135034, consistent with previous findings [2] and was the only one of these specific haplotype associations to withstand correction for multiple testing (Benjamini and Hochberg FDR; α = 0.0036). Haplotype block 4, encompassing the *HLA-DPA1* and *HLA-DPB1* loci, consisted of seven haplotypes >5%. Of these only one (4-B) was more frequent in T-ALL cases (18.14%) than controls (11.52%; uncorrected P = 0.04). PHASE analysis predicted that *HLA-DPB1*06:01*, which we reported is associated with childhood ALL [13], would be carried on this haplotype. Ninety per cent of ALL cases with this haplotype were positive for *DPB1*06:01* (Table 2), consistent with our earlier finding that *HLA-DPB1*06:01* is significantly associated with T-ALL (Odds ratio, 95% confidence interval 10.0, 3.3–30.2; [13]), but not supportive of an association of this allele with BCP-ALL. In addition, the 4-G haplotype was marginally less common among BCP-ALL cases than controls (3.36 vs 4.86%; P = 0.03). Eighty five per cent of cases positive for the *HLA-DPB1*01:01* allele were predicted by PHASE predicts to carry haplotype 4-G (Table 2).

Case-control comparison of recombination rates

We observed that the number of case haplotypes in each block differed from the number in controls when we used control groups containing the same number of individuals as each case group. For BCP-ALL vs controls (n = 447 in each group) 1040 vs. 991 haplotypes, respectively, were predicted whereas for T-ALL vs controls (n = 44 in each group) 250 vs. 527 haplotypes, respectively, were predicted (Table S2). We suspected that these differences could be due to different recombination rates across the 92 SNP interval in cases compared with controls. This is supported by the observation that the T-ALL group showed a lower (23 x), whilst BCP-ALL had a much higher (228 x), recombination rate at the strongest hotspot, *DNA3*, compared with controls (117 x background) (Figure 1).

Since the number of PHASE-predicted haplotypes in a group (here cases or controls) is not only a function of the recombination rate but also of the number of individuals included in the group, we tested different numbers of randomly selected controls as comparators. We found that where the number of controls (447 or 44) matched the number of cases in each ALL sub-type, this did not significantly affect recombination rate estimates (Figure 2).

We carried out permutation tests to determine if the observed differences in case-control recombination rates were significant, and found that differences in recombination rates at the *DNA3* hotspot were significant (BCP ALL, P = 0.02; T-ALL, P = 0.048). Although case-control differences in recombination rates detected by PHASE were observed at three other hotspots (*DNA2*, *DPA1*, and *VPS52*) they were not significant (P>0.18); however, the rates at *DPA1* and *VPS52* showed the same trend as *DNA3* (ie BCP-ALL > Control > T-ALL). Median recombination rates at *DNA2* were

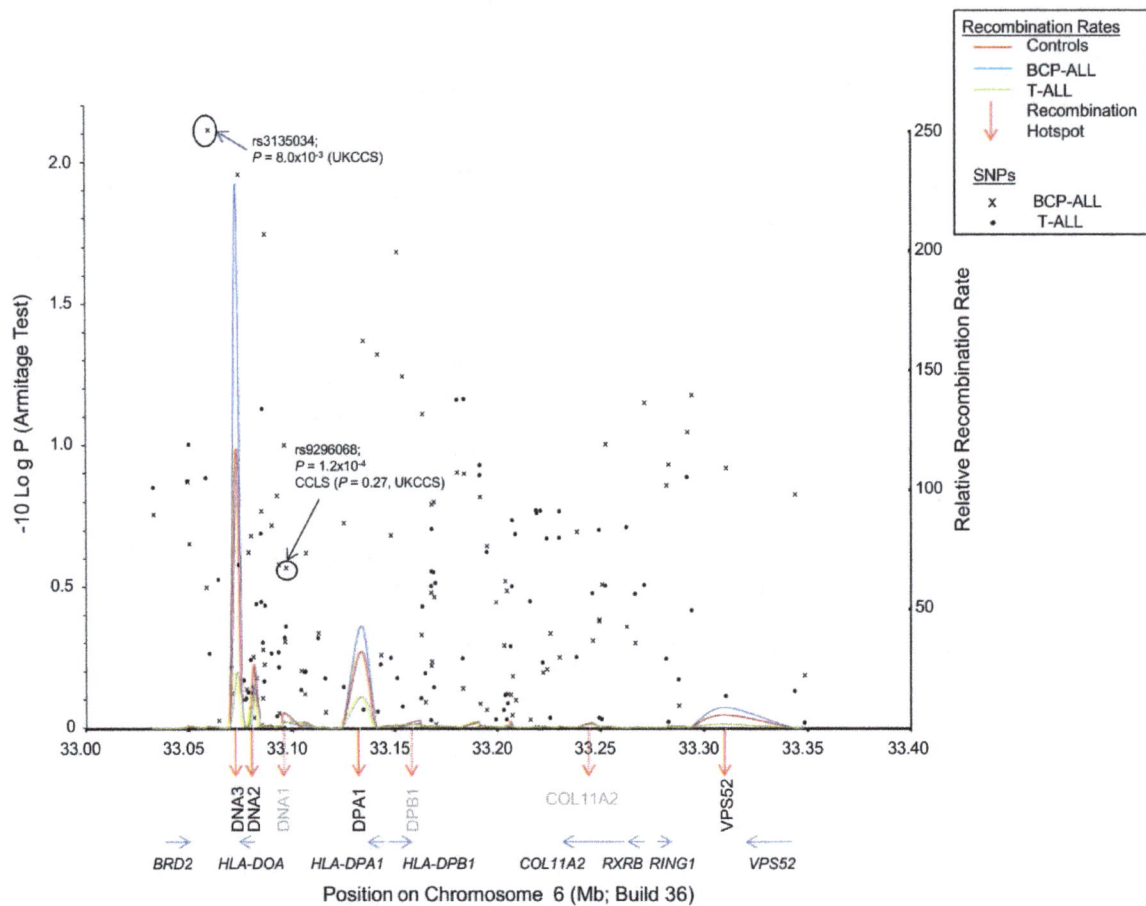

Figure 1. Relative recombination rates (right Y axis) at *DNA3* and flanking hotspots in Controls (red line), BCP-ALL cases (blue line), and T-ALL cases (green line), estimated using PHASE plotted over –Log P values (linear regression; left Y axis) for SNP associations. SNPs identified in array-based association studies of childhood ALL, rs3135034 (UKCCS [18]) and rs9296068 (CCLS)[19] are indicated. Recombination at *DNA3* is significantly higher in BCP-ALL cases than controls (P = 0.02), and significantly lower in T-ALL cases (P = 0.048). There is no significant difference at flanking hotspots.

similar in all three study groups though marginally higher in controls than in BCP-ALL and T-ALL (Figure 1). Although the previously identified '*DNA1*' locus [20] did not meet our definition of a recombination hotspot (ie. recombination rate >10 x background), there was evidence of increased recombination at this locus (between rs3128931 and rs1044429) with similar rates of 8.0, 5.0, and 9.3 x background in T-ALL, BCP-ALL, and Controls, respectively.

As polymorphisms at the gene *PRDM9*, which encodes a meiosis specifc histone methyltransferase, are known to specify hotspot location and intensity [26], we plotted publically available data from an Icelandic population [27] to investigate whether genotype at *PRDM9* is likely to influence recombination rates in the region of chromosome 6 investigated in this study. The results indicated that recombination rates, including those at *DNA3*, are likely to be strongly affected by the numbers of zinc fingers in PRDM9 (Figure S1).

Table 1. Overall comparison of haplotype frequencies at four blocks in the MHC Class II region between childhood ALL cases and controls.

Haplotype Block	*P*, BCP-ALL Cases v Controls*	*P*, T-ALL Cases v Controls*
1	**0.002**	0.534
2	0.230	0.442
3	0.097	0.501
4	0.58	**0.049**

*P values were calculated by permutation testing (1000 permutations) within PHASE. Bold indicates P<0.05.

Table 2. Frequencies of specific haplotypes in blocks 1 and 4 in Controls, BCP-ALL and T-ALL.

Haplotype ID	Associated *HLA-DPB1* allele(s)	Control av. Freq (n = 2699)	BCP-ALL av. Freq (n = 447)	BCP-ALL, P	T-ALL av. Freq (n = 44)	T-ALL, P
1-A		27.05%	28.24%	0.2645	21.07%	0.1528
1-B		25.15%	27.17%	0.1063	32.86%	0.0679
1-C		9.91%	7.04%	**0.0032***	7.88%	0.3481
1-D		9.90%	11.58%	0.0690	14.04%	0.1835
1-E		9.72%	7.42%	**0.0135**	6.71%	0.2386
1-F		9.03%	8.84%	0.4586	9.09%	0.6016
1-G		5.55%	4.77%	0.2040	4.56%	0.4567
4-A	*04:01 (62%)	25.75%	28.15%	0.0702	20.58%	0.1572
4-B	*06:01 (90%) *03:01 (85%)	11.52%	11.14%	0.4104	18.14%	**0.0404**
4-C	*04:02 (52%) *04:01 (2%)	8.03%	9.04%	0.1590	12.98%	0.1127
4-D	*02:01 (8%) *04:01 (14%)	7.65%	8.39%	0.2561	6.90%	0.4868
4-E	*02:01 (55%) *02:02 (88%) *04:02 (16%) *04:01 (1%)	7.38%	8.66%	0.1046	6.75%	0.5235
4-F	*04:01 (10%)	5.36%	4.43%	0.1553	4.58%	0.4901
4-G	*01:01 (85%)	4.86%	3.36%	**0.0261**	8.39%	0.1385

P values are the results of two-tailed Fisher's Exact tests comparing control with either BCP-ALL or T-ALL frequency; bold format indicates uncorrected P<0.05. *P withstands Benjamini and Hochberg FDR correction for 14 haplotypes (α = 0.0036). *HLA-DPB1* alleles predicted by PHASE to be carried on each Block 4 haplotype are also shown (percentages in brackets indicate the proportion of each *DPB1* allele predicted to be carried on the haplotype.

Association of SNPs flanking *DNA3* with hotspot intensity

Recent work using the LDsplit program [28,29] to analyze population genetic data has shown that *cis*-acting loci are associated with recombination hotspot activity. This confirms results obtained using traditional sperm-typing methodology [20]. In an effort to identify these *cis*-acting loci affecting recombination rates at *DNA3*, we used LDsplit to compare recombination rates associated with SNP alleles at flanking polymorphic sites. Thirty-five tag SNPs (MAF>0.07; Table S3.) in the region (chr6:33058028–33097923; GRCh36) were identified in the European (CEU) population, using the algorithm Tagger (pairwiseTagging)[30] and phased haplotypes, available from the HapMap website, were used as input data for LDsplit. LDsplit did not identify any single SNP as having a dominant *cis*-influence

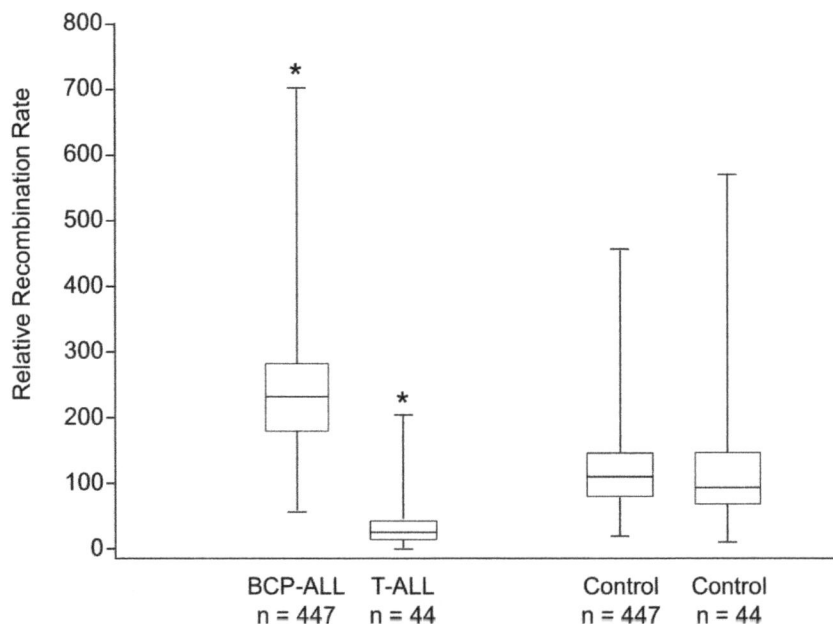

Figure 2. Box and whisker plots illustrating medians, quartiles, and ranges of recombination rates estimated using PHASE software between rs176248 and rs206767 (*DNA3* hotspot) in childhood leukemia cases and controls. Sample size (n = 447 and n = 44) of randomly selected controls did not significantly affect recombination rate estimates. Relative recombination rates (y- axis) are significantly higher in BCP-ALL (n = 447; P = 0.02) and significantly lower in T-ALL (n = 44; P = 0.048) cases than controls.

over recombination rates at *DNA3*. However, using a Bonferroni corrected P value of 1.4×10^{-3}, 13 of the 35 tag SNPs were associated with levels of recombination at *DNA3* (P values for all 10 replicate analyses $<1.4 \times 10^{-3}$). The SNPs identified in the UKCCS (rs3135034) and NCCLS (rs9296068) were among those linked to hotspot intensity, with P values ranging from 2.2×10^{-9}–2.7×10^{-5} and 5.5×10^{-5}–1.1×10^{-3}, respectively (Figure 3.). rs3135034 is ~14 kb centromeric and rs9296068 is ~23 kb telomeric from the centre of *DNA3*, with the major and minor alleles at these loci, respectively, being associated with increased hotspot intensity. These results suggest that several *cis*-acting loci in this region, including those identified in studies of childhood ALL, may influence recombination rates at *DNA3*.

Discussion

Haplotype analysis in this study differed from that of both Hosking et al [18] and Urayama et al [19] as we used the PHASE algorithm (Stephens et al. 2001; Li and Stephens 2003) which has the advantage of taking into account similarities in haplotypes, rather than simply comparing frequencies of identical haplotypes, so that, even if every individual case and control carried a different combination of alleles, if they are more similar within than between groups, this can be detected. Haplotype associations identified here using this method are of a similar magnitude to those previously reported for the UKCCS data in single SNP analyses [18]; however, rather than a simple association of the major allele of rs3135034 with leukemia risk, our data suggests the possible presence of two haplotypes protective for leukemia, one

carrying the major, and the other being the only common haplotype carrying the minor, allele at rs3135034. This would translate into an uncorrected odds ratio, 95% confidence interval of 1.26, 1.06–1.51 (P = 0.004) for BCP-ALL development in patients carrying the major allele on one of the remaining five common haplotypes. This haplotype block spans the *BRD2* locus, which has been associated with Juvenille Epilepsy, and is not an obvious candidate risk factor for ALL, despite its relatively wide expression pattern [31]. Taken in combination with published data from the California Childhood Leukemia study [19], and the results of LDsplit analyses which indicate multiple cis-acting sequences, including loci identified in the SNP association studies, contributing to recombination at *DNA3*, this is suggestive of an association of these haplotypes and recombination events affecting *HLA-DOA*, with BCP-ALL. *HLA-DOA* encodes one component of the heterodimeric HLA-DO molecule, a non-classical HLA molecule which contributes to the antigen-recognition repertoire of CD4+ T-cells through influencing intracellular peptide loading by HLA-DM by acting as a substrate mimic [32]. HLA-DO expression is restricted to professional antigen presenting cells, including B-cells and those of the thymic epithelium [33]. The modulation of MHC II antigen presentation is of vital importance in immune regulation, providing a potential link between genetic susceptibility to childhood ALL and postulated immune system dysregulation [34].

The data presented in this paper provide evidence of alterations in ancestral recombination rates in the MHC Class II region in childhood ALL populations compared to ethnically matched controls, with lower and higher rates than controls at the *DNA3*

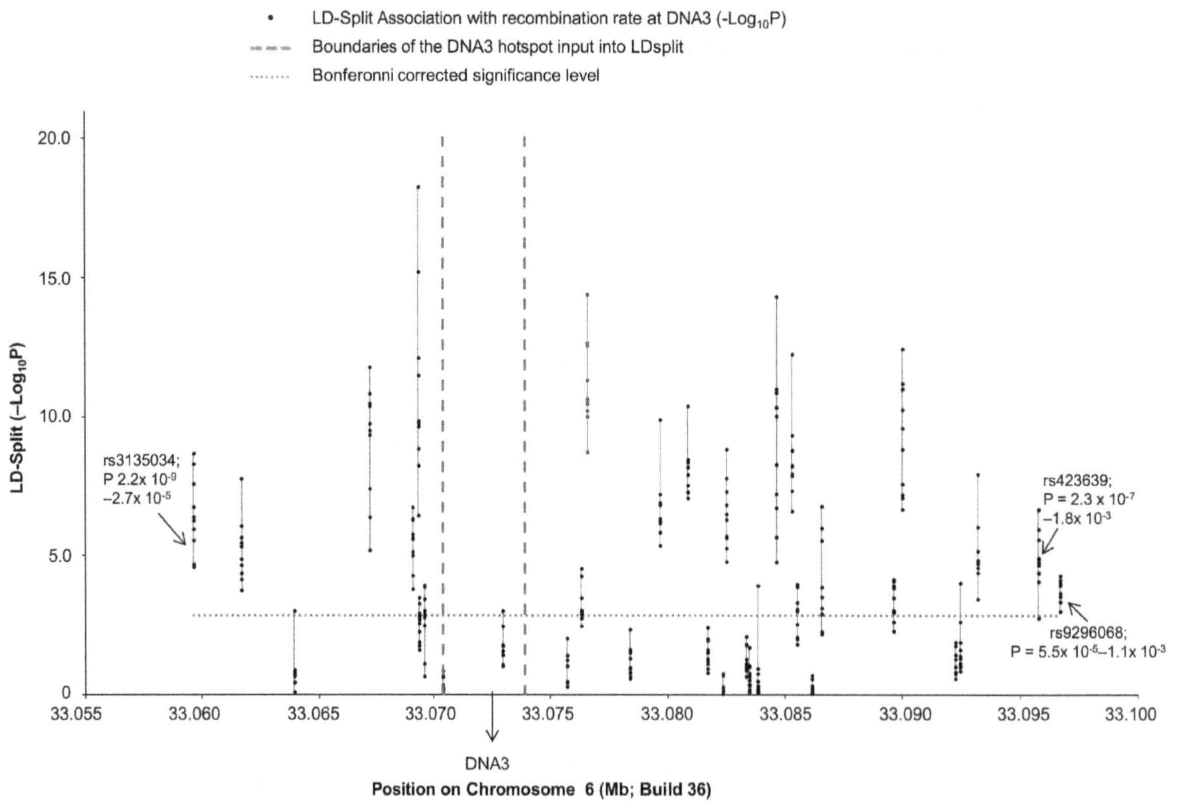

Figure 3. Results of LDsplit analysis for association of SNPs flanking *DNA3* with hotspot intensity. For each SNP included in the HAPMAP-CEU phased haplotypes (Table S3), ten estimates of -Log10P values for association with hotspot intensity are plotted (black spots joined by lines). P values of SNPs identified in association studies of childhood ALL are indicated. The boundaries of the *DNA3* hotspot used for the analysis are indicated by vertical dashed lines and the corrected P value cut-off is shown by a horizontal dotted line.

hotspot in populations of children who developed T-ALL and BCP-ALL, respectively. Our results are consistent with those of recent family studies, which uncovered a substantial overrepresentation of rare *PRDM9* alleles in the parents of children with BCP-ALL compared to ethnically matched controls in two North American populations [35]. Furthermore, our data indicate that differences in recombination rates may be detectable by analysis of Western European population genetic data, representing ancestral meiotic crossover events through many generations, suggesting that some populations carrying these alleles are at increased risk for development of childhood leukemias. However, as discussed by Hussin et al., [35], the relatively high frequency among Africans [26,36] of the rare *PRDM9* alleles associated with childhood ALL in Caucasian populations, along with a proportionally low incidence of childhood leukemias among African-Americans [37] indicates that variant alleles of *PRDM9* are insufficient to predispose to leukemia and suggestive of further contributory parental genetic background factors. Moreover, another plausible interpretation of our results is that recombination rates in ancestors of ALL patients are the same as those of ancestors of controls, with the observed changes being due to association of disease with interacting alleles in different haplotype blocks, such that associated allele combinations are selected for in the disease groups, leading to the appearance of increased recombination. Given the recent reports of an association of rare *PRDM9* alleles with ALL [35], we favour the hypothesis that altered recombination rates are also associated with this disease. However, further work to distinguish between these possibilities will be required.

Disease associations coinciding with recombination hotspots are rare, due to the statistical methods employed in genetic susceptibility studies; indeed it has been noted that etiological variants within a recombination hot spot may be impossible to identify using standard association strategies [38]. However, a schizophrenia locus within a recombination hotspot has been described [39] and a Type 1 Diabetes susceptibility locus has also been mapped in mouse [40]. In both studies, mechanisms of locus-specific disease etiology effects were shown to be dependent on sequence variation mediated by recombination events. Given the identification in two studies of childhood ALL of SNPs flanking a recombination hotspot coinciding with the *HLA-DOA* coding sequence, and the observed apparent variations in recombination rates at this locus among our study groups, we speculate that similar recombination mechanisms may functionally influence *HLA-DOA* sequence in childhood leukemia, although this will require experimental verification. Although a previous study of sperm recombinants indicated that recombination events at the *DNA3* hotspot invariably resulted in fully reciprocal crossovers [20], it is not clear if this will also be true of female recombination, or whether the unusual distribution of *PRDM9* genotypes among the parents of children with ALL [35] may influence the nature of crossovers at *DNA3*.

Among our patient samples, the 4-G haplotype was moderately less frequent among BCP-ALL cases than controls (3.36 vs 4.86%; P = 0.03); this is the predominant carrier of the *HLA-DPB1* allele *DPB1*01:01* (in 85% of ALL cases typed *DPB1*01:01*, PHASE predicted that the allele would be carried on the 4-G haplotype) (Table 2). *HLA-DPB1*01:01* has previously been reported to be underrepresented among UKCCS ALL patients [41] and was recently reported to be associated with an increased risk for ALL in the NCCLS [14]. In addition, our results are suggestive that this haplotype may be overrepresented among T-ALL patients in the UK population (8.39%; P = 0.1). As childhood T-ALL is relatively rare compared to BCP-ALL, this study was underpowered to detect associations of the expected magnitude; however, our results

strongly support a specific association of T-ALL with haplotypes carrying the *HLA-DPB1*0601* locus. Further investigations of combined data from different studies will be highly desirable for T-ALL.

In conclusion, this study provides evidence of potentially significant population level differences in meiotic recombination at the *HLA-DOA* locus in BCP- and T-ALL, with increased and decreased activity, respectively. These findings will require replication in other sample sets and at other hotspots, and as discussed above, may alternatively reflect interactions between disease associated loci in this region. However, the intensity of this hotspot is strongly influenced by variation at *PRDM9* (Figure S1) and our data should be interpreted in the context of the recent discovery of substantial overrepresentation of rare PRDM9 alleles in parents of children with ALL, combined with unusual recombination patterns [35]. Hence our results suggest that differences in hotspot magnitude, in addition to location, can be observed, and that these are detectable by population-based methods, raising the possibility of genetically defined sub-populations with increased susceptibility to childhood leukemia.

Materials and Methods

Patients and Controls

The UKCCS was a population-based case control study of childhood malignant disease, carried out in the UK between 1992 and 1998. Case diagnoses were classified as previously described [42] as B cell precursor (BCP-) ALL, and T-ALL and validated by the UKCCS data centre at the University of York, UK. We used SNP data generated from cases and controls as part of a previously described GWAS [2]. Data were available from 447 cases of BCP-ALL, 44 cases of T-ALL, and 2699 control (Wellcome Trust Case Control 1958 Birth Cohort) samples. Only data from individuals confirmed by principal component analysis to be of Western European ancestry were included in the analyses [2].

Comparison of Case and Control allele and haplotype frequencies

Single SNP allele frequencies were compared using SNP & Variation Suite v7.5.5 (Golden Helix, Inc., Bozeman, MT, www. goldenhelix.com), using linear regression analysis (additive model), with correction for stratification by principal component analysis (eigenvalues).

To identify haplotype blocks, case and control SNP data from all 92 observed loci in the region chr6:32924583–33240505 (GRCh37) genotyped in the UKCCS GWAS were input into the PHASE (v2.1.1) program [21,23,24,25] and run using the flags -MR, -S*, and -X10; where −MR specifies the use of the recombination model for estimation of haplotypes (this takes account of the presence of recombination hotspots), -X10 sets the number of iterations performed in the final run to be 10x greater than the default (recommended by the software authors to increase confidence in output data, particularly where recombination rates are estimated), and −S the specification of a randomly generated seed (*). The analysis was performed four times, using a different seed each time, for each set of cases and controls, also to increase confidence in output data, in accordance with the recommendations of the software authors.

Haplotype blocks were defined as contiguous groups of SNPs where recombination rates did not exceed 5x background rate. Of the 92 SNPs those excluded from haplotype blocks by these criteria were rs176248, rs2395300, rs1044429, rs2581, rs2284191, rs2395309, rs213220, rs213199, and rs464921, which either defined recombination hotspots, or were isolated at the telomeric end of the region under investigation (Table S1).

To compare overall haplotype frequencies between case and control groups input files consisting of both cases and controls (indicated by their identifiers) were run in PHASE v2.1.1 [21,23,24,25] using the flag –c1000 to specify comparison between the two groups using 1000 permutations. The statistical significance of differences between case and control frequencies of specific haplotypes in each block was calculated using the Fisher's Exact test.

For determination of associations between individual haplotypes and *HLA-DPB1* alleles, coded *HLA-DPB1* types [13] were included in PHASE input data (between rs3135021 and rs9277535) before calculation of haplotypes (N.B. This was not done for case-control haplotype comparison analysis as *HLA-DPB1* types are not available for the control samples) and the percentage of each *HLA-DPB1* allele predicted to occur in a specific haplotype (frequency occurring on haplotype/frequency in the population) calculated. The number of samples with available *HLA-DPB1* types included in this analysis was 453.

Estimation of the location and strength of Recombination Hotspots

Recombination hotspot locations (defined as relative recombination rate >10x background rate across the region, ρ [25] in cases or controls, were identified from PHASE *.out_recom files, which also provided estimates of recombination rates between each pair of adjacent loci included. Each run generated 1000 estimates of recombination rates between adjacent SNPs and the results of 4 runs were combined to give estimated values based on the median of 4000 values generated for each pair of loci.

The significance of differences between predicted case and control recombination rates were tested by performing 250 permutation tests (a number chosen as the maximum practicable, given the computing time involved) using input data where case and control samples were randomly assigned pseudo-case or pseudo-control status. As for the actual case and control data, analyses were performed four times using different seeds. Medians of each set of 4000 values generated were calculated and the difference between these for 250 pseudo-case/pseudo-control pairs calculated for SNPs flanking hotspots defined by the initial PHASE analysis (rs176248 and rs206767; rs2395300 and rs176248; rs2581 and rs1044429; rs2395309 and rs375912).

Association of hotpots with proximal SNPs

CEU-phased haplotypes (Utah residents with ancestry from northern and western Europe; HapMap Phase 3, release 2), available from the HapMap website, were used as input data for the program LDsplit, which was previously used to confirm the association of the SNP 'FG11' (rs416622; [43]) with recombination at *DNA2*. CEU phased haplotypes were used in preference to the case and control data generated in this study due to the higher density of SNPs included in the HapMap data, compared to our GWAS-generated information. Thirty-five tag SNPs (MAF>0.07; Table S2) were identified for the population CEU in the region (chr6:33058028–33097923; GRCh36), using the algorithm Tagger (pairwise Tagging)[30]. Ten estimates of P values for association of each SNP with recombination rates at *DNA3* were generated by LDsplit. For SNPs with MAF>0.1, these were generated using a different randomly selected 190 CEU haplotypes as input for each

estimate, and for SNPs with MAF<0.1, all haplotypes which carried the minor allele were included in each replicate, combined with randomly selected haplotypes carrying the major allele to a total of 160. LDsplit parameters were set as follows: -iteration, 2000000; -burn, 5000; -sample, 200; -random permutations; 200.

Supporting Information

Figure S1   Recombination Rates in Icelandic Population Data According to PRDM9 Genotype. Plots of male (A) and female (B) recombination rates (chr6:33,000,000–33,400,000) in Icelandic parent-child pairs stratified by PRDM9 ZnF variants (data obtained from supplementary tables associated with [27]). Red line, recombination rate with 12–13 ZnF motifs. Blue line, recombination rate with 14–15 ZnF motifs. There are two female specific hotspots in this region, one of which (COL11A2) is ablated in individuals with 14–15 ZnF motifs and the other (*DPB1*) is enhanced. Of three other visible hotspots (*DNA1-3*, *DPA1* and *VPS52*), which occur in both males and females, all are ablated in males carrying 14–15 ZnF motifs, whereas, although both the *DNA1-3* and *VPS52* hotspots are absent, there appears to be little effect of the presence of this variant on recombination at *DPA1* in females.

Table S1   Association tests for 92 single SNPs in the MHC Class II region from *HLA-DMB* to *COL11A2* and haplotype block definitions. Results shown are P values of linear regression analysis (additive mode), corrected for stratification by principal component analysis using SNP and Variation Suite (v 7.7.5). SNPs identified in previous studies (rs3135034 and rs9296068) [18,19] are highlighted in bold. SNPs included in haplotype blocks 1–4 are shaded.

Table S2   Haplotype Numbers Predicted by PHASE. Average numbers of predicted haploytpes using matched numbers of cases and controls (BCP-ALL, 447; T-ALL, 44) based on output data from four replicate PHASE analyses using different seed values.

Table S3   Tagger Selected SNPs. Thirty five SNPs, selected using Tagger [44] for haplotype analysis with LDsplit [28], showing chromosomal location and minor allele frequency (MAF) in the CEU population.

Acknowledgments

would like to thank Fay Hosking and Richard Houlston for providing the chromosome 6 SNP data, Alec Jeffreys and Celia May for helpful advice and critical appraisal of the manuscript, and Matthew Stephens and Peter Donnelly for their advice and for allowing us to access the PHASE software. We are grateful to participants in the UK Childhood Cancer Study.

Author Contributions

Conceived and designed the experiments: PT KU JZ PY MF PB AC TL MT. Performed the experiments: PT PY MF MT. Analyzed the data: PT KU JZ PY MF MT. Contributed reagents/materials/analysis tools: JZ PY MF PB TL. Wrote the paper: PT KU JZ PY MF PB AC TL MT.

References

1. Coebergh JWW, Reedijk AMJ, de Vries E, Martos C, Jakab Z, et al. (2006) Leukaemia incidence and survival in children and adolescents in Europe during 1978–1997. Report from the Automated Childhood Cancer Information System project. European Journal of Cancer 42: 2019–2036.

2. Papaemmanuil E, Hosking FJ, Vijayakrishnan J, Price A, Olver B, et al. (2009) Loci on 7p12.2, 10q21.2 and 14q11.2 are associated with risk of childhood acute lymphoblastic leukemia. Nat Genet 41: 1006–1010.

3. Sherborne AL, Hosking FJ, Prasad RB, Kumar R, Koehler R, et al. (2010) Variation in CDKN2A at 9p21.3 influences childhood acute lymphoblastic leukemia risk. Nat Genet 42: 492–494.

4. Trevino LR, Yang W, French D, Hunger SP, Carroll WL, et al. (2009) Germline genomic variants associated with childhood acute lymphoblastic leukemia. Nat Genet 41: 1001–1005.

5. Georgopoulos K, Winandy S, Avitahl N (1997) The Role of the Ikaros Ggene in Lymphocyte Development and Homeostasis. Annual Review of Immunology 15: 155–176.

6. Lahoud MH, Ristevski S, Venter DJ, Jermiin LS, Bertoncello I, et al. (2001) Gene Targeting of Desrt, a Novel ARID Class DNA-Binding Protein, Causes Growth Retardation and Abnormal Development of Reproductive Organs. Genome Research 11: 1327–1334.

7. Akasaka T, Balasas T, Russell LJ, Sugimoto K-j, Majid A, et al. (2007) Five members of the CEBP transcription factor family are targeted by recurrent IGH translocations in B-cell precursor acute lymphoblastic leukemia (BCP-ALL). Blood 109: 3451–3461.

8. Mullighan CG, Downing JR (2009) Genome-wide profiling of genetic alterations in acute lymphoblastic leukemia: recent insights and future directions. Leukemia 23: 1209–1218.

9. Migliorini G, Fiege B, Hosking FJ, Ma Y, Kumar R, et al. (2013) Variation at 10p12.2 and 10p14 influences risk of childhood B-cell acute lymphoblastic leukemia and phenotype. Blood 122: 3298–3307.

10. Eden T (2010) Aetiology of childhood leukaemia. Cancer Treatment Reviews 36: 286–297.

11. Lilly F, Boyse EA, Old LJ (1964) GENETIC BASIS OF SUSCEPTIBILITY TO VIRAL LEUKÆMOGENESIS. The Lancet 284: 1207–1209.

12. Khor CC, Hibberd ML (2012) Host–pathogen interactions revealed by human genome-wide surveys. Trends in Genetics 28: 233–243.

13. Taylor GM, Hussain A, Urayama K, Chokkalingam A, Thompson P, et al. (2009) The human major histocompatibility complex and childhood leukemia: an etiological hypothesis based on molecular mimicry. Blood Cells Mol Dis 42: 129–135.

14. Urayama KY, Chokkalingam AP, Metayer C, Ma X, Selvin S, et al. (2012) HLA-DP genetic variation, proxies for early life immune modulation and childhood acute lymphoblastic leukemia risk. Blood 120: 3039–3047.

15. Dorak MT, Oguz FS, Yalman N, Diler AS, Kalayoglu S, et al. (2002) A male-specific increase in the HLA-DRB4 (DR53) frequency in high-risk and relapsed childhood ALL. Leuk Res 26: 651–656.

16. Taylor GM, Dearden S, Ravetto P, Ayres M, Watson P, et al. (2002) Genetic susceptibility to childhood common acute lymphoblastic leukaemia is associated with polymorphic peptide-binding pocket profiles in HLA-DPB1*0201. Hum Mol Genet 11: 1585–1597.

17. Taylor M, Bergemann TL, Hussain A, Thompson PD, Spector L (2011) Transmission of HLA-DP variants from parents to children with B-cell precursor acute lymphoblastic leukemia: Log-linear analysis using the case parent design. Human Immunology 72: 897–903.

18. Hosking FJ, Leslie S, Dilthey A, Moutsianas L, Wang Y, et al. (2011) MHC variation and risk of childhood B-cell precursor acute lymphoblastic leukemia. Blood 117: 1633–1640.

19. Urayama KY, Chokkalingam AP, Metayer C, Hansen H, May S, et al. (2013) SNP Association Mapping across the Extended Major Histocompatibility Complex and Risk of B-Cell Precursor Acute Lymphoblastic Leukemia in Children. PLoS One 8: e72557.

20. Jeffreys AJ, Kauppi L, Neumann R (2001) Intensely punctate meiotic recombination in the class II region of the major histocompatibility complex. Nat Genet 29: 217–222.

21. Stephens M, Smith NJ, Donnelly P (2001) A new statistical method for haplotype reconstruction from population data. Am J Hum Genet 68: 978–989.

22. Taylor GM, Hussain A, Verhage V, Thompson PD, Fergusson WD, et al. (2009) Strong association of the HLA-DP6 supertype with childhood leukaemia is due to a single allele, DPB1*0601. Leukaemia 23: 863–869.

23. Li N, Stephens M (2003) Modeling linkage disequilibrium and identifying recombination hotspots using single-nucleotide polymorphism data. Genetics 165: 2213–2233.

24. Crawford DC, Bhangale T, Li N, Hellenthal G, Rieder MJ, et al. (2004) Evidence for substantial fine-scale variation in recombination rates across the human genome. Nat Genet 36: 700–706.

25. Stephens M, Donnelly P (2003) A comparison of bayesian methods for haplotype reconstruction from population genotype data. Am J Hum Genet 73: 1162–1169.

26. Berg IL, Neumann R, Sarbajna S, Odenthal-Hesse L, Butler NJ, et al. (2011) Variants of the protein PRDM9 differentially regulate a set of human meiotic recombination hotspots highly active in African populations. Proc Natl Acad Sci U S A 108: 12378–12383.

27. Kong A, Thorleifsson G, Gudbjartsson DF, Masson G, Sigurdsson A, et al. (2010) Fine-scale recombination rate differences between sexes, populations and individuals. Nature 467: 1099–1103.

28. Zheng J, Khil PP, Camerini-Otero RD, Przytycka TM (2010) Detecting sequence polymorphisms associated with meiotic recombination hotspots in the human genome. Genome Biol 11: R103.

29. Yang P, Wu M, Guo J, Kwoh C, Przytycka T, et al. (2014) LDsplit: screening for cis-regulatory motifs stimulating meiotic recombination hotspots by analysis of DNA sequence polymorphisms. BMC Bioinformatics 15: 48.

30. de Bakker PIW, Yelensky R, Pe'er I, Gabriel SB, Daly MJ, et al. (2005) Efficiency and power in genetic association studies. Nat Genet 37: 1217–1223.

31. Shang E, Cui Q, Wang X, Beseler C, Greenberg DA, et al. (2011) The bromodomain-containing gene BRD2 is regulated at transcription, splicing, and translation levels. Journal of Cellular Biochemistry 112: 2784–2793.

32. Guce AI, Mortimer SE, Yoon T, Painter CA, Jiang W, et al. (2013) HLA-DO acts as a substrate mimic to inhibit HLA-DM by a competitive mechanism. Nat Struct Mol Biol 20: 90–98.

33. Karlsson L, Surh CD, Sprent J, Peterson PA (1991) A novel class II MHC molecule with unusual tissue distribution. Nature 351: 485–488.

34. Greaves M (2006) Infection, immune responses and the aetiology of childhood leukaemia. Nat Rev Cancer 6: 193–203.

35. Hussin J, Sinnett D, Casals F, Idaghdour Y, Bruat V, et al. (2013) Rare allelic forms of PRDM9 associated with childhood leukemogenesis. Genome Res 23: 419–430.

36. Hinch AG, Tandon A, Patterson N, Song Y, Rohland N, et al. (2011) The landscape of recombination in African Americans. Nature 476: 170–175.

37. Gurney JG, Severson RK, Davis S, Robison LL (1995) Incidence of cancer in children in the United States. Sex-, race-, and 1-year age-specific rates by histologic type. Cancer 75: 2186–2195.

38. Kauppi L, Jeffreys AJ, Keeney S (2004) Where the crossovers are: recombination distributions in mammals. Nat Rev Genet 5: 413–424.

39. Ng SK, Lo WS, Pun FW, Zhao C, Yu Z, et al. (2010) A recombination hotspot in a schizophrenia-associated region of GABRB2. PLoS One 5: e9547.

40. Tan IKL, Mackin L, Wang N, Papenfuss AT, Elso CM, et al. (2010) A recombination hotspot leads to sequence variability within a novel gene (AK005651) and contributes to type 1 diabetes susceptibility. Genome Research 20: 1629–1638.

41. Taylor GM, Hussain A, Lightfoot TJ, Birch JM, Eden TO, et al. (2008) HLA-associated susceptibility to childhood B-cell precursor ALL: definition and role of HLA-DPB1 supertypes. Br J Cancer 98: 1125–1131.

42. Investigators UCCS (2000) The United Kingdom Childhood Cancer Study: objectives, materials and methods. UK Childhood Cancer Study Investigators. Br J Cancer 82: 1073–1102.

43. Jeffreys AJ, Neumann R (2002) Reciprocal crossover asymmetry and meiotic drive in a human recombination hot spot. Nat Genet 31: 267–271.

44. de Bakker PI, Yelensky R, Pe'er I, Gabriel SB, Daly MJ, et al. (2005) Efficiency and power in genetic association studies. Nat Genet 37: 1217–1223.

7

The Diagnostic Value of DNA Methylation in Leukemia: A Systematic Review and Meta-Analysis

Danjie Jiang[1], Qingxiao Hong[1], Yusheng Shen[1], Yan Xu[1], Huangkai Zhu[1], Yirun Li[1], Chunjing Xu[1], Guifang Ouyang[2]*, Shiwei Duan[1]*

1 Zhejiang Provincial Key Laboratory of Pathophysiology, School of Medicine, Ningbo University, Ningbo, Zhejiang, China, 2 Department of Hematology, Ningbo First Hospital, Ningbo, Zhejiang, China

Abstract

Background: Accumulating evidence supports a role of DNA methylation in the pathogenesis of leukemia. The aim of our study was to evaluate the potential genes with aberrant DNA methylation in the prediction of leukemia risk by a comprehensive meta-analysis of the published data.

Methods: A series of meta-analyses were done among the eligible studies that were harvested after a careful filtration of the searching results from PubMed literature database. Mantel-Haenszel odds ratios and 95% confidence intervals were computed for each methylation event assuming the appropriate model.

Results: A total of 535 publications were initially retrieved from PubMed literature database. After a three-step filtration, we harvested 41 case-control articles that studied the role of gene methylation in the prediction of leukemia risk. Among the involving 30 genes, 20 genes were shown to be aberrantly methylated in the leukemia patients. A further subgroup meta-analysis by subtype of leukemia showed that *CDKN2A, CDKN2B, ID4* genes were significantly hypermethylated in acute myeloid leukemia.

Conclusions: Our meta-analyses identified strong associations between a number of genes with aberrant DNA methylation and leukemia. Further studies should be required to confirm the results in the future.

Editor: Osman El-Maarri, University of Bonn, Institut of experimental hematology and transfusion medicine, Germany

Funding: The research was supported by the grants from National Natural Science Foundation of China (31100919 and 81371469), Natural Science Foundation of Zhejiang Province (LR13H020003), K. C. Wong Magna Fund in Ningbo University, and Ningbo Social Development Research Projects (2010C50019 and 2012C50032). The funders had no role in study design, data collection and analysis, decision to publish, or preparation of the manuscript.

Competing Interests: The authors have declared that no competing interests exist.

* E-mail: duanshiwei@nbu.edu.cn (SD); ouyangguifang2000@aliyun.com (GO)

Introduction

Leukemia is a common malignant disease of hematopoietic system, caused by unbalanced hematopoietic cells proliferation and death [1]. The development and progression of leukemia is complex. Based on the speed of disease progression and the types of affected white blood cell, leukemia can be divided into four most common types of leukemia, which comprise acute myeloid leukemia (AML), chronic myeloid leukemia (CML), acute lymphocytic leukemia (ALL) and chronic lymphocytic leukemia (CLL) (http://www.nlm.nih.gov/medlineplus/leukemia.html).

Although tremendous efforts have been made in the identification of susceptible factors of leukemia [2,3], the pathogenesis of leukemia is not fully clarified [4]. Environmental factors, such as high benzene exposure, radiation, electrical work, are shown to be associated with the development of leukemia [5,6]. Meanwhile, leukemia is known to be associated with the accumulation of defects in a wide range of cancer genes [7].

Many genetic and epigenetic alternations were found to play an important role in leukemia pathogenesis [8,9]. Previous study has indicated aberrant DNA methylation associated with leukemogenesis [10]. As a typical epigenetic modifications, aberrant DNA methylation was observed in lymphoid/hematopoietic malignancies, including AML [4,11], CML [12,13], ALL [1,14], and CLL [15,16].

These aberrant patterns of DNA methylation in leukemia can be useful for cancer risk prediction. Recent advances attest to the great promise of DNA methylation markers as powerful tools in the clinic [17–19]. Meta-analysis can generate a more objective evaluation of candidate genes DNA methylation and the risks of leukemia, based on the conclusions of uncertainty and disagreements. Here we perform comprehensive meta-analyses based on the accumulating leukemia association studies on DNA methylation to better identify biomarkers with aberrant DNA methylation in leukemia. The goal of our study was to summarize the genes with aberrant DNA methylation as promising biomarkers for leukemia risk prediction.

Materials and Methods

Search Strategy

A systematic literature search was performed in PubMed by using "leukemia" and "DNA methylation" as the search terms for articles updated until December 25, 2013. The search was limited to articles published in English and Chinese. Articles in the search output were surveyed according to their titles and abstracts. Studies were selected if they met the following criteria: 1) they were case-control associations of gene methylation with the risk of leukemia in humans; 2) they had sufficient methylation information to calculate the odd ratios (ORs) and 95% confidential intervals (CIs) for the meta-analysis. The selection procedures of studies were illustrated in the flow chart of Figure 1.

Data Extraction

For the eligible articles, we extracted the following information: first author's name, published year, PubMed ID, disease category (AML, ALL, CML, CLL or others), the numbers of cases and controls. All the data were extracted by four authors (DJ, YX, HZ and CX). A consensus was reached through a rigorous discussion when there existed conflicting evaluations.

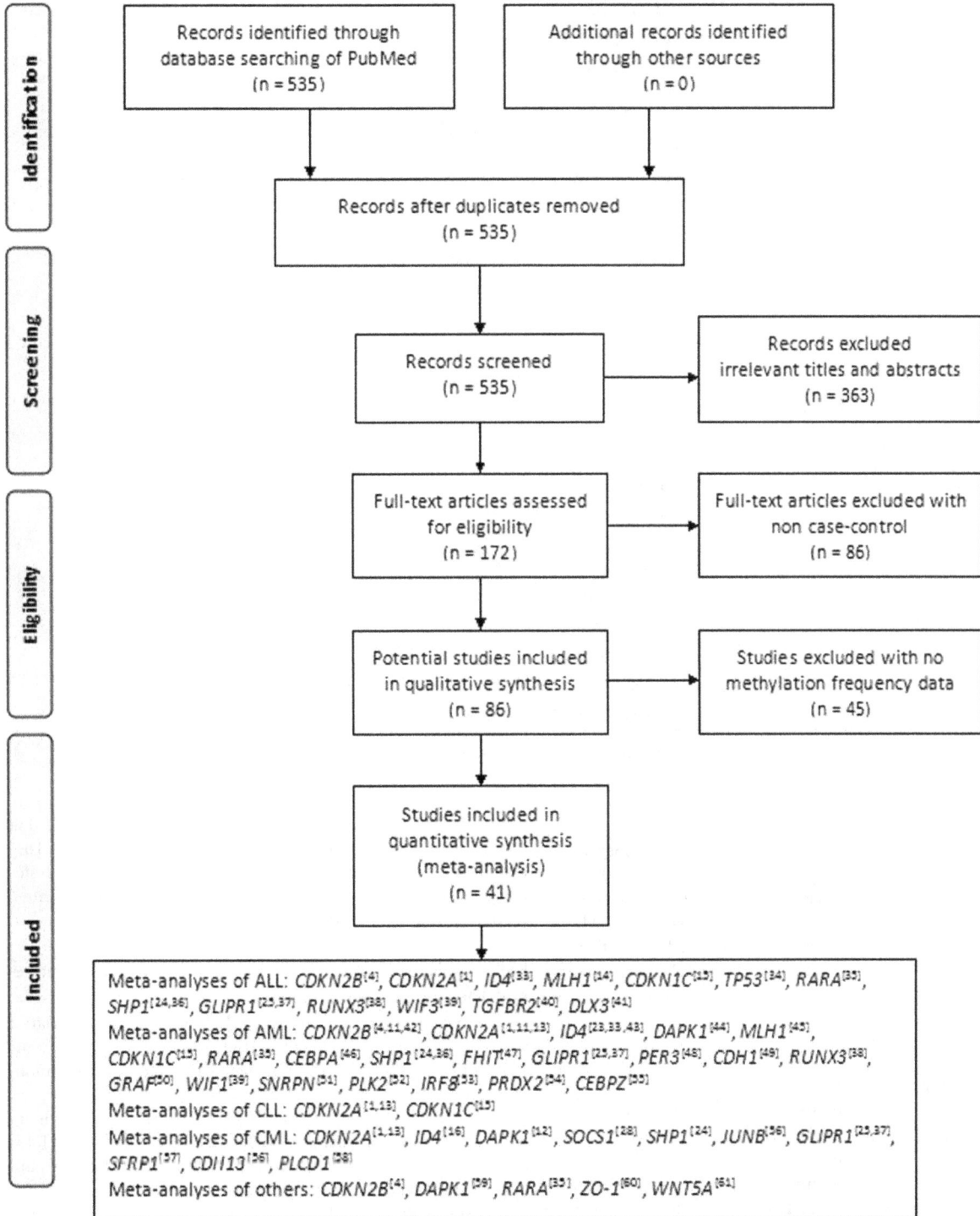

Figure 1. Flow diagram of the stepwise selection from relevant studies.

Table 1. Genes differently methylated in case-control studies from leukemia subjects.

Gene	Studies	Overall OR (95% CI)[a]	P value
CDKN2A	12	3.53[1.43, 8.73]	<0.01
GLIPR1	6	5.96 [2.29, 15.46]	<0.01
CDKN2B	5	9.67 [2.48, 37.75]	<0.01
SHP1	5	29.27 [6.80, 125.99]	<0.01
ID4	5	45.24 [11.02, 185.78]	<0.01
DAPK1	3	28.85 [5.54, 150.14]	<0.01
CDKN1C	3	6.16 [0.66, 57.72]	0.11
RARA	3	3.46 [0.65, 18.39]	0.15
RUNX3	2	11.91 [1.45, 97.86]	0.02
WIF1	2	14.15 [1.78, 112.81]	0.01
MLH1	2	5.93 [0.27, 130.34]	0.26
SOCS1	1	0.10 [0.01, 0.78]	0.03
JUNB	1	55.00 [1.86, 1622.60]	0.02
ZO-1	1	45.00 [2.01, 1006.75]	0.02
WNT5A	1	121.51 [7.08, 2085.83]	<0.01
PER3	1	104.27 [6.33, 1718.74]	<0.01
CDH1	1	33.00 [1.78, 610.61]	0.02
GRAF	1	81.54 [4.82, 1379.56]	<0.01
SNRPN	1	25.00 [1.39, 449.48]	0.03
PLK2	1	67.34 [3.77, 1204.54]	<0.01
PRDX2	1	22.32 [1.32, 377.72]	0.03
PLCD1	1	39.38 [2.21, 702.41]	0.01
CEBPZ	1	35.84 [2.12, 604.80]	0.01
TP53	1	3.40 [0.16, 73.57]	0.44
CEBPA	1	2.53 [0.14, 47.18]	0.53
FHIT	1	4.80 [0.27, 85.35]	0.29
SFRP1	1	1.54 [0.17, 14.09]	0.70
CDH13	1	11.00 [0.46, 263.53]	0.14
DLX3	1	1.66 [0.48, 5.65]	0.42
IRF8	1	6.41 [0.34, 120.24]	0.21

[a]Odds ratio (OR) describes the likelihood of gene methylation observed in leukemia cases compared to controls.

Meta-analysis

Review manager 5 was used for meta-analysis. Mantel-Haenszel ORs and their 95% CIs were computed for each gene to evaluate the contribution of gene methylation to the risk of leukemia. Heterogeneity of the studies in the meta-analysis was evaluated by I^2 metric [20,21]. A random-effect model was used when there existed heterogeneity in the meta-analysis ($I^2>50\%$), otherwise a fixed-effect model was applied for the meta-analysis [22].

Results

Study Characteristics

A total of 535 studies were retrieved from the PubMed literature database after searching the keywords of "leukemia" and "DNA methylation". After a series of selection procedure shown in Figure 1, we excluded 363 irrelevant studies, 86 non-case-control studies, and 45 studies without methylation data. Finally, 41 case-control studies were qualified for our meta-analyses. These comprised 15 ALL studies, 31 AML studies, 4 CLL studies, 13 CML studies, and 5 other studies (including 1 on acute

promyelocytic leukemia, and 4 on undefined leukemia). The 41 case-control studies were involved with 30 genes among 1640 healthy individuals and 2587 leukemia patients. Among the tested genes, there were 19 genes with only one report, 3 genes with 2 reports, and 8 genes with 3 or more reports (Table 1).

Meta-analysis of the Association Studies between Gene and the Risk of Leukemia

As shown in Figure 2, the meta-analysis of CDKN2A methylation was involved with 12 case-control studies among 576 controls and 167 cases. Our results showed a significant heterogeneity among the 12 studies ($I^2 = 65\%$). In addition, the meta-analysis indicated that hypermethylation of CDKN2A gene was associated with the increased risk of leukemia (P = 0.006, OR = 3.53, 95% CI = 1.43–8.73). Meta-analysis between GLIPR1 methylation and leukemia was involved with 6 case-control studies among 384 controls and 309 cases (Figure 2). The meta-analysis showed a significant heterogeneity ($I^2 = 83\%$) among these studies, and revealed that GLIPR1 hypermethylation was associated with the increased risk of leukemia (P = 0.0002, OR = 5.96, 95% CI = 2.29–15.46). Meta-

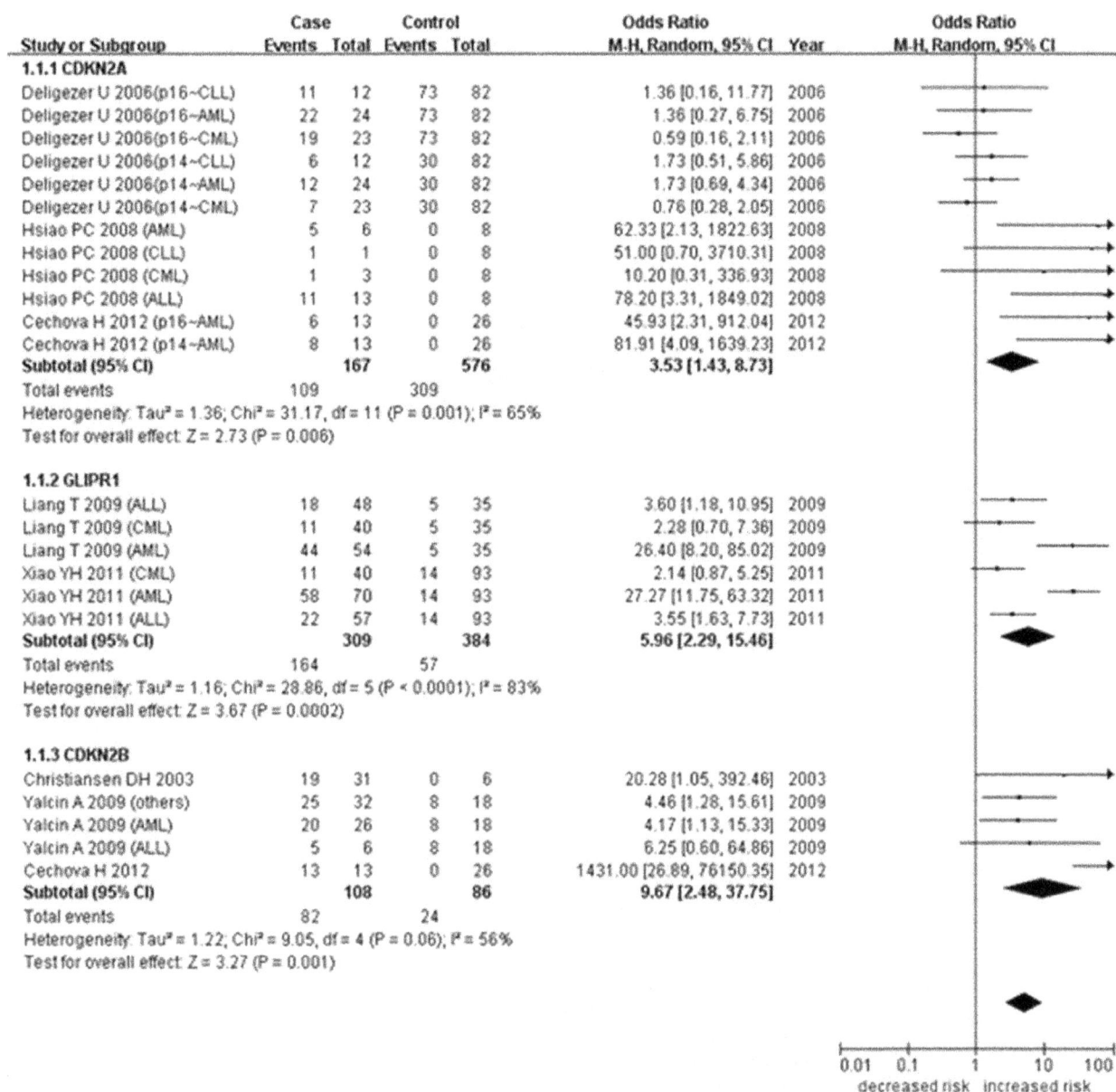

Study or Subgroup	Case Events	Total	Control Events	Total	Odds Ratio M-H, Random, 95% CI	Year	Odds Ratio M-H, Random, 95% CI
1.1.1 CDKN2A							
Deligezer U 2006(p16~CLL)	11	12	73	82	1.36 [0.16, 11.77]	2006	
Deligezer U 2006(p16~AML)	22	24	73	82	1.36 [0.27, 6.75]	2006	
Deligezer U 2006(p16~CML)	19	23	73	82	0.59 [0.16, 2.11]	2006	
Deligezer U 2006(p14~CLL)	6	12	30	82	1.73 [0.51, 5.86]	2006	
Deligezer U 2006(p14~AML)	12	24	30	82	1.73 [0.69, 4.34]	2006	
Deligezer U 2006(p14~CML)	7	23	30	82	0.76 [0.28, 2.05]	2006	
Hsiao PC 2008 (AML)	5	6	0	8	62.33 [2.13, 1822.63]	2008	
Hsiao PC 2008 (CLL)	1	1	0	8	51.00 [0.70, 3710.31]	2008	
Hsiao PC 2008 (CML)	1	3	0	8	10.20 [0.31, 336.93]	2008	
Hsiao PC 2008 (ALL)	11	13	0	8	78.20 [3.31, 1849.02]	2008	
Cechova H 2012 (p16~AML)	6	13	0	26	45.93 [2.31, 912.04]	2012	
Cechova H 2012 (p14~AML)	8	13	0	26	81.91 [4.09, 1639.23]	2012	
Subtotal (95% CI)		167		576	3.53 [1.43, 8.73]		
Total events	109		309				
Heterogeneity: Tau² = 1.36; Chi² = 31.17, df = 11 (P = 0.001); I² = 65%							
Test for overall effect: Z = 2.73 (P = 0.006)							
1.1.2 GLIPR1							
Liang T 2009 (ALL)	18	48	5	35	3.60 [1.18, 10.95]	2009	
Liang T 2009 (CML)	11	40	5	35	2.28 [0.70, 7.36]	2009	
Liang T 2009 (AML)	44	54	5	35	26.40 [8.20, 85.02]	2009	
Xiao YH 2011 (CML)	11	40	14	93	2.14 [0.87, 5.25]	2011	
Xiao YH 2011 (AML)	58	70	14	93	27.27 [11.75, 63.32]	2011	
Xiao YH 2011 (ALL)	22	57	14	93	3.55 [1.63, 7.73]	2011	
Subtotal (95% CI)		309		384	5.96 [2.29, 15.46]		
Total events	164		57				
Heterogeneity: Tau² = 1.16; Chi² = 28.86, df = 5 (P < 0.0001); I² = 83%							
Test for overall effect: Z = 3.67 (P = 0.0002)							
1.1.3 CDKN2B							
Christiansen DH 2003	19	31	0	6	20.28 [1.05, 392.46]	2003	
Yalcin A 2009 (others)	25	32	8	18	4.46 [1.28, 15.61]	2009	
Yalcin A 2009 (AML)	20	26	8	18	4.17 [1.13, 15.33]	2009	
Yalcin A 2009 (ALL)	5	6	8	18	6.25 [0.60, 64.86]	2009	
Cechova H 2012	13	13	0	26	1431.00 [26.89, 76150.35]	2012	
Subtotal (95% CI)		108		86	9.67 [2.48, 37.75]		
Total events	82		24				
Heterogeneity: Tau² = 1.22; Chi² = 9.05, df = 4 (P = 0.06); I² = 56%							
Test for overall effect: Z = 3.27 (P = 0.001)							

0.01 0.1 1 10 100
decreased risk   increased risk

Figure 2. Correlation between *CDKN2A/GLIPR1/CDKN2B* **methylation and leukemia in the meta-analysis.**

analysis of *CDKN2B* methylation with leukemia was carried out in 5 studies among 86 controls and 108 cases (Figure 2). Our results showed a significant heterogeneity among the 5 case-control studies ($I^2 = 56\%$), and revealed that hypermethylation of *CDKN2B* gene was associated with the increased risk of leukemia (P = 0.001, OR = 9.67, 95% CI = 2.48–37.75).

Table 2. Genes differently methylated in case-control studies from different kinds of leukemia subjects.

Gene~Disease	Studies	Overall OR (95% CI)[a]	P value
CDKN2A~AML	5	8.63 [1.52, 48.91]	0.01
CDKN2B~AML	3	31.92 [1.37, 742.18]	0.03
CDKN2A~CML	3	0.82 [0.38, 1.74]	0.6
CDKN2A~CLL	3	2.04 [0.74, 5.59]	0.17
ID4~AML	3	87.52 [16.05, 477.38]	<0.01

[a]Odds ratio (OR) describes the likelihood of gene methylation observed in leukemia cases compared to controls.

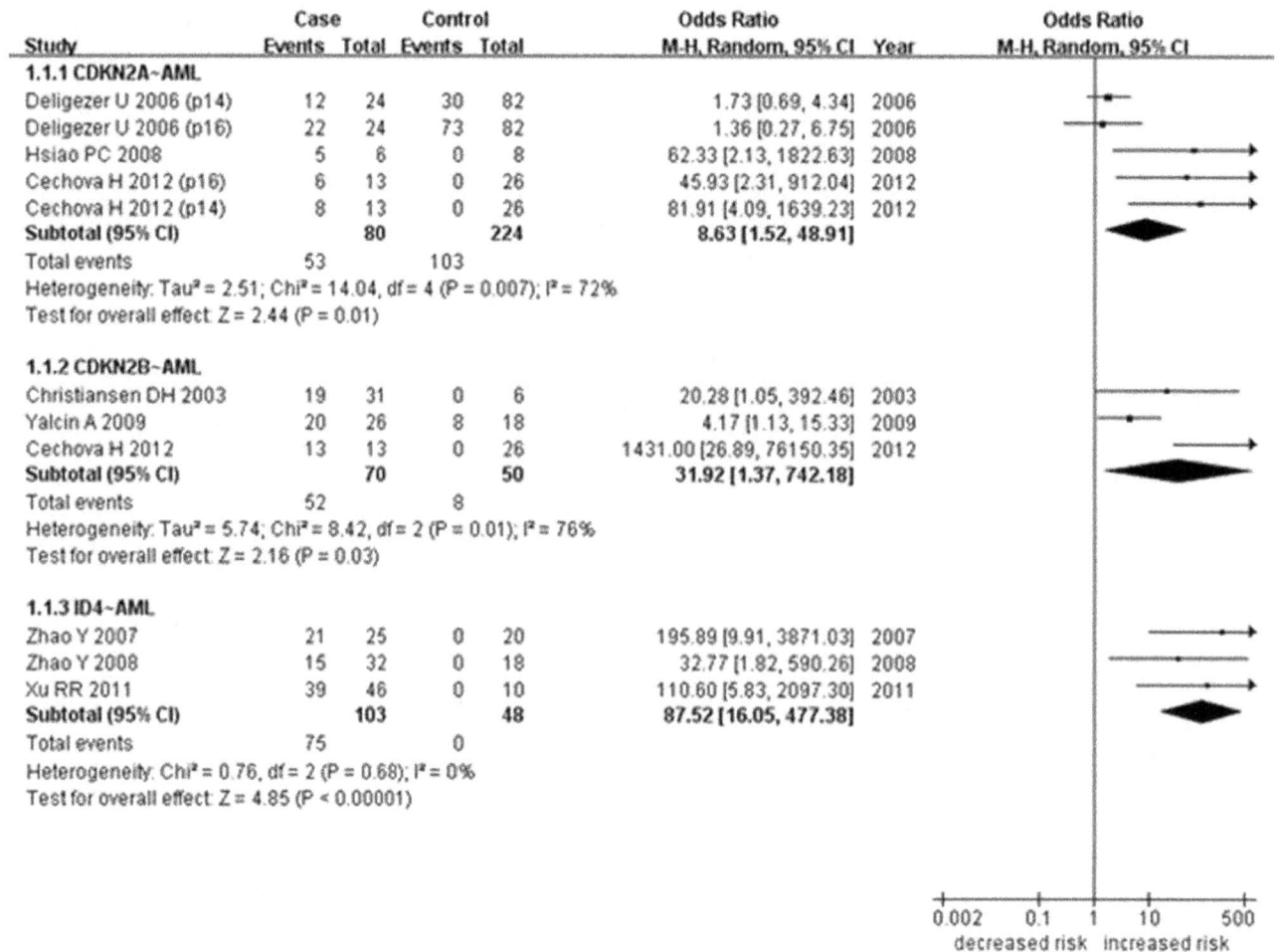

Figure 3. Correlation between *CDKN2A/CDKN2B/ID4* methylation and AML in the meta-analysis.

Meta-analysis of *SHP1* methylation was involved with 5 case-control studies among 46 controls and 104 cases. Our results indicated that hypermethylation of SHP1 gene was associated with the increased risk of leukemia (P<0.00001, OR = 29.27, 95% CI = 6.80–125.99). Meta-analysis between *ID4* methylation and leukemia was involved with 5 case-control studies among 78 controls and 165 cases. The results revealed that *ID4* hypermethylation was associated with the increased risk of leukemia (P< 0.00001, OR = 45.24, 95% CI = 11.02–185.78). Meta-analysis of *DAPK1* methylation with leukemia was carried out in 3 studies among 29 controls and 169 cases. Our results showed that hypermethylation of *DAPK1* gene was associated with the increased risk of leukemia (P<0.0001, OR = 28.85, 95% CI = 5.54–150.14). In addition, our results were unable to observe significant association of the methylation of *CDKN1C* and *RARA* genes with leukemia.

Meta-analysis of the Association Studies between Gene and the Risk of AML

We further performed a breakdown meta-analysis by leukemia subtypes in the above-mentioned studies (Table 2). As shown in Figure 3, meta-analysis of *CDKN2A* methylation in AML was involved with 5 case-control studies among 80 cases and 224 controls. A significant heterogeneity was observed among the 5 studies ($I^2 = 72\%$). Our results showed that *CDKN2A* hypermethy-

lation was associated with the increased risk of AML (P = 0.01, OR = 8.63, 95% CI = 1.52–48.91). The meta-analysis between *CDKN2B* methylation and AML was involved with 3 studies among 70 cases and 50 controls (Figure 3). There existed significant heterogeneity among the 3 studies in the meta-analysis of *CDKN2B* methylation ($I^2 = 76\%$). Our results showed *CDKN2B* hypermethylation was associated with the increased risk of AML (P = 0.03, OR = 31.92, 95% CI = 1.37–742.18). As shown in Figure 3, the meta-analysis of *ID4* methylation was involved with 3 studies among 103 cases and 48 controls. The results showed that *ID4* hypermethylation was associated with the increased risk of AML (P<0.00001, OR = 87.52, 95% CI = 16.05–477.38).

Discussion

Numerous studies have found that DNA methylation of different genes was associated with the risk of leukemia [11–13,23–25], which implicated a potential role of DNA methylation in the prediction and prognostication for leukemia.

De novo methylation of the 5′CpG island has been reported as an alternative mechanism of inactivation for tumor suppressor genes *CDKN2A* and *CDKN2B* [26]. De novo methylation of *CDKN2B* and *CDKN2A* CpG islands is frequent in malignant transformation [11]. According to the results of our meta-analysis, the aberrant DNA methylation at *CDKN2A* gene and *CDKN2B* gene were risk factors for leukemia, especially for AML. In the subgroup analysis, we found that DNA methylation of *CDKN2A* gene was significantly associated with AML, but not with CML or CLL. A microarray analysis in 2011 identified that glioma pathogenesis-related protein 1 (*GLIPR1*) was a methylation-silenced gene in the AML patients, and might serve as a marker to monitor the therapeutic effect of AML [25]. Our analysis also demonstrated that DNA methylation of *GLIPR1* gene was a risk factor for leukemia. *GLIPR1* is a pleiotropic protein involved in cell proliferation, tumor growth and apoptosis, and it may affect G protein signaling and cell cycle regulation [27]. *SOCS1* is an important protein in the JAK/STAT pathway, and plays a key role in the downstream regulation of BCR-ABL protein kinase [28]. Our results showed that DNA methylation of *SOCS1* gene was a protective factor for leukemia. *SHP1* is tumor suppressor gene involved in the regulation of cell cycle control and apoptosis [29]. *SHP1* is negative regulator of the Jak/STAT signaling pathway that is implicated in leukemogenesis. Promoter methylation of *SHP1* gene is able to silence its gene expression, and was frequently detected in various kinds of leukemias and lymphoma [24]. Our results showed that aberrant DNA methylation of *SHP1* gene was a risk factor for leukemia. Inhibitor of DNA binding protein 4 (*ID4*) is a member of the dominant-negative basic helix-loop-helix transcription factor family that lacks DNA binding activity and has tumor suppressor function. Promoter of *ID4* is consistently methylated to various degrees in CLL cells, and increased promoter methylation in a univariable analysis was shown to be correlated with shortened patient survival [30]. In our results of analysis, the aberrant DNA methylation at *ID4* gene was a risk factor for leukemia, especially for AML. Death-associated protein kinase 1 (*DAPK1*), a tumor suppressor, is a rate-limiting effecter in an endoplasmic reticulum stress-dependent apoptotic pathway [31]. Aberrant DNA methylation and concomitant transcriptional silencing of *DAPK1* have been demonstrated to be key pathogenic events in CLL [32]. Our study identified the aberrant DNA methylation at *DAPK1* gene was a risk factor for leukemia.

The current meta-analysis has some limitations. Firstly, selection bias is inevitable due to the search strategy restricted to articles published in English or Chinese. Secondly, some large between-study heterogeneity existed in our meta-analyses. This phenomenon may be caused by the facts that different subtypes of leukemia were not separated in the first place due to the limited studies, and that different regions of the same gene were tested for methylation in the involved studies. Thirdly, this analysis was performed at the study level, which limited ability to explore the potential for confounding by various demographic and clinical factors (e.g. ethnicity, hormone, different treatments). Fourthly, most of the studies we selected were performed with Methylation-Specific PCR (MSP) and the status of DNA methylation was qualitative (M+ or M−), and it also limited the scope of our analysis. Finally, the efficiency and accuracy of statistical analysis may be influenced by the moderate amount of subjects. We expect more samples being tested in the future to draw a more reliable conclusion.

In conclusion, the results of this study indicated that certain genes DNA methylation was independently associated with the risk of leukemia, especially some kinds of leukemia. Also more studies should be required to confirm the results in the future. DNA methylation has a very strong potential to be a useful biomarker for predicting, prognostication and prediction of response to chemotherapy of leukemia.

Supporting Information

Checklist S1   PRISMA Checklist.

Author Contributions

Conceived and designed the experiments: SD GO. Analyzed the data: DJ QH YS YX HZ YL CX. Contributed reagents/materials/analysis tools: SD GO. Wrote the paper: DJ SD.

References

1. Hsiao PC, Liu MC, Chen LM, Tsai CY, Wang YT, et al. (2008) Promoter methylation of p16 and EDNRB gene in leukemia patients in Taiwan. Chin J Physiol 51: 27–31.
2. Olme CH, Finnon R, Brown N, Kabacik S, Bouffler SD, et al. (2013) Live cell detection of chromosome 2 deletion and Sfpi1/PU1 loss in radiation-induced mouse acute myeloid leukaemia. Leuk Res 37: 1374–1382.
3. Lupo PJ, Nousome D, Kamdar KY, Okcu MF, Scheurer ME (2012) A case-parent triad assessment of folate metabolic genes and the risk of childhood acute lymphoblastic leukemia. Cancer Causes Control 23: 1797–1803.
4. Yalcin A, Serin MS, Emekdas G, Tiftik N, Aslan G, et al. (2009) Promoter methylation of P15(INK4B) gene is possibly associated with parvovirus B19 infection in adult acute leukemias. Int J Lab Hematol 31: 407–419.
5. Rushton L, Schnatter AR, Tang G, Glass DC (2014) Acute myeloid and chronic lymphoid leukaemias and exposure to low-level benzene among petroleum workers. Br J Cancer 110: 783–787.
6. Flodin U, Fredriksson M, Persson B, Hardell L, Axelson O (1986) Background radiation, electrical work, and some other exposures associated with acute myeloid leukemia in a case-referent study. Arch Environ Health 41: 77–84.
7. Balmain A, Gray J, Ponder B (2003) The genetics and genomics of cancer. Nat Genet 33 Suppl: 238–244.
8. Chen C, Liu Y, Lu C, Cross JR, Morris JPt, et al. (2013) Cancer-associated IDH2 mutants drive an acute myeloid leukemia that is susceptible to Brd4 inhibition. Genes Dev 27: 1974–1985.
9. Kanno S, Maeda N, Tomizawa A, Yomogida S, Katoh T, et al. (2012) Characterization of cells resistant to the potent histone deacetylase inhibitor spiruchostatin B (SP-B) and effect of overexpressed p21waf1/cip1 on the SP-B resistance or overexpression of human leukemia cells. Int J Oncol 41: 862–868.
10. Issa JP, Baylin SB, Herman JG (1997) DNA methylation changes in hematologic malignancies: biologic and clinical implications. Leukemia 11 Suppl 1: S7–11.
11. Cechova H, Lassuthova P, Novakova L, Belickova M, Stemberkova R, et al. (2012) Monitoring of methylation changes in 9p21 region in patients with myelodysplastic syndromes and acute myeloid leukemia. Neoplasma 59: 168–174.
12. Qian J, Wang YL, Lin J, Yao DM, Xu WR, et al. (2009) Aberrant methylation of the death-associated protein kinase 1 (DAPK1) CpG island in chronic myeloid leukemia. Eur J Haematol 82: 119–123.
13. Deligezer U, Erten N, Akisik EE, Dalay N (2006) Methylation of the INK4A/ARF locus in blood mononuclear cells. Ann Hematol 85: 102–107.
14. Matsushita M, Takeuchi S, Yang Y, Yoshino N, Tsukasaki K, et al. (2005) Methylation of the MLH1 gene in hematological malignancies. Oncol Rep 14: 191–194.
15. Li Y, Nagai H, Ohno T, Yuge M, Hatano S, et al. (2002) Aberrant DNA methylation of p57(KIP2) gene in the promoter region in lymphoid malignancies of B-cell phenotype. Blood 100: 2572–2577.
16. Wang XR, Kang HY, Cen J, Li YH, Wang LL, et al. (2010) [Methylation status of id4 gene promoter in patients with chronic myeloid leukemia]. Zhongguo Shi Yan Xue Ye Xue Za Zhi 18: 1402–1404.
17. Laird PW (2003) The power and the promise of DNA methylation markers. Nat Rev Cancer 3: 253–266.
18. Jiang D, Zheng D, Wang L, Huang Y, Liu H, et al. (2013) Elevated PLA2G7 gene promoter methylation as a gender-specific marker of aging increases the risk of coronary heart disease in females. PLoS One 8: e59752.
19. Zhang LN, Liu PP, Wang L, Yuan F, Xu L, et al. (2013) Lower ADD1 gene promoter DNA methylation increases the risk of essential hypertension. PLoS One 8: e63455.
20. DerSimonian R (1996) Meta-analysis in the design and monitoring of clinical trials. Stat Med 15: 1237–1248; discussion 1249–1252.
21. Higgins JP, Thompson SG, Deeks JJ, Altman DG (2003) Measuring inconsistency in meta-analyses. BMJ 327: 557–560.
22. Bax L, Ikeda N, Fukui N, Yaju Y, Tsuruta H, et al. (2009) More than numbers: the power of graphs in meta-analysis. Am J Epidemiol 169: 249–255.
23. Zhao Y, Wang QS, Li HH, Bo J, Dou LP, et al. (2008) [Significance of id4 promoter methylation in monitoring AML patients with completely remission]. Zhongguo Shi Yan Xue Ye Xue Za Zhi 16: 476–478.

24. Oka T, Ouchida M, Koyama M, Ogama Y, Takada S, et al. (2002) Gene silencing of the tyrosine phosphatase SHP1 gene by aberrant methylation in leukemias/lymphomas. Cancer Res 62: 6390–6394.

25. Xiao YH, Li XH, Tan T, Liang T, Yi H, et al. (2011) Identification of GLIPR1 tumor suppressor as methylation-silenced gene in acute myeloid leukemia by microarray analysis. J Cancer Res Clin Oncol 137: 1831–1840.

26. Martel V, Guerci A, Humbert JC, Gregoire MJ, Chery M, et al. (1997) De novo methylation of tumour suppressor genes CDKN2A and CDKN2B is a rare finding in B-cell chronic lymphocytic leukaemia. Br J Haematol 99: 320–324.

27. Capalbo G, Mueller-Kuller T, Koschmieder S, Klein HU, Ottmann OG, et al. (2013) Endoplasmic reticulum protein GliPR1 regulates G protein signaling and the cell cycle and is overexpressed in AML. Oncol Rep 30: 2254–2262.

28. Hatirnaz O, Ure U, Ar C, Akyerli C, Soysal T, et al. (2007) The SOCS-1 gene methylation in chronic myeloid leukemia patients. Am J Hematol 82: 729–730.

29. Gauffin F, Diffner E, Gustafsson B, Nordgren A, Wingren AG, et al. (2009) Expression of PTEN and SHP1, investigated from tissue microarrays in pediatric acute lymphoblastic, leukemia. Pediatr Hematol Oncol 26: 48–56.

30. Chen SS, Claus R, Lucas DM, Yu L, Qian J, et al. (2011) Silencing of the inhibitor of DNA binding protein 4 (ID4) contributes to the pathogenesis of mouse and human CLL. Blood 117: 862–871.

31. Shanmugam R, Gade P, Wilson-Weekes A, Sayar H, Suvannasankha A, et al. (2012) A noncanonical Flt3ITD/NF-kappaB signaling pathway represses DAPK1 in acute myeloid leukemia. Clin Cancer Res 18: 360–369.

32. Claus R, Hackanson B, Poetsch AR, Zucknick M, Sonnet M, et al. (2012) Quantitative analyses of DAPK1 methylation in AML and MDS. Int J Cancer 131: E138–142.

33. Zhao Y, Wang QS, Dou LP, Bo J, Li HH, et al. (2007) [Methylation of Id4 gene promoter in acute leukemia]. Zhongguo Shi Yan Xue Ye Xue Za Zhi 15: 1156–1160.

34. Agirre X, Vizmanos JL, Calasanz MJ, Garcia-Delgado M, Larrayoz MJ, et al. (2003) Methylation of CpG dinucleotides and/or CCWGG motifs at the promoter of TP53 correlates with decreased gene expression in a subset of acute lymphoblastic leukemia patients. Oncogene 22: 1070–1072.

35. Chim CS, Wong SY, Pang A, Chu P, Lau JS, et al. (2005) Aberrant promoter methylation of the retinoic acid receptor alpha gene in acute promyelocytic leukemia. Leukemia 19: 2241–2246.

36. Chim CS, Wong AS, Kwong YL (2004) Epigenetic dysregulation of the Jak/STAT pathway by frequent aberrant methylation of SHP1 but not SOCS1 in acute leukaemias. Ann Hematol 83: 527–532.

37. Liang T, Tan T, Xiao Y, Yi H, Li C, et al. (2009) [Methylation and expression of glioma pathogenesis-related protein 1 gene in acute myeloid leukemia]. Zhong Nan Da Xue Xue Bao Yi Xue Ban 34: 388–394.

38. Lin DJ, Fan RF, Liu XF (2008) [Significance of DNA methylation status of runx3 gene promoter region in acute leukemia]. Zhongguo Shi Yan Xue Ye Xue Za Zhi 16: 263–266.

39. Wang Y, Zhu CS, Bi KH, Xu WW, Dong L, et al. (2011) [Study of WIF-1 promoter methylation with expressions of beta-catenin in acute leukemia]. Zhonghua Yi Xue Za Zhi 91: 2858–2860.

40. Scott S, Kimura T, Ichinohasama R, Bergen S, Magliocco A, et al. (2003) Microsatellite mutations of transforming growth factor-beta receptor type II and caspase-5 occur in human precursor T-cell lymphoblastic lymphomas/leukemias in vivo but are not associated with hMSH2 or hMLH1 promoter methylation. Leuk Res 27: 23–34.

41. Campo Dell'Orto M, Banelli B, Giarin E, Accordi B, Trentin L, et al. (2007) Down-regulation of DLX3 expression in MLL-AF4 childhood lymphoblastic leukemias is mediated by promoter region hypermethylation. Oncol Rep 18: 417–423.

42. Christiansen DH, Andersen MK, Pedersen-Bjergaard J (2003) Methylation of p15INK4B is common, is associated with deletion of genes on chromosome arm 7q and predicts a poor prognosis in therapy-related myelodysplasia and acute myeloid leukemia. Leukemia 17: 1813–1819.

43. Xu RR, Liu F, Cui X, Zhang XW, Wang Y (2011) [ID4 promoter methylation in acute myeloid leukemia]. Zhongguo Shi Yan Xue Ye Xue Za Zhi 19: 582–584.

44. Qian J, Yao DM, Lin J, Chen Q, Li Y, et al. (2010) [Alteration of methylation status of death-associated protein kinase (dapk) gene promoter in patients with acute myeloid leukemia]. Zhongguo Shi Yan Xue Ye Xue Za Zhi 18: 1390–1394.

45. Seedhouse CH, Das-Gupta EP, Russell NH (2003) Methylation of the hMLH1 promoter and its association with microsatellite instability in acute myeloid leukemia. Leukemia 17: 83–88.

46. Jost E, do ON, Wilop S, Herman JG, Osieka R, et al. (2009) Aberrant DNA methylation of the transcription factor C/EBPalpha in acute myelogenous leukemia. Leuk Res 33: 443–449.

47. Iwai M, Kiyoi H, Ozeki K, Kinoshita T, Emi N, et al. (2005) Expression and methylation status of the FHIT gene in acute myeloid leukemia and myelodysplastic syndrome. Leukemia 19: 1367–1375.

48. Wang YK, Zhou JH, Zhou SQ, Fang GA, Li YW, et al. (2011) [Promoter methylation status of hPer3 gene in AML patients and the in vitro effect of decitabine on the status]. Zhonghua Xue Ye Xue Za Zhi 32: 317–321.

49. Gao F, Li Y, Liu W, Lu XL, Li X, et al. (2006) [Studies on gene expression and the 5' CpG islands methylation status of E-cadherin in acute myeloid leukemia]. Zhonghua Xue Ye Xue Za Zhi 27: 25–27.

50. Qian J, Qian Z, Lin J, Yao DM, Chen Q, et al. (2011) Abnormal methylation of GRAF promoter Chinese patients with acute myeloid leukemia. Leuk Res 35: 783–786.

51. Benetatos L, Hatzimichael E, Dasoula A, Dranitsaris G, Tsiara S, et al. (2010) CpG methylation analysis of the MEG3 and SNRPN imprinted genes in acute myeloid leukemia and myelodysplastic syndromes. Leuk Res 34: 148–153.

52. Benetatos L, Dasoula A, Hatzimichael E, Syed N, Voukelatou M, et al. (2011) Polo-like kinase 2 (SNK/PLK2) is a novel epigenetically regulated gene in acute myeloid leukemia and myelodysplastic syndromes: genetic and epigenetic interactions. Ann Hematol 90: 1037–1045.

53. Otto N, Manukjan G, Gohring G, Hofmann W, Scherer R, et al. (2011) ICSBP promoter methylation in myelodysplastic syndromes and acute myeloid leukaemia. Leukemia 25: 1202–1207.

54. Agrawal-Singh S, Isken F, Agelopoulos K, Klein HU, Thoennissen NH, et al. (2012) Genome-wide analysis of histone H3 acetylation patterns in AML identifies PRDX2 as an epigenetically silenced tumor suppressor gene. Blood 119: 2346–2357.

55. Yao DM, Qian J, Lin J, Wang YL, Chen Q, et al. (2011) Aberrant methylation of CCAAT/enhancer binding protein zeta promoter in acute myeloid leukemia. Leuk Res 35: 957–960.

56. Wang XJ, Li J, Fu BJ, Guo LL, Zhang JH, et al. (2009) [Methylation status of JunB and CDH13 gene promoter in CD34(+)CD38(−) chronic myelogenous leukemia cells]. Zhongguo Shi Yan Xue Ye Xue Za Zhi 17: 1405–1408.

57. Pehlivan M, Sercan Z, Sercan HO (2009) sFRP1 promoter methylation is associated with persistent Philadelphia chromosome in chronic myeloid leukemia. Leuk Res 33: 1062–1067.

58. Song JJ, Liu Q, Li Y, Yang ZS, Yang L, et al. (2012) Epigenetic inactivation of PLCD1 in chronic myeloid leukemia. Int J Mol Med 30: 179–184.

59. Nakatsuka S, Takakuwa T, Tomita Y, Hoshida Y, Nishiu M, et al. (2003) Hypermethylation of death-associated protein (DAP) kinase CpG island is frequent not only in B-cell but also in T- and natural killer (NK)/T-cell malignancies. Cancer Sci 94: 87–91.

60. Dou LP, Liu JH, Wang C, Zhao Y, Wang QS, et al. (2009) [Study on the involvement of ZO-1 gene in leukemogenesis]. Zhonghua Xue Ye Xue Za Zhi 30: 473–476.

61. Deng G, Li ZQ, Zhao C, Yuan Y, Niu CC, et al. (2011) WNT5A expression is regulated by the status of its promoter methylation in leukaemia and can inhibit leukemic cell malignant proliferation. Oncol Rep 25: 367–376.

8

Proteinase-Activated Receptor 1 (PAR1) Regulates Leukemic Stem Cell Functions

Nicole Bäumer[1], Annika Krause[1], Gabriele Köhler[2], Stephanie Lettermann[1], Georg Evers[1], Antje Hascher[5], Sebastian Bäumer[1], Wolfgang E. Berdel[1], Carsten Müller-Tidow[1,3,4]*◗, Lara Tickenbrock[1,5]*◗

1 Department of Medicine, Hematology/Oncology, University of Muenster, Muenster, Germany, 2 Gerhard Domagk Institute for Pathology, University of Muenster, Muenster, Germany, 3 Interdisciplinary Center for Clinical Research IZKF, University of Muenster, Muenster, Germany, 4 Dept. of Medicine IV, Hematology and Oncology, University of Halle, Halle, Germany, 5 Hochschule Hamm-Lippstadt, University of Applied Science, Hamm, Germany

Abstract

External signals that are mediated by specific receptors determine stem cell fate. The thrombin receptor PAR1 plays an important role in haemostasis, thrombosis and vascular biology, but also in tumor biology and angiogenesis. Its expression and function in hematopoietic stem cells is largely unknown. Here, we analyzed expression and function of PAR1 in primary hematopoietic cells and their leukemic counterparts. AML patients' blast cells expressed much lower levels of PAR1 mRNA and protein than CD34$^+$ progenitor cells. Constitutive *Par1*-deficiency in adult mice did not affect engraftment or stem cell potential of hematopoietic cells. To model an AML with *Par1*-deficiency, we retrovirally introduced the oncogene MLL-AF9 in wild type and *Par1*$^{-/-}$ hematopoietic progenitor cells. *Par1*-deficiency did not alter initial leukemia development. However, the loss of *Par1* enhanced leukemic stem cell function *in vitro* and *in vivo*. Re-expression of PAR1 in *Par1*$^{-/-}$ leukemic stem cells delayed leukemogenesis *in vivo*. These data indicate that Par1 contributes to leukemic stem cell maintenance.

Editor: Wolfgang Wagner, RWTH Aachen University Medical School, Germany

Funding: This work was supported by grants from the Deutsche Forschungsgemeinschaft GZ TI 693/2-1 and SFB1009 A07 (www.dfg.de). The funders had no role in study design, data collection and analysis, decision to publish, or preparation of the manuscript.

Competing Interests: The authors have declared that no competing interests exist.

* E-mail: Carsten.Mueller-Tidow@UK-Halle.de (CMT); lara.tickenbrock@hshl.de (LT)

◗ These authors contributed equally to this work.

Introduction

The four Proteinase-Activated Receptors (PAR1 to PAR4) belong to a superfamily of seven transmembrane, G-protein coupled cell-surface receptors [1]. PARs receive various extracellular signals and mediate them to intracellular responses and play a prominent role in a variety of physiological processes [2,3]. Activation of PARs occurs usually via proteolytic cleavage of their N-terminal exodomain through extracellular proteases like thrombin. Cleavage creates a new N-terminus that serves as tethered ligand and allows the activation of intracellular signal cascades [4,5].

PAR1 as the prototype of this group is a high-affinity thrombin receptor and it is therefore critical e.g. in thrombosis [3,6], inflammation [7,8,9] and angiogenesis [10]. PAR1 can also be activated by MMP-1, a matrix metalloprotease [2,11]. Absence of Par1 is partially incompatible with embryonic development, since at least half of *Par1*-deficient mice die around embryonic day E9.5 due to severe bleeding that could be rescued by the introduction of Par1 expression in embryonic endothelial cells [10]. The surviving mice do not exhibit obvious abnormalities [12,13]. Yue *et al.* recently demonstrated that Par1 plays a role in the *in vitro* differentiation of mouse embryonic stem cells into hematopoietic progenitors and in endothelial-to-hematopoietic transition in zebrafish [14]. However, the function of Par1 in adult hematopoiesis has not yet been addressed.

High PAR1 expression was found in tumors including malignant melanoma [15] and breast cancer [16,17] and correlated with invasiveness and motility of numerous cancer cell lines [18,19,20,21], indicating that PAR1 might act as an oncogene. Since the function of PAR1 in leukemia is yet unknown, we here present the first report about PAR1 in adult hematopoiesis and leukemogenesis. In particular, we identify PAR1 as a novel regulator of leukemic stem cells in AML in an *in vivo* mouse model.

Materials and Methods

Patient samples and ethics statement

The study was reviewed and approved by the ethics committee of the medical association and the medical faculty of the University of Muenster (2007-524-f-S and 2007-390-f-S) before the study began. AML samples were obtained from bone marrow of patients with acute myeloid leukemia at the time of initial diagnosis. The median blast count was 80%. For microarray analysis and RT-PCR, CD34$^+$ cells were obtained from the peripheral blood of healthy donors who were stimulated with G-CSF using standard protocols. Informed written consent was obtained from all patients.

Microarray analysis and data from the Leukemia Gene Atlas

Published microarray data from human bone marrow and blood cells were analyzed using the Leukemia Gene Atlas at http://www.leukemia-gene-atlas.org (accessed 2014 Mar 25) [22,23]. The analyzed cells were obtained from human umbilical cord blood or from peripheral blood samples [23].

For comparison of control and AML patient samples, the mRNA of 5 healthy CD34$^+$ progenitor specimens and 67 AML patient samples was hybridized on Whole Genome Microarrays. Microarray data and the patient cohort were analyzed previously [24]. Informed consent was obtained from all patients and donors.

RNA isolation and real-time quantitative RT-PCR

RNA isolation from patient samples and murine cells was performed using RNeasy Micro Kit (Qiagen, Hilden, Germany) according to the manufacturer's protocol.

Reverse transcription and real-time quantitative RT-PCR were performed as described [25]. The probes were labeled at the 5' end with the fluorescent dye FAM (PAR1) or VIC (GAPDH) and at the 3' end with the quencher TAMRA. Primer/Probe sets were obtained from Life Technologies (Darmstadt, Germany; "Mm00438851_m1 F2r" for murine and "Hs00169258_m1 F2R" for human samples).

Flow cytometry, mice, colony assays, limiting dilution transplantation, and competitive transplantations

FACS analyses of blood were performed as described [26]. HSC FACS and sorting for HSC subpopulations was performed as described [27].

Par1-Knockout (−/−) mice were obtained from Jackson laboratory (Stock Number: 002862) [12] and genotyped as published. Par1$^{-/-}$ mice survived with a lower frequency than expectable according to Mendelian ratio, since we obtained only 32 Par1$^{-/-}$ mice out of 269 pubs (12% instead of expected 25%) from matings of heterozygous parents.

All animal experiments in this study were carried out in strict accordance with the recommendations of the Institutional Animal Care and Use Committee "Landesamt fuer Natur, Umwelt und Verbraucherschutz NRW". This study was performed with permission of the Institutional Animal Care and Use Committee and of the local veterinary administration of Muenster (Permit Numbers: G15/2005, 8.87-51.04.20.09.322, and 8.87-51.04.2011.A005).

For colony formation assays, bone marrow cells from three age-matched Par1-wild type and − knockout mice were flushed from femur and tibia of both hind legs using PBS/2% FCS and the red cells were lysed by AKC shock as described [26]. 10,000 cells from the total unsorted bone marrow or from c-kit$^+$ bone marrow cells and sorted by FACS as described above were seeded in M3434 methylcellulose (StemCell Technologies, Inc.) and counted after 7–8 days. Replating was performed by resolving the colonies in PBS, seeding again 10,000 cells per ml methylcellulose and counting as above.

For limiting dilution analysis, limiting amounts of donor cells (100, 1000 or 10000 total bone marrow cells) from 3 pairs of Par1$^{+/+}$ (total of n = 44) vs. Par1$^{-/-}$ mice (total of n = 45) were transplanted into irradiated (9 Gy) B6.SJL recipients along with 1×10^5 wild type B6.SJL cells. Analysis of engraftment of competitive repopulating units (CRU) was determined by FACS analysis as the percentage of CD45.2 donor cells in the peripheral blood 4 and 16 weeks after transplantation. Mice were scored positive for CRU engraftment when the percentage of CD45.2 peripheral blood cells exceeded 0.1% and the percentage of CD45.2$^+$/CD11b$^+$, CD45.2$^+$/B220$^+$, and CD45.2$^+$/CD3$^+$ cells exceeded 0.02%. CRU frequencies in the blood were calculated by applying Poisson statistics to the proportion of positive recipients at different dilutions using Limiting Dilution Analyses software L-Calc (StemCell Technologies Inc.).

Overexpression of PAR1 in murine cells

Human PAR1 cDNA was cloned into pEntry vector for gateway system (Invitrogen) and then switched from pEntry vector into the retroviral pMY-RFB destination vector, that contains a green fluorescence (GFP) expressed from an internal ribosomal entry site (IRES), by recombination reaction with LR-Clonase (Invitrogen).

Retroviral supernatants were collected as described [26]. For transduction, viruses were bound to retronectin-coated plates by centrifugation as described [28]. Lineage-depleted bone marrow cells were stimulated overnight, transduced by growth on the virus-coated plates for 24 h and sorted by FACS for EGFP-positivity. For colony assays, 1000 EGFP-positive cells per ml methylcellulose M3434 (Stem Cell Technologies) were plated. The total number of GFP-positive colonies was determined on day 10 after plating.

A total of 50,000 GFP-positive freshly transduced and FACS sorted cells were injected with 50,000 wild type bone marrow cells into the lateral tail vein of lethally irradiated (8.5 Gy) C57Bl/6N mice. Fraction of GFP-positive cells was determined by FACS in blood samples at the indicated time points after transplantation.

Tissue array construction and immunohistochemistry analyses

Tissue array construction was performed of formalin-fixed and paraffin embedded trephine bone marrow biopsies of 152 patients diagnosed with primary, untreated AML and 7 samples of CD34$^+$ cells was performed as described [29]. Informed consent was obtained from all patients and donors. For PAR1 detection, sections were incubated with the primary antibody (Thrombin R antibody (H-111), sc-5605, Santa Cruz Biotechnology Inc., Dallas, Texas, USA; dilution 1:100). PAR1 expression was regarded as negative or positive.

Retroviral transduction and transplantations

Retroviral transduction with MSCV2.2-MLL-AF9-IRES-GFP was performed as described [26,28]. Briefly, bone marrow cells of wild type and Par1-knockout recipients were isolated, AKC-lysed and transduced as described previously [26]. 90.000 (MLL-AF9) GFP-positive cells were transplanted by tail-vein injection into C57Bl/6N wild type recipients, which were lethally irradiated with 8 Gy.

For secondary transplantation, bone marrow cells of leukemic mice were isolated of three independent donors of each genotype and 1×10^6 MLL-AF9/GFP-positive cells of each donor were intravenously injected into irradiated secondary C57Bl/6N wild type mice.

Tertiary C57Bl/6N recipient mice were irradiated with 8 Gy and transplanted with 100 or 1000 ckit$^+$ MLL-AF9 blasts isolated from six secondary recipients (three of each genotype). Frequencies of leukemia initiating cells (LICs) from tertiary transplanted mice were calculated using the L-Calc program (StemCell technologies, Inc.).

For the rescue experiment, leukemic spleen cells were retrovirally transduced as described above with an empty vector MSCV2.2-IRES-mCherry or with MSCV2.2-PAR1-IRES-mCherry, which contained blunt-ended human PAR1 cDNA cloned into a blunted XhoI site 5′ of the IRES. Cells were stained with a c-kit-APC antibody and sorted by FACS for c-kit, GFP and mCherry expression. 1,000 triple positive cells were transplanted into six irradiated recipient mice per group.

All transplanted mice were dosed with Cotrim (100 mg/l) (Ratiopharm, Ulm, Germany) until two weeks after transplantation. The results of the survival experiments were analysed with the log-rank non-parametric and represented as Kaplan-Meier survival curves.

Cloning efficiency assays of murine leukemic blasts

To determine the cloning efficiency of bone marrow cells, different concentrations of bone marrow cells of untreated mice or leukemic blasts of mice that were transplanted with leukemic blasts from the primary transplantation experiment were FACS-sorted. 1, 10, 30, 100 and 300 c-kit-and, GFP-positive cells of $Par1^{+/+}$; MLL-AF9 or $Par1^{-/-}$;MLL-AF9 bone marrow cells were then seeded in 200 μl methylcellulose in 14 wells of a 48-well plate. 7 days later wells with one or more colonies were classified as positive. The stem cell frequency was determined by Poisson statistical analysis (L-calc software, StemCell Technologies).

Results

PAR1 expression profile in hematopoietic cells

Recent studies hint at a role for PAR1 in the hematopoietic system [14]. To address a potential role for PAR1 in hematopoiesis, we used published microarray data [22] to analyse PAR1 expression in multiple human hematopoietic cell types. As expected, PAR1 expression was high in cells of the erythroid/megakaryocytic lineage (Fig. 1A). Moreover, PAR1 was prominently expressed in hematopoietic stem cells (HSC), while its expression decreased upon differentiation in myeloid and lymphoid progenitor cells (Fig. 1A). Such a distinct expression pattern could not be detected for the other three proteinase-activated receptors PAR2, PAR3 or PAR4 (Fig. S1A-C).

To analyse the function of Par1 especially in the adult mice, which was not addressed yet [12], we determined Par1 expression in subpopulations of mouse bone marrow. We sorted primary cells by flow cytometry (Fig. 1B) and isolated RNA. In line with the microarray results of human hematopoietic cells (Fig. 1A), real-time RT-PCR demonstrated that Par1 mRNA was most abundant in the stem cell compartment (Fig. 1B, upper right panel). Par1 expression was also present in multipotent progenitor (MPPs, Fig. 1B, upper right panel) and common lymphoid progenitor (CLP). PAR1 was also expressed in CD3-positive T-cells in peripheral blood (Fig. 1B, lower right panel). Expression of PAR1 was notably absent in the more differentiated B220$^+$, Ter119$^+$ or CD11b$^+$ bone marrow cells (Fig. 1B, lower right panel).

Absence of Par1 does not interfere with normal hematopoiesis

Since Par1 was mostly expressed in stem cell fractions of primary bone marrow mouse cells, a function of Par1 in undifferentiated hematopoietic cells could be possible. We analyzed adult hematopoiesis in a previously generated Par1-knockout mouse model [12]. As published, we also faced a more than 50% underrepresentation of $Par1^{-/-}$ adult mice (see Materials and Methods).

We determined the function of Par1 in the regulation of stem cell growth by comparing the phenotype of wild type and Par1-deficient mice. We determined a spectrum of blood parameters such as white blood cells count, composition of the blood

according to surface markers and hemoglobin (Table 1) and found out that the blood composition was not altered in Par1-deficient mice in any parameter tested. Also, the number of hematopoietic stem and progenitor cells was similar (Fig. 2A). To determine the potential of $Par1^{-/-}$ bone marrow cells to form colonies in methylcellulose, we performed colony assays using total bone marrow and c-kit$^+$ bone marrow cells. The colony formation potential was not altered by Par1 deficiency (Fig. 2B). Also, differentiation of these colonies was unchanged between both genotypes (data not shown). Moreover, two serial replatings of the colonies formed from $Par1^{+/+}$ and $Par1^{-/-}$ cells did not reveal differences (data not shown).

Although the phenotypic number of HSCs was unchanged in Par1-deficient bone marrow, these cells could potentially behave differently in vivo and reveal a function of Par1 in hematopoietic stem/progenitor cell differentiation or proliferation after transplantation. Therefore, we transplanted wild type and Par1-knockout bone marrow cells in different concentrations as limiting dilution assay into wild type recipients (Fig. 2C). No significant differences were observed at 4 or 16 weeks that would indicate altered short- and long-term hematopoietic stem cell functions, respectively. Par1-deficient cells tended to perform better than wild type cells upon transplantation since the frequency of Par1-deficient cells that were detectable in the blood was higher than the frequency of wild type cells without reaching statistical significance (Fig. 2C, right-hand side).

Interestingly, bone marrow cells that retrovirally overexpressed PAR1 as depicted schematically in Fig. 2D were significantly less abundant four weeks after transplantation in wild type recipients than control cells transduced with the empty vector (Fig. 2F). These cells were not impaired in their colony formation ability (Fig. 2E). Contribution to blood cell formation was not changed (data not shown). Remarkably, Par1 did not induce a proliferative advantage in non-transformed cells.

In conclusion, neither loss nor overexpression of Par1 interferes with normal hematopoiesis.

PAR1 expression is significantly decreased in blasts of AML patients

Thrombin receptors have long been implicated in the development of malignant diseases [16]. Especially PAR1 expression was correlated to cell migration and metastasis in different tumor entities [15,17,18,19,20,21] but its expression and function in leukemia was unknown.

Although the activity of receptors is tightly regulated on protein levels, PAR1 recovery might also rely on new protein synthesis and therefore on the abundance of its mRNA in some cell types including cells from the hematopoietic system [30]. Hence, we analyzed the expression of PAR1 in a large set of leukemia patient samples using Gene expression microarrays for mRNA analyses (Fig. 3) and real-time RT-PCR (Fig. 3) and a tissue microarray for protein expression (Fig. 4).

The mRNA analysis of five CD34$^+$ cells of healthy donors and 64 AML patients revealed that PAR1 expression was markedly lower in AML blasts than in CD34$^+$ progenitor cells (Fig. 3A), whereas the expression of the other three family members did not differ (Fig. 3B-D). Detailed analysis of PAR1 expression demonstrated its significant downregulation in all FAB subtypes of AML (Fig. S2A). AML patients with high PAR1 expression (level > 9 log arbitrary units in this microarray analysis) did not reveal changes in hemoglobin, LDH, number of platelets, white blood cells or blasts in the blood or bone marrow at the time of diagnosis compared to patients with lower PAR1 expression (level < 9 log arbitrary units in this microarray; data not shown). PAR1

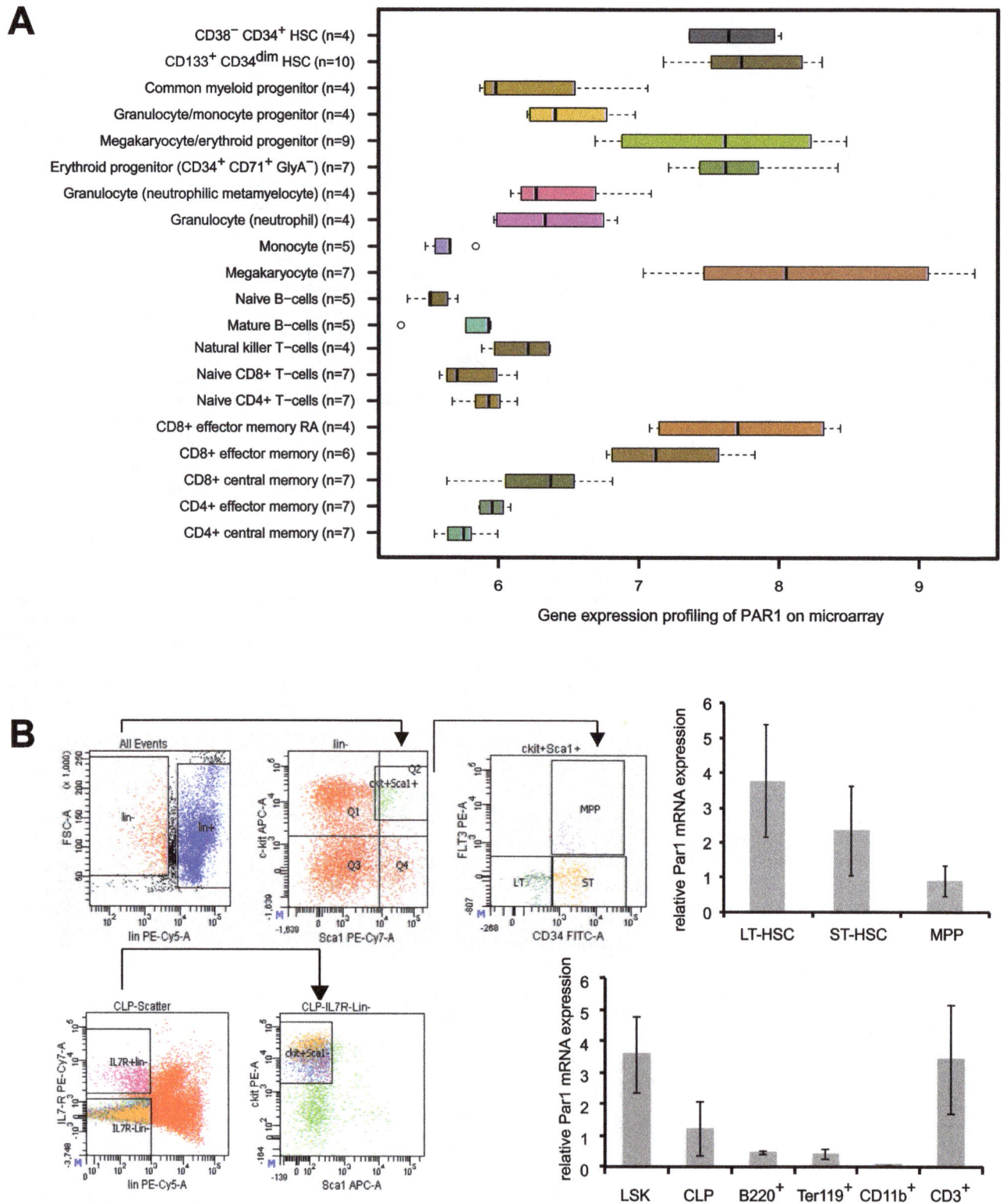

Figure 1. PAR1 is expressed in hematopoietic cells. 1A. PAR1 was analyzed in mRNA microarray expression data from FACS sorted bone marrow cells [22,23]. Highest expression was found in hematopoietic stem cells (HSC) and cells of the erythroid/megakaryocyte and of the T-cell lineage. Shown here are log arbitrary units. **1B.** Left-hand side: To sort for the different murine bone marrow subpopulation, total bone marrow was stained with lineage-markers, sca1 and c-kit. Lineage-negative, sca1+, c-kit+ (LSK) cells were further divided into long-term (LT)-HSCs as Flt3−CD34− population, short-term (ST)-HSCs as Flt3−CD34+ cells and multipotent progenitors (MPPs) as Flt3+CD34+ cells (upper panel). Common lymphoid progenitors (CLPs) were defined as lineage-negative, IL7R+c-kit+ cells. Upper and lower right panel: *Par1* mRNA expression was determined by real-time quantitative RT-PCR using cDNA from the FACS-sorted murine bone marrow subpopulations and Par1 expression was normalized to GAPDH expression. Par1 was expressed in all hematopoietic stem/progenitor subpopulations and CD3+ T-cells whereas monocytes/macrophages/granulocytes (CD11b+) or erythrocytic (Ter119+) or B-cells (B220+) expressed low or no Par1.

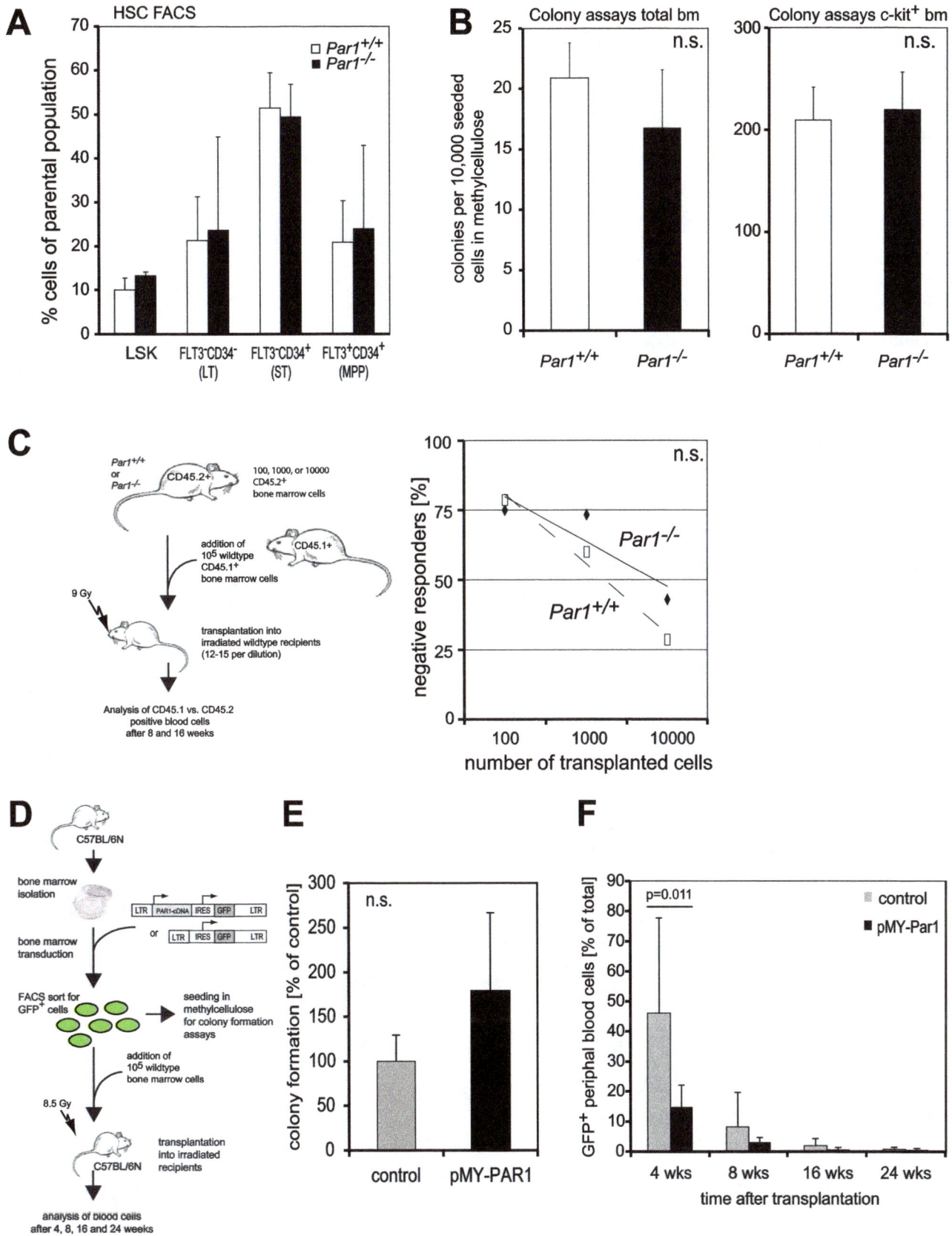

Figure 2. PAR1 function in proliferation and differentiation. 2A. Stem cell FACS analysis revealed similar numbers of stem and progenitor subpopulations (n = 3 mouse pairs for each FACS). Shown here are the percentage of lin⁻sca1⁺c-kit⁺ (LSK) cells from the lineage-negative parental population and the percentage of longterm (LT)-HSCs, shortterm (ST)-HSCs and multipotent progenitors (MPP) from the parental LSK population. **2B**. Colony assays of cells from *Par1*⁺/⁺ and *Par1*⁻/⁻ total bone marrow (left-hand side) and c-kit+ bone marrow cells (right-hand side; n = 3 mouse pairs

for each experiments). No significant changes in the ability of forming colonies were observed in any cell population. **2C**. Left-hand side: Bone marrow cells from CD45.2$^+$ Par1$^{-/-}$ or Par1$^{+/+}$ mice were mixed with Par1$^{+/+}$ bone marrow from congenic CD45.1$^+$ as depicted in the schematic overview. Right-hand side: At 16 weeks after transplantation, the number of negative responders, which were transplanted with Par1$^{-/-}$ bone marrow, did not differ from wild type transplanted mice. Therefore, the stem cell frequency was comparable in the bone marrow of both genotypes. **2D**. Schematic outline of the transplantation experiment using PAR1-overexpressing lineage-negative bone marrow cells compared to control cells transduced with the empty vector. **2E**. Colony formation of bone marrow cells transduced with empty vector ("control") or with a PAR1 expressing retroviral vector ("pMY-PAR1") was not significantly different between the two groups. **2F**. Transplantation of cells as depicted in Figure 2D lead to a significantly lower ratio of PAR1-overexpressing cells after four weeks.

expression also did not influence overall survival or relapse-free survival (data not shown). Of note, the expression of the main upstream regulator of PAR1 function, the ligand Thrombin, was unchanged (Fig. 3E).

We confirmed PAR1 expression by quantitative real-time RT-PCR in CD34-positive cells from healthy patients and samples from AML patients (Fig. 3F) in an independent cohort of patients. Compared to CD34$^+$ cells, PAR1 expression was again significantly decreased in all AML subtypes (Fig. 3F).

To analyze the protein expression of PAR1 in control and AML patient samples, we used immunohistochemical detection of PAR1 on a tissue array that included CD34-positive cells as well as sections of bone marrow punches. Remarkably, tissue array analysis of PAR1 expression revealed that PAR1 was more prominently expressed in CD34$^+$ cells from healthy volunteers compared to AML blasts (Fig. 4A and B). Only 30 out of 119 AML patient samples showed PAR1-expression (25%), whereas 5 out of 7 samples of CD34$^+$ cells were positive for PAR1-expression (71%; Fig. 4B) (p = 0.008, Chi-square test [31]). The finding of PAR1 protein expressing AML samples (Fig. 3F) suggest that PAR1 protein might be present although mRNA levels were very low in most AML patients. Immunohistochemistry staining might also pick up other PAR proteins, which might be expressed in certain AML samples (Fig. 3C and D). Nonetheless, PAR1 mRNA and protein data are highly concordant with loss of expression in most of the specimens. Also, these results were in accordance with the observed differences in the Par1 expression in sorted mouse bone marrow cells, in which Par1 was highly expressed in the stem cell compartment and in progenitor cells (Fig. 1B). In line with the results obtained in the microarray analysis, PAR1 expression did

not correlate with hemoglobin, number of platelets, white blood cells or blasts in the blood or the bone marrow at the time of diagnosis (data not shown). Also, different PAR1 levels were not associated with the overall survival time or the relapse-free survival of the patients (data not shown). Interestingly, in this analysis PAR1 expression was especially low in AML M2, M4 and M5 (Fig. 4C).

PAR1-deficiency enhances leukemic stem cell potential

The observation that PAR1 expression differed significantly in human acute myeloid leukemia and especially in AML M4 and M5 (Fig. 4C) led us to analyze Par1 functions in murine leukemogenesis. To model AML *in vivo*, wild type or Par1-knockout ($-/-$) bone marrow cells were retrovirally transduced with the leukemogenic MLL-AF9, which occurs in human AML M5 [32] and reliably induces an AML in mice [33,34,35].

Transplantation of 90.000 positive cells as assessed by GFP expression (Fig. 5A) of bone marrow cells retrovirally transduced with the oncogene MLL-AF9 induced myeloid leukemia both in wild type and Par1$^{-/-}$ bone marrow cells with comparable latency, penetrance, and morphology (Fig. 5B and data not shown). Acute myeloid leukemia in mouse models is defined by transplantability into secondary recipients [36]. Transplantation into secondary recipients assesses leukemic stem cell function. Interestingly, Par1-deficiency significantly accelerated the leukemic disease in secondary recipients (Fig. 5C; p<0.001). Of note, this finding was cell intrinsic, since all recipients were of Par1 wild type genotype. Both genotypes generated an acute myeloid leukemia after secondary transplantation (Fig. 5D).

Table 1. Blood parameters of wild type and Par1$^{-/-}$ mice.

Parameters	3 months		6 months	
	Par1$^{+/+}$	Par1$^{-/-}$	Par1$^{+/+}$	Par1$^{-/-}$
WBC [10^3/µl]	9.6±1.7	9.2±2.9	6.9±1.9	7.2±3.1
RBC [10^6/µl]	8.8±0.5	9.0±0.8	8.5±0.5	8.4±1.6
HGB [g/dl]	14.0±0.9	14.2±1.1	13.3±0.6	13.1±2.4
HCT [%]	45.8±2.8	46.7±4.2	43.9±2.4	42.7±8.4
MCV [fL]	52.2±0.6	51.9±0.9	51.7±0.7	50.9±0.7
MCH [pg]	15.9±0.2	15.8±0.5	15.7±0.4	15.7±0.4
MCHC [g/dl]	30.5±0.4	30.4±0.9	30.4±0.5	30.8±1.0
PLT [10^3/µl]	914.4±204.4	780.6±176.0	736.6±174.3	765.3±359.5
FACS				
B220$^+$ [%]	54.1±3.0	55.6±5.3	50.3±6.1	42.5±11.8
CD3$^+$ [%]	23.0±7.9	26.6±6.7	25.5±3.8	26.3±6.1
CD11b$^+$ [%]	18.8±6.0	16.9±3.1	14.8±5.0	17.6±12.8

The data show mean values of 11 wild type and 11 Par1$^{-/-}$ blood analyses at the age of three months and mean values of 10 wild type and 10 Par1$^{-/-}$ blood preparations at the age of 6 months. WBC, white blood cell count; RBC, red blood cell count; HGB, haemoglobin; HCT, hematocrit; MCV, mean corpuscular volume; MCH, mean corpuscular haemoglobin; MCHC; mean corpuscular haemoglobin concentration; PLT, platelets. B220$^+$, B-cells; CD3$^+$, T-cells; CD11b$^+$, myeloid cells.

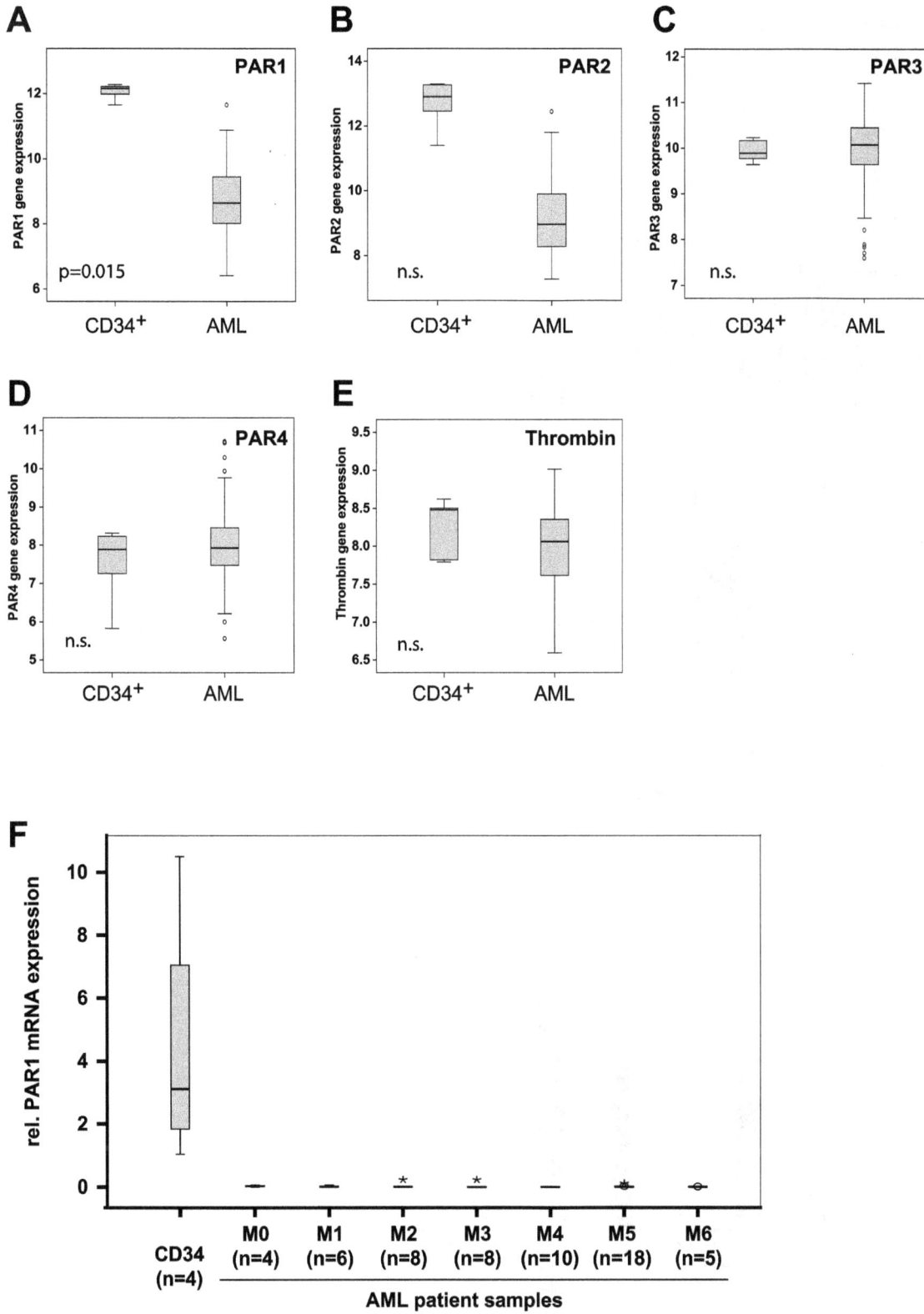

Figure 3. PAR1 mRNA expression in primary patient samples. PAR1 expression (**3A**) was significantly down-regulated in bone marrow cells from human Acute Myeloid Leukemia (AML, n = 67) patients compared to sorted CD34+ cells (n = 5) in microarray analysis, while the expression of PAR2 only showed a non-significant trend (**3B**), and the expression of PAR3 (**3C**), PAR4 (**3D**) and Thrombin (**3E**) was unchanged. Shown here are log arbitrary units. **3E**. PAR1 expression was significantly downregulated in bone marrow cells from human Acute Myeloid Leukemia (AML) patients compared to CD34-positive bone marrow cells. PAR1 expression was determined by qRT-PCR and normalized to GAPDH expression level.

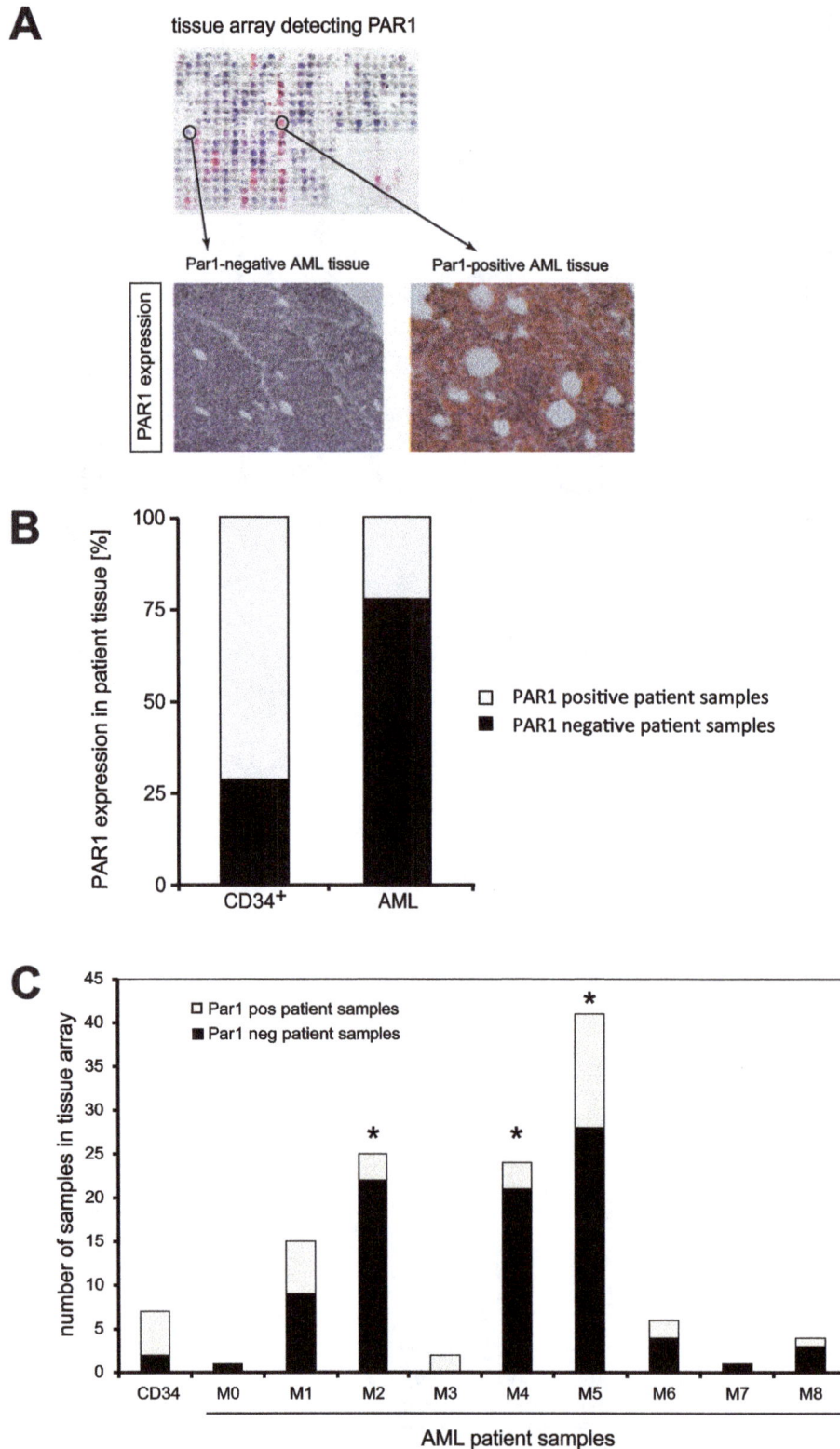

A tissue array detecting PAR1

Par1-negative AML tissue   Par1-positive AML tissue

PAR1 expression

B

PAR1 expression in patient tissue [%]

□ PAR1 positive patient samples
■ PAR1 negative patient samples

CD34⁺   AML

C

number of samples in tissue array

□ Par1 pos patient samples
■ Par1 neg patient samples

CD34 M0 M1 M2 M3 M4 M5 M6 M7 M8

AML patient samples

Figure 4. PAR1 expression in primary patient samples. 4A. Micrographs of Tissue Array analysis from NBM and AML patients stained with anti-PAR1 antibody and Fast-Red secondary antibody contrasted with hematoxylin and eosin. Overview (upper panel) and magnification of one example of CD34⁺ and AML samples that were defined PAR1-negative (lower left) and PAR1-positive (lower right). **4B.** Quantitative Tissue Array analysis of PAR1 expression using categories of staining intensity as positive or negative. Significantly more AML patient samples were negative for PAR1 expression than CD34⁺ healthy patient samples (p = 0.003, Chi-square test). **4C.** PAR1 protein was significantly less abundant in bone marrow cells from human Acute Myeloid Leukemia (AML) patients compared to CD34-positive bone marrow cells in Tissue Array samples. *p<0.05, Chi-square test.

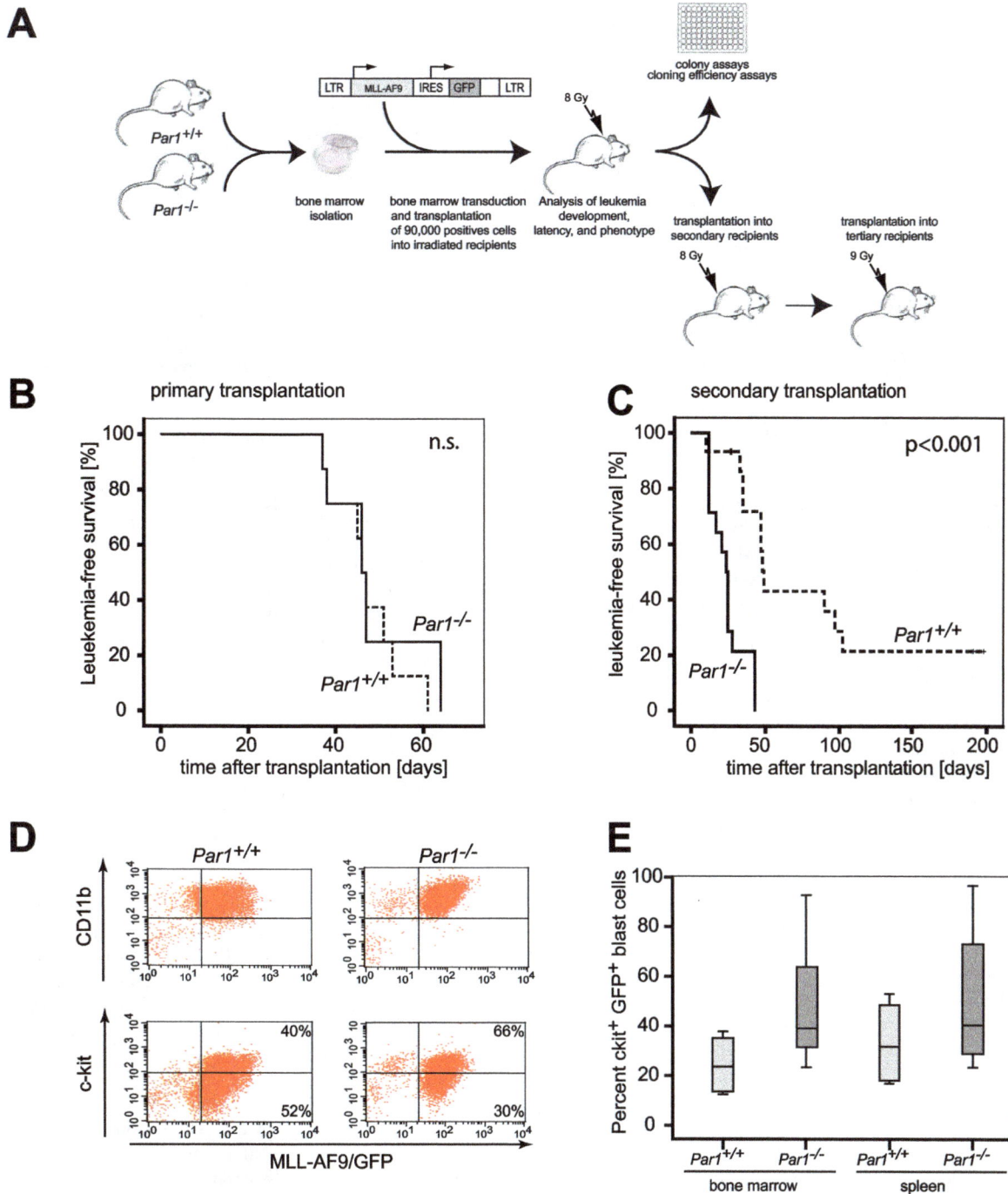

Figure 5. Absence of *Par1* accelerates MLL-AF9 driven murine leukemogenesis. 5A. Schematic overview about the performed transduction and transplantation experiments. Bone marrow isolated from *Par1*[+/+] or *Par1*[−/−] mice was retrovirally transduced with MLL-AF9/GFP. Equal numbers of positive cells were transplanted into lethally irradiated recipients, which were then subjected to different analyses and subsequent serial transplantations. **5B.** Survival curves of recipient mice which were transplanted with bone marrow cells of *Par1*[+/+] or *Par1*[−/−] mice that were retrovirally transduced with MLL-AF9 (n = 8 of each genotype). Cells of both genotypes led to a fatal leukemic disease with comparable latency. **5C.** Survival curves of secondary recipient mice which were transplanted with bone marrow cells of leukemic mice derived from the primary transplantation shown in Fig. 5B. The secondary recipients of *Par1*[−/−];MLL-AF9 cells (n = 14) died after a significantly shorter latency than mice transplanted with *Par1*[+/+];MLL-AF9 primary blasts (n = 15; p<0.001). **5D.** The phenotypic analysis of blasts of the secondary leukemic mice did not reveal differences in CD11b expression between *Par1*[+/+];MLL-AF9 and *Par1*[−/−];MLL-AF9 cells. **5E.** *Par1*[−/−];MLL-AF9 transplanted mice (n = 8) exhibited a strong tendency towards higher percentages of c kit expressing cells in spleens (p = 0.055, t test) and bone marrow (p = 0.22, t test) compared to *Par1*[+/+];MLL-AF9 transplanted mice (n = 4).

In murine MLL-AF9 leukemias, the c-kit positive fraction contains the leukemic stem cells [33]. We determined the fraction of c-kit$^+$ blasts within the GFP$^+$ cells to determine whether the phenotypic stem cell fraction was altered. In spleen as well as in bone marrow, the fraction of c-kit$^+$ stem cells was increased in the $Par1^{-/-}$ blasts (Fig. 5E). In spleen, the mean percentage of c-kit positive cells was 24.3% in wild type leukemias but 48.1% in leukemias with $Par1$-deficiency. Also, half of the leukemias with wild type Par1 showed less than 20% c-kit positive cells whereas all $Par1$-deficient leukemias harbored more than 20% of c-kit positive cells (Fig. 5E).

Par1 restricts the leukemic stem cell pool size and function

We hypothesized that loss of $Par1$ led to an expansion of the leukemic stem cell pool with enhanced stem cell activity. To test this hypothesis, we performed cloning efficiency experiments of c-kit$^+$GFP$^+$ bone marrow cells (as depicted in Fig. 5A) from leukemic mice after secondary transplantation to determine the fraction of MLL-AF9 expressing cells that could give rise to clonal growth. MLL-AF9-positive cells from secondary transplanted mice were sorted according to their c-kit- and GFP-positivity and seeded in cell numbers from 1 to 300 cells per well in methylcellulose in 48-well plates and the clone forming efficiency was determined according to Poisson-statistics. $Par1^{-/-}$;MLL-AF9 cells exhibited a cloning efficiency of 1/1.7, while the cloning efficiency of $Par1^{+/+}$;MLL-AF9 cells (1/3.4) was two times lower (Fig. 6A; p = 0.047). Interestingly, non-transduced c-kit$^+$ $Par1^{-/-}$ bone marrow cells, which were seeded in the same way to determine their cloning efficiency capacity, did not form more clones than wild type bone marrow cells (data not shown).

To determine the frequency of leukemia initiating cells (LICs) *in vivo*, we transplanted 100 and 1000 c-kit$^+$ cells of secondary transplanted leukemic mice serially into irradiated tertiary recipients as depicted in Fig. 6B. Recipients that received $Par1^{+/+}$ blasts survived significantly longer than those that received $Par1^{-/-}$ cells (Fig. 6C, left-hand side). From this transplantation, we determined the frequency of LICs in both genotypes according to the positive responder mice that died due to leukemia by Poisson-statistics (Fig. 6C, right-hand side). The frequency of LICs was about four times higher in absence of $Par1$ (1/56) than in presence of $Par1$ (1/256; p = 0.0166), which most likely contributed to the shortened latency and higher penetrance in this transplantation.

Re-expression of Par1 restricts leukemic stem cell function

Since the absence of Par1 enhanced leukemogenesis, we hypothesized that re-introduction of Par1 expression in $Par1$-deficient leukemic blasts could decelerate the disease. Hence, we used MLL-AF9 positive splenic wild type and $Par1^{-/-}$ blasts from primary transplanted mice (Fig. 5B) and transduced them with a retroviral construct that expressed human PAR1 and the red fluorescent protein mCherry or as a control the empty vector only expressing mCherry. Cells were sorted by flow cytometry for their expression of MLL-AF9 (GFP), mCherry and c-kit as a marker for MLL-AF9 LICs. Each mouse received 1,000 triple-positive cells (Fig. 6D, left-hand side; n = 6 for each group). As expected from the results obtained from transplantation of 1,000 c-kit$^+$ MLL-AF9 splenic cells before (Fig. 6C), blasts of both genotypes transduced with the control vector led to a rapid disease with comparable latency (Fig. S3). In contrast, overexpression of PAR1 in $Par1^{-/-}$ blasts significantly extended the survival time of recipient mice compared to mice transplanted with PAR1-overexpressing wild

type MLL-AF9 blasts (Fig. 6D, right-hand side; p = 0.013). Moreover, overexpressing of PAR1 in cells with wild type levels of endogenous Par1 do not exhibit a significantly altered survival time compared to the control groups (Fig. S3).

In conclusion, Par1 acts as controller of leukemic stem cells in MLL-AF9 triggered murine leukemia and leukemic mice lacking $Par1$-expression in their blasts benefit from recovery of Par1 function.

Discussion

Our study reveals that PAR1 is especially expressed in healthy hematopoietic stem cells, whereas PAR1 expression is markedly lost in acute myeloid leukemia. The loss of Par1 leads to enhanced leukemic stem cell function *in vivo*.

Members of the hematopoietic serine protease superfamily that activate PARs, such as cathepsin G, neutrophile elastase and proteinase 3, may play an important role in myeloid biology [37]. Patients, who suffer from hematological disorder or congenital neutropenia frequently exhibit mutations in genes for neutrophil serine-proteases or show alterations in its expression, localisation or activity [38]. Nonetheless, PAR1 is not required in normal hematopoiesis and HSC function. The dispensability of Par1 in these processes might rely on redundant action of other proteinase-activated receptors, as it was already assumed for Par2 in thrombin-induced responses in $Par1^{-/-}$ platelets [12]. Moreover, persistent thrombin signalling in Par3-deficient platelets led to the identification of Par4 [39]. To determine the role of other PAR family members in hematopoiesis will require further experiments like the generation of Par1/Par2-double deficient mice, which might be difficult using the straight knockout mice due to the limited survival of both single-mutant mouse models [12,40]. For this kind of experiments, the generation of conditional knockout mouse lines might be necessary.

Up to now, PAR1 was assigned to oncogenic function in many tumor entities [2,16,18,19,41]. We were intrigued by the widespread loss of PAR1 in AML blasts by integrating the expression levels of PAR1 in three different leukemia patient cohorts on mRNA and protein levels. We therefore tested the role of $Par1$-deficiency in mouse leukemia. The oncogenic translocation product MLL-AF9 is frequently found in human leukemias [42,43]. We took advantage of the fact that PAR1 protein expression was downregulated in human AML patient samples of FAB subtypes M4 and M5 in our tissue arrays (Fig. 5C) and that these AML subtypes can be modelled by the retroviral introduction of MLL-AF9 in hematopoietic progenitors [34]. The AML-like phenotype is readily induced by MLL-AF9 in mice, either as a stable knockin [44] or by transient retroviral transduction and transplantation [34]. The widely-accepted concept of leukemic stem cells [45] can be recapitulated very consistently in this leukemia model, since predominantly the c-kit$^+$ fraction of MLL-AF9 positive leukemic blasts is transplantable and capable of self-renewal comparable to normal HSCs [34,35].

We discovered that Par1 expression restricted the pool of functional leukemic stem cells, rather than promoting it as an oncogene. Many receptors have been assigned as oncogenes, also in leukemogenesis. Prominent examples are the receptor-tyrosine kinases like FLT3 [46] and c-KIT [47]. But usually, these receptors are overexpressed or constitutively active due to mutations, which lead to overactivation of downstream targets, or to misactivation of other targets. In the case of PAR1, the mechanism of action in leukemogenesis might be different. Absence of Par1 enhances leukemia development, which might indicate *vice versa* that wild type expression of Par is able to suppress

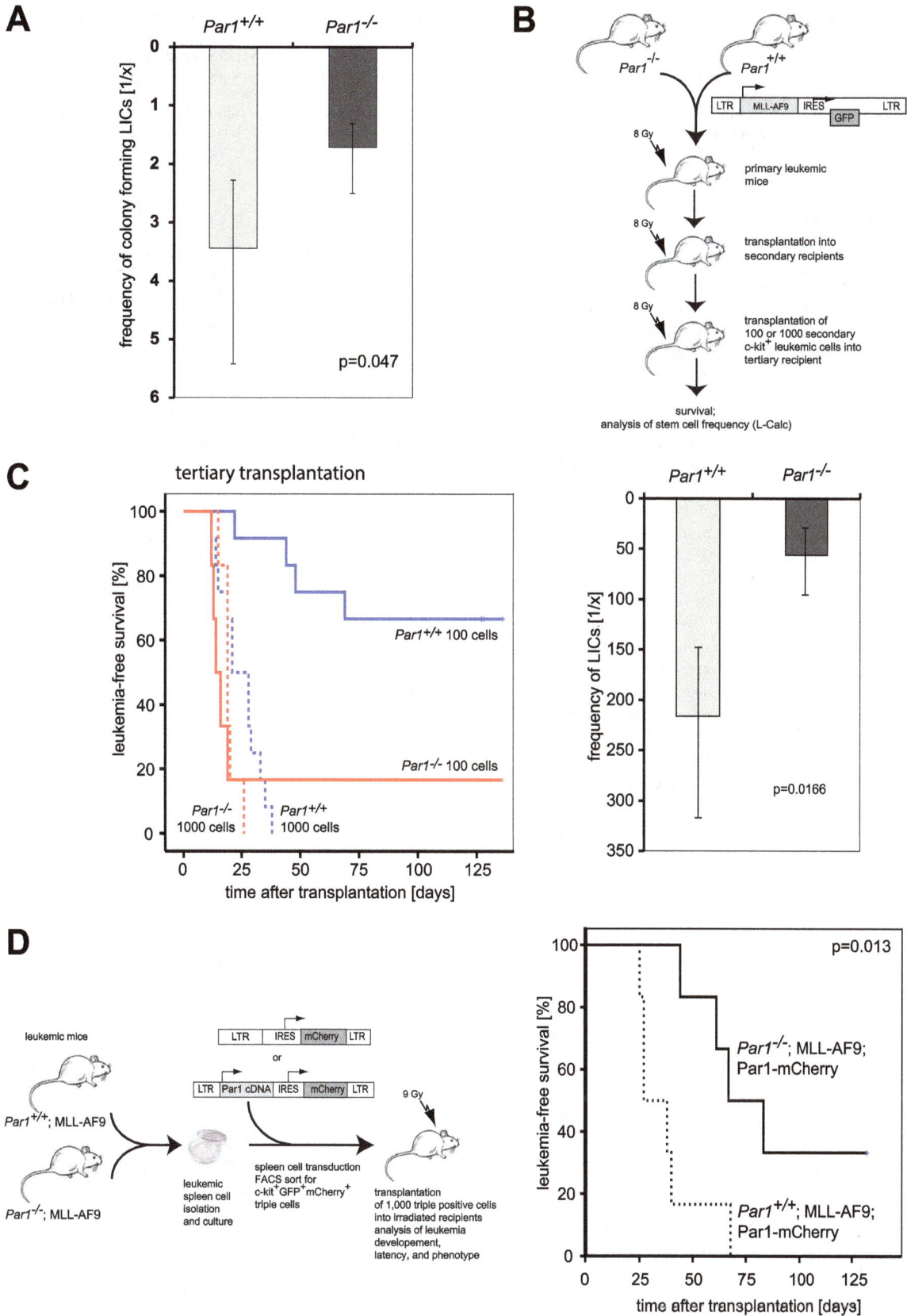

Figure 6. Leukemia initiating cells are regulated by Par1. 6A. For a cloning efficiency assay, *Par1*[+/+];MLL-AF9 or *Par1*[−/−];MLL-AF9 bone marrow cells from leukemia-transplanted mice were FACS-sorted and 1 to 300 c-kit[+]GFP[+] cells were seeded in semi-solid medium in a 48-well plate. *Par1*[+/+] cells had a clone forming frequency of 1/3.4, while the frequency was much higher in *Par1*[−/−] cells (1/1.7; p = 0.047). Shown here are the mean results of three independent experiments. **6B.** Schematic overview about the serial transplantations performed with MLL-AF9 leukemic blasts.

6C. Left-hand side: Kaplan-Meier plot illustrates the leukemia-free survival of tertiary transplanted mice. After tertiary transplantation, transplantation of 100 MLL-AF9 c-kit$^+$ leukemic blasts revealed a significant elongated life span of mice transplanted with Par1$^{+/+}$ cells (n = 12) compared to Par1$^{-/-}$ cells (n = 6; p = 0.002). Transplantation of 1000 cells did not reveal significant difference concerning the overall survival. Right-hand side: The frequency of leukemia-initiating cell was calculated according to the results shown in the left-hand plot by using the program L-Calc. Par1$^{+/+}$ leukemia-initiating cells appeared with a frequency of 1/216, while the frequency was much higher in Par1$^{-/-}$ cells (1/56; p = 0.0166). **6D**. Overexpression of PAR1 in Par1$^{-/-}$ MLL-AF9 leukemic spleen cells extents the life time of transplanted mice. Left-hand side: Schematic outline of the experimental of the transplantation. Right-hand side: Kaplan-Meier plot reveals the significant longer latency of leukemia in mice transplanted with Par1-deficient compared to wild type MLL-AF9 c-kit$^+$ blasts overexpressing PAR1.

leukemogenesis to a certain extent. Recently, it was shown that Par1 signal transduction might occur via the RhoA/ROCK1 pathway [14,48], which is also implicated to influence hematopoietic stem cells [49]. It will be interesting to investigate to which extent an alteration in this or another signal pathway in involved in the phenotype of Par1-deficient MLL-AF9 leukemic mice.

Although it was somewhat surprising that Par1 acted as a suppressor of stem cell function in leukemia, whereas it is implicated as an oncogene in other cancer entities, several other prominent factors also display such divergent functions. One example is the polycomb complex protein EZH2 that acts as an oncogene i.e. in prostate and breast cancer [50,51], while it suppresses T-cell leukemia development in mice [52]. In addition, Notch1 signalling is intensively studied and discussed as oncogene in different tumors and as tumor suppressor in leukemias [53,54,55]. Therefore, it is quite possible that Par1 acts with divergent outcome in different cancers. In addition, also its close relative Par2 was already identified as tumor suppressor in a model for skin carcinogenesis [56], although Par2 was also mostly accepted as oncogene [57,58], which illustrates the diverse functions that can be expected in this receptor family.

Finally, the fact that mice transplanted with Par1-deficient MLL-AF9 blasts benefit from the re-activation of Par1-expression might suggest that this could also help as a therapy for patients initially expressing very low or no PAR1. Rendering leukemic stem cells responsive to leukemia therapy is still a big task with the goal to be able to ultimately eradicate the disease (reviewed in [59]). Further studies on the role of Par1 in different leukemias might help to understand leukemic stem cell function and to develop molecular therapies to target these cells.

Supporting Information

Figure S1 PAR2, PAR3 and PAR4 expression in hematopoietic cells. Expression of PAR2 (S1A), PAR3 (S1B) and PAR4 (S1C) was analyzed in published microarray data from FACS sorted bone marrow cells (22, 23). None of them was prominently expressed in hematopoietic stem cells (HSC). Shown here are log arbitrary units.

Figure S2 PAR1 expression determined in microarray analysis according to FAB subtypes. PAR1 is significantly less expressed in all FAB subtypes tested by microarray analysis.

Figure S3 Empty vector controls to PAR1-overexpression transplantation. Survival curve of mice that were transplanted with MLL-AF9-induced Par1-wt and -ko leukemic spleen blasts that were additionally transduced with MSCV-IRES-mCherry empty vector. Mice that were transplanted with these cells exhibited leukemia initiation with comparable latency.

Acknowledgments

We are grateful to Frank Berkenfeld for excellent technical assistance. We thank Frank Rosenbauer for providing constructs.

Author Contributions

Performed the experiments: NB AK GK SL GE LT. Analyzed the data: NB GK SL GE AH SB CMT LT. Contributed reagents/materials/analysis tools: NB GK WEB CMT LT. Wrote the paper: NB SB AH WEB CMT LT.

References

1. Coughlin SR (2005) Protease-activated receptors in hemostasis, thrombosis and vascular biology. J Thromb Haemost 3: 1800–1814.
2. Austin KM, Covic L, Kuliopulos A (2013) Matrix metalloproteases and PAR1 activation. Blood 121: 431–439.
3. Coughlin SR (2000) Thrombin signalling and protease-activated receptors. Nature 407: 258–264.
4. Seeley S, Covic L, Jacques SL, Sudmeier J, Baleja JD, et al. (2003) Structural basis for thrombin activation of a protease-activated receptor: inhibition of intramolecular liganding. Chem Biol 10: 1033–1041.
5. Vu TK, Hung DT, Wheaton VI, Coughlin SR (1991) Molecular cloning of a functional thrombin receptor reveals a novel proteolytic mechanism of receptor activation. Cell 64: 1057–1068.
6. Leger AJ, Covic L, Kuliopulos A (2006) Protease-activated receptors in cardiovascular diseases. Circulation 114: 1070–1077.
7. Ossovskaya VS, Bunnett NW (2004) Protease-activated receptors: contribution to physiology and disease. Physiol Rev 84: 579–621.
8. Shpacovitch V, Feld M, Hollenberg MD, Luger TA, Steinhoff M (2008) Role of protease-activated receptors in inflammatory responses, innate and adaptive immunity. J Leukoc Biol 83: 1309–1322.
9. Steinhoff M, Buddenkotte J, Shpacovitch V, Rattenholl A, Moormann C, et al. (2005) Proteinase-activated receptors: transducers of proteinase-mediated signaling in inflammation and immune response. Endocr Rev 26: 1–43.
10. Griffin CT, Srinivasan Y, Zheng YW, Huang W, Coughlin SR (2001) A role for thrombin receptor signaling in endothelial cells during embryonic development. Science 293: 1666–1670.
11. Trivedi V, Boire A, Tchernychev B, Kaneider NC, Leger AJ, et al. (2009) Platelet matrix metalloprotease-1 mediates thrombogenesis by activating PAR1 at a cryptic ligand site. Cell 137: 332–343.
12. Connolly AJ, Ishihara H, Kahn ML, Farese RV Jr, Coughlin SR (1996) Role of the thrombin receptor in development and evidence for a second receptor. Nature 381: 516–519.
13. Darrow AL, Fung-Leung WP, Ye RD, Santulli RJ, Cheung WM, et al. (1996) Biological consequences of thrombin receptor deficiency in mice. Thromb Haemost 76: 860–866.
14. Yue R, Li H, Liu H, Li Y, Wei B, et al. (2012) Thrombin receptor regulates hematopoiesis and endothelial-to-hematopoietic transition. Dev Cell 22: 1092–1100.
15. Massi D, Naldini A, Ardinghi C, Carraro F, Franchi A, et al. (2005) Expression of protease-activated receptors 1 and 2 in melanocytic nevi and malignant melanoma. Hum Pathol 36: 676–685.
16. Even-Ram S, Uziely B, Cohen P, Grisaru-Granovsky S, Maoz M, et al. (1998) Thrombin receptor overexpression in malignant and physiological invasion processes. Nat Med 4: 909–914.
17. Hernandez NA, Correa E, Avila EP, Vela TA, Perez VM (2009) PAR1 is selectively over expressed in high grade breast cancer patients: a cohort study. J Transl Med 7: 47.
18. Arora P, Cuevas BD, Russo A, Johnson GL, Trejo J (2008) Persistent transactivation of EGFR and ErbB2/HER2 by protease-activated receptor-1 promotes breast carcinoma cell invasion. Oncogene 27: 4434–4445.
19. Boire A, Covic L, Agarwal A, Jacques S, Sherifi S, et al. (2005) PAR1 is a matrix metalloprotease-1 receptor that promotes invasion and tumorigenesis of breast cancer cells. Cell 120: 303–313.
20. Kaufmann R, Rahn S, Pollrich K, Hertel J, Dittmar Y, et al. (2007) Thrombin-mediated hepatocellular carcinoma cell migration: cooperative action via proteinase-activated receptors 1 and 4. J Cell Physiol 211: 699–707.

21. Nierodzik ML, Chen K, Takeshita K, Li JJ, Huang YQ, et al. (1998) Protease-activated receptor 1 (PAR-1) is required and rate-limiting for thrombin-enhanced experimental pulmonary metastasis. Blood 92: 3694–3700.

22. Hebestreit K, Grottrup S, Emden D, Veerkamp J, Ruckert C, et al. (2012) Leukemia gene atlas-a public platform for integrative exploration of genome-wide molecular data. PLoS One 7: e39148.

23. Novershtern N, Subramanian A, Lawton LN, Mak RH, Haining WN, et al. (2011) Densely interconnected transcriptional circuits control cell states in human hematopoiesis. Cell 144: 296–309.

24. Isken F, Steffen B, Merk S, Dugas M, Markus B, et al. (2008) Identification of acute myeloid leukaemia associated microRNA expression patterns. Br J Haematol 140: 153–161.

25. Diederichs S, Baumer N, Ji P, Metzelder SK, Idos GE, et al. (2004) Identification of interaction partners and substrates of the cyclin A1-CDK2 complex. J Biol Chem 279: 33727–33741.

26. Bäumer N, Tickenbrock L, Tschanter P, Lohmeyer L, Diederichs S, et al. (2011) Inhibitor of cyclin-dependent kinase (CDK) interacting with cyclin A1 (INCA1) regulates proliferation and is repressed by oncogenic signaling. J Biol Chem 286: 28210–28222.

27. Schemionek M, Spieker T, Kerstiens L, Elling C, Essers M, et al. (2011) Leukemic spleen cells are more potent than bone marrow-derived cells in a transgenic mouse model of CML. Leukemia 26: 1030–1037.

28. Agrawal S, Koschmieder S, Baumer N, Reddy NG, Berdel WE, et al. (2008) Pim2 complements Flt3 wild-type receptor in hematopoietic progenitor cell transformation. Leukemia 22: 78–86.

29. Worch J, Tickenbrock L, Schwable J, Steffen B, Cauvet T, et al. (2004) The serine-threonine kinase MNK1 is post-translationally stabilized by PML-RARalpha and regulates differentiation of hematopoietic cells. Oncogene 23: 9162–9172.

30. Hoxie JA, Ahuja M, Belmonte E, Pizarro S, Parton R, et al. (1993) Internalization and recycling of activated thrombin receptors. J Biol Chem 268: 13756–13763.

31. Preacher KJ (2001l) Calculation for the Chi-Square test: An interactive calculation tool for chi-square tests of goodness of fit and independence (Computer software). Available from http://quantpsy.org.

32. Ibrahim S, Estey EH, Pierce S, Glassman A, Keating M, et al. (2000) 11q23 abnormalities in patients with acute myelogenous leukemia and myelodysplastic syndrome as detected by molecular and cytogenetic analyses. Am J Clin Pathol 114: 793–797.

33. Bröske AM, Vockentanz L, Kharazi S, Huska MR, Mancini E, et al. (2009) DNA methylation protects hematopoietic stem cell multipotency from myeloerythroid restriction. Nat Genet 41: 1207–1215.

34. Somervaille TC, Cleary ML (2006) Identification and characterization of leukemia stem cells in murine MLL-AF9 acute myeloid leukemia. Cancer Cell 10: 257–268.

35. Somervaille TC, Matheny CJ, Spencer GJ, Iwasaki M, Rinn JL, et al. (2009) Hierarchical maintenance of MLL myeloid leukemia stem cells employs a transcriptional program shared with embryonic rather than adult stem cells. Cell Stem Cell 4: 129–140.

36. Kogan SC, Ward JM, Anver MR, Berman JJ, Brayton C, et al. (2002) Bethesda proposals for classification of nonlymphoid hematopoietic neoplasms in mice. Blood 100: 238–245.

37. Garwicz D (2006) Neutrophil serine proteases: future therapeutic targets in patients with severe chronic neutropenia and leukemia? Stem Cells 24: 2158–2159.

38. Dale DC, Person RE, Bolyard AA, Aprikyan AG, Bos C, et al. (2000) Mutations in the gene encoding neutrophil elastase in congenital and cyclic neutropenia. Blood 96: 2317–2322.

39. Kahn ML, Zheng YW, Huang W, Bigornia V, Zeng D, et al. (1998) A dual thrombin receptor system for platelet activation. Nature 394: 690–694.

40. Damiano BP, Cheung WM, Santulli RJ, Fung-Leung WP, Ngo K, et al. (1999) Cardiovascular responses mediated by protease-activated receptor-2 (PAR-2) and thrombin receptor (PAR-1) are distinguished in mice deficient in PAR-2 or PAR-1. J Pharmacol Exp Ther 288: 671–678.

41. Lopez-Pedrera C, Barbarroja N, Dorado G, Siendones E, Velasco F (2006) Tissue factor as an effector of angiogenesis and tumor progression in hematological malignancies. Leukemia 20: 1331–1340.

42. Swansbury GJ, Slater R, Bain BJ, Moorman AV, Secker-Walker LM (1998) Hematological malignancies with t(9;11)(p21-22;q23)—a laboratory and clinical study of 125 cases. European 11q23 Workshop participants. Leukemia 12: 792–800.

43. Moorman AV, Hagemeijer A, Charrin C, Rieder H, Secker-Walker LM (1998) The translocations, t(11;19)(q23;p13.1) and t(11;19)(q23;p13.3): a cytogenetic and clinical profile of 53 patients. European 11q23 Workshop participants. Leukemia 12: 805–810.

44. Corral J, Lavenir I, Impey H, Warren AJ, Forster A, et al. (1996) An Mll-AF9 fusion gene made by homologous recombination causes acute leukemia in chimeric mice: a method to create fusion oncogenes. Cell 85: 853–861.

45. Bonnet D, Dick JE (1997) Human acute myeloid leukemia is organized as a hierarchy that originates from a primitive hematopoietic cell. Nat Med 3: 730–737.

46. Leung AY, Man CH, Kwong YL (2013) FLT3 inhibition: a moving and evolving target in acute myeloid leukaemia. Leukemia 27: 260–268.

47. Jiao B, Wu CF, Liang Y, Chen HM, Xiong SM, et al. (2009) AML1-ETO9a is correlated with C-KIT overexpression/mutations and indicates poor disease outcome in t(8;21) acute myeloid leukemia-M2. Leukemia 23: 1598–1604.

48. Vouret-Craviari V, Bourcier C, Boulter E, van Obberghen-Schilling E (2002) Distinct signals via Rho GTPases and Src drive shape changes by thrombin and sphingosine-1-phosphate in endothelial cells. J Cell Sci 115: 2475–2484.

49. Fonseca AV, Freund D, Bornhauser M, Corbeil D (2010) Polarization and migration of hematopoietic stem and progenitor cells rely on the RhoA/ROCK I pathway and an active reorganization of the microtubule network. J Biol Chem 285: 31661–31671.

50. Varambally S, Dhanasekaran SM, Zhou M, Barrette TR, Kumar-Sinha C, et al. (2002) The polycomb group protein EZH2 is involved in progression of prostate cancer. Nature 419: 624–629.

51. Simon JA, Lange CA (2008) Roles of the EZH2 histone methyltransferase in cancer epigenetics. Mutat Res 647: 21–29.

52. Simon C, Chagraoui J, Krosl J, Gendron P, Wilhelm B, et al. (2012) A key role for EZH2 and associated genes in mouse and human adult T-cell acute leukemia. Genes Dev 26: 651–656.

53. Klinakis A, Lobry C, Abdel-Wahab O, Oh P, Haeno H, et al. (2011) A novel tumour-suppressor function for the Notch pathway in myeloid leukaemia. Nature 473: 230–233.

54. Lobry C, Ntziachristos P, Ndiaye-Lobry D, Oh P, Cimmino L, et al. (2013) Notch pathway activation targets AML-initiating cell homeostasis and differentiation. J Exp Med 210: 301–319.

55. Ranganathan P, Weaver KL, Capobianco AJ (2011) Notch signalling in solid tumours: a little bit of everything but not all the time. Nat Rev Cancer 11: 338–351.

56. Rattenholl A, Seeliger S, Buddenkotte J, Schon M, Schon MP, et al. (2007) Proteinase-activated receptor-2 (PAR2): a tumor suppressor in skin carcinogenesis. J Invest Dermatol 127: 2245–2252.

57. Darmoul D, Gratio V, Devaud H, Laburthe M (2004) Protease-activated receptor 2 in colon cancer: trypsin-induced MAPK phosphorylation and cell proliferation are mediated by epidermal growth factor receptor transactivation. J Biol Chem 279: 20927–20934.

58. Shi X, Gangadharan B, Brass LF, Ruf W, Mueller BM (2004) Protease-activated receptors (PAR1 and PAR2) contribute to tumor cell motility and metastasis. Mol Cancer Res 2: 395–402.

59. Misaghian N, Ligresti G, Steelman LS, Bertrand FE, Basecke J, et al. (2009) Targeting the leukemic stem cell: the Holy Grail of leukemia therapy. Leukemia 23: 25–42.

9

A New Prognostic Score for Elderly Patients with Diffuse Large B-Cell Lymphoma Treated with R-CHOP: The Prognostic Role of Blood Monocyte and Lymphocyte Counts Is Absent

Vít Procházka[1], Robert Pytlík[2], Andrea Janíková[3], David Belada[4], David Šálek[3], Tomáš Papajík[1], Vít Campr[5], Tomáš Fürst[6], Jana Furstova[6]*, Marek Trněný[2]

1 Department of Hemato-Oncology, Faculty of Medicine and Dentistry, Palacký University, Olomouc, Czech Republic, 2 First Internal Department, Charles University General Hospital, Prague, Czech Republic, 3 Department of Internal Medicine-Hematooncology, University Hospital Brno, and Faculty of Medicine, Masaryk University, Brno, Czech Republic, 4 Second Department of Medicine, Department of Hematology, University Hospital and Faculty of Medicine, Hradec Králové, Czech Republic, 5 Department of Pathology and Molecular Medicine, Charles University, and Second Medical School and Faculty Hospital in Motol, Prague, Czech Republic, 6 Department of Mathematical Analysis and Applications of Mathematics, Faculty of Science, Palacký University, Olomouc, Czech Republic

Abstract

Background: Absolute lymphocyte count (ALC) and absolute monocyte count (AMC) have been documented as independent predictors of survival in patients with newly diagnosed Diffuse Large B-cell Lymphoma (DLBCL). Analysis of the prognostic impact of ALC and AMC in the context of International Prognostic Index (IPI) and other significant variables in elderly population treated in the R-CHOP regime has not been carried out yet.

Methodology/Principal Findings: In this retrospective study, a cohort of 443 newly diagnosed DLBCL patients with age ≥ 60 was analyzed. All patients were treated with the R-CHOP therapy. An extensive statistical analysis was performed to identify risk factors of 3-year overall survival (OS). In multivariate analysis, only three predictors proved significant: Eastern Cooperative Oncology Group performance status (ECOG), age and bulky disease presence. These predictors were dichotomized (ECOG ≥1, age ≥70, bulk ≥7.5) to create a novel four-level score. This score predicted 3-year OS of 94.0%, 77.4%, 62.7% and 35.4% in the low-, low-intermediate, high-intermediate and high-risk groups, respectively (P<0.001). Further, a three-level score was tested which stratifies the population better (3-year OS: 91.9%, 67.2%, 36.2% in the low, intermediate and high-risk groups, respectively) but is more difficult to interpret. Both the 3- and 4-level scores were compared to standard scoring systems and, in our population, were shown to be superior in terms of patients risk stratification with respect to 3-year OS prediction. The results were successfully validated on an independent cohort of 162 patients of similar group characteristics.

Conclusions: The prognostic role of baseline ALC, AMC or their ratio (LMR) was not confirmed in the multivariate context in elderly population with DLBCL treated with R-CHOP. The newly proposed age-specific index stratifies the elderly population into risk groups more precisely than the conventional IPI and its existing variants.

Editor: William Tse, West Virginia University School of Medicine, United States of America

Funding: This work was supported by grants from Czech Ministry of Health (MZČR IGA NT 12193, http://www.mzcr.cz/) and Faculty of Medicine and Dentistry, Palacky University Olomouc (LF-2014-001, http://www.lf.upol.cz/). Tomas Fürst and Jana Furstova gratefully acknowledge the support of the J. W. Fulbright Commission (http://www.fulbright.cz/). The funders had no role in study design, data collection and analysis, decision to publish, or preparation of the manuscript.

Competing Interests: The authors have declared that no competing interests exist.

* Email: jana.furstova@email.cz

Introduction

Diffuse large B-cell lymphoma (DLBCL) is one of the most frequent subtypes of lymphoma of the Western Hemisphere [1]. The median age at diagnosis is about 65 years and the majority of patients are sixty or older. Novel treatment with rituximab-containing regimens and better supportive care markedly improved the outcomes in elderly patients [2–4]. The improved prognosis of DLBCL in elderly patients may also be related to intrinsic biological features of the tumor [5]. In addition to clinical conditions related to age, the role of the conventional prognostic variables, included in the International Prognostic Index (IPI) [6] or novel revised IPI (R-IPI) [7], may be altered in this population. The IPI was postulated in the pre-rituximab era and some retrospective analyses show its limited predictive value: Despite being a four-level score, the IPI usually identifies only two risk subgroups. Analyses published by Ziepert et al. [8] confirm IPI as a valid predictor when analyzing data from prospective trials with rituximab-based regimens. A subanalysis of older patient population (the RICOVER-60 study) [9] showed overlaps between the high-intermediate and high IPI categories. Moreover, two of the IPI variables (ECOG, and Ann Arbor stage) did not reach statistical significance in the Cox regression model for progression-free survival (PFS) and overall survival (OS). The novel "recalculated" R-IPI is a more powerful tool for the whole population, however with a limited information value for patients older than sixty years. No patients over sixty are considered low risk due to their age. This fact, together with an increasing proportion of elderly patients in good physical conditions, advocates for age-specific prognostic tools. Advani et al. [10] published an analysis of patients older than 60 treated with R-CHOP in US intergroup studies. Their elderly IPI (E-IPI) considered age over 70 as a negative prognostic marker, and it showed a superior discrimination power compared to IPI and age-adjusted IPI (AA-IPI) [6] scores. Unfortunately, no extensive multivariate analysis of predictor variables was done. Prognostic stratification in older population should be more focused on the real "biological" age of patients and on primary variables that reflect tumor aggressiveness and immune interaction between the tumor and host. There is growing evidence of a strong predictive role of the absolute lymphocyte count (ALC), absolute monocyte count (AMC) or their ratio (lymphocyte to monocyte ratio, LMR). This supports the hypothesis that host innate immunity is critical in tumor growth control and it is a limiting factor for the efficacy of immunochemotherapy in patients with DLBCL [11–13]. The optimal cut-off levels of ALC and AMC may be different in various populations [14–15]. This fact should be taken into account when designing new ALC/AMC-based prognostic schemes [16–18].

This retrospective study analyzes the role of conventional clinical and laboratory parameters in an unselected cohort of elderly patients with DLBCL treated in the Czech Republic with rituximab-based chemotherapy. The original focus was on modifying the IPI score for elderly population, by incorporating the prognostic roles of AMC, ALC, and LMR. However, no prognostic role of baseline ALC, AMC or their ratio (LMR) was found in the multivariate context in elderly population with

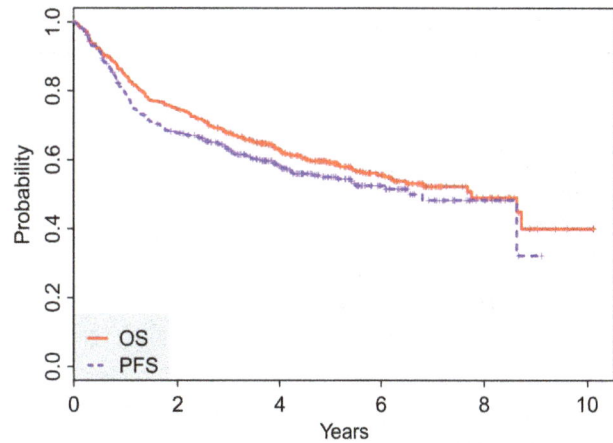

Figure 1. Overall survival (OS) and Progression-free survival (PFS) curves for the entire cohort. Complete follow-up.

DLBCL treated with R-CHOP. On the other hand, two variants of a novel prognostic score were postulated for this population. The scores are based on age, performance status according to WHO (ECOG), and the presence of bulky disease. Both the novel scores are found to be superior to previously published schemes. The novel scores were successfully validated on an independent cohort of similar group characteristics.

Materials and Methods

Ethics Statement

The study was performed in accordance with the 2008 revision of the Declaration of Helsinki. All patients provided an informed written consent to anonymous processing of data on their disease. The study was approved by the ethical committee of the Faculty Hospital in Prague.

Table 1. Summary of all the prognostic factors.

Prognostic factor	OS univariate analysis		Descriptive statistics		
	HR (95% CI)	P-value	Min–Max	Median	N (%)
Age [years]	1.07 (1.04, 1.10)	<0.0001	60–88	70	
ALC [$\times 10^9$ /l]	0.67 (0.54, 0.84)	0.0006	0.01–16.64	1.41	
AMC [$\times 10^9$ /l]	1.16 (0.83, 1.63)	0.3740	0.02–5.04	0.60	
LMR [–]	0.89 (0.81, 0.98)	0.0146	0.03–81.00	2.43	
Hemoglobine [g/l]	0.69 (0.52, 0.92)	0.0123	15–171	126	
No. of extranodal regions	1.20 (1.01, 1.43)	0.0357	0–5	1	
ECOG score	1.66 (1.41, 1.96)	<0.0001	0–4	1	
Ann Arbor stage	1.40 (1.20, 1.64)	<0.0001	1–4	3	
Sex (male)	1.32 (0.94, 1.84)	0.1050			186 (49.1)
Bulky disease (≥7.5 cm)	2.22 (1.55, 3.17)	<0.0001			136 (35.9)
Systemic symptoms present	2.44 (1.75, 3.41)	<0.0001			138 (37.1)
Bone marrow affected	1.69 (1.08, 2.66)	0.0228			49 (18.7)
LDH (≥ limit)	2.29 (1.56, 3.36)	<0.0001			226 (60.4)
B2M (≥ limit)	2.29 (1.47, 3.55)	0.0002			165 (56.5)

Results of the univariate 3-year overall survival (OS) analyses: hazard rate (HR) with its 95% confidence interval (CI) and P-value based on the Cox regression model. Descriptive statistics of all the prognostic factors.

Table 2. Multivariate model results.

Prognostic factor	OS multivariate analysis	
	HR (95% CI)	P-value
Age [years]	1.08 (1.04, 1.11)	<0.0001
Bulky disease (≥7.5 cm)	1.76 (1.21, 2.57)	0.0033
ECOG score (0–4)	1.61 (1.33, 1.95)	<0.0001

Results of the final multivariate 3-year overall survival (OS) model: Hazard rate (HR) with its 95% confidence interval (CI) and P-value based on the Cox regression model.

Subjects

The Czech Lymphoma Study Group (CLSG) is a national scientific organization which provides a platform for cooperation among Czech hematologists, oncologists and hematopathologists. The Lymphoma Registry (LR) is a prospective online database founded and operated by the CLSG which collects data from newly diagnosed lymphoma patients since 2000. The CLSG database covers up to 68% of all newly diagnosed lymphoma cases [19]. It currently contains 11,122 patients with lymphoma, including 627 DLBCL patients sixty years and older treated in the rituximab era. A cohort was selected to include all patients with a histologically confirmed diagnosis of DLBCL who were sixty years or older at the time of diagnosis and were treated with the R-CHOP regime [20]. The cohort included all patients with newly diagnosed DLBCL recorded in LR between April 2002 and May 2010, to allow for at least three-year follow-up. Patients with central nervous system involvement were excluded from the study. All biopsies were reviewed by a reference hematopathologist and the final diagnosis was provided in compliance with the published World Health Organization (WHO) classification. A central review of all final diagnosis reports was carried out [21]. The cohort consists of 443 patients (clinical data summarized in Table 1). On this cohort, all univariate and multivariate statistical analyses (see below) were performed. Before constructing the predictive score, further 64 patients were excluded because of missing data (i.e. at least one of the predictors used in the final

score was missing). Consequently, the comparison with existing scores and assessment of the score performance was done on a group of 379 patients. In the original CLSG query, only patients with complete data on ALC and AMC were selected. However, no prognostic role of these predictors was found (see Results). This enabled us to repeat the query without this constraint and thereby obtain a validation cohort of 162 patients from the same population. The validation cohort was selected about 1 year later than the original one.

Data

The following dichotomous predictors were considered for each subject at the time of the diagnosis: sex, bulky disease presence (limit 7.5 cm) [9], bone marrow affected, presence of systemic symptoms, lactate dehydrogenase level exceeding upper limit (LDH), beta-2-microglobulin level exceeding upper limit (B2M). The following categorical predictors were considered: number of extranodal regions affected, performance status according to WHO/ECOG (0–4), and Ann Arbor stage (1–4). The following continuous predictors were considered: age, absolute lymphocyte count (ALC, $\times 10^9/l$), absolute monocyte count (AMC, $\times 10^9/l$), lymphocyte to monocyte ratio (LMR = ALC/AMC), hemoglobin level (g/l).

Follow-up

OS was defined as the time from diagnosis of DLBCL to death from any cause. PFS was defined as time from diagnosis to lymphoma relapse, progression or death of any cause. Analyses were fitted to detect differences in survival times after 3 years of follow-up. All living patients' OS and PFS were censored three years from the diagnosis. This was done because the prognostic factors allow for the best discrimination of the population at around three years from the diagnosis. In later years, DLBCL unrelated factors may start outweighing the DLBCL-related ones in the OS and PFS.

Statistical methods

First, univariate analysis was performed to find out which of the risk factors are significant independent predictors of the 3-year OS. The Cox proportional hazards model was used. All independently significant predictors were consequently used in multivariate Cox regression analysis. By stepwise elimination, the least significant predictors were excluded to arrive at the final model. Only non-significant predictors were excluded. The predictors included in the final model were further dichotomized to allow for the construction of a simple predictive score (see Results). Performance of the newly proposed score was compared to existing predictive scores by means of the concordance measure and Akaike's information criterion (AIC). Concordance measures the probability of agreement for any pair of patients, where

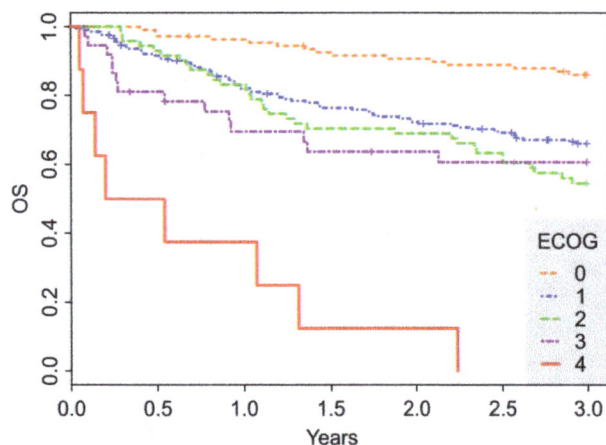

Figure 2. 3-year overall survival (OS) curves for the entire cohort stratified by the ECOG score. The hazard rates of groups 1, 2, 3, 4 relative to group ECOG = 0 are 2.85, 3.89, 3.82, 24.58, respectively. Notice the clear separation of the group ECOG = 4 from the rest of the population. However, group ECOG = 4 contains only 8 patients. Optimal stratification of the population into two groups thus separates group ECOG = 0 (109 patients) from the rest of the population (334 patients).

Table 3. Construction of the ABE4-Score.

Group	ABE4-Score	Risk factors present			N (%)	HR	P-value
		Age ≥70	Bulk ≥7.5	ECOG ≥1			
i	0	0	0	0	51 (13.5)		
ii	I	1	0	0	22 (5.8)	1.52	0.6444
iii		0	1	0	14 (3.7)	2.56	0.3028
iv		0	0	1	89 (23.5)	5.17	0.0073
v	II	1	1	0	7 (1.8)	14.77	0.0004
vi		1	0	1	81 (21.4)	8.17	0.0005
vii		0	1	1	61 (16.1)	6.61	0.0023
viii	III	1	1	1	54 (14.2)	18.90	<0.0001

Presence (1) or absence (0) of the three risk factors stratifies the population into eight groups (Group i–viii). The ABE4-Score is defined as the number of risk factors present in the patient. Results of the univariate Cox regression analysis: hazard rate (HR) and P-value with reference group being Group i (ABE4-Score = 0).

agreement means that the patient with the shorter survival time also has the larger risk score. Comparison of survival times was performed by the Kaplan-Meier survival curve plots and log-rank tests. All statistical analyses were performed using the R software [22]. The significance level of all tests was set to 0.05. Validation was performed by means of the concordance measure and by comparing the proportional hazards of the respective risk groups in the training and the validation cohorts.

Results

Treatment response and survival analysis

Treatment response was available in 400 out of the 443 patients (90.3%) in the training cohort. Complete response (CR), partial response (PR), stable (SD) and progressive disease (PD) were observed in 326 (81.5%), 42 (10.5%), 3 (0.8%) and 29 (7.3%) of the patients, respectively. During the follow-up (a median of 5.06 years for the surviving patients), 188 patients died (42.4%). The 3-year OS was 67.9% (95% CI: 0.64–0.72) and the median OS was 7.8 years (95% CI: 6.2–8.7 years). 3-year PFS reached 61.1% (95% CI: 0.56–0.66), median PFS was 5.4 years (95% CI: 4.1–6.6 years), see Figure 1.

Regression analysis

Univariate Cox regression analysis was performed on all prognostic factors listed in Table 1. The regression analysis revealed that all the considered risk factors are significant individual predictors of 3-year OS, except for the sex and AMC. In the multivariate analysis, we started by including all significant univariate predictors in a Cox proportional hazards model, and then gradually eliminated the insignificant ones. The final model contains only age, bulky disease presence (dichotomous) and ECOG performance status (0–4) (see Table 2). The AMC has no prognostic impact and the significance of ALC disappeared in the multivariate context.

Predictive score construction

The construction of a simple predictive score was based on the multivariate analysis results. In order to construct a simple score out of the three significant multivariate predictors, it is necessary to further discretize age and ECOG. Otherwise, the score would stratify the population into too many groups. Thus, we propose the following scheme: A patient gets one point for having age ≥70, one point for having bulky disease (bulk ≥7.5 cm) and one point for having ECOG ≥1. The cut-off level for age (70 years) was determined so that the hazard rate of the high risk group (age ≥ 70) relative to the low risk group (age below 70) is comparable to the hazard rates of the two remaining predictors. Moreover, the median age of the cohort is 70 years, and the E-IPI prognostic score [10] uses the same cut-off. The ECOG score was discretized according to Figure 2 which clearly differentiates patients with ECOG = 0 from the rest of the population. The three dichotomized predictors remain significant: the hazard rates (HR) for age ≥70, bulky disease and ECOG ≥1 are 2.20 (95% CI: 1.52–3.19, P<0.0001), 2.00 (95% CI: 1.39–2.87, P = 0.0002) and 3.18 (95% CI: 1.70–5.95, P = 0.0003), respectively.

Presence or absence of these three binary predictors (risk factors) stratifies the entire population into eight groups (see Table 3). It is convenient to define a four-level prognostic score (here denoted as ABE4-Score to remember that it is derived from Age, Bulk, and ECOG), analogously to IPI, as the number of risk factors present in the patient. Thus, patients without any risk factor ('Group I') are assigned ABE4-Score = 0 (N = 51) and represent the low risk group, patients with 1 risk factor ('Groups ii–iv') are assigned

Table 4. Summary of the scoring systems.

Group	N (%)	Estimated 3-year OS [%] (95% CI)	HR (95% CI)	P-value
Four-level scores				
ABE4				
Low (0)	51 (13.5)	94 (88, 100)		
Low-intermediate (I)	125 (33.0)	77 (70, 85)	4.15 (1.26, 13.66)	0.0191
High-intermediate (II)	149 (39.3)	63 (55, 71)	7.75 (2.42, 24.78)	0.0006
High (III)	54 (14.2)	35 (24, 52)	18.86 (5.78, 61.58)	<0.0001
IPI				
Low	90 (24.1)	83 (76, 91)		
Low-intermediate	93 (24.9)	75 (66, 84)	1.58 (0.83, 3.03)	0.1663
High-intermediate	98 (26.2)	65 (56, 75)	2.37 (1.29, 4.36)	0.0053
High	93 (24.9)	51 (41, 62)	3.86 (2.14, 6.93)	<0.0001
Age-adjusted IPI				
Low	83 (22.3)	82 (74, 91)		
Low-intermediate	117 (31.5)	77 (70, 85)	1.29 (0.68, 2.43)	0.4357
High-intermediate	106 (28.5)	64 (56, 74)	2.19 (1.20, 3.99)	0.0106
High	66 (17.7)	40 (29, 54)	4.80 (2.64, 8.73)	<0.0001
Elderly IPI				
Low	142 (38.2)	82 (76, 89)		
Low-intermediate	80 (21.5)	72 (63, 83)	1.78 (1.01, 3.16)	0.0484
High-intermediate	91 (24.4)	59 (50, 70)	2.64 (1.59, 4.40)	0.0002
High	59 (15.9)	41 (30, 56)	5.23 (3.10, 8.81)	<0.0001
Three-level scores				
ABE3				
Low	87 (23.0)	92 (86, 98)		
Intermediate	231 (61.0)	67 (61, 74)	4.75 (2.19, 10.30)	<0.0001
High	61 (16.0)	36 (26, 51)	13.33 (5.93, 29.95)	<0.0001
RIPI				
Very good	5 (1.3)	80 (51, 100)		
Good	178 (47.6)	79 (73, 85)	1.01 (0.14, 7.35)	0.9930
Poor	191 (51.1)	58 (51, 65)	2.37 (0.33, 17.06)	0.3900
ALC/RIPI				
Low	164 (43.9)	80 (74, 87)		
Intermediate	141 (37.7)	63 (56, 72)	2.12 (1.36, 3.30)	0.0009
High	69 (18.4)	50 (39, 64)	3.14 (1.93, 5.12)	<0.0001

Distribution and outcome of patients according to the compared risk scoring systems. Results of the univariate 3-year overall survival analysis: estimated 3-year overall survival (OS) with its 95% confidence interval (CI), hazard rate (HR) with its 95% CI and P-value based on the Cox regression model. Reference group in all regression models is the lowest risk group.

ABE4-Score = I (N = 125) and represent the low-intermediate risk group, patients with 2 risk factors ('Groups v–vii') are assigned ABE4-Score = II (N = 149) and represent the high-intermediate risk group, and patients with all three risk factors ('Group viii') are assigned ABE4-Score = III (N = 54) and represents the high risk group. Table 4 shows the hazard rates of the individual ABE4-Score groups calculated by means of the Cox proportional hazards model with the ABE4-Score as the only predictor.

This prognostic score is easy to interpret (it represents the number of risk factors present), however, it is interesting to note that 'Group v' has significantly worse 3-year OS (HR with respect to 'Group I' is 14.8, P = 0.0004) than 'Group vi' (HR = 8.1, P = 0.0005) and 'Group vii' (HR = 6.6, P = 0.0022). The HR of 'Group v' is even comparable to the HR of the worst prognosis

'Group viii' (HR = 18.9, P<0.0001). Thus, it seems that the combination of age ≥70 and bulky disease, despite ECOG = 0, has comparably pessimistic prognosis as the group where all the risk factors are present. This suggests defining another prognostic score, this time a three-level one: according to the results of the Cox regression analysis (see Table 3), there is no significant difference in HR of Groups i, ii and iii. Thus, Groups i, ii and iii are pooled into the low risk group and are assigned ABE3-Score = 0 (N = 87), Groups iv, vi, and vii represent the intermediate risk group and are assigned ABE3-Score = I (N = 231), and Groups v and viii are assigned ABE3-Score = II (N = 61) and represent the high risk group of patients (see Table 5). The Cox proportional hazards model provides the following results with respect to the ABE3-Score low risk group (see Table 4): HR of

Table 5. Construction of the ABE3-Score.

| Group | ABE3-Score | Risk factors present | | |
		Age ≥70	Bulk ≥7.5	ECOG ≥1
i	0	0	0	0
ii		1	0	0
iii		0	1	0
iv	I	0	0	1
vi		1	0	1
vii		0	1	1
v	II	1	1	0
viii		1	1	1

Presence (1) or absence (0) of the three risk factors stratifies the population into eight groups (Group i–viii). The ABE3-Score pools certain groups to stratify the population into three risk groups. Note that the Groups i–viii (the first column) do not appear in ascending order in contrast to Table 3.

ABE3-Score intermediate risk group is 4.75 (P<0.0001), HR of ABE3-Score high risk group is 13.33 (P<0.0001). The estimated 3-year OS with ABE3-Score stratification is: 0.92 (95% CI: 0.86–0.98) for ABE3-Score low risk group, 0.67 (95% CI: 0.61–0.74) for ABE3-Score intermediate risk group and 0.36 (95% CI: 0.26–0.51) for ABE3-Score high risk group. The ABE3-Score model stratifies the cohort in a more reasonable way (see the 'Comparison' section), however, the group sizes are not well balanced, and it is not as easily interpreted as the 4-category ABE4-Score model.

Comparison to existing scoring systems

Let us now compare the ABE4-Score and ABE3-Score systems to existing scoring systems, namely the four-level scores IPI, age-adjusted IPI (AA-IPI), and elderly-IPI (E-IPI), and the three-level scores revised IPI (R-IPI) [6] and its ALC/RIPI form. We fitted a Cox proportional hazards model with each of the scores as the only predictor and calculated the measure of concordance and AIC for each model. Both the ABE4-Score and the ABE3-Score are superior to the existing scoring systems because the ABE4-Score and the ABE3-Score have the highest measures of concordance, which indicate better discrimination. Apart from E-IPI, the ABE4 and ABE3-Scores also have the lowest AIC values in their group which indicate better fit (see the results in Table 6). The estimated 3-year OS by risk groups of individual

scoring systems are provided in Table 4 as well as the HR using the lowest risk group as the reference group. These results show better stratification of the risk groups by the ABE4-Score and the ABE3-Score as well. For each of the scoring systems, the estimated OS distribution using the Kaplan-Meier curves are shown in Figures 3 and 4.

Validation

Validation was performed on an independent cohort selected from the same population approximately a year later than collecting the data for the ABE scores construction (see Methods). There is no overlap between the training and validation cohorts. The descriptive statistics of the validation cohort are shown in Table 7. The characteristics of the validation cohort are very similar to the training cohort except for bone marrow involvement, which is notably less present in the validation group (8.8% in the validation group compared to 18.7% in the training group). Also, the median follow-up is significantly lower (3.53 years for the surviving patients) in the validation cohort because it was selected about a year later than the training one. Most of the patients with a long follow-up had already been included in the training group consequently, the validation cohort is biased towards patients with shorter follow-ups. Table 8 compares the hazard rates and the measures of concordance of the ABE3 and ABE4-Score groups in

Table 6. Comparison of the novel scores with the existing ones.

	Concordance (95% CI)	AIC
Four-level scores		
ABE4	0.686 (0.637, 0.735)	1304
IPI	0.635 (0.584, 0.686)	1336
Age-adjusted IPI	0.650 (0.599, 0.701)	1325
Elderly IPI	0.665 (0.614, 0.716)	1292
Three-level scores		
ABE3	0.676 (0.631, 0.721)	1299
RIPI	0.605 (0.558, 0.652)	1340
ALC/RIPI	0.619 (0.570, 0.668)	1337

Results from comparison of newly constructed scores (ABE4-Score and ABE3-Score) with several existing scoring systems. The measure of concordance compares the model discrimination, the Akaike Information Criterion (AIC) compares the model fit.

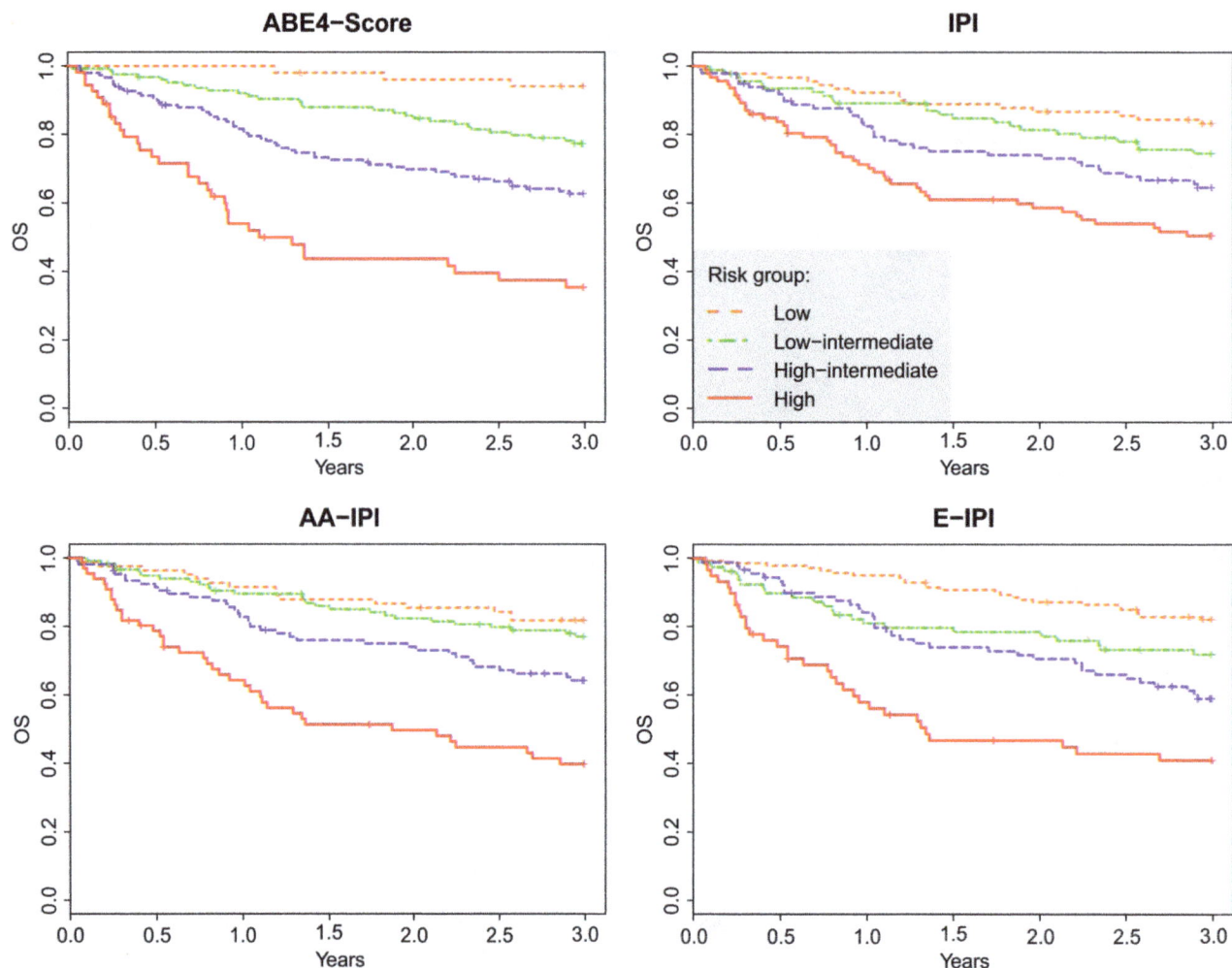

Figure 3. Overall survival (OS) curves for the entire cohort stratified by the 4-level scoring systems: the proposed novel ABE4-Score, and the classical IPI, AA-IPI, and E-IPI scores.

the training and validation cohorts. For ABE4, the validation hazard rates are well within the confidence intervals of the HR in the training cohort. For ABE3, the validation hazard rates are significantly lower. The measure of concordance for ABE4-Score (resp. ABE3-Score) on the validation cohort reads 0.66 (resp. 0.65). Both these values are well within the CI of the respective concordance measures on the training cohort.

Discussion

Recent years have brought a lot of information about prognostic role of the absolute lymphocyte count (ALC) and absolute monocyte count (AMC), together with their ratio, LMR. Lymphocytopenia was found to be a strong negative prognostic marker which correlates strongly with the disease burden, patients' fitness and overall outcome. Negative prognostic roles of low ALC and, inversely, high AMC were explained as results of impaired host-tumor immunosurveillance mechanisms and probably also by the weakening of ADCC activity. Unfortunately, none of these studies used large classes of prognostic factors not included in the conventional IPI score [17], [23], [24]. The present study shows that, if more prognostic factors are included, the role of ALC, AMC, and LMR is overshadowed by different factors.

Diffuse large B-cell lymphoma is a disease of elderly patients, with median age at diagnosis of about 70 years [25]. Despite this fact, most of the predictive scores use the cut-off age of 60 and cover the whole population of DLBCL. Elderly population is markedly different from the younger patients who tend to be in a better physical condition. Consequently, some prognostic factors may have different impact on the overall outcome in the elderly population.

This study attempts to establish the roles of ALC and AMC in an unselected DLBCL population aged over 60, when the role of (at least) all IPI-related factors is taken into account. Analysis of the fourteen clinical and laboratory parameters found only three of them to be sufficient (multivariate) predictors of survival: age ≥ 70 years, bulk ≥ 7.5 cm and ECOG ≥ 1. Surprisingly, ALC, AMC, or LMR were not found to add any predictive power to the multivariate model. Even when tested in the univariate context (each factor as the only predictor of the OS), AMC was found insignificant. The analyses were performed both with continuous values of these variables and with dichotomized values (with the cut-off set to the median of each variable). We suggest that the lack of predictive power of the AMC and ALC can be explained by their close correlation with the bulk and ECOG predictors. These two predictors possibly overshadow the role of AMC and ALC in the final model.

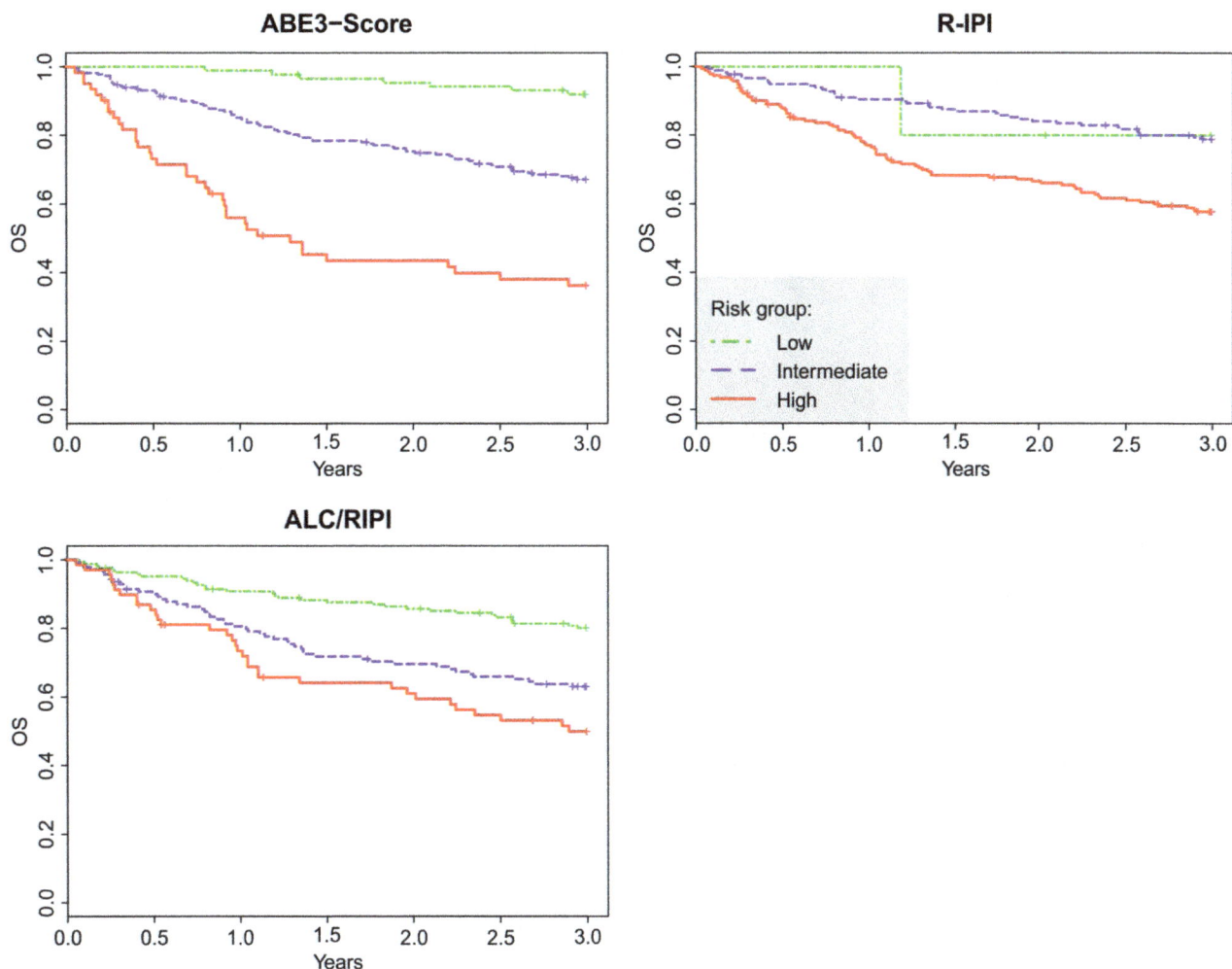

Figure 4. Overall survival (OS) curves for the entire cohort stratified by the 3-level scoring systems: the proposed novel ABE3-Score, and the classical R-IPI, and ALC/RIPI scores.

Table 7. Summary of the prognostic factors in the validation and training cohorts.

Prognostic factor	Validation cohort			Training cohort		
	Min–Max	Median	N (%)	Min–Max	Median	N (%)
Age [years]	60–85	69		60–88	70	
Hemoglobine [g/l]	11–169	128		15–171	126	
No. of extranodal regions	0–4	1		0–5	1	
ECOG score	0–3	1		0–4	1	
Ann Arbor stage	1–4	3		1–4	3	
Sex (male)			76 (46.9)			186 (49.1)
Bulky disease (≥7.5 cm)			58 (35.8)			136 (35.9)
Systemic symptoms present			63 (39.1)			138 (37.1)
Bone marrow affected			14 (8.8)			49 (18.7)
LDH (≥ limit)			98 (62.4)			226 (60.4)
B2M (≥ limit)			68 (54.4)			165 (56.5)

Comparison of the distribution of the prognostic factors in the validation and the training cohorts.

Table 8. Summary of the validation of the ABE scoring systems.

Score group	HR (95% CI)	P-value	Concordance
ABE4 in training cohort			0.686 (0.637, 0.735)
Low (0)			
Low-intermediate (I)	4.15 (1.26, 13.66)	0.0191	
High-intermediate (II)	7.75 (2.42, 24.78)	0.0006	
High (III)	18.86 (5.78, 61.58)	<0.0001	
ABE4 in validation cohort			0.656
Low (0)			
Low-intermediate (I)	5.3 (0.68, 41.05)	0.1105	
High-intermediate (II)	7.18 (0.95, 54.40)	0.0564	
High (III)	13.36 (1.72, 103.53)	0.0131	
ABE3 in training cohort			0.676 (0.631, 0.721)
Low			
Intermediate	4.75 (2.19, 10.30)	<0.0001	
High	13.33 (5.93, 29.95)	<0.0001	
ABE3 in validation cohort			0.650
Low			
Intermediate	2.12 (0.79, 5.67)	0.1357	
High	4.81 (1.73, 13.38)	0.0026	

Results of the univariate 3-year overall survival analysis in the training and the validation data sets: hazard rate (HR) with its 95% CI and P-value based on the Cox regression model. Reference group in all regression models is the lowest risk group. The measure of concordance compares the model discrimination.

On the other hand, IPI-related factors were found to be strong predictors of OS. First, the cut-off for age was set to the median value of 70 years, in agreement with previously published data [10]. Second, the overall fitness of the patients seems to be more important in the elderly population. In contrast to IPI, patients with only a moderate performance status decrease (ECOG ≥ 1) showed significantly decreased survival times. Figure 2 shows that the standard dichotomization (ECOG≤ 1 and ECOG ≥ 2) does not seem appropriate for the elderly population. Consequently, both the newly proposed ABE scores dichotomize ECOG $= 0$ and ECOG ≥ 1. Another important finding is the strong prognostic role of the tumor bulk. This predictor is not included in the IPI score but its relevance has already been confirmed in younger DLBCL patients but not in older population treated with dose-dense regimens [9], [26].

According to the measure of concordance, the four-level ABE4-Score is superior to IPI, AA-IPI, and E-IPI in our dataset. Analogously, the ABE3-Score is superior to both R-IPI and ALC/RIPI. We advise caution when using the measure of concordance to compare a four-level score to a three-level score, however, even in this comparison, the ABE3-Score outperforms all the standard four-level scores (IPI, AA-IPI, and E-IPI). This interpretation is confirmed by the AIC that shows the ABE3-Score to be superior to all other scores except for the E-IPI. However, the stratification of the cohort according to E-IPI lacks the power of the ABE4-Score, because the hazard rates of the E-IPI groups are much lower than the hazard rates of the ABE4 groups. From the practical point of view, both ABE4 and ABE3 scores show the highest span (highest discrimination power) between low- and high-risk groups (59% and 56% difference in OS at 3 years, respectively) compared to all other scores tested. This fact is well captured in the Kaplan-Meier curves (see Figures 3 and 4). IPI, AA-IPI, E-IPI, R-IPI, and ALC/RIPI scores all exhibit some degree of overlapping among the Kaplan-Meier curves for the various risk groups but ABE4 and ABE3 scores show markedly differing outcomes.

It is important to understand the way in which our scores are "fitted" to the data. When fitting a regression model (i.e. tuning its parameters) it comes as no surprise that the fitted model outperforms many other models which were fitted on different datasets. However, in our case, there are no "tunable" parameters that can be fitted to our data. Our training dataset was used only to identify the important predictors and, in case of ECOG, make a decision about their dichotomization. The ABE4-Score was successfully validated on an independent cohort selected from the same population. The score was shown to retain its high discriminatory power and high concordance measure. In case of the ABE3-Score, the validation revealed significantly lower hazard rates in the intermediate and high risk groups. This, together with the simpler interpretation of the ABE4-Score (it represents the number of risk factors present) advocates for the use of the ABE4-Score.

Conclusions

Prognostic stratification in lymphoma is a "moving target" [16] and our tools should be under continuous revalidation process. Elderly patients are an extremely heterogeneous population and optimal treatment strategy must be adapted with respect to comorbidities and should reflect the true biological age. On the other hand, DLBCL is a curable disease even in the elderly population. Our goal was to postulate a simple, valid and robust prognostic tool for population above the "arbitrary" age limit of sixty years, treated with R-CHOP. We have constructed two variants (three- and four level) of a novel prognostic score. For the routine practice, we recommend the four level ABE4-Score, which is simple to interpret (it represents the number of risk factors present) and robust (it was validated successfully). In conclusion, this study represents the first large analysis of a wide spectrum of prognostic factors in elderly, homogenously treated population with DLBCL. Predictive value of lymphocyte or monocyte count has not been confirmed. The proposed scores based on age, bulk and ECOG were found to be superior to previously published schemes. Other researchers are invited to validate our findings on different populations of elderly patients, homogeneously treated for DLBCL.

Author Contributions

Conceived and designed the experiments: VP MT. Analyzed the data: VP TF JF. Contributed reagents/materials/analysis tools: VP RP AJ DB DS TP VC MT. Wrote the paper: TF JF VP. Proof reading: RP AJ DB DS TP VC MT.

References

1. Morton LM, Wang SS, Devesa SS, Hartge P, Weisenburger DD, et al. (2006) Lymphoma incidence patterns by WHO subtype in the United States, 1992–2001. Blood. 107: 265–276.
2. Peyrade F, Gastaud L, Ré D, Pacquelet-Cheli S, Thyss A (2012) Treatment decisions for elderly patients with haematological malignancies: a dilemma. Lancet Oncol. 13: 344–352.
3. Coiffier B, Thieblemont C, Van Den Neste E, Lepeu G, Plantier I, et al. (2010) Long-term outcome of patients in the LNH-98.5 trial, the first randomized study comparing rituximab-CHOP to standard CHOP chemotherapy in DLBCL patients: a study by the Groupe d'Etudes des Lymphomes de l'Adulte. Blood. 116: 2040–2045.
4. Peyrade F, Jardin F, Thieblemont C, Thyss A, Emile J-F, et al. (2011) Attenuated immunochemotherapy regimen (R-miniCHOP) in elderly patients older than 80 years with diffuse large B-cell lymphoma: a multicentre, single-arm, phase 2 trial. Lancet Oncol. 12: 460–468.
5. Mareschal S, Lanic H, Ruminy P, Bastard C, Tilly H, et al. (2011) The proportion of activated B-cell like subtype among de novo diffuse large B-cell lymphoma increases with age. Haematologica. 96: 1888–1890.
6. The International Non-Hodgkin's Lymphoma Prognostic Factors Project (1993) A Predictive Model for Aggressive Non-Hodgkin's Lymphoma. N Engl J Med. 329: 987–994.
7. Sehn LH, Berry B, Chhanabhai M, Fitzgerald C, Gill K, et al. (2007) The revised International Prognostic Index (R-IPI) is a better predictor of outcome than the standard IPI for patients with diffuse large B-cell lymphoma treated with RCHOP. Blood. 109: 1857–1861.
8. Ziepert M, Hasenclever D, Kuhnt E, Glass B, Schmitz N, et al. (2010) Standard International Prognostic Index Remains a Valid Predictor of Outcome for Patients With Aggressive CD20+ B-Cell Lymphoma in the Rituximab Era. Journal of Clinical Oncology. 28: 2373–2380.
9. Pfreundschuh M, Schubert J, Ziepert M, Schmits R, Mohren M, et al. (2008) Six versus eight cycles of bi-weekly CHOP-14 with or without rituximab in elderly patients with aggressive CD20+ B-cell lymphomas: a randomised controlled trial (RICOVER-60). German High-Grade Non-Hodgkin Lymphoma Study Group (DSHNHL). Lancet Oncol. 9: 105–116.
10. Advani RH, Chen H, Habermann TM, Morrison VA, Weller EA, et al. (2010) Comparison of conventional prognostic indices in patients older than 60 years with diffuse large B-cell lymphoma treated with R-CHOP in the US Intergroup Study (ECOG 4494, CALGB 9793): consideration of age greater than 70 years in an elderly prognostic index (E-IPI). British Journal of Haematology. 151: 143–151.
11. Cox MC, Nofroni I, Ruco L, Amodeo R, Ferrari A, et al. (2008) Low absolute lymphocyte count is a poor prognostic factor in diffuse-large-b-cell-lymphoma. Leuk Lymphoma. 49: 1745–1751.
12. Talaulikar D, Choudhury A, Shadbolt B, Brown M (2008) Lymphocytopenia as a prognostic marker for diffuse large B cell lymphomas. Leuk Lymphoma. 49: 959–964.
13. Mociková H (2010) Prognostic significance of absolute lymphocyte count and lymphocyte subsets in lymphomas. Prague Med Rep. 111: 5–11.
14. Porrata LF, Rsitow K, Inwards DJ, Ansell SM, Micallef IN, et al. (2010) Lymphopenia assessed during routine follow-up after immunochemotherapy (R-CHOP) is a risk factor for predicting relapse in patients with diffuse large B-cell lymphoma. Leukemia. 24: 1343–1349.
15. Oki Y, Yamamoto K, Kato H, Kuwatsuka Y, Taji H, et al. (2008) Low absolute lymphocyte count is a poor prognostic marker in patients with diffuse large B-cell lymphoma and suggests patients' survival benefit from rituximab. Eur J Haematol. 81: 448–453.
16. Bari A, Marcheselli L, Sacchi S, Marcheselli R, Pozzi S, et al. (2010) Prognostic models for diffuse large B-cell lymphoma in the rituximab era: a never-ending story. Ann Oncol. 21: 1486–1491.
17. Tadmor T, Bari A, Sacchi S, Marcheselli L, Liardo EV, et al. (2013) Monocyte count at diagnosis is a prognostic parameter in diffuse large B-cell lymphoma: a large multicenter study involving 1191 patients, in the pre and post rituximab era. Haematologica. 99: 125–130.
18. Porrata LF, Ristow K, Habermann TM, Ozsan N, Dogan A, et al. (2012) Absolute monocyte/lymphocyte count prognostic score is independent of immunohistochemically determined cell of origin in predicting survival in diffuse large B-cell lymphoma. Leuk Lymphoma. 53: 2159–2165.
19. Cancer Incidence 2010 in the Czech Republic (2010) UZIS, NOR, ISBN 978-80-7472-034-5. Available: www.uzis.cz/system/files/novot2010.pdf. Accessed 2014 May 21.
20. Fisher RI, Gaynor ER, Dahlberg S, Oken MM, Grogan TM, et al. (1993) Comparison of a standard regimen (CHOP) with three intensive chemotherapy regimens for advanced non-Hodgkin's lymphoma. N Engl J Med. 328: 1002–1006.
21. Swerdlow SH (2008) WHO Classification of Tumours of Haematopoietic and Lymphoid Tissues. Lyon, France: International Agency for Research on Cancer.
22. R Core Team (2013) R: A language and environment for statistical computing. R Foundation for Statistical Computing, Vienna, Austria. Available: http://www.R-project.org/. Accessed 2013 July 30.
23. Aoki K, Tabata S, Yonetani N, Matsushita A, Ishikawa T (2013) The Prognostic Impact of Absolute Lymphocyte and Monocyte Counts at Diagnosis of DiffuseLarge B-Cell Lymphoma in the Rituximab Era. Acta Haematol. 130: 242–246.
24. Li ZM, Huang JJ, Xia Y, Sun J, Huang Y, et al. (2012) Blood Lymphocyte-to-Monocyte Ratio Identifies High-Risk Patients in Diffuse Large B-Cell Lymphoma Treated with R-CHOP. PLoS ONE 7(7): e41658. doi:10.1371/journal.pone.0041658.
25. Smith A, Howell D, Patmore R, Jack A, Roman E (2011) Incidence of haematological malignancy by sub-type: A report from the Haematological Malignancy Research Network. British Journal of Cancer 105: 1684–1692.
26. Pfreundschuh M, Kuhnt E, Trümper L, Österborg A, Trneny M, et al. (2011) MabThera International Trial(MInT) Group. CHOP-like chemotherapy with or without rituximab in young patients with good-prognosis diffuse large-B-cell lymphoma: 6-year results of an open-label randomised study of the MabThera International Trial (MInT) Group. Lancet Oncol. 12: 1013–1022.

10

Ubiquitous Expression of *MAKORIN-2* in Normal and Malignant Hematopoietic Cells and Its Growth Promoting Activity

King Yiu Lee[1], Kathy Yuen Yee Chan[1], Kam Sze Tsang[2], Yang Chao Chen[3], Hsiang-fu Kung[3], Pak Cheung Ng[1], Chi Kong Li[1], Kam Tong Leung[1], Karen Li[1]*

1 Department of Paediatrics, The Chinese University of Hong Kong, Hong Kong, **2** Department of Anatomical and Cellular Pathology, The Chinese University of Hong Kong, Hong Kong, **3** Centre for Emerging Infectious Diseases, Department of Medicine and Therapeutics, The Chinese University of Hong Kong, Hong Kong

Abstract

Makorin-2 (MKRN2) is a highly conserved protein and yet its functions are largely unknown. We investigated the expression levels of *MKRN2* and *RAF1* in normal and malignant hematopoietic cells, and leukemia cell lines. We also attempted to delineate the role of *MKRN2* in umbilical cord blood CD34$^+$ stem/progenitor cells and K562 cell line by over-expression and inhibition of *MKRN2* through lentivirus transduction and shRNA nucleofection, respectively. Our results provided the first evidence on the ubiquitous expression of *MKRN2* in normal hematopoietic cells, embryonic stem cell lines, primary leukemia and leukemic cell lines of myeloid, lymphoid, erythroid and megakaryocytic lineages. The expression levels of *MKRN2* were generally higher in primary leukemia samples compared with those in age-matched normal BM cells. In all leukemia subtypes, there was no significant correlation between expression levels of *MKRN2* and *RAF1*. sh-MKRN2-silenced CD34$^+$ cells had a significantly lower proliferation capacity and decreased levels of the early stem/progenitor subpopulation (CFU-GEMM) compared with control cultures. Over-expression of *MKRN2* in K562 cells increased cell proliferation. Our results indicated possible roles of *MKRN2* in normal and malignant hematopoiesis.

Editor: Kevin D. Bunting, Emory University, United States of America

Funding: This project was supported by the Earmarked Grant 470507 and Direct Grant 2041293 of the Research Grant Council of Hong Kong to The Chinese University of Hong Kong. The funders had no role in the study design, data collection and analysis, decision to publish, or preparation of the manuscript.

Competing Interests: The authors have declared that no competing interests exist.

* E-mail: lipang@cuhk.edu.hk

◑ These authors contributed equally to this work.

Introduction

Makorin-2 (HSPC070; MKRN2) belongs to the *MKRN* gene family of which the ribonucleoproteins are characterized by a variety of zinc-finger motifs [1,2]. MKRN2 holds four C$_3$H zinc fingers and a signature C$_3$HC$_4$ RING zinc finger domain. *MKRN2* is a highly conserved gene [1] yet its function remains largely unknown. Previous studies reported that mkrn2 in *Xenopus laevis* acted upstream of glucogen synthase kinase-3β in the phosphatidylinositol 3-kinase/Akt pathway. The third C$_3$H zinc finger and the RING motif are required for the anti-neurogenesis activity [3,4]. *MKRN2* was first identified in human CD34$^+$ stem/progenitor cells, as well as in some leukemic cell lines [2,5,6]. In chromosome 3p25, *MKRN2* is located next to the proto-oncogene *RAF1*. Interestingly, they share a sequence of 105 bp in the 3' UTR in a reversed transcription orientation [2]. This antisense sequence-overlapping of *MKRN2* with *RAF1* suggested that these two genes may regulate each other and be involved in normal hematopoietic and leukemic development. In this study, we investigated the expression levels of *MKRN2* and *RAF1* in normal and malignant hematopoietic cells, and leukemic cell lines. We also attempted to explore the role of *MKRN2* in umbilical cord blood CD34$^+$ stem/progenitor cells and K562 cell line by over-expression and inhibition of *MKRN2* through lentivirus transduc-

tion and shRNA nucleofection, respectively. Our results demonstrated ubiquitous mRNA expression of *MKRN2* and *RAF1* in normal hematopoietic cells, embryonic stem cell lines, primary leukemia and leukemic cell lines. We also showed *MKRN2* functions on promoting cell proliferation of primary CD34$^+$ progenitor cells and K562 cells, indicating its possible involvement in normal and malignant hematopoiesis.

Materials and Methods

Ethics statement

Written informed consents were obtained for collection of all human samples. For minors/children enrolled in the study, written consents were obtained from their parents on their behalf. This study was approved by the Ethics Committee for Clinical Research of The Chinese University of Hong Kong. All necessary permits were obtained for the described study, which complied with all relevant regulations.

Patients and samples

Primary leukemic cells (over 70% blast cells) were obtained from the bone marrow of children (age ≤19 years) who were newly diagnosed with chronic myeloid leukemia (CML), acute lymphoid (ALL) or acute myeloid (AML) leukemia at the Prince of Wales

Hospital, The Chinese University of Hong Kong. Age-matched normal subjects were siblings of patients who donated bone marrow for transplantation.

Peripheral blood samples were collected from normal adult volunteers. Mononuclear cells (MNC) were enriched by Ficoll-Hypaque density gradients (Amersham, Piscataway, NJ, USA). Human umbilical cord blood (CB) MNC and enriched CD34$^+$ cells were obtained from full-term deliveries as described previously [7].

Human leukemic cell lines and culture condition

Leukemic cell lines of B-cell lymphoid (RS411, 697, REH, Raji, IM9), T-cell lymphoid (HSB2, CEM119, Jurkat, Molt 3, SupT1), myeloid (KG1a, Kasumi-1, HL60, K562), natural killer (NK-92) lineages, and myeloma NCIH929 line were obtained from the American Type Culture Collection (ATCC; Manassas, VA, USA). These cell lines were cultured in Iscove modified Dulbeccco medium (IMDM; Invitrogen, Carlsbad, CA, USA) or RPMI 1640 medium (Invitrogen) containing 10% fetal bovine serum (FBS; Invitrogen) (20% for Kasumi-1 cells), 1 x Penicillin-Streptomycin (Invitrogen) accordingly to the manufacturer's instruction. Mega-karyoblastic cell lines (MEG01, MO7e, CHRF288) were obtained and maintained as previous described [8]. The human embryonic stem cell (ESC) lines H9 (P48-53) and H14 (P44-68) were products of Wicell (Madison, WI, USA) and maintained as previously described [9].

Over-expression of MKRN2 in CD34$^+$ and K562 cells by lentivirus transduction

Full length makorin cDNA was subcloned into lentiviral vector (pLEF1αIG-MKRN2) (Fig A in File S1). The empty vector (pLEF1α-IG) was used as a control. The VSV-G pseudotyped lentivirus was produced by cotransfecting 293T cells with the transfer vector and three packaging vectors [10]. CD34$^+$ or K562 cells were infected by the lentivirus at the multiplicity of infection (MOI) of 30. K562 cells were selected as the study model because K562 blasts are multipotential, hematopoietic malignant cells that could spontaneously differentiate into recognizable progenitors of the erythrocytic, granulocytic and monocytic lineages. In addition, we observed that MKRN2 and RAF1 were consistently and highly expressed in K562 and in primary myelocytic leukemia cells. Cells were first transduced for 16 hr, followed by 12 hr recovery in medium with 10% FBS and then transduced for a further 16 hr. Analysis and further manipulation was conducted 48 hr post transduction. The percentage of GFP expressing cells was monitored by flow cytometry using FACS Calibur flow cytometer and the CellQuest software (BD Biosciences), with 7-amino-actinomycin D (7-AAD) staining to gate out dead cells.

Silencing of MKRN2 by nucleofection using shRNA

A set of 29 mer shRNA constructs targeting MKRN2 (pGFP-V-RS-MKRN2, 4 unique sh cassettes in retroviral GFP vector) was introduced to inhibit the expression of MKRN2 in primary CD34$^+$ cells and K562 cells. pGFP-V-RS (retroviral GFP vector) and pGFP-V-RS-NE (non-effective 29-mer sh GFP cassette retroviral GFP vector) were used as control experiments. All Hush constructs were purchased from OriGene Technologies (Rockville, MD, USA). Briefly, 200 ug of each of the shRNA plasmids were used for nucleofection. Enriched CB CD34$^+$ cells (2×10^4/mL) and K562 cells (1×10^5/mL) were transfected using the Human CD34$^+$ Cell Nucleofection Kit and K562 Nucleofection Kit (Amaxa Biosystems, Koeln, Germany), respectively. After nucleofection, cells were allowed to grow for 48 hr prior to measurement of

readout parameters. The stable suppression of MKRN2 in K562 cells was maintained using Puromycin treatment (1 μg/mL; Invitrogen).

Cell viability

Transduced cells from each treatment were plated in duplicate wells (12-well plates, Corning) with the appropriate culture conditions (starting at 2×10^4 cells/mL) and splitted at a ratio of 1:3 on day 6. Cells were counted daily by a hematocytometer under light-microscope, with trypan-blue staining (0.4%; Bio-Rad, Hercules, CA, USA) to exclude dead cells.

Ex vivo expansion of transfected CD34$^+$ cells

Enriched CD34$^+$ cells at 2×10^4/mL were expanded in IMDM containing 10% FBS (StemCell Technology, Vancouver, Canada), 0.1% BSA, thrombopoietin (TPO; 50 ng/mL), stem cell factor (SCF; 50 ng/mL) and Flt-3 ligand (FL; 80 ng/mL). All cytokines were products of Peprotech (Rocky Hill, NJ, USA). After 8 days, multilineage stem/progenitor cells in the expansion culture were quantified by further culture for 14 days in cytokine-enriched methylcellulose medium (StemCell Technology). The number of colony forming units (CFU) of the erythroid (BFU-E, CFU-E), myeloid (CFU-GM) and early mixed (CFU-GEMM) lineages was counted under a microscope.

MTT assay

Effects of over-expression and inhibition of MKRN2 on proliferation of K562 cells were assessed by the methabenzthia-zuron (MTT) method. Cells (5×10^4 per well) were seeded in duplicates onto a 24-well plate (Corning, NY, USA) and incubated with 100 μL MTT (5 mg/mL; Invitrogen) for 30 min at 37°C. The insoluble violet formazan crystals and cells were collected by centrifugation at $18,300 \times g$ for 10 min and dissolved in 100 μL dimethylsulphoxide (DMSO, Invitrogen). Absorbance was read at 570 nm. Duplicate measurements were determined in 3 independent experiments and expressed as percentage of the control.

Reverse transcription and qPCR

Total RNA was extracted from cell cultures (1×10^6/samples), peripheral blood MNC or bone marrow samples using Trizol reagent (Invitrogen). cDNA was synthesized from 1 μg of total RNA using the High Capacity cDNA Reverse Transcription Kit (Applied Biosystems, Foster City, CA, USA). qPCR analysis was carried out using human specific Taqman Gene Expression Assays (Applied Biosystems). These primer and probe sets (MKRN2, Hs00274055_m1 and RAF1, Hs00234119_m1) have been recommended for specific gene expression experiments because they detect the maximum number of transcripts for target genes. Results were expressed as relative to glyceraldehyde-3-phosphate dehydrogenase (GAPDH).

Statistical analysis

The significance of growth or inhibitory effects exerted by over-expression or shRNA suppression of MKRN2 in CD34$^+$ cells and K562 cell line were determined by the paired-samples t test. The differences in MKRN2 and RAF-1 mRNA expression levels between normal and malignant hematopoietic cells, and leukemic cell lines were determined by independent samples t test. Correlations of MKRN2 and RAF-1 in primary leukemic samples and normal bone marrow samples were analyzed by the Pearson Correlation test. All analyses were performed using SPSS for Windows 17 software (SPSS, Chicago, IL, USA). A P value of

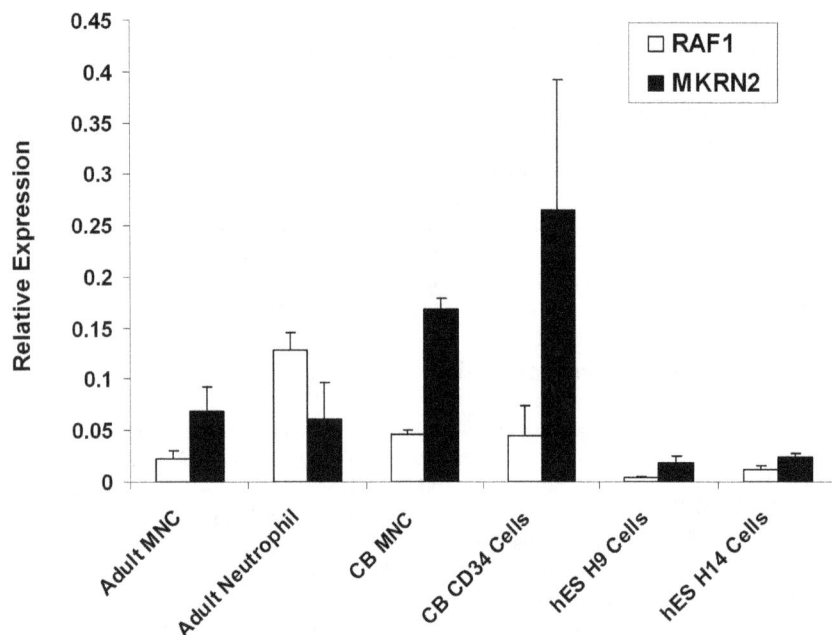

Figure 1. Expression of *MKRN2* and *RAF1* in primary hematopoietic cells and embryonic stem cell lines. Expression levels of *MKRN2* and *RAF1* mRNA were measured in adult and CB hematopoietic cells, enriched CD34+ stem/progenitor cells and human embryonic cell lines H9 and H14 by qPCR (n = 2–6). The Y-axis represents the expression level relative to *GAPDH*.

≤ 0.05 was considered significant. Results are expressed as mean ± standard error of the mean (SEM).

Results

mRNA expression of MKRN2 in normal and malignant hematopoietic cells

By qPCR analysis, we observed ubiquitous expressions of *MKRN2* and *RAF1* in primary hematopoietic cells including adult MNC, neutrophils, cord blood MNC, enriched CD34+ cells, and human embryonic stem cell lines H9 and H14 (n = 2–6) (Fig 1).

The expression levels are represented as relative to *GAPDH* (Y-axis, Fig 1–3). We also demonstrated expressions of *MKRN2* and *RAF1* in leukemia cell lines of B-ALL, T-ALL, AML, CML, NK and MK lineages (n = 2–3) (Fig 2). In primary leukemia samples obtained from BM of patients, we showed positive expressions of *MKRN2* and *RAF1* in B-ALL Philadelphia chromosome (*BCR/ABL* or Ph) positive and negative, T-ALL, AML and CML samples (n = 5–22) (Fig 3). The expression levels of *MKRN2* were generally higher in leukemia samples (*P*<0.05 in Ph–B-ALL, Ph+B-ALL, T-ALL and AML samples) compared with those in age-matched normal BM cells (n = 9), whilst *RAF1* was higher in Ph–B-ALL and

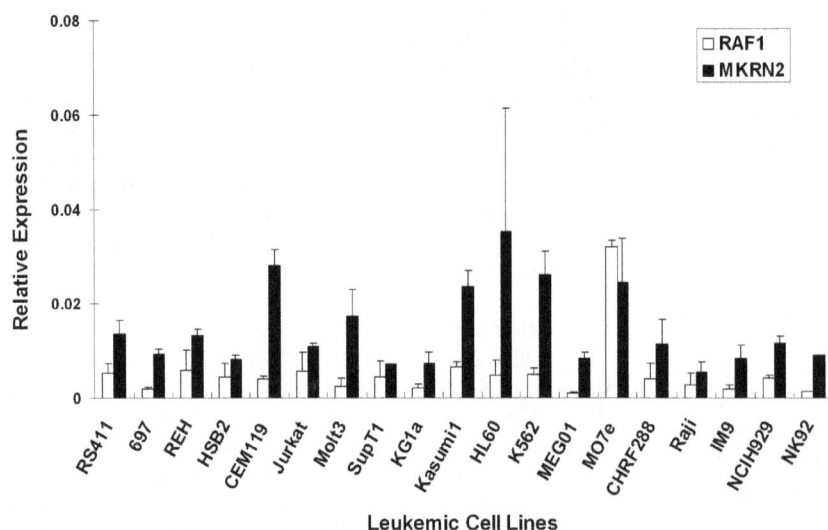

Figure 2. Expression of *MKRN2* and *RAF1* in leukemic cell lines. Expression levels of *MKRN2* and *RAF1* mRNA were measured by qPCR in leukemic cell lines of specific lineage subtypes. The Y-axis represents the expression level relative to *GAPDH*.

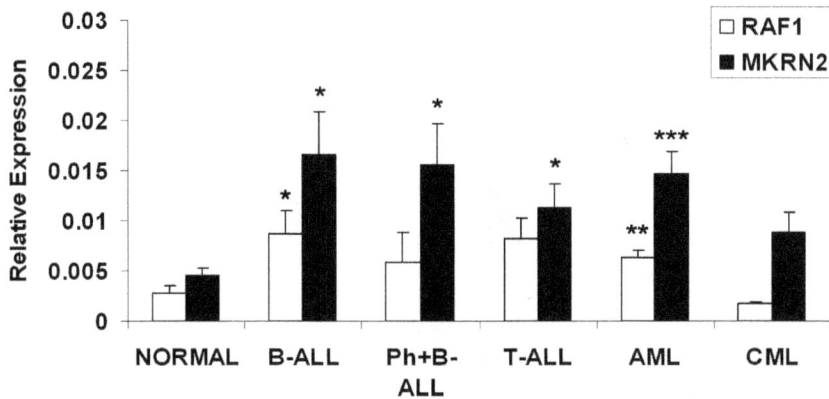

Figure 3. Expression of *MKRN2* and *RAF1* in primary human leukemic cells. Expression levels of *MKRN2* and *RAF1* mRNA were measured by qPCR in bone marrow cells collected from leukemic patients (Ph–B-ALL, n = 8; Ph+B-ALL, n = 7; T-ALL, n = 5; AML, n = 22 and CML, n = 11). The Y-axis represents the expression level relative to *GAPDH*. Expression levels of *MKRN2* and *RAF1* were compared with those of age-matched normal bone marrow cells (n = 9) (* $P<0.05$, ** $P<0.01$ and *** $P<0.001$). Ph = Philadelphia chromosome or *BCR/ABL* translocation.

AML samples ($P<0.05$). In all leukemia subtypes, there was no significant correlation between expression levels of *MKRN2* and *RAF1* (Fig B in File S1). In CML samples, there was no notable difference between *BCR/ABL* major (n = 8) and *BCR/ABL* minor samples (n = 3) in terms of *MKRN2* or *RAF1* mRNA expression (Fig C in File S1).

Over-expression of MKRN2 in cord blood CD34$^+$ cells

Lentiviral transduction of *MKRN2* resulted in 1.14±0.09 fold change of *MKRN2* mRNA and 0.93±0.27 fold change of *RAF1* in total CD34$^+$ cells, relative to their respective levels in control cells containing the empty vector (n = 3). There were trends of increased cell expansion (Fig 4) and the number of multilineage stem/progenitor cells (Fig 5) after *ex vivo* culture of transfected cell in the presence of cytokine supplement. However, the differences were not statistically significant.

ShRNA-silencing of MKRN2 in cord blood CD34$^+$ cells

ShRNA inhibition of *MKRN2* resulted in reduction of *MKRN2* expression (0.66±0.12 fold vs. pGFP-V-RS; and 0.79±0.07 fold

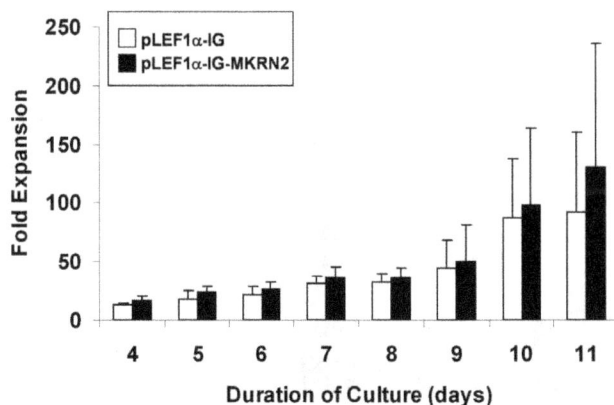

Figure 4. *Ex vivo* expansion of CD34$^+$ cells overexpressing *MKRN2*. CD34$^+$ cells were transduced with *MKRN2* cDNA subcloned into lentiviral vector (pLEF1α-IG-MKRN2) and cultured in expansion medium for 11 days (n = 3). The kinetics of expansion was not different between the *MKRN2*-transduced and control cells containing the empty vector (pLEF1α-IG).

vs. pGFP-V-RS-NE) (Fig 6). *RAF1* expression in *MKRN2*-silenced cells was 1.28±0.31 fold compared with that in control pGFP-V-RS cells. CD34$^+$ cells expressing pGFP-V-RS-MKRN2 had significantly lower proliferation capacity as shown in day 7 culture ($P=0.005$) and a trend of reduced expansion at day 2 and day 8 cultures (n = 3), when compared with either non-effective sh cassette (pGFP-V-RS-NE) or empty vector (pGFP-V-RS) control cultures. The early stem/progenitor cells (CFU-GEMM) were also decreased in the pGFP-V-RS-MKRN2 nucleofected cell expansion culture (Fig 7).

Over-expression of MKRN2 in K562 cells

Lentiviral transduction of *MKRN2* in K562 cells resulted in 1.54±0.21 fold change of *MKRN2* mRNA expression compared with pLEF1α-IG control cells (n = 3). *RAF1* expression in *MKRN2*-tranduced cells was 1.06±0.03 fold of control cells. By flow cytometric analysis, 83±15.3% (range 52–98%) of pLEF1α-IG and 90±4.79% (80.1–95.2%) of pLEF1α-IG-MKRN2 transduced K562 cells expressed GFP (n = 3) (Fig D in File S1). MTT assay of pLEF1α-IG-MKRN2 transduced cells showed a significantly increased proliferation in culture, compared with that of the pLEF1-IG control cells ($P=0.05$) (Fig 8).

ShRNA-silencing of MKRN2 in K562 cells

At 2 days post-nucleofection, Sh-MKRN2-silenced K562 had 0.86±0.02 fold change of *MKRN2* expression and 1.39±0.27 fold change of RAF1 expression (n = 3). GFP positive cells ranged 62.2 – 85.3% of the total cell population. However, shRNA silencing of *MKRN2* did not reduce cell proliferation of K562 cells in culture (MTT assay).

Discussion

Our data provided the first evidence on the ubiquitous expression of *MKRN2* in multi-lineage normal hematopoietic and leukemic cells, as well as its function on promoting CD34$^+$ and K562 cell proliferation. In spite of the known conservation of the *MKRN2* gene through evolution, little has been reported on its role in any organism other than the anti-neurogenic activity in *Xenopus laevis* [3,4]. Using shRNA silencing, we demonstrated the activity of *MKRN2* on promotion of CD34$^+$ cell expansion to early progenitor cells, indicating its role on normal hematopoiesis. However, over-expression of *MKRN2* in CD34$^+$ cells did not

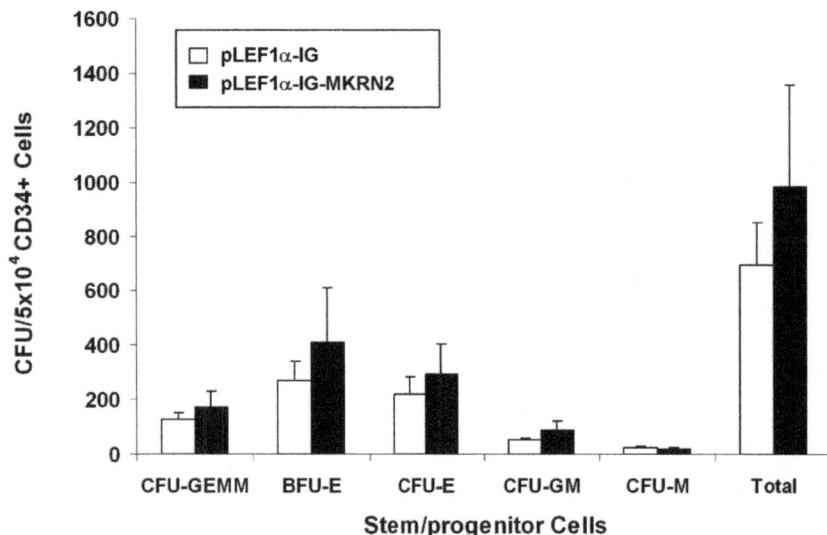

Figure 5. Colony forming capacity of *ex vivo* expanded CD34$^+$ cells over-expressing *MKRN2*. CD34$^+$ cells were transduced with *MKRN2* cDNA subcloned into lentiviral vector (pLEF1α-IG-MKRN2) and expanded for 8 days, and subjected to CFU culture for 14 days (n = 3). There was no difference between *MKRN2*-transduced cells and control cells containing the empty vector (pLEF1α-IG).

significantly affect cell expansion and lineage development, possibly because endogenous levels of MKRN2 protein were sufficient for its cell promoting functions. Upregulated expressions of *MKRN2* in primary leukemia cells prompted us to further investigate the effects of forced expression and silencing of *MKRN2* in the leukemic cell line K562. Again, we observed the stimulating activity of over-expressing *MKRN2* on K562 proliferation. In contrast to CD34$^+$ cells, sh-silencing of *MKRN2* in K562 did not affect cell proliferation, indicating possible differences between the regulatory mechanism of *MKRN2* in CD34$^+$ cells and leukemic cell line K562. Further evaluation of *MKRN2* gene manipulation on cell cycle regulation might reveal its specific mechanism on hematopoietic cell proliferation.

Due to the common sequence between *MKRN2* and *RAF1* in the antisense orientation, we suspected existence of a mutual regulatory mechanism between the two genes [11,12]. RAF1, a protein closely associated with the RAP1, RAS, ERK and AKT pathways, plays multiple roles in hematopoietic cells [13]. It is required for growth factor-induced proliferation of normal hematopoietic and leukemic cells [14]. RAF1 is also implicated in drug resistance of *BCR/ABL* expressing leukemic cells [15]. In normal and leukemic cells, however, we only observed ubiquitous expressions of *MKRN2* and *RAF1*. They did not exhibit any convincingly significant correlation in their expression patterns. It is anticipated that a larger sample size of each leukemia subtype would be required to accurately address the relationship between *MKRN2* and *RAF1*, as well as between specific translocations such as *BCR-ABL*.

To our knowledge, there have been very few reports on the involvement of *MKRN2* in malignancy, except some microarray

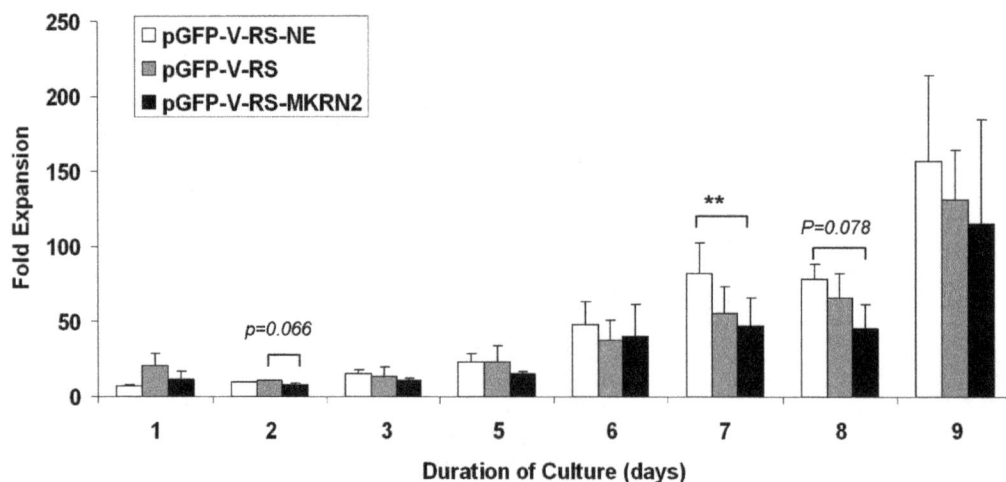

Figure 6. ShRNA-silencing of MKRN2 in cord blood CD34$^+$ cells. *MKRN2* expression was down-regulated in CD34$^+$ cells by nucleofection of shRNA. CD34$^+$ cells expressing pGFP-V-RS-MKRN2 had lower expansion capacity in day 7 culture (*P* = 0.005; n = 4) and a trend of reduced expansion at days 2 and 8, compared with cells transfected with non-effective sh-pGFP-V-RS-NE or empty vector (pGFP-V-RS).

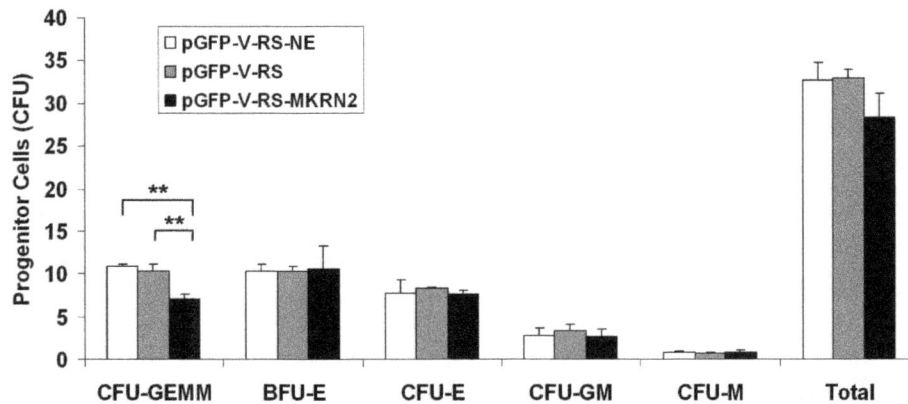

Figure 7. Colony forming capacity of *ex vivo* expanded CD34$^+$ cells with silenced *MKRN2*. *MKRN2* expression was down-regulated in CD34$^+$ cells by nucleofection of shRNA. CD34$^+$ cells expressing pGFP-V-RS-MKRN2 had a lower level of CFU-GEMM, compared with cells transfected with non-effective sh-pGFP-V-RS-NE or empty vector (pGFP-V-RS) (** $P<0.01$; n = 3).

screening data on papillary thyroid cancer [16]. *MKRN1*, the most studied member of the *MKRN* family has been shown to participate in a variety of mechanisms such as RNA-II-dependent transcription [17], Oct-4 signaling in mouse embryonic stem cells [18], telomere length homeostasis in cancer cell lines [19,20], polycystic kidney [21], ubiquitinase activity [22], and p14ARF-associated cellular senescence and gastric tumorigenesis [23]. Based on the ubiquitous expression and proliferative promoting activity of *MKRN2* in the various developmental windows of hematopoiesis, we suggest that *MKRN2* may play a house-keeping role on normal hematopoiesis. Our study has provided evidence that *MKRN2* might also be involved in the proliferation of human leukemic cells. Further knowledge on *MKRN2* interaction with known proto-oncogenes and involvement in leukemogenesis may lead to development of alternative treatment for the malignancy.

Supporting Information

File S1 Figure A: *MKRN2* construct for lentiviral transduction. Figure B: Correlation of *MKRN2* and *RAF1* Expression in Leukemia Samples. Expression levels of *MKRN2* and *RAF1* mRNA, relative to *GAPDH*, in bone marrow cells collected from leukemic patients (Ph−B-ALL, n = 8; Ph+B-ALL, n = 7; T-ALL, n = 5; AML, n = 22 and CML, n = 11) and age-matched normal bone marrow donors (n = 9) were measured by qPCR and analyzed by Pearson correlation test. A positive correlation ($P = 0.042$) was observed in Ph+B-ALL samples. However, the correlation became insignificant when the one sample with extremely high expressions of both *MKRN2* and *RAF1* was excluded from analysis. Ph = Philadelphia chromosome or *BCR/ABL* translocation. Figure C: Expression of *MKRN2* and *RAF1* in CML patients with Major or Minor *BCR/ABL*. Expression levels of *MKRN2* and *RAF1* mRNA, relative to *GAPDH*, in bone marrow cells collected from CML *BCR/ABL* Major (n = 8) and Minor (n = 3) leukemic patients were measured by qPCR. There were no significant differences between the mRNA expression of either genes in the 2 subgroups of CML patients. Ph = Philadelphia chromosome or *BCR/ABL* translocation. Figure D: Flow cytometric analysis of K562 transduction with MKRN2-GFP. Representative flow cytometric scatter plots of K562 cells lentiviral transduced with MKRN2-GFP. The empty vector GFP-IGV was used as a control. (A) Forward-scatter (x-axis) and side-scatter (y-axis) plot of K562 cells. R1 was gated for GFP expression analysis. (B) GFP expression (x-axis) and 7-AAD (y-axis, representing dead cells) of non-transduced cells. (C) K562 cells transduced with GFP-IGV control vector, showing 91.8% cells with GFP expression. (D) K562 cells transduced with MKRN2-GFP, showing 90.4% GFP-positive expression. (DOC)

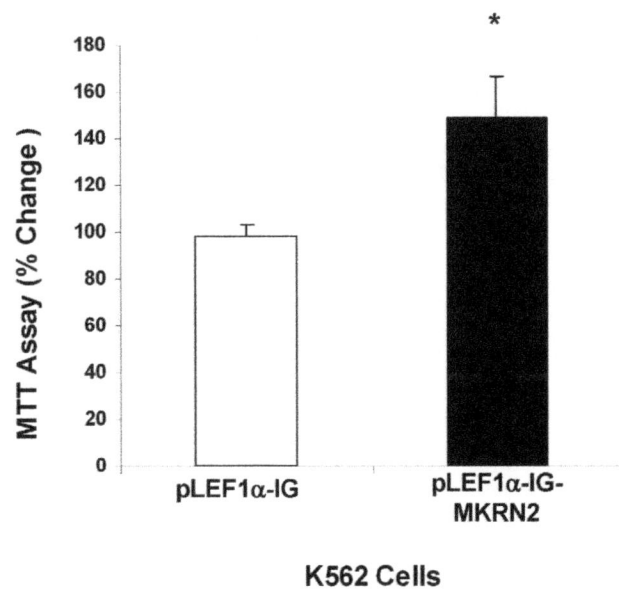

Figure 8. Proliferation capacity of K562 cells over-expressing *MKRN2*. K562 cells were transduced with *MKRN2* cDNA subcloned into lentiviral vector (pLEF1α-IG-MKRN2). MTT assay of pLEF1α-IG-MKRN2-transduced cells showed a significantly increased proliferation in culture, compared with pLEF1α-IG (empty vector) control cells (*$P = 0.05$; n = 3).

Author Contributions

Conceived and designed the experiments: KL KYYC HK YCC CKL PCN. Performed the experiments: KYL KYYC KTL KST. Analyzed the data: KYL KYYC KST KTL. Contributed reagents/materials/analysis tools: KST CKL KYYC PCN. Wrote the paper: KL KYYC KYL.

References

1. Gray TA, Hernandez L, Carey AH, Schaldach MA, Smithwick MJ, et al. (2000) The ancient source of a distinct gene family encoding proteins featuring RING and C(3)H zinc-finger motifs with abundant expression in developing brain and nervous system. Genomics 66: 76–86.

2. Gray TA, Azama K, Whitmore K, Min A, Abe S, et al. (2001) Phylogenetic conservation of the makorin-2 gene, encoding a multiple zinc-finger protein, antisense to the RAF1 proto-oncogene. Genomics 77: 119–126.

3. Cheung WK, Yang PH, Huang QH, Chen Z, Chen SJ, et al. (2010) Identification of protein domains required for makorin-2-mediated neurogenesis inhibition in Xenopus embryos. Biochem Biophys Res Commun 394: 18–23.

4. Yang PH, Cheung WK, Peng Y, He ML, Wu GQ, et al. (2008) Makorin-2 is a neurogenesis inhibitor downstream of phosphatidylinositol 3-kinase/Akt (PI3K/Akt) signal. J Biol Chem 283: 8486–8495.

5. Mao M, Fu G, Wu JS, Zhang QH, Zhou J, et al. (1998) Identification of genes expressed in human CD34(+) hematopoietic stem/progenitor cells by expressed sequence tags and efficient full-length cDNA cloning. Proc Natl Acad Sci U S A 95: 8175–8180.

6. Zhang QH, Ye M, Wu XY, Ren SX, Zhao M, et al. (2000) Cloning and functional analysis of cDNAs with open reading frames for 300 previously undefined genes expressed in CD34+ hematopoietic stem/progenitor cells. Genome Res 10: 1546–1560.

7. Leung KT, Chan KY, Ng PC, Lau TK, Chiu WM, et al. (2011) The tetraspanin CD9 regulates migration, adhesion, and homing of human cord blood CD34+ hematopoietic stem and progenitor cells. Blood 117: 1840–1850.

8. Li K, Yang M, Lam AC, Yau FW, Yuen PM (2000) Effects of flt-3 ligand in combination with TPO on the expansion of megakaryocytic progenitors. Cell Transplant 9: 125–131.

9. Lee KY, Fong BS, Tsang KS, Lau TK, Ng PC, et al. (2011) Fetal stromal niches enhance human embryonic stem cell-derived hematopoietic differentiation and globin switch. Stem Cells Dev 20: 31–38.

10. Chen Y, Lin MC, Yao H, Wang H, Zhang AQ, et al. (2007) Lentivirus-mediated RNA interference targeting enhancer of zeste homolog 2 inhibits hepatocellular carcinoma growth through down-regulation of stathmin. Hepatology 46: 200–208.

11. Krystal GW, Armstrong BC, Battey JF (1990) N-myc mRNA forms an RNA-RNA duplex with endogenous antisense transcripts. Mol Cell Biol 10: 4180–4191.

12. Yelin R, Dahary D, Sorek R, Levanon EY, Goldstein O, et al. (2003) Widespread occurrence of antisense transcription in the human genome. Nat Biotechnol 21: 379–386.

13. Stork PJ, Dillon TJ (2005) Multiple roles of Rap1 in hematopoietic cells: complementary versus antagonistic functions. Blood 106: 2952–2961.

14. Muszynski KW, Ruscetti FW, Heidecker G, Rapp U, Troppmair J, et al. (1995) Raf-1 protein is required for growth factor-induced proliferation of hematopoietic cells. J Exp Med 181: 2189–2199.

15. Demidenko ZN, An WG, Lee JT, Romanova LY, McCubrey JA, et al. (2005) Kinase-addiction and bi-phasic sensitivity-resistance of Bcr-Abl- and Raf-1-expressing cells to imatinib and geldanamycin. Cancer Biol Ther 4: 484–490.

16. Jarzab B, Wiench M, Fujarewicz K, Simek K, Jarzab M, et al. (2005) Gene expression profile of papillary thyroid cancer: sources of variability and diagnostic implications. Cancer Res 65: 1587–1597.

17. Omwancha J, Zhou XF, Chen SY, Baslan T, Fisher CJ, et al. (2006) Makorin RING finger protein 1 (MKRN1) has negative and positive effects on RNA polymerase II-dependent transcription. Endocrine 29: 363–373.

18. Du Z, Cong H, Yao Z (2001) Identification of putative downstream genes of Oct-4 by suppression-subtractive hybridization. Biochem Biophys Res Commun 282: 701–706.

19. Kim JH, Park SM, Kang MR, Oh SY, Lee TH, et al. (2005) Ubiquitin ligase MKRN1 modulates telomere length homeostasis through a proteolysis of hTERT. Genes Dev 19: 776–781.

20. Salvatico J, Kim JH, Chung IK, Muller MT (2010) Differentiation linked regulation of telomerase activity by Makorin-1. Mol Cell Biochem 342: 241–250.

21. Yoshida N, Yano Y, Yoshiki A, Ueno M, Deguchi N, et al. (2003) Identification of a new target molecule for a cascade therapy of polycystic kidney. Hum Cell 16: 65–72.

22. Joazeiro CA, Weissman AM (2000) RING finger proteins: mediators of ubiquitin ligase activity. Cell 102: 549–552.

23. Ko A, Shin JY, Seo J, Lee KD, Lee EW, et al. (2012) Acceleration of gastric tumorigenesis through MKRN1-mediated posttranslational regulation of p14ARF. J Natl Cancer Inst 104: 1660–1672.

11

Single-Nucleotide Polymorphism Array-Based Karyotyping of Acute Promyelocytic Leukemia

Inés Gómez-Seguí¹, Dolors Sánchez-Izquierdo², Eva Barragán³, Esperanza Such¹, Irene Luna¹, María López-Pavía¹, Mariam Ibáñez¹, Eva Villamón¹, Carmen Alonso¹, Iván Martín¹, Marta Llop³, Sandra Dolz³, Óscar Fuster³, Pau Montesinos¹, Carolina Cañigral¹, Blanca Boluda¹, Claudia Salazar¹, Jose Cervera¹,⁴⁹*, Miguel A. Sanz¹,⁵⁹*

1 Hematology Department, Hospital Universitari i Politècnic La Fe, Valencia, Spain, 2 Array's Unit. Instituto Investigación Sanitaria Fundación La Fe, Valencia, Spain, 3 Laboratory of Molecular Biology, Department of Clinical Chemistry, University Hospital La Fe, Valencia, Spain, 4 Genetics Unit, Hospital Universitari i Politècnic La Fe, Valencia, Spain, 5 Department of Medicine, University of Valencia, Valencia, Spain

Abstract

Acute promyelocytic leukemia (APL) is characterized by the t(15;17)(q22;q21), but additional chromosomal abnormalities (ACA) and other rearrangements can contribute in the development of the whole leukemic phenotype. We hypothesized that some ACA not detected by conventional techniques may be informative of the onset of APL. We performed the high-resolution SNP array (SNP-A) 6.0 (Affymetrix) in 48 patients diagnosed with APL on matched diagnosis and remission sample. Forty-six abnormalities were found as an acquired event in 23 patients (48%): 22 duplications, 23 deletions and 1 Copy-Neutral Loss of Heterozygocity (CN-LOH), being a duplication of 8(q24) (23%) and a deletion of 7(q33-qter) (6%) the most frequent copy-number abnormalities (CNA). Four patients (8%) showed CNAs adjacent to the breakpoints of the translocation. We compared our results with other APL series and found that, except for dup(8q24) and del(7q33-qter), ACA were infrequent (≤3%) but most of them recurrent (70%). Interestingly, having CNA or *FLT3* mutation were mutually exclusive events. Neither the number of CNA, nor any specific CNA was associated significantly with prognosis. This study has delineated recurrent abnormalities in addition to t(15;17) that may act as secondary events and could explain leukemogenesis in up to 40% of APL cases with no ACA by conventional cytogenetics.

Editor: William B. Coleman, University of North Carolina School of Medicine, United States of America

Funding: This work was supported by the Grant "Rio Hortega" (CM10/00321, CM11/00343), the Health Research Program (PI12/01047), the program "Red Temática de Investigación Cooperativa en Cáncer" (RD12/0036/0014) and the "Red Cooperativa de Biobancos Hospitalarios" (RD09/0076/00021) from "Instituto de Salud Carlos III", Ministry of Science and Innovation, Spain, (www.isciii.es); the research grant 2013/0327 from the "Instituto Investigación Sanitaria Hospital La Fe", (www.iislafe.es); and the Excellence Research Project (PROMETEO/2011/025) granted by Generalitat Valenciana, (www.cece.gva.es). The funders had no role in study design, data collection and analysis, decision to publish, or preparation of the manuscript.

Competing Interests: The authors have declared that no competing interests exist.

* Email: gomez_ine@gva.es (IGS); sanz_mig@gva.es (MAS)

⑨ These authors contributed equally to this work and should be considered joint senior authors.

Introduction

Acute promyelocytic leukemia (APL) is characterized by the t(15;17)(q22;q21) and the corresponding fusion gene *PML-RARA*. Additional chromosomal abnormalities (ACA) have been traditionally analyzed by conventional cytogenetics and fluorescence *in situ* hybridization (FISH). In the last decade, the single-nucleotide polymorphism array (SNP-A) has become a powerful tool to perform what has been called "molecular karyotyping", because it increases the resolution of conventional cytogenetics and detects a wider spectrum of abnormalities than FISH and other targeted techniques. Moreover, SNP-A are able to uncover regions of copy-neutral loss of heterozygosity (CN-LOH), a known phenomenon that occurs in cancer and which is not detectable by conventional cytogenetics.[1]

Most reports studying ACA in APL with SNP-A have used low resolution arrays or have not systematically matched tumor and germline sample,[2,3] which is the only certain way to rule out copy-number variations (CNV).[4] Our interest in the clinical impact of ACA in APL was addressed in previous studies,[5,6] but these were performed with conventional cytogenetics and FISH. We hypothesize that there may be some ACA not detected by conventional techniques that could be detected by high resolution SNP-A karyotype.

In this report, we have performed SNP-A in a series of APL patients to learn the incidence of cryptic ACA, as well as to study any possible clinical or biologic association.

Methods

Ethics Statement

In accordance with the Declaration of Helsinki, this study was approved by the Research Ethics Board of our hospital (CEIB; *Comité Ético de Investigación Biomédica*). According to the Spanish law, written informed consent was obtained from all patients to participate in this study.

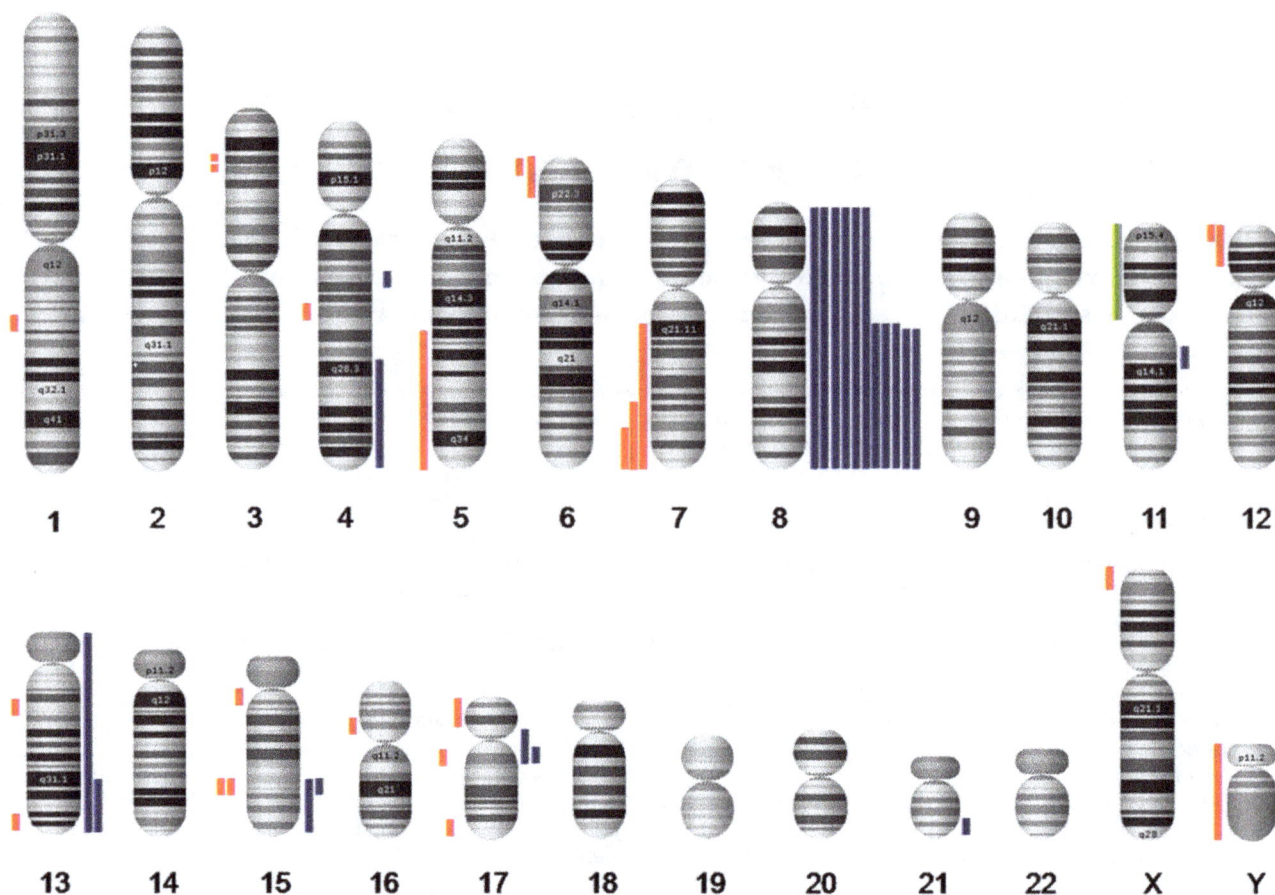

Figure 1. Karyogram of APL according to SNP-A analysis in our series. Coloured bars depict the extension of abnormalities. Gains appear in blue at the right of each chromosome; losses in red and CN-LOH in green, at the left side of it.

Patients and samples

Patients consecutively diagnosed with APL between November 1998 and February 2011 in the Hospital Universitari i Politècnic La Fe with available tumor and germline DNA sample were selected for this study. DNA was provided by Biobank La Fe. Tumor DNA was obtained from bone marrow cells at diagnosis. Matched germline DNA was obtained from bone marrow or peripheral blood when qRT-PCR was negative for PML-RARA rearrangement. Conventional cytogenetics, FISH or RT-PCR for the detection of PML-RARA fusion were performed in every case, as well as tests for mutation detection of *FLT3-ITD* and D835 as previously described.[7] Patients were enrolled in three consecutive multicenter PETHEMA trials (LPA96, LPA99, and LPA2005).[8,9] Clinical data as well as treatment outcome and follow-up were collected prospectively.

SNP-A

Samples (500ng) were genotyped with Affymetrix GeneChip Human Mapping 6.0 according to manufacturer's protocol (Affymetrix Santa Clara, C.A., U.S.A.). DNA copy number and paired LOH analysis were performed using the Genotyping Console and the Chromosome Analysis Suite (ChAS) software (Affymetrix). Filters applied for the detection of segmental copy-number abnormalities (CNA) were ≥10 consecutive markers in a region of at least 10Kb, and for regions of CN-LOH, ≥50 markers in at least 100Kb. All abnormalities found in the remission sample were ruled out and assumed as non-somatic. In addition, every

potential abnormality was checked in the Database of Genomic Variants (http://projects.tcag.ca/variation). Size, position, and location of genes were identified with UCSC Genome Browser (http://genome.ucsc.edu/). The human reference sequence used for alignment was the GRCh37/hg19assembly.

SNP-A data from other APL series

We compared our results with other APL series, namely APL cases from The Cancer Genome Atlas (TCGA) Network with publicly available SNP-A data (n = 20), the series of Akagi *et al.* (n = 47) and the series of Nowak *et al.* (n = 93).[2,3] Lesions found in the TCGA cohort are listed in Table S1 in Appendix S1. Lesions found in the series of Akagi *et al.* and Nowak *et al.* were listed in the corresponding report.[2,3]

Conversion of hg18 to version hg19 was done in these cases using the "Batch Coordinate Conversion (liftOver)" Tool from the UCSC Genome Browser, with a minimum ratio of bases that remapped >0.95.

Statistical analysis

Chi-square and Fisher's exact tests were used to analyze differences in the distribution of categorical variables. Mann–Whitney U-test was used to analyze differences in mean ranks. Unadjusted time-to-event analyses were performed using the Kaplan–Meier estimate and for comparisons, log-rank tests. Last update on clinical data was performed on March 2012. Median follow-up of patients alive was 77 months (range 13–151 mo.).

Table 1. Main characteristics of our series.

Characteristics	Median (range)
Age	43 (17–76)
Leukocyte count (×10⁹/L)	2.2 (0–59)
Hemoglobin(g/dL)	9.0 (4.2–15.2)
Platelet count (x10⁹/L)	24.5 (2–168)
Bone marrow blasts (%)	90 (53–100)
	n (%)
Male gender	26 (54)
Therapy-related APL	3 (6)
Mophologic variant	
Classical	35 (73)
Hypogranular	13 (28)
Risk group (Sanz et al)²	
Low	9 (19)
Intermediate	26 (54)
High	13 (27)
Cytogenetics	
t(15;17)(q22;q21)	28 (58)
t(15;17)(q22;q21) and additional chromosomal abnormalities	7 (15)
Cryptic translocation*	5 (10)
Non-evaluable*	8 (17)
PML-RARA isoform type	
Bcr-1	28 (58)
Bcr- 2	2 (4)
Bcr- 3	18 (38)
FLT3 mutational status	
FLT3-ITD	9 (19)
FLT3-D835	1 (2)
Treatment Protocol	
LPA-96	3 (6)
LPA-99	22 (46)
LPA-2005	23 (48)

*PML-RARA was diagnosed by FISH or RT-PCR.

To investigate any possible association of the SNP-A abnormalities with clinical and biological characteristics, patients were divided according to the presence or not of CNA, the number of CNA and any recurrent CNA with n>3, such as +8/8q and CNA adjacent to the translocation breakpoints. Regarding the other APL series, we had available data for overall survival (OS) analysis from TCGA (n = 20) and Nowak *et al.* cohort (n = 89), and for relapse-free survival (RFS) from Nowak *et al.* cohort (n = 72 patients who achieved complete remission).

All computations were performed using the statistical package SPSS, version 17.0 (SPSS Inc., Chicago, IL, USA). A two-sided *P* value below .05 was considered significant.

Results

Identification of CNA and CN-LOH by SNP-A analysis

A total of 48 patients were included in this study. Main clinical and genetic characterization of our cohort is summarized in Table 1. Conventional cytogenetic studies were successful in 40

patients (83%). Seven of these patients (18%) had ACA (Table 1). SNP-A analysis revealed 46 abnormalities in 23 patients (48%). These consisted of 23 heterozygous deletions, 22 duplications and 1 CN-LOH (Figure 1). Ten (21%), 7 (15%) and 5 (12%) patients had one, two, and three or more anomalies, respectively.

A detailed list of the CNA and CN-LOH found in our series is shown in Table 2 and Figure 1. Median size of interstitial and telomeric CNA was 0.30 Mb (range, 0.11–19.38) and 77.48 Mb (range 3.45–146.36), respectively (Figure S1 in Appendix S1). No statistical difference in size was found for interstitial CNA (median size 0.46 Mb for duplications *vs.* 0.15 Mb for deletions).

Recurrent SNP-A lesions

The most common abnormality was a duplication of +8/8q (11 patients, 23%), followed by a deletion of 7q (3 patients, 6%). Of note, 7 out of 11 +8/8q had not been detected by conventional cytogenetics. Four cases (8%) showed CNA adjacent to the breakpoints of the t(15;17) translocation (Figure 2). In case APL_20, two partial deletions were 0.5 Mb telomeric to *PML*

Table 2. Detailed list of abnormalities found in our series (n = 48).

APL_ID	Copy Number State	Chr	Cytoband	Start Position	End Position	Size (Mb)
Duplication of chr. 8						
6	3	8	complete	0	146364022	146.36
23	3	8	complete	0	146364022	146.36
37	3	8	complete	0	146364022	146.36
1	1	6	p25.1–p24.3	4883499	7409514	2.53
	3	8	complete	0	146364022	146.36
11	3	8	q13.2-qter	68579063	146364022	77.48
	1	X	p22.33	0	3454962	3.45
26	3	8	complete	0	146364022	146.36
	3	11	q13.4	72283371	72418939	0.14
	1	12	p13.33	1027361	1134264	0.11
33	1	7	q21.11-qter	82589142	159119708	76.53
	3	4	q27-qter	123059206	191020138	67.96
	3	8	q12.3-qter	65285149	146364022	81.08
40	1	7	q31.32-qter	121167520	159138663	37.97
	3	8	q12.3-qter	65108706	146364022	81.26
46	1	5	q21.3-qter	107659808	180915260	73.26
	3	8	q12.3-qter	63759284	146364022	82.6
47	1	7	q33-qter	137199691	159138663	21.94
	3	8	q13.2-qter	68825854	146364022	77.54
CNA in t(15;17) breakpoints						
7	3	15	q24.1	74168174	74304138	0.14
20	1	15	q24.1	74691249	75117832	0.43
	1	17	q12	37959105	38079219	0.12
	3	21	q22.13–q22.2	39661746	39772776	0.11
32	1	17	pter-p11.2	0	19050914	19.05
	1	Y	complete	0	59373566	59.37
	3	15	q24.1-qter	74326556	102459244	28.13
	3	17	p11.2–q21.2	19093472	38477259	19.38
36	3	8	complete	0	146364022	146.36
	3	13	complete	0	115169878	115.17
	3	15	q24.1	74145053	74314995	0.17
	3	17	q21.2	38505591	38673928	0.17
Others						
3	1	16	p12.1	24507155	24661476	0.15
9	1	1	q24.2	167718498	168149489	0.43
10	1	4	q24	105743315	105897864	0.15
13	1	12	pter-p12.3	0	18489408	18.49
	3	13	q31.1-qter	85060629	115169878	30.11
21	1	17	q25.3	76335284	76796083	0.46
22	3	4	q21.3	87551324	87700668	149.34
25	1	6	p25.1-p22.3	5544745	15635655	10.09
	1	15	q11.2-q12	23641501	27343875	3.7
28	CN-LOH	11	p15.5-p12	198509	42278838	42.08
29	1	3	p24.2	24782029	28427029	3.65
	1	3	p22.3	34388000	35859690	1.47
	1	13	q14.11	40282116	40786721	0.5
	1	13	q33.2-q33.3	105672486	109302864	3.63
	1	13	q33.3	109671057	109798831	0.13

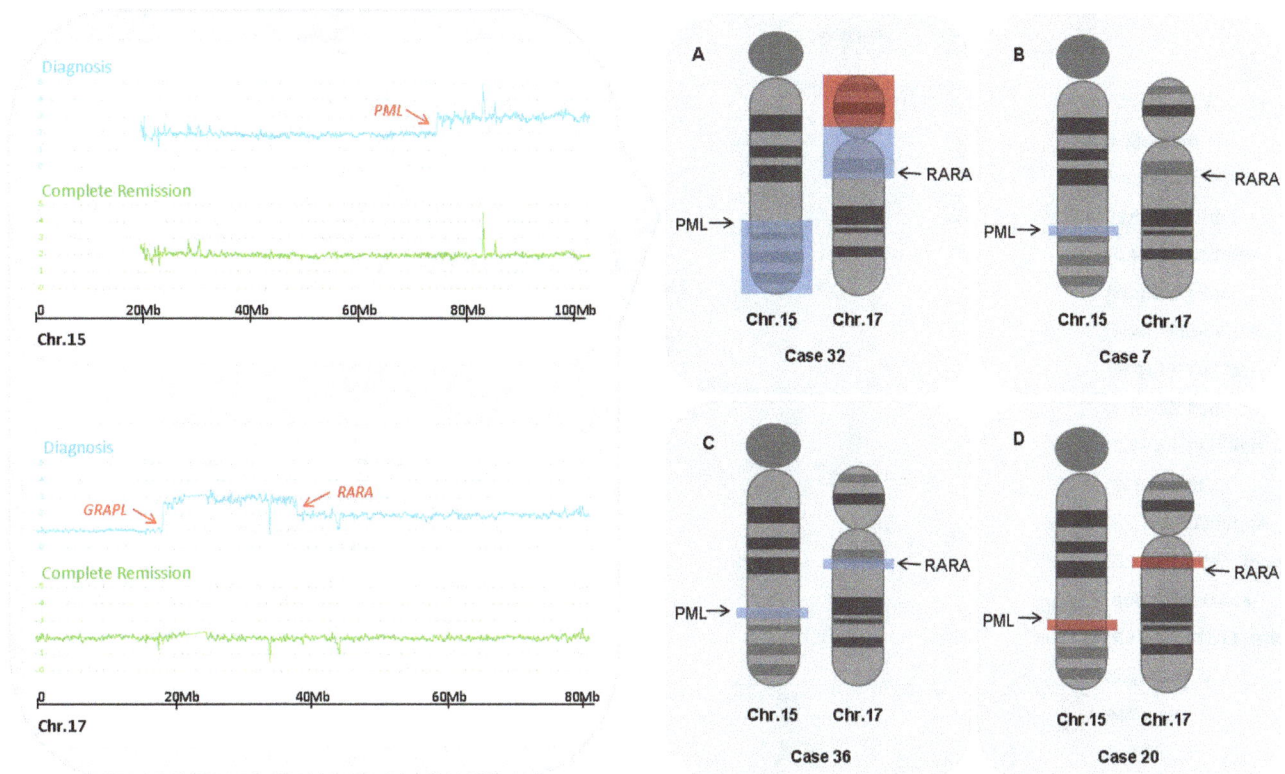

Figure 2. Schematic representation of CNA adjacent to the translocation breakpoints found in our series. On the left panel, the Smooth Signal of chromosome 15 and 17 from case APL_32 are represented. Results from diagnosis sample are shown in blue and from complete remission sample, in green. On the right, chromosomes 15 and 17 are depicted with G-banding and arrows pointing the location of the *PML* and *RARA* genes. Areas shaded in blue show regions duplicated and in red, deleted. Panel (A) corresponds to isochromosome der(17)t(15;17); Panel (B) shows a small duplication of the *PML* gene, and in panel (C) both the *PML* and the *RARA* genes are duplicated. These two cases had a cryptic t(15;17) by CC, that was revealed by FISH. In panel (D) two small deletions are found distally to the translocation breakpoints.

and 0.5 Mb centromeric to *RARA*. In case APL_32, the SNP-A showed two large amplifications adjacent to the *PML* and the *RARA* gene and, additionally, a heterozygous partial deletion of 17p contiguous to the amplification. The breakpoint was in the coding region of *GRAPL* gene instead of the centromere. This event corresponds to an isochromosome of the derivative chromosome 17 of the translocation t(15;17) [ider(17)(q10)t(15;17)], which is occasionally seen in some APL cases by conventional cytogenetics. We could not confirm it in this case because no evaluable metaphases were obtained. In case APL_36, two small amplifications were found involving the *PML* and the *RARA* genes, and in case APL_7, a small amplification included part of the coding region of the *PML* gene. These 2 cases were among the 5 patients with cryptic translocation by conventional cytogenetics of our series.

Except for the 3 patients that had del(7q) and +8/8q concomitantly, no other association with clinical or biologic variables was observed. Conventional cytogenetics and *FLT3* mutation analysis revealed a secondary event to t(15;17) in 16 cases (33%). SNP-A uncovered cryptic additional abnormalities in 15 additional cases (31%). One third of cases still had no known secondary event (Figure 3). Patients carrying *FLT3-ITD* mutations had less frequently SNP-A anomalies (32% of mutations in patients without CNA *vs.* 4% in patients with at least one CNA; *P* = .016).

Comparison with other series

The analysis of the type, size and number of lesions in each series is shown in Table 3. The series of Nowak *et al.* had fewer cases without CNA (17% in Nowak's series *vs.* 52%, 65% and 60% in our series, TCGA' and Akagi's series, respectively; *P*.001 in all three pairwise comparisons) and more abnormalities per case (median of 2 abnormalities in Nowak's series *vs.* 0 in all other report; *P*<.001 in all three pairwise comparisons). They also reported more deletions than duplications (65% of deletions in Nowak's series *vs.* 50% in this report and 29% in Akagi's series; *P* = .027 and .002, respectively) and a smaller size of each lesion (median size of 0.19 Mb *vs.* 18.77 Mb, 9.53 Mb and 45.11 Mb in this report, TCGA' and Akagi's series; *P*<.001, = .018 and <.001, respectively). Akagi *et al.* reported more CN-LOH (21% of CN-LOH *vs.* 2% and 3% in this report and Nowak's series; *P* = .009 and <.001, respectively).

The common deleted region (CDR) or the common gained region (CGR) of the CNA found in our series were delineated taking into account the boundaries reported by us and the other APL series (Table 4). Many CDR/CGR harbored well-known genes implicated in leukemia, such as *MYC*, *NF1*, *TP53* or *EZH2*. In every series, CGR 8(q24) was, by far, the most frequent abnormality (ranging from 10% to 25%), followed by CDR 7(q33-qter) (ranging from 2% to 6%). The remaining CDR/CGR were present in a lower frequency (≤3% of patients). One third (n = 68 out of 208) of the whole cohort carried at least one of the recurrent CDR/CGR. Most of the abnormalities found in our series (70%;

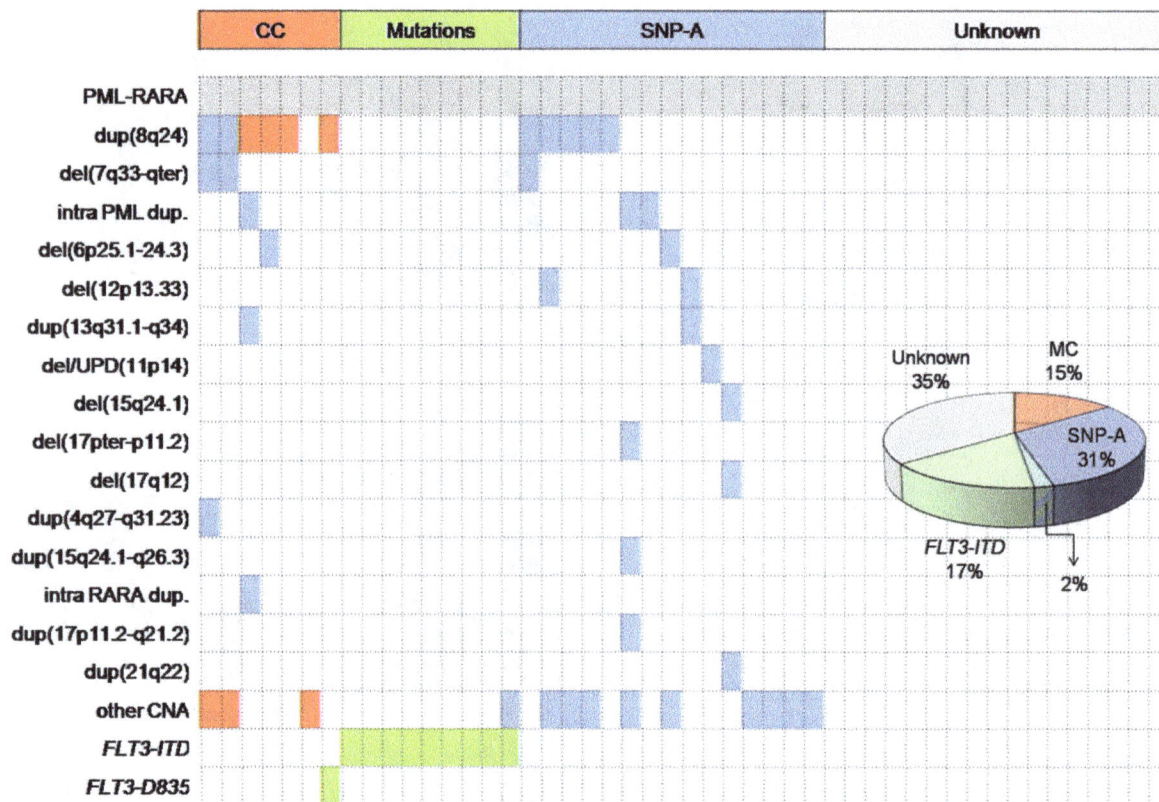

Figure 3. Heatmap and pie chart depicting abnormalities found in our series in addition to the t(15;17). Each column represents one patient. Abnormalities are listed in the Y axis and coloured in the corresponding row of the heatmap. Abnormalities detected by Conventional Cytogenetics (CC) (red) and *FLT3* mutations (green) are frequent events; however, SNP-A revealed an important proportion of patients with potentially leukemogeneic abnormalities (blue). Dup: duplication: del: deletion; CNA: copy-number abnormality.

n = 32) were recurrent in the other series, and the remaining CNA were known abnormalities in myeloid neoplasms, such as 5q- and −Y.

Two patterns of CNAs adjacent to the t(15;17) breakpoints were found recurrently. The first one was the pattern corresponding to ider(17)(q10)t(15;17) (5 cases, 2%). The breakpoint leading to deletion of 17p was found within the coding region of the *GRAPL* gene, the *GRAP* gene, or even more centromeric. The second recurrent pattern was the duplication of the *PML* locus without reciprocal duplication of the *RARA* locus, (5 cases, 2%).

We observed again that CGR 8(q24) and CDR 7(q33-qter) appeared concomitantly [80% of deletions in 7(q33-qter)] in patients with dup(8q24) *vs.* 18% in patients without dup(8q24); P <.001].

Correlation with clinical data

No single CNA showed an association with clinical variables or a prognostic impact in terms of OS and RFS, as was also the case of those cases with cryptic CNA that were not observed by conventional cytogenetics, and those with 0, 1 or ≥2 CNAs revealed by SNP-A.

We analyzed next every recurrent CDR/CGR in the series with available survival data. All three series had independent similar OS and RFS. No recurrent CDR/CGR showed a prognostic value; however, patients who carried ≥1 recurrent CDR/CGR showed a shorter 3-year OS (86% *vs.* 75%; P = .05), and RFS (90% *vs.* 78% in patients having 0 *vs.* ≥1 recurrent lesion; P = .05) (Figure S2 in Appendix S1).

Discussion

This study shows that high-resolution SNP-A analysis reveals ACA in roughly half the patients with APL (48%). Most of them (90%) had not been properly detected by conventional cytogenetics. Systematic use of matched diagnosis and molecular remission sample in every single case has allowed us to ascertain the somatic nature of these lesions. Moreover, the majority of them were recurrent (70%) but of low frequency (≤3%), and accounted for a secondary event in up to 40% of APL cases with no ACA by conventional cytogenetics.

Our analysis showed a low burden of CNA in our series, which is in line with previous reports of core-binding factor acute myeloid leukemia (AML),[10] and even lower than AML of any kind,[11] suggesting that few additional lesions are needed in this type of leukemias. These findings differ widely from the results reported by Nowak *et al.*,[3] where they found three times more lesions per case and with a much smaller size. It could be possible that these differences are due to the lack of systematic use of germline sample and assumption of some CNV as somatic when not reported in public CNV databases.

Among the SNP-A abnormalities, +8/8q was the most frequent in our series and the other reports.[2,3] Trisomy 8 is known to be the most frequent chromosomal abnormality in APL [5] and very common in myeloid neoplasms. However, SNP-A analysis allowed for a three-fold detection of duplications in chromosome 8 in our series. Of note, the CGR had a size of 9.5Mb and comprised few genes, including *MYC* as the most probable candidate gene, which has been shown to be deregulated and amplified in several types of

Table 3. Comparison of type, size and number of SNP-A abnormalities in reported APL series.

	Akagi *et al.*	TCGA	Nowak *et al.*	This Report
Number of patients	**n = 47**	**n = 20**	**n = 93**	**n = 48**
Array type	50 k & 250 K	SNP 6.0	SNP 6.0	SNP 6.0
Use of germline sample	7 (15%)	0 (0%)	3 (3%)	48 (100%)
Patient's abnormalities				
No CNA	28 (60%)	13 (65%)	16 (17%)	25 (52%)
Trisomy 8/8q+	8 (17%)	2 (10%)	25 (27%)	11 (23%)
Others	11 (23%)	5 (25%)	52 (56%)	12 (25%)
CNA types				
Duplications	17 (50%)	7 (54%)	83 (32%)	22 (48%)
Deletions	10 (29%)	6 (46%)	171 (65%)	23 (50%)
CN-LOH	7 (21%)	1 (5%)*	7 (3%)	1 (2%)
Total	34 (100%)	13 (100%)	261 (100%)	46 (100%)
CNA per case				
median	0	0	2	0
media	0.72	0.75	2.78	0.96
range	0–4	0–4	0–14	0–5
Size (Mb)				
median	45.11	9.53	0.19	18.77
media	55.06	25.65	16.38	41.72
range	0.02–146.36	0.13–146.36	0.001–191.15	0.11–146.36

*one Uniparental Tetrasomy has been included both in duplication and CN-LOH group.
CNA: Copy-Number Abnormality. CN-LOH: Copy-Neutral Loss of Heterozygocity.

leukemias and lymphomas.[12,13] The second most recurrent abnormality was del(7q), which appeared in association with dup(8q24), both common CNA in myeloid neoplasms. Regarding CN-LOH, most series of APL and other translocation-associated leukemias have reported a very low rate (<5%),[3,10,14] which is in line with our findings and suggest a very low frequency of this event in APL.

CNA in the boundaries of t(15;17) breakpoints were disclosed in some patients. This also occurs in other supposedly balanced translocations in an even higher frequency (around 25% of core binding factor AML and 10% in CML).[10,14] Two patterns seemed to be recurrent: the first one corresponded to an isochromosome derivative of chromosome 17(t15;17). Isochromosome 17q [i(17q)] is not monocentric but a dicentric chromosome. It has a breakpoint cluster region located at 17p11.2, which is a genetically unstable region that contains multiple low-copy repeats and segmental duplications.[15] We located the breakpoint region at the *GRAPL* gene. Other authors have located the breakpoint at the *GRAP* gene [3] or more centromeric in a non-coding region,[2] but all of them are within this breakpoint cluster region. This region has shown susceptibility to rearrangement and explains the relative high frequency of i(17q) in hematologic and non-hematologic cancers, as well as deletions in this area in Smith-Magenis syndrome.[15,16] The fact that the i(17q) harbours the t(15;17) indicates that the i(17q) occurs as a secondary event, that in addition will produce an extra RARA-PML transcript.[17]

Cases with duplication of the *PML* gene were recurrent, and also similar cases have been reported before.[18] It is interesting that some of these cases had a cryptic t(15;17) according to conventional cytogenetics. APL cases with cryptic t(15;17) may be due to small interstitial insertions of *PML* or *RARA* genes one

beside the other [19] or even ectopic to the natural gene loci. [18,20,21] Small deletions very close to the translocated genes have been reported in 10-30% of patients with CBF-AML [t(8;21) and inv(16)] and CML [t(9;22)], usually involving the translocated genes.[10,14] Less frequently (~1%), some cases have been described in such leukemias with deletions located in more telomeric or centromeric regions from the translocated gene, [10,14] resembling our case APL_20. The study of such cases with imbalanced translocations may help to elucidate the mechanisms that give rise to the t(15;17).

The parallel study of *FLT3-ITD* mutations and CNA by SNP-A showed a mutually exclusive association of these events. This is in agreement with previous studies [2] and supports the hypothesis that tyrosin kinase activation through *FLT3-ITD* mutations is a sufficient cooperating event to produce APL and therefore, other genomic aberrations such as CNAs are not needed. In our series, *FLT3* mutations and conventional cytogenetics revealed an additional abnormality in one third of patients. Interestingly, SNP-A analysis uncovered one additional third of patients from this cohort that carried acquired CNA/CN-LOH in the leukemic blasts. Most of those abnormalities were infrequent (≤3% of patients) but recurrent, indicating a role of these lesions in the development of APL and therefore the capability of high-resolution SNP-A karyotype to reveal hidden leukemogenic events. The majority of these recurrent CNAs and also some non-recurrent are well-known abnormalities in myeloid neoplasms. This suggests that additional events which occur after the t(15;17) are not necessarily exclusive of APL, but common with acute myeloid leukemia and other hematologic neoplasms. Likewise, these facts highlight the wide degree of heterogeneity seen in the cooperating events that contribute to APL.

Table 4. Minimal deleted or gained regions found in APL series, their frequency and the genes included in each region.

Minimal deleted region (MDR)	Proximal	Distal	Size (Mb)	Akagi et al. (n = 47)	TCGA (n = 20)	Nowak et al. (n = 93)	This Report (n = 48)	Total n = 208	Genes
del(6p25.1–24.3)	5600438	7409514	1,81	1 (2%)	0	0	2 (4%)	3 (1%)	*FARS2, NRN1, F13A1, LY86, RREB1, CAGE1.*
del(6p24.1)	12278913	13386241	1,11	0	0	1 (1%)	1 (1%)	2 (1%)	*EDN1, PHACTR1, TBC1D7, GF0D1.*
del(7q33-qter)	137199691	158861884	21,66	1 (2%)	1 (5%)	5 (5%)	3 (6%)	10 (5%)	several genes including *LUC7L2, EZH2.*
del/UPD(11p14)	22936456	30671304	7,73	3 (6%)	1 (5%)	0	1 (1%)	5 (2%)	*LUZP2, ANO3, MUC15, SLC5A12, BBPX1, CCDC34, LGR4, LIN7C, BDNF, METTL15, KCNA4, FSHB, MPPED2.*
del(12p13.33)	1027361	1134264	0,11	0	0	0	2 (4%)	2 (1%)	*RAD52, ERC1.*
del(15q24.1)	74691249	75117832	0,43	0	0	1 (1%)	1 (1%)	2 (1%)	*SEMA7A, UBL7, ARID3B, CLK3, EDC3, CYP1A1, CSK, LMAN1L.*
del(17pter-p11.2)	0	18935523	18,94	1 (2%)	0	3 (3%)	1 (1%)	5 (2%)	several genes including *TP53.*
del(17q12)	37959105	38079219	0,12	0	0	1 (1%)	1 (1%)	2 (1%)	*IKZF3, GSDMB, ZPBP2, ORMDL3.*
Minimal gained region (MGR)									
dup(4q27–q31.23)	123059206	150420462	27,36	0	0	5 (5%)	1 (1%)	6 (3%)	several genes.
dup(8q24)	122538604	132023578	9,48	8 (17%)	2 (10%)	23 (25%)	11 (23%)	44 (21%)	several genes including *MYC.*
dup(13q31.1–q34)	85060629	115108397	30,05	1 (2%)	0	1 (1%)	2 (4%)	4 (2%)	several genes.
dup(15q24.1) intra *PML*	74262253	74304138	0,04	0	0	4 (4%)	2 (4%)	6 (3%)	*PML.*
dup(15q24.1–q26.3)	74326556	102364660	28,04	2 (4%)	0	3 (3%)	1 (1%)	6 (3%)	several genes including *PML.*
dup(17q21.2) intra *RARA*	38505591	38673928	0,17	0	0	1 (1%)	1 (1%)	2 (1%)	*RARA.*
dup(17p11.2–q21.2)	21550542	38477259	16,93	1 (2%)	0	3 (3%)	1 (1%)	5 (2%)	several genes including *NF1, RARA*
dup(21q22)	39661746	39772776	0,11	2 (4%)	0	1 (1%)	1 (1%)	5 (2%)	*KCNJ15, ERC.*

Still another third of patients had neither *FLT3* mutations nor ACA. Probably, more advanced technologies such as next-generation sequencing will help to elucidate the abnormalities acquired in these cases.

No independent association with prognosis could be established for any recurrent CNA, although we are aware of the small size of our series for this type of analysis. Even the most frequent CNA, dup(8q24), that has been assigned a prognostic value in certain hematologic neoplasms,[22,23] was not related to the patient's outcome, as was also the case in previous reports of APL.[3,5] However, patients who lacked an available remission sample, such as those who died before achieving complete remission, were not included in this study. This last fact may constitute a selection bias.

Carrying one or more CDR/CGR showed a trend towards a worse prognosis, although our cohort was heterogeneous for survival analysis and besides, multivariate analysis could not be performed. More solid evidence will therefore be required to confirm this finding. However, it is true that similar results have been reported before in other hematologic neoplasms [24-26] revealing that the more lesions in the cell's genome, the more complexity and poorer prognosis the disease has.

In summary, these data demonstrate an acquired lesion in leukemic blasts in 40% of patients with no ACA by conventional cytogenetics. The low frequency and recurrence of these ACA indicate the broad spectrum of abnormalities that can occur after

the t(15;17) and are required for the leukemic transformation. Whether this picture can be fully explained using more comprehensive technology remains to be seen.

Supporting Information

Appendix S1 Supporting Information file. Table S1. Lesions found in the 20 APL cases of the TCGA cohort. Figure S1. Graphic representation of the size and type of Copy Number Abnormalities (CNA) in our series. Figure S2. Survival curves of the reported APL series according to the number of CDR/CGR.

Acknowledgments

We would like to thank Ana Martín, Elena Bellmunt and Raquel Amigó from "Biobank La Fe" for their help in sample processing and supply. We also thank the TCGA Research Network for access to the SNP-A results and associated clinical data described in the text.

Author Contributions

Conceived and designed the experiments: IGS DSI JC MAS. Performed the experiments: IGS DSI EB IM. Analyzed the data: IGS DSI ES. Contributed reagents/materials/analysis tools: IL MLP MI ML SD OF PM CS CC BB. Wrote the paper: IGS EV CA JC MAS.

References

1. O'Keefe C, McDevitt MA, Maciejewski JP (2010) Copy neutral loss of heterozygosity: a novel chromosomal lesion in myeloid malignancies. Blood 115: 2731–2739.
2. Akagi T, Shih LY, Kato M, Kawamata N, Yamamoto G, et al. (2009) Hidden abnormalities and novel classification of t(15;17) acute promyelocytic leukemia (APL) based on genomic alterations. Blood 113: 1741–1748.
3. Nowak D, Klaumuenzer M, Hanfstein B, Mossner M, Nolte F, et al. (2012) SNP array analysis of acute promyelocytic leukemia may be of prognostic relevance and identifies a potential high risk group with recurrent deletions on chromosomal subband 1q31.3. Genes Chromosomes Cancer 51: 756–767.
4. Heinrichs S, Li C, Look AT (2010) SNP array analysis in hematologic malignancies: avoiding false discoveries. Blood 115: 4157–4161.
5. Cervera J, Montesinos P, Hernandez-Rivas JM, Calasanz MJ, Aventin A, et al. (2010) Additional chromosome abnormalities in patients with acute promyelocytic leukemia treated with all-trans retinoic acid and chemotherapy. Haematologica 95: 424–431.
6. Hernandez JM, Martin G, Gutierrez NC, Cervera J, Ferro MT, et al. (2001) Additional cytogenetic changes do not influence the outcome of patients with newly diagnosed acute promyelocytic leukemia treated with an ATRA plus anthracyclin based protocol. A report of the Spanish group PETHEMA. Haematologica 86: 807–813.
7. Barragan E, Montesinos P, Camos M, Gonzalez M, Calasanz MJ, et al. (2011) Prognostic value of FLT3 mutations in patients with acute promyelocytic leukemia treated with all-trans retinoic acid and anthracycline monochemotherapy. Haematologica 96: 1470–1477.
8. Sanz MA, Martín G, González M, León A, Rayón C, et al. (2004) Risk-adapted treatment of acute promyelocytic leukemia with all-trans-retinoic acid and anthracycline monochemotherapy: a multicenter study by the PETHEMA group. Blood 103: 1237–1243.
9. Sanz MA, Montesinos P, Rayón C, Holowiecka A, de la Serna J, et al. (2010) Risk-adapted treatment of acute promyelocytic leukemia based on all-trans retinoic acid and anthracycline with addition of cytarabine in consolidation therapy for high-risk patients: further improvements in treatment outcome. Blood 115: 5137–5146.
10. Kuhn MW, Radtke I, Bullinger L, Goorha S, Cheng J, et al. (2012) High-resolution genomic profiling of adult and pediatric core-binding factor acute myeloid leukemia reveals new recurrent genomic alterations. Blood 119: e67–75.
11. Walter MJ, Payton JE, Ries RE, Shannon WD, Deshmukh H, et al. (2009) Acquired copy number alterations in adult acute myeloid leukemia genomes. Proc Natl Acad Sci U S A 106: 12950–12955.
12. Delgado MD, Albajar M, Gomez-Casares MT, Batlle A, Leon J (2013) MYC oncogene in myeloid neoplasias. Clin Transl Oncol 15: 87–94.
13. Slack GW, Gascoyne RD (2011) MYC and aggressive B-cell lymphomas. Adv Anat Pathol 18: 219–228.
14. Huh J, Jung CW, Kim JW, Kim HJ, Kim SH, et al. (2011) Genome-wide high density single-nucleotide polymorphism array-based karyotyping improves

detection of clonal aberrations including der(9) deletion, but does not predict treatment outcomes after imatinib therapy in chronic myeloid leukemia. Ann Hematol 90: 1255–1264.
15. Barbouti A, Stankiewicz P, Nusbaum C, Cuomo C, Cook A, et al. (2004) The breakpoint region of the most common isochromosome, i(17q), in human neoplasia is characterized by a complex genomic architecture with large, palindromic, low-copy repeats. Am J Hum Genet 74: 1–10.
16. Chen KS, Manian P, Koeuth T, Potocki L, Zhao Q, et al. (1997) Homologous recombination of a flanking repeat gene cluster is a mechanism for a common contiguous gene deletion syndrome. Nat Genet 17: 154–163.
17. Manola KN, Karakosta M, Sambani C, Terzoudi G, Pagoni M, et al. (2010) Isochromosome der(17)(q10)t(15;17) in acute promyelocytic leukemia resulting in an additional copy of the RARA-PML fusion gene: report of \ases and review of the literature. Acta Haematol 123: 162–170.
18. Koshy J, Qian YW, Bhagwath G, Willis M, Kelley TW, et al. (2012) Microarray, gene sequencing, and reverse transcriptase-polymerase chain reaction analyses of a cryptic PML-RARA translocation. Cancer Genet 205: 537–540.
19. Goldschmidt N, Yehuda-Gafni O, Abeliovich D, Slyusarevsky E, Rund D (2010) Interstitial insertion of RARalpha gene into PML gene in a patient with acute promyelocytic leukemia (APL) lacking the classic t(15;17). Hematology 15: 332–337.
20. Haraguchi K, Ohno N, Tokunaga M, Itoyama T, Gotoh M, et al. (2009) Masked t(15;17) APL with the insertion of PML-RARalpha fusion gene in 4q21. Leuk Res 33: 1552–1555.
21. Garcia-Casado Z, Cervera J, Valencia A, Pajuelo JC, Mena-Duran AV, et al. (2006) A t(17;20)(q21;q12) masking a variant t(15;17)(q22;q21) in a patient with acute promyelocytic leukemia. Cancer Genet Cytogenet 168: 73–76.
22. Such E, Cervera J, Costa D, Solé F, Vallespí T, et al. (2011) Cytogenetic risk stratification in chronic myelomonocytic leukemia. Haematologica 96: 375–383.
23. Greenberg PL, Tuechler H, Schanz J, Sanz G, Garcia-Manero G, et al. (2012) Revised International Prognostic Scoring System for Myelodysplastic Syndromes. Blood 120: 2454–2465.
24. Parkin B, Erba H, Ouillette P, Roulston D, Purkayastha A, et al. (2010) Acquired genomic copy number aberrations and survival in adult acute myelogenous leukemia. Blood 116: 4958–4967.
25. Tiu RV, Gondek LP, O'Keefe CL, Huh J, Sekeres MA, et al. (2009) New lesions detected by single nucleotide polymorphism array-based chromosomal analysis have important clinical impact in acute myeloid leukemia. J Clin Oncol 27: 5219–5226.
26. Schweighofer CD, Coombes KR, Majewski T, Barron LL, Lerner S, et al. (2013) Genomic Variation by Whole-Genome SNP Mapping Arrays Predicts Time-to-Event Outcome in Patients with Chronic Lymphocytic Leukemia: A Comparison of CLL and HapMap Genotypes. The Journal of molecular diagnostics: JMD 15: 196–209.

12

Pterostilbene Simultaneously Induced G0/G1-Phase Arrest and MAPK-Mediated Mitochondrial-Derived Apoptosis in Human Acute Myeloid Leukemia Cell Lines

Pei-Ching Hsiao[1,2], Ying-Erh Chou[3], Peng Tan[4], Wei-Jiunn Lee[5], Shun-Fa Yang[3,6], Jyh-Ming Chow[7], Hui-Yu Chen[3], Chien-Huang Lin[8], Liang-Ming Lee[5]*, Ming-Hsien Chien[4,9]*

1 School of Medicine, Chung Shan Medical University, Taichung, Taiwan, 2 Department of Internal Medicine, Chung Shan Medical University Hospital, Taichung, Taiwan, 3 Institute of Medicine, Chung Shan Medical University, Taichung, Taiwan, 4 Graduate Institute of Clinical Medicine, Taipei Medical University, Taipei, Taiwan, 5 Department of Urology, Wan Fang Hospital, Taipei Medical University, Taipei, Taiwan, 6 Department of Medical Research, Chung Shan Medical University Hospital, Taichung, Taiwan, 7 Department of Internal Medicine, Wan Fang Hospital, Taipei Medical University, Taipei, Taiwan, 8 Graduate Institute of Medical Sciences, Taipei Medical University, Taipei, Taiwan, 9 Wan Fang Hospital, Taipei Medical University, Taipei, Taiwan

Abstract

Background: Pterostilbene (PTER) is a dimethylated analog of the phenolic phytoalexin, resveratrol, with higher anticancer activity in various tumors. Herein, the molecular mechanisms by which PTER exerts its anticancer effects against acute myeloid leukemia (AML) cells were investigated.

Methodology and Principal Findings: Results showed that PTER suppressed cell proliferation in various AML cell lines. PTER-induced G0/G1-phase arrest occurred when expressions of cyclin D3 and cyclin-dependent kinase (CDK)2/6 were inhibited. PTER-induced cell apoptosis occurred through activation of caspases-8-9/-3, and a mitochondrial membrane permeabilization (MMP)-dependent pathway. Moreover, treatment of HL-60 cells with PTER induced sustained activation of extracellular signal-regulated kinase (ERK)1/2 and c-Jun N-terminal kinase (JNK)1/2, and inhibition of both MAPKs by their specific inhibitors significantly abolished the PTER-induced activation of caspases-8/-9/-3. Of note, PTER-induced cell growth inhibition was only partially reversed by the caspase-3-specific inhibitor, Z-DEVE-FMK, suggesting that this compound may also act through a caspase-independent pathway. Interestingly, we also found that PTER promoted disruption of lysosomal membrane permeabilization (LMP) and release of activated cathepsin B.

Conclusion: Taken together, our results suggest that PTER induced HL-60 cell death via MAPKs-mediated mitochondria apoptosis pathway and loss of LMP might be another cause for cell apoptosis induced by PTER.

Editor: Ferenc Gallyas Jr, University of Pecs Medical School, Hungary

Funding: This study was supported by no. 103 swf03 and 103 TMU-WFH-04 from Wan Fang Hospital-Taipei Medical University. This study was also supported by a grant (CSH-2014-C-020) from Chung Shan Medical University Hospital, Taiwan. The funders had no role in study design, data collection and analysis, decision to publish, or preparation of the manuscript.

Competing Interests: The authors have declared that no competing interests exist.

* Email: mhchien1976@gmail.com (MHC); lm@tmu.edu.tw (LML)

Introduction

Acute myeloid leukemia (AML) is an aggressive malignancy characterized by the rapid growth of abnormal white blood cells (WBCs). AML is primarily treated by chemotherapy, with radiotherapy rarely being applied [1]. Although conventional chemotherapy of AML with either cytarabine or daunorubicin given as a single agent induces complete remission in around 30%~40% of patients, and combination treatment with both agents induces complete remission in more than 50% of patients [2], only 20%~30% of patients enjoy long-term disease-free survival [2], and these chemotherapeutic drugs can also affect normal cells causing unpleasant side effects such as anemia, bleeding, and infection. Thus, there is a need for new agents to treat AML.

Over the years, stilbene-based compounds have attracted the attention of many researchers due to their wide range of biological activities. One of the most relevant and extensively studied stilbenes is resveratrol (RESV), a phytoalexin present in grapes and other foods, which is capable of acting as a cancer chemopreventive agent [3,4]. Indeed, several in vitro and in vivo studies showed that RESV has powerful growth-inhibitory and apoptosis-inducing effects on various solid tumor cells, including colon, breast, prostate, cervical, and pancreatic cancers [5–9]. As to the effects of RESV on non-solid tumors, several studies also indicated that RESV is particularly active in continuous leukemic cells, and it is capable of suppressing the colony-forming cell proliferation of fresh AML marrow cells from patients with AML [10,11]. Despite its promising properties, RESV's rapid metabolism and low bioavailability have precluded its advancement to clinical use [12]. Limitations of RESV prompted our interest in natural and synthetic analogues with improved pharmacokinetics and superior pharmacological potencies that hold greater potential as natural anticancer drugs.

Pterostilbene (PTER) (trans-3,5-dimethoxy-4-hydroxystilbene, Figure. 1A), a natural dimethylated analog of RESV, was proposed to have similar properties as RESV including anticancer, anti-inflammation, antioxidant, apoptosis, antiproliferation, and analgesic potential [13]. Under most circumstances, PTER is either equally or significantly more potent than RESV [14,15]. Most importantly, following equimolar oral dosing in rats, plasma levels of PTER were markedly greater than those of RESV [16]. The greater bioavailability of PTER indicates that PTER could potentially be developed for clinical applications. Indeed, many studies confirmed that PTER exerts antiproliferative and proapoptotic effects in both solid (e.g., lung, gastric, prostate, colon, and breast cancers) [15,17–20] and non-solid tumors (e.g., chronic myelogenous leukemia and lymphoblastic leukemia) [21,22]. However, the mechanisms of PTER activity in cancer cell lines, especially against leukemic cells, have not been fully elucidated.

In this study, we examined the antitumor activities of PTER in five different human AML cell types. Furthermore, we explored the effects of PTER on the mitochondrial and lysosomal apoptotic pathways and cell cycle-related proteins in AML cells.

Materials and Methods

Materials

PTER of 98% purity was purchased from Enzo Life Sciences (Lausen, Switzerland). A 100 mM stock solution of PTER was made in dimethyl sulfoxide (DMSO) (Sigma, St. Louis, MO) and stored at $-20°C$. The final concentration of DMSO for all treatments was <0.5%. Antibodies, specifically of cleaved caspase-3, caspase-8, caspase-9, poly(ADP-ribose) polymerase (PARP), heat shock protein 70 (HSP70), p-extracellular signal-regulated kinase (ERK)1/2, p-p38, p-c-Jun N-terminal kinase (JNK), ERK1/2, p38, JNK1/2, CDK 2, cathepsin B, C23, and β-actin (for the Western blot analysis), were purchased from Santa Cruz Biotechnology (Santa Cruz, CA). Antibodies against cyclin-dependent kinase (CDK)6, p21 Cip1, p27 Kip1, p15 INK4B, and cyclin D3 were purchased from Cell Signaling Technology (Danvers, MA). Anti-cyclin A2 and anti-cyclin E2 antibodies were purchased from Epitomic (Burlingame, CA). 4′-6-Diamidino-2-phenylindole (DAPI) was purchased from Sigma. The p38 mitogen-activated protein kinase (MAPK) inhibitor, SB202190, the ERK1/2 inhibitor, U0126, and the JNK1/2 inhibitors, SP600125 and JNK-IN-8, were purchased from Calbiochem (San Diego, CA). The caspase-3 inhibitor, Z-DEVE-FMK, was purchased from BioVision (Mountain View, CA). Unless otherwise specified, other chemicals used in this study were purchased from Sigma.

Cell Culture

The human MV4-11 HL-60, U937, and THP-1 AML cell lines were purchased from the American Type Culture Collection (Manassas, VA), while the OCI-AML3 cell line was purchased from DSMZ (Braunschweig, Germany). All cell lines were cultured in RPMI 1640 medium supplemented with 10% heat-inactivated fetal bovine serum (FBS; Gibco, Grand Island, NY), 2 mM L-glutamine, 100 U/ml penicillin, and 100 μg/ml streptomycin.

In Vitro Cytotoxicity Assay

AML cells (OCI-AML3, MV4-11, HL-60, U937, and THP-1) were plated in 96-well microtiter plates and treated with various concentrations (0, 12.5, 25, 50, 75, 100, and 150 μM) of PTER for 24 h, and cell viabilities were assessed using an MTS (Promega, Madison, WI) assay. The absorbance (A) was read at 490 nm using an enzyme-linked immunosorbent assay (ELISA) reader (MQX200; Bio-Tek Instruments, Winooski, VT). The cell viability rate (multiple) was determined by the formula: $A_{490, PTER}/A_{490, vehicle}$.

Cell Proliferation Assay

The proliferation of AML cells was measured by directly counting cells with a hemocytometer. Briefly, cells were seeded at a density of 10^5 cells/well in a 12-well culture plate, grown in RPMI containing 10% FBS and then treated with 0.5% DMSO without (control) or with various concentrations of PTER. Medium without or with PTER was changed daily until cells were counted.

Flow Cytometric Analysis

HL-60 cells (2×10^6/ml) were treated with 0.5% DMSO or PTER (0~100 μM) for 24 h. At the end of incubation, cells were collected and fixed with 70% ethanol. Cells were stained with propidium iodide (PI) buffer (4 μg/ml PI, 1% Triton X-100, and 0.5 mg/ml RNase A in phosphate-buffered saline (PBS)) for 30 min in the dark at room temperature and then filtered through a 40-μm nylon filter (Falcon, San Jose, CA). The cell cycle distribution was analyzed for 10,000 collected cells by a FACS Vantage flow cytometer that uses the Cellquest acquisition and analysis program (Becton-Dickinson FACS Calibur, San Jose, CA). The proportion of nuclei in each phase of the cell cycle was determined, and apoptotic cells with hypodiploid DNA content were detected in the sub-G_1 region. All results were obtained from three independent experiments.

Annexin-V/PI Staining Assay

Apoptosis-mediated cell death of tumor cells was examined using a double-staining method with an FITC-labeled Annexin-V/PI Apoptosis Detection kit (BD Biosciences, San Jose, CA). For PI and Annexin-V double-staining, cells were suspended in 100 μl of binding buffer (10 mM HEPES/NaOH, 140 mM NaCl, and 2.5 mM $CaCl_2$ at pH 7.4) and stained with 5 μl of FITC-conjugated Annexin-V and 5 μl of PI (50 μg/ml) for 30 min at room temperature in the dark, and then 400 μl of binding buffer was added. Apoptotic cells were analyzed via flow cytometry, with a FACScan system flow cytometer. Data were acquired and analyzed in a Becton-Dickinson FACS Calibur flow cytometer using Cell Quest software.

DAPI Staining

HL-60 cells were treated with 100 μM PTER for 24 h and were then seeded on a slide via cytospinning. Apoptotic morphological changes were assessed using DAPI staining, as previously described [23].

Western Blot Analysis

Total cell lysates and cytosolic protein extraction were prepared as previously described [24]. Equal amounts of protein extracts (2~0 μ 30 g) were subjected to 10% or 12% sodium dodecylsulfate polyacrylamide gel electrophoresis (SDS-PAGE) and blotted onto polyvinylidene fluoride membranes (Millipore, Belford, MA). After blocking, membranes were incubated with primary antibodies for CDK 2, CDK6, cyclin A2, cyclin D3, cyclin E2, p15 INK4B, p21 Cip1, p27 Kip1, caspases-9, -3, and -8, PARP, HSP70, ERK1/2, p-ERK1/2, p38, p-p38, JNK1/2, p-JNK1/2, cathepsin B, and β-actin. Blots were then incubated with a horseradish peroxidase (HRP)-conjugated anti-mouse or anti-rabbit antibody. Signals were detected via enhanced chemiluminescence using Immobilon Western HRP Substrate (Millipore, Billerica, MA).

Mitochondrial Membrane Potential (MMP) Measurement

Breakdown of the mitochondrial membrane potential was assessed by FACS analyses or epifluorescent microscopy (Zeiss Axioplan) using JC-1 (5,5',6,6'-tetra-chloro-1,1',3,3'-tetra-ethyl-benzimidazol-carbocyanine iodide), which allows detection of changes in the MMP. For this purpose, a Mitochondrial Membrane Potential Detection Kit (Immunochemistry, Bloomington, MN) was used, as described in the manufacturer's instructions. HL60 cells at 10^6 were treated for 24 h with PTER. After PBS washing, cells were incubated for 15 min in freshly prepared JC-1 solution (10 μg/ml in culture medium) at 37°C. Spare dye was removed by PBS washing, and cell-associated fluorescence was measured with FACS and fluorescent microscopy, respectively.

Lysosome Membrane Permeability (LMP) Analysis

Acridine orange (AO) was used to determine changes in LMP [25]. In brief, 10^6 HL60 cells were treated for 12 h with PTER. AO was then added (at a final concentration of 5 μg/ml), and cells were incubated for another 15 min. Cells were washed twice with PBS and examined with an epifluorescence microscope (Zeiss Axioplan). The excitation and emission wavelengths of red fluorescence were 555 and 617 nm and those of green fluorescence were 490 and 528 nm, respectively. A previous study demonstrated that AO concentrated in lysosomes emits granular red fluorescence, whereas AO in the cytosol emits diffuse green fluorescence. Following a change in lysosome permeability, increased diffuse cytosolic green fluorescence can be observed, indicating a relocation of AO from the lysosomes to the cytosol [25].

Measurement of ROS Production

HL-60 cells were treated with PTER for the indicated time; then ROS production was measured by staining with ROS probes (5 μM DCFDA) in RPMI 1640 medium for 30 min. After being washed with PBS or medium, the ROS production of DCFDA-preloaded cells was measured by FACS.

Statistical Analysis

Values are shown as the mean ± standard error (SE). Statistical analyses were performed using the Statistical Package for Social Science software, vers. 16 (SPSS, Chicago, IL). Data comparisons between two groups were performed with Student's t-test. A one-way analysis of variance (ANOVA) followed by Tukey's post-hoc test was used when more than three groups were analyzed. Differences were considered significant at the 95% confidence level when $p < 0.05$.

Results

Effect of PTER on Cell Proliferation of AML Cell Lines

The chemical structure of PTER is shown in Figure 1A. To determine the in vitro efficacy of PTER in AML cells, we treated several AML cell lines with PTER. The cytotoxic effects of PTER were examined in five AML cell lines which represent different French-American-British (FAB) types (M2: HL-60; M4: OCI-AML3; and M5: MV4-11, U937, and THP-1). As shown in Figure 1B, after treatment for 24 h, PTER significantly reduced cell proliferation in a concentration-dependent manner, and 50% growth inhibitory concentration (IC_{50}) values were around 20~80 μM for the five AML cell lines. In these five AML cell lines, HL-60 cells were the most sensitive to PTER treatment (IC_{50}: 23.4 M). We further studied the antiproliferative activity of PTER against HL-60 cells by counting cells. As illustrated in Figure 1C, PTER time- and concentration-dependently decreased the number of cultured HL-60 cells. These results indicated that PTER can potently inhibit the proliferation of different AML FAB types.

PTER Simultaneously Induces HL-60 Cell Apoptosis and Cell Cycle Arrest

Physiological cell death is characterized by apoptotic morphology, including chromatin condensation, membrane blebbing, internucleosomal degradation of DNA, and apoptotic body formation. To investigate the mode of cell death induced by PTER, HL-60 cells were treated with PTER (0~100 μM) for 24 h. It was shown that PTER induced concentration-dependent increases of the sub-G_1 population (Figure 2A). Similarly, as shown in Figure 2B, we assessed the translocation of phosphatidylserine (PS) using Annexin-V and PI double-staining. Apoptotic cells (PI-negative/Annexin-V-positive and PI-positive/Annexin-V-positive) increased from 8.45% to 14.74%, 16.06%, 20.01%, and 33.27% after respectively treating HL-60 cells with 25, 50, 75, and 100 μM PTER. Actually, we can't exclude the possibility that the necrotic cells also involved in PI-positive/Annexin-V-positive populations. Next, the effect of PTER on cell morphology was further examined using fluorescence microscopy. Cells treated with 100 μM PTER for 24 h demonstrated morphologies characteristic of apoptosis, such as chromatin condensation and formation of apoptotic bodies (Figure 2C, arrows). These results are all hallmarks of apoptotic cell death and demonstrated the ability of PTER to induce apoptosis in HL-60 cells. Moreover, the similar effect of PTER on the translocation of PS was also observed in another AML cell line, U937 (Figure S1A in File S1). In addition to apoptosis induction by PTER, we further found another mechanism responsible for the growth inhibition induced by PTER. As shown in Figure 2A, more cells were arrested at the G_0/G_1 phase of the cell-cycle after PTER (50~100 μM) exposure for 24 h (Figure 2A).

Effect of PTER on Alterations of Cell-cycle Regulatory Proteins

To investigate the molecular mechanisms underlying PTER-induced G_0/G_1 arrest, cells were cultured in media supplemented with 10% FBS and 0.5% DMSO without or with PTER (100 μM), and at 24 h, they were harvested for protein extraction and a Western blot analysis. As shown in the Figure 3A and 3B, levels of cyclin D3, CDK2, and CDK6 proteins had significantly decreased in PTER-treated HL-60 cells. Because CDK activity can be controlled by a group of cyclin-dependent kinase inhibitors (CKIs), we examined protein levels of p15 INK4B, p21Cip1, and p27Kip1, three known CKIs, in PTER-treated HL-60 cells. However, levels of p15 INK4B, p21Cip1, and p27Kip1 proteins exhibited no significant change in PTER-treated HL-60 cells compared to DMSO-treated cells (Figure 3C). Moreover, expression of cyclin D3, CDK2, and CDK6 proteins can also be suppressed significantly by lower concentration of PTER (50 μM) in HL-60 cells (Figure 3D).

A

Pterostilbene

B

C

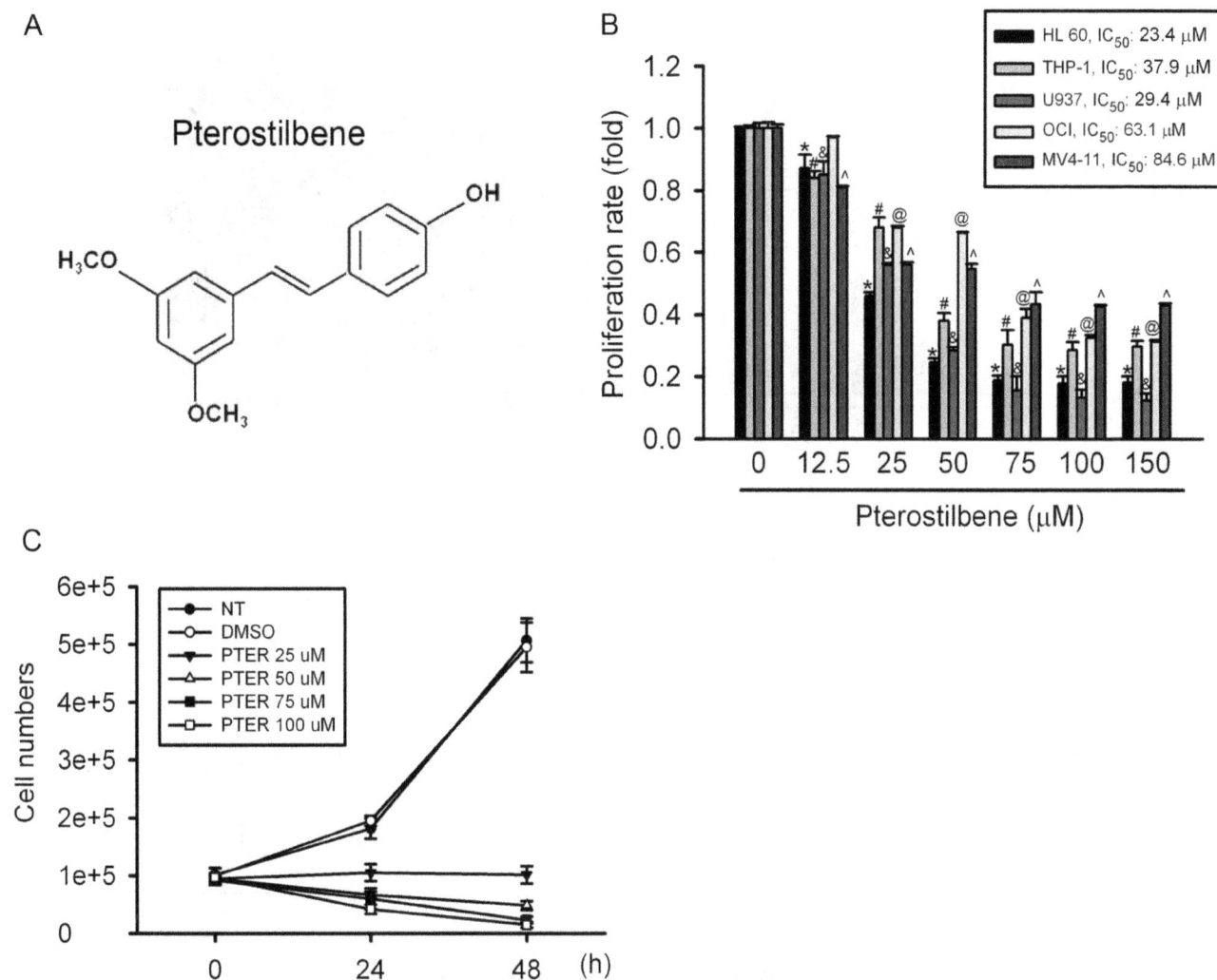

Figure 1. Effect of pterostilbene (PTER) on the cell proliferation of acute myeoloid leukemia (AML) cell lines. (A) The chemical structure of PTER. (B) Five AML cell lines were treated with the vehicle (DMSO) or PTER (12.5~150 μM) in serum-containing medium for 24 h. Cell proliferation was determined by an MTS assay. Results are expressed as multiples of cell proliferation rate. Values represent the mean ± SE of 3 independent experiments. *, #, &, @, ∧ $p < 0.05$, compared to the vehicle groups. (C) HL-60 cells were treated with different concentrations of PTER (0~150 μM) for 24 and 48 h and analyzed by a trypan blue exclusion assay. Quantitative assessment of the mean number of cells is expressed as the mean ± SE.

PTER Induces Caspase Activation and Changes in the MMP in HL-60 Cells

The apoptotic process is executed by a member of the highly conserved caspases, and modulation of the mechanisms of caspase activation and suppression is a critical molecular target in chemoprevention, since these processes lead to apoptosis [26]. To identify the mechanisms underlying PTER-induced apoptosis in HL-60 cells, activation of caspases-8, -9, and -3 and cleavage of PARP were detected. Figure 4A shows that exposure of HL-60 cells to PTER (0~150 μM for 24 h) caused concentration-dependent increases in the activation of caspases-8, -9, and -3, and cleaved PARP. PTER treatment at 50, 100, and 150 μM for 24 h significantly increased expression levels of cleaved PARP by 3.81, 11.83-, and 26.98-fold, respectively, compared to the control (Figure 4B). Moreover, treatment of HL-60 cells with PTER (100 μM) also resulted in a time-dependent increase in activated caspases-8, -9, and -3, with a maximal effect at 24 h (Figure 4C). In addition, the PTER (100 μM)-mediated activation of caspases-8, -9, and -3 was also observed in U937 cells (Figure S1B in File

S1). In order to further explore the significance of caspase activation in PTER-induced apoptosis, a specific inhibitor of executioner caspase-3, Z-DEVE-FMK, was used to suppress the effect of PTER. Pretreatment with Z-DEVE-FMK partially attenuated PTER-induced inhibition of proliferation (Figure 4D), suggesting that PTER-mediated anti-proliferative effect partially occurs through a caspase-dependent apoptosis pathway.

To further detect whether PTER-induced apoptotic cell death involves a mitochondrial pathway, the fluorescent cationic dye, JC-1, was used to detect the mitochondrial permeability transition. Collapse of the MMP is an early step in the induction of apoptosis by the intrinsic pathway [27]. In healthy, non-apoptotic cells, the dye accumulates and aggregates within mitochondria, resulting in bright-red staining. In apoptotic cells, due to the collapse of the membrane potential, JC-1 cannot accumulate within mitochondria and remains in the cytoplasm in its green-fluorescent monomeric form. FACS and immunofluorescence analyses of JC-1-stained HL60 cells treated with PTER for 24 h are shown in Figure 4E and 4F. PTER induced concentration-dependent collapse of the MMP (Figure 4E). Moreover, our results showed

A

C

B

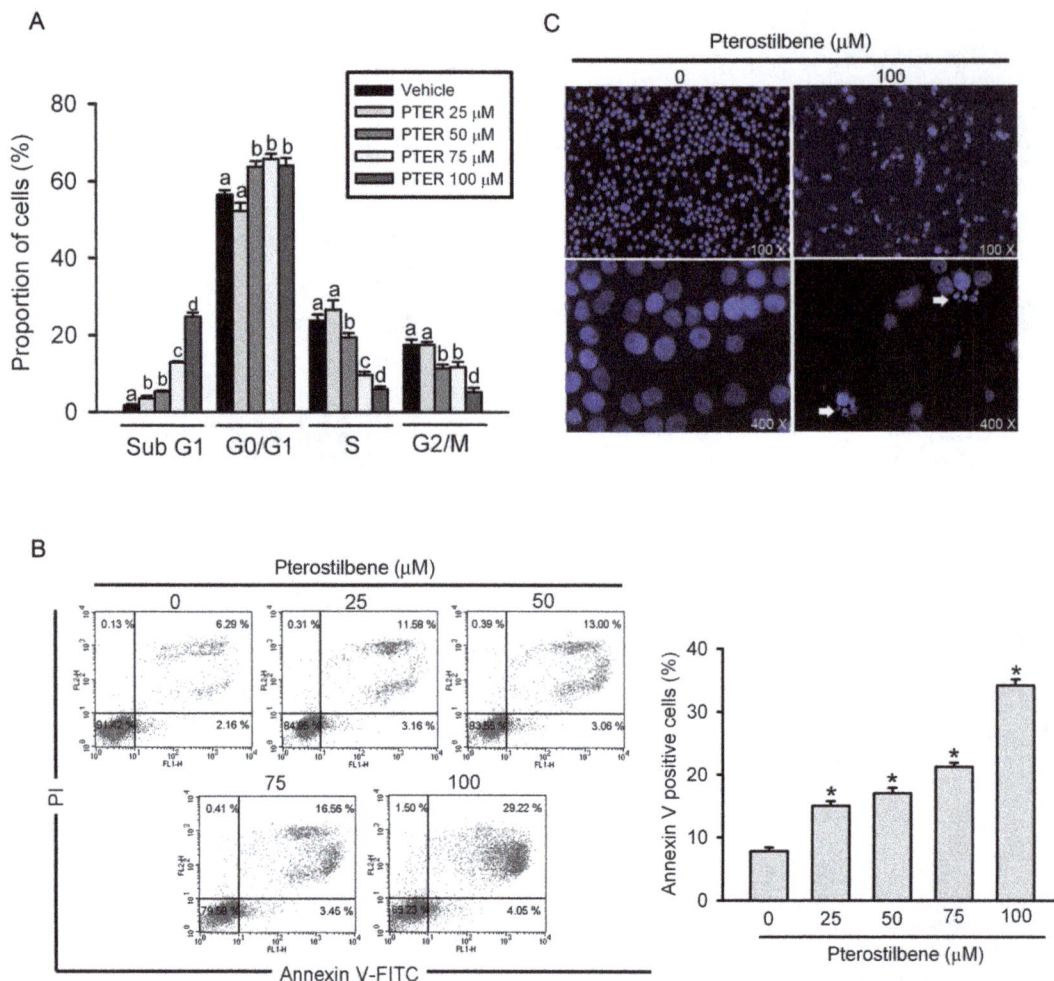

Figure 2. Effect of pterostilbene (PTER) on HL-60 cell-cycle regulation and apoptosis. (A) HL-60 cells were treated with different concentrations of PTER (0~100 μM) for 24 h, and flow cytometry was used to detect the cell cycle phase distribution and cell death in the sub-G$_1$ phase. Data are presented as the mean ± SE of three independent experiments. Results were analyzed using one-way ANOVA with Tukey's post hoc tests at 95% confidence intervals. Different letters represent significantly different, $p<0.05$. (B) Quantitative analysis of cell apoptosis by Annexin-V and propidium iodide (PI) double-staining flow cytometry. Values represent the mean ± SE of three independent experiments. *$p<0.05$, compared to the vehicle group. (C) HL-60 cells were treated with 100 μM PTER for 24 h and analyzed by fluorescence microscopy after DAPI staining. White arrows indicate apoptotic HL-60 cells.

that treatment of cells with PTER in earlier stages (4 and 6 h) also can induce the changes of mitochondrial membrane potential (Figure S2 in File S1).

ERK1/2 and JNK1/2 Are Essential for Caspase-8, -9, and -3 Activation Induced by PTER

Previous studies showed that the MAPK signaling pathway plays an important role in the action of chemotherapeutic drugs [28]. Therefore, we determined whether MAPKs were activated in PTER-treated HL-60 cells, and found that PTER induced activation of JNK1/2 and ERK1/2, but not p38 MAPK in dose-dependent manners (Figure 5A–C). Next, we further investigated relationships among PTER-induced activation of caspases-8, -9, and -3, and MAPKs. HL-60 cells were pretreated with 20 μM U0126 (an ERK inhibitor), SP600125 (a JNK inhibitor), or SB202190 (a p38 inhibitor) for 1 h, treated with 100 μM PTER for another 24 h, and then analyzed by Western blotting. The concentrations of U0126 and SP600125 we used here showed significant inhibitory effects on PTER-induced ERK1/2 and JNK

activation (Figure S3 in File S1). As shown in Figure 5D, both U0126 and SP600125 significantly attenuated PTER-induced caspase-8, -9, and -3 activation. To consider the specificity of SP600125, we further used another selective inhibitor of JNK, JNK-IN-8, and found pretreatment of JNK-IN-8 (1 μM) with HL-60 cells also suppressed PTER-induced caspase-8, -9, and -3 activation obviously (Figure S4 in File S1). Moreover, we also found that JNK1/2 and ERK1/2 activation occurred at earlier time than caspases-8, -9, and -3 activation after PTER treatment (Figure 4C and Figure S5 in File S1). These findings suggest that activation of ERK1/2 and JNK1/2 might play critical roles in PTER-mediated caspases activation in HL-60 cells.

PTER Induces Lysosomal Membrane Alterations

Notably, our results showed that the caspase-3 inhibitor, Z-DEVE-FMK, only partially reversed PTER-induced cell death (Figure 3C). This result suggests that caspase-independent mechanisms might also play a role in PTER-induced cytotoxicity. Lysosomal leakage was described as an inducer of cell death [29], and lysosomal destabilization was shown to be a common

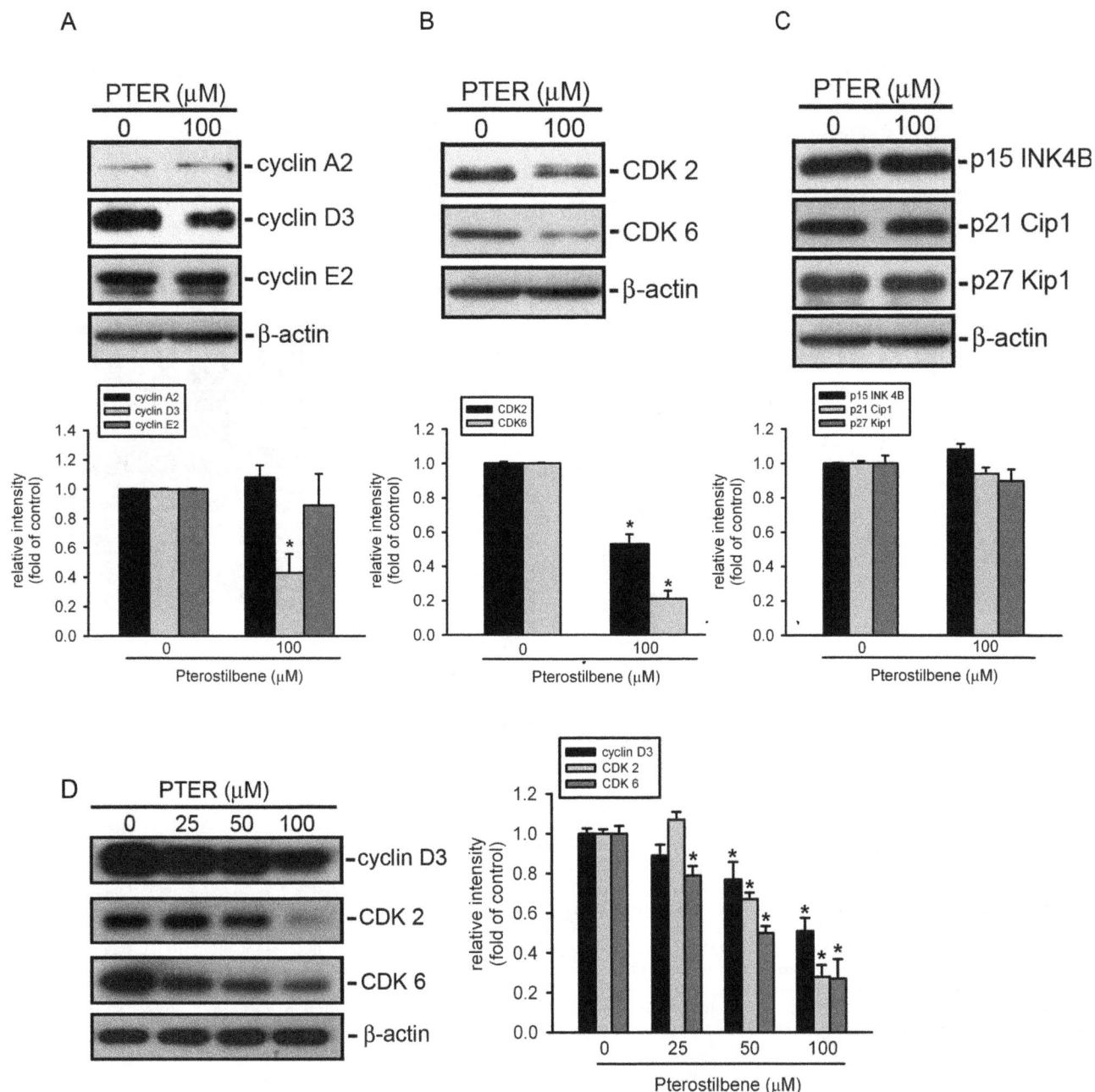

Figure 3. Effect of pterostilbene (PTER) on alterations of cell-cycle regulatory proteins in HL-60 cells. Proteins were extracted from cultured HL-60 cells at 24 h after PTER treatment and probed with proper dilutions of specific antibodies. (A and B) PTER at a concentration of 100 µM induced significant decreases in protein levels of cyclin D3, CDK2, and CDK6. Upper panels: Representative results of cyclins and cyclin-dependent kinase (CDK) protein levels as determined by a Western blot analysis. Lower panels: Quantitative results of cyclin and CDK protein levels, which were adjusted to the β-actin protein level and expressed as multiples of induction beyond its own control. Values are presented as the mean ± SE of three independent experiments. *$p < 0.05$, compared to the vehicle control group. (C) There were no significant differences in protein levels of p15 INK4B, p21 Cip1, or p27 Kip1 between control and PTER-treated HL-60 cells. Upper panel: Representative results of p15, p21, and p27 protein levels as determined by a Western blot analysis. Lower panel: Quantitative results of p15, p21, and p27 protein levels, which were adjusted with the β-actin protein level and expressed as multiples of induction beyond its own control. (D) Cyclin D3, CDK2, and CDK6 peotein expression were downregulated in a concentration-dependent fashion after PTER treatment in HL-60 cells. Left panel: Representative results of cyclin D3, CDK2, and CDK6 protein levels as determined by a Western blot analysis. Right panel: Quantitative results of cyclin D3, CDK2, and CDK6 protein levels, which were adjusted with the β-actin protein level and expressed as multiples of induction beyond its own control. *$p < 0.05$, compared to the vehicle control group.

consequence of microtubule-targeting drugs [30]. Thus, to further elucidate the mechanisms underlying PTER-induced cancer cell death, we studied its possible effects on lysosomes. Lysosomal permeability was examined using AO staining. AO is a metachromatic fluorescent cationic dye that emits red light at high concentrations inside lysosomes, and green light in the cytosol. Following a change in lysosomal permeability, increased diffuse cytosolic green fluorescence can be observed, indicating a

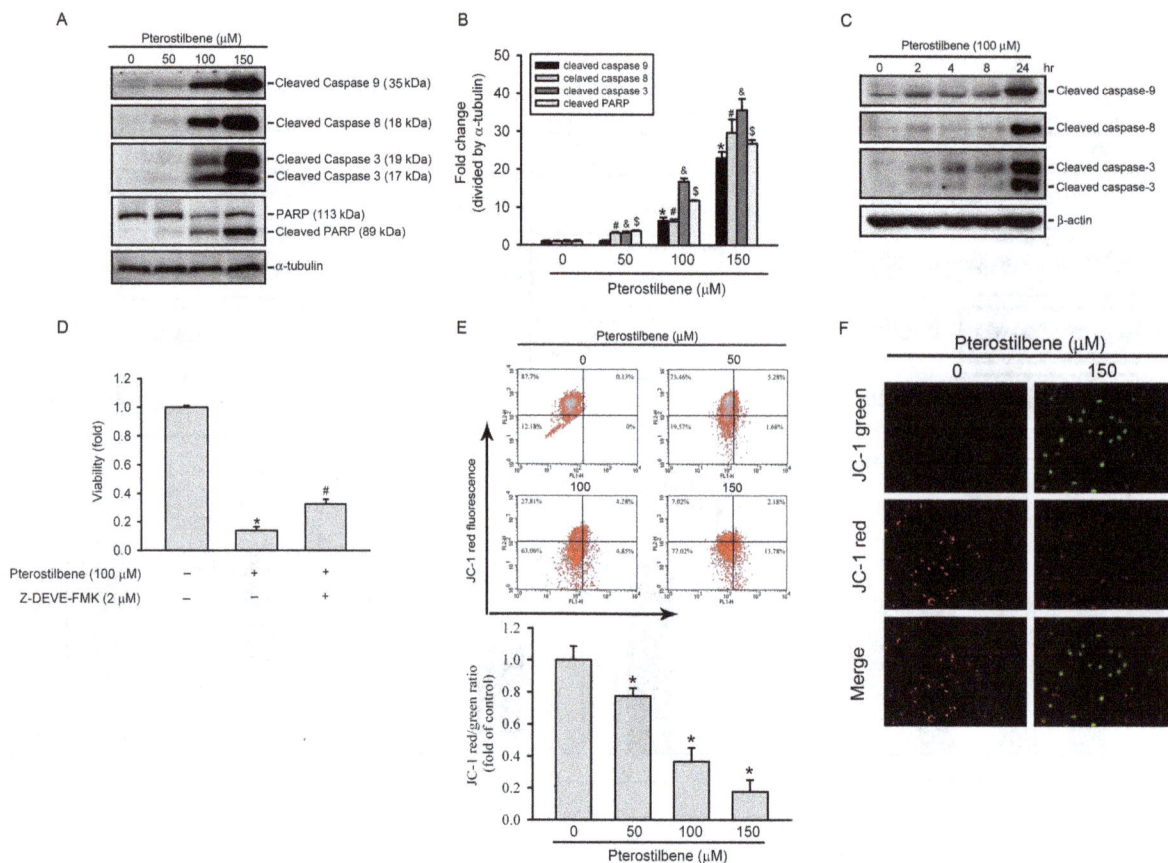

Figure 4. Effect of pterostilbene (PTER) on caspase activation and mitochondrial membrane permeability (MMP) in HL-60 cells. (A) Expression levels of cleaved caspases-3, -8, and -9, and poly (ADP-ribose polymerase (PARP) were assessed by a Western blot analysis after treatment with various concentrations of PTER (0~150 μM) for 24 h. (B) Quantitative results of cleaved caspase-3, -8, and -9, and PARP protein levels, which were adjusted to the α-tubulin protein level and expressed as multiples of induction beyond each respective control. Values are presented as the mean ± SE of three independent experiments. *, #, &, $ $p<0.05$, compared to the vehicle control groups. (C) Activated caspase-9, -8, and -3 protein expression were upregulated in a time-dependent fashion after PTER 100 μM) treatment, peaking at 24 h in HL-60 cells. (D) Effect of a caspase-3 inhibitor on PTER-induced cell death. Cells were treated with 100 μM PTER for 24 h in the presence or absence of 2 μM Z-DEVE-FMK. Cell proliferation was determined by an MTS assay. Data are presented as the mean ± SE of three independent experiments performed in triplicate. *$p<0.05$, control vs. PTER; #$p<0.05$, PTER vs. Z-DEVE-FMK plus PTER. (E and F) Loss of the MMP after 24 h of treatment with PTER as determined by FACS and immunofluorescence analyses of JC-1 staining. (E) From the FACS analysis, increased percentages of green fluorescent apoptotic (FL 1) populations of HL-60 at the indicated drug concentrations (cells in the lower right field) are indicated (upper panel). The red-to-green fluorescence ratio indicates functional mitochondria with membrane potential. Data are presented as the mean ± SE of three independent experiments performed in triplicate. *$p<0.05$, control vs. PTER (F) Immunofluorescence analysis showed that green-fluorescent monomeric form increases in HL-60 cells after treatment with 100 μM PTER for 24 h. Original magnification, 200×.

relocation of AO from lysosomes to the cytosol [25]. As shown in Figure 6A, dramatic increases in the diffuse cytosolic green fluorescence were observed in PTER-treated HL-60 cells. Next, we analyzed the release of lysosomal cathepsin B to the cytosol as a marker of lysosomal membrane permeabilization (LMP). Remarkably, PTER caused a concentration-dependent increase in activated cathepsin B in the cytosol in HL-60 cells after 24 h of PTER treatment (Figure 6B). These results indicated that PTER can induce changes in lysosomal permeability. Several studies reported that reactive oxygen species (ROS) production induces permeabilization of lysosomes [31]. To determine whether ROS are induced by PTER in HL-60 cells, cellular ROS were monitored with the redox-sensitive dyes, H₂DCFDA. Our results showed that in compared to the control group, treatment of cells with 100 μM PTER significantly increased ROS production (Figure 6C). To investigate the role of ROS in PTER-induced lysosomal permeability and cathepsin B release, HL-60 cells were pretreated with the ROS scavenger, NAC. The immunofluores-

cence and Western blot results showed that NAC did not affect PTER-induced lysosomal permeability (Figure 6D) or cathepsin B release to the cytosol (Figure 6E). To further explore the significance of activated cathepsin B release in PTER-induced apoptosis, the cathepsin B-specific inhibitor, CA-074 Me, was used to suppress the effect of PTER. As shown in Figure 6F, PTER induced the same effect in the presence or absence of the cathepsin B inhibitor.

Discussion

AML is a non-solid tumor with high mortality rates, for which novel strategies are needed to improve current treatment standards [2]. To improve clinical outcomes, identification and evaluation of novel therapeutic agents that have less toxicity in normal cells for treatment of AML are important and challenging tasks.

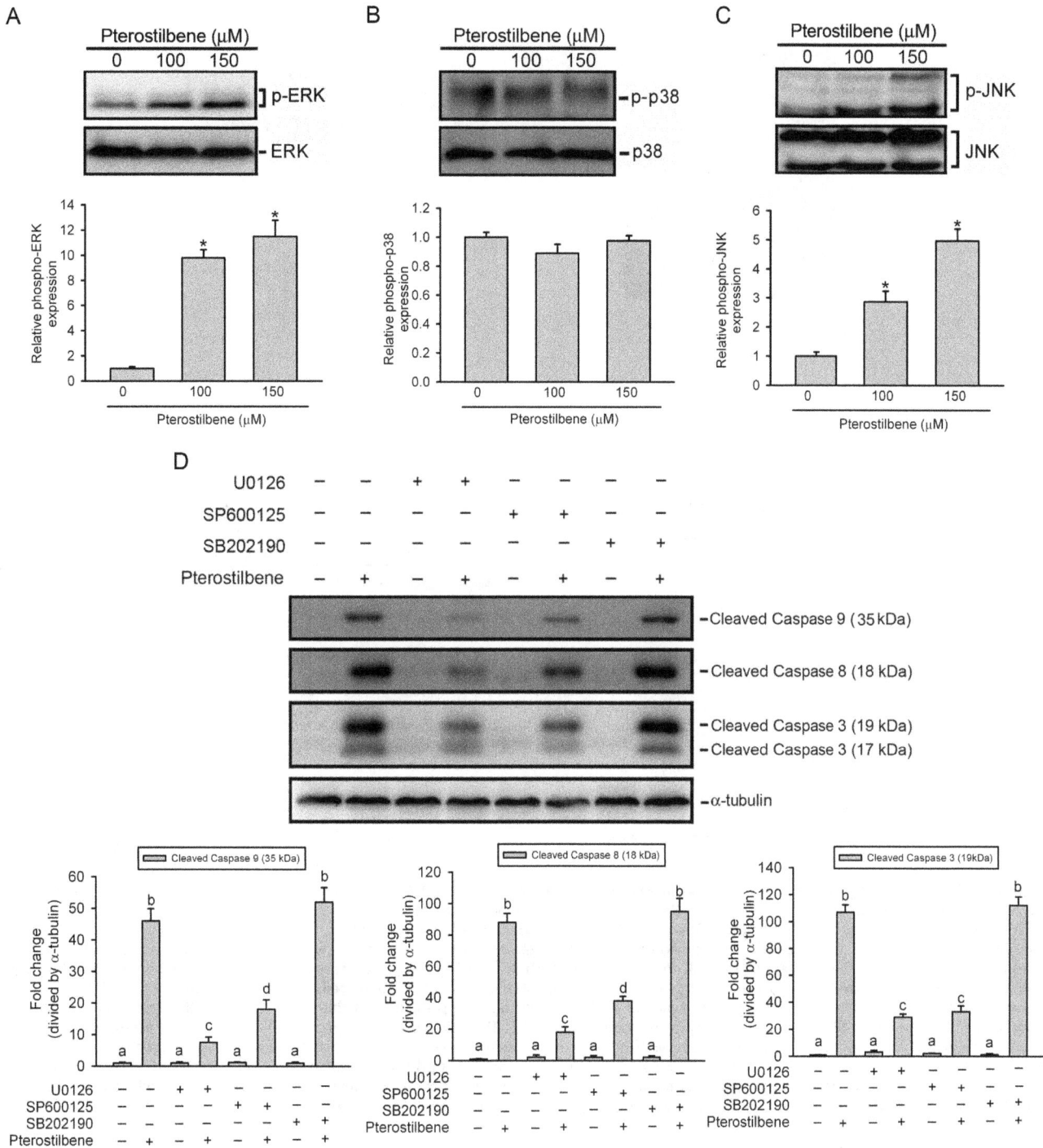

Figure 5. Role of mitogen-activated protein kinase (MAPKs) in pterostilbene (PTER)-induced activation of caspases-8, -9, and -3. (A–C, upper panel) Phosphorylation levels of extracellular signal-regulated kinase (ERK)1/2, p38, and c-Jun N-terminal kinase (JNK)1/2 were assessed by a Western blot analysis after treatment with various concentrations of PTER (0~150 μM M) for 24 h. (A–C, lower panel) Quantitative results of phopho-ERK1/2, p38, and JNK1/2 protein levels, which were adjusted with the total ERK1/2, p38, and JNK1/2 protein levels and expressed as multiples of induction beyond each respective control. Values represent the mean ± SE of three independent experiments. *$p < 0.05$, compared to the vehicle control group. (D, upper panel) HL-60 cells were pretreated with or without 20 μM U0126, SP600125, or SB202190 for 1 h followed by PTER (100 μM) treatment for an additional 24 h. Expression levels of cleaved caspase-3, -8, and -9 were determined by a Western blot analysis. (D, lower panel) Quantitative results of cleaved caspase-3, -8, and -9 protein levels, which were adjusted to the α-tubulin protein level and expressed as multiples of induction beyond each respective control. Values represent the mean ± SE of three independent experiments. Data were analyzed using a one way ANOVA with Tukey's post-hoc tests at 95% confidence intervals; different letters represent different levels of significance. Different letters represent significantly different, $p < 0.05$.

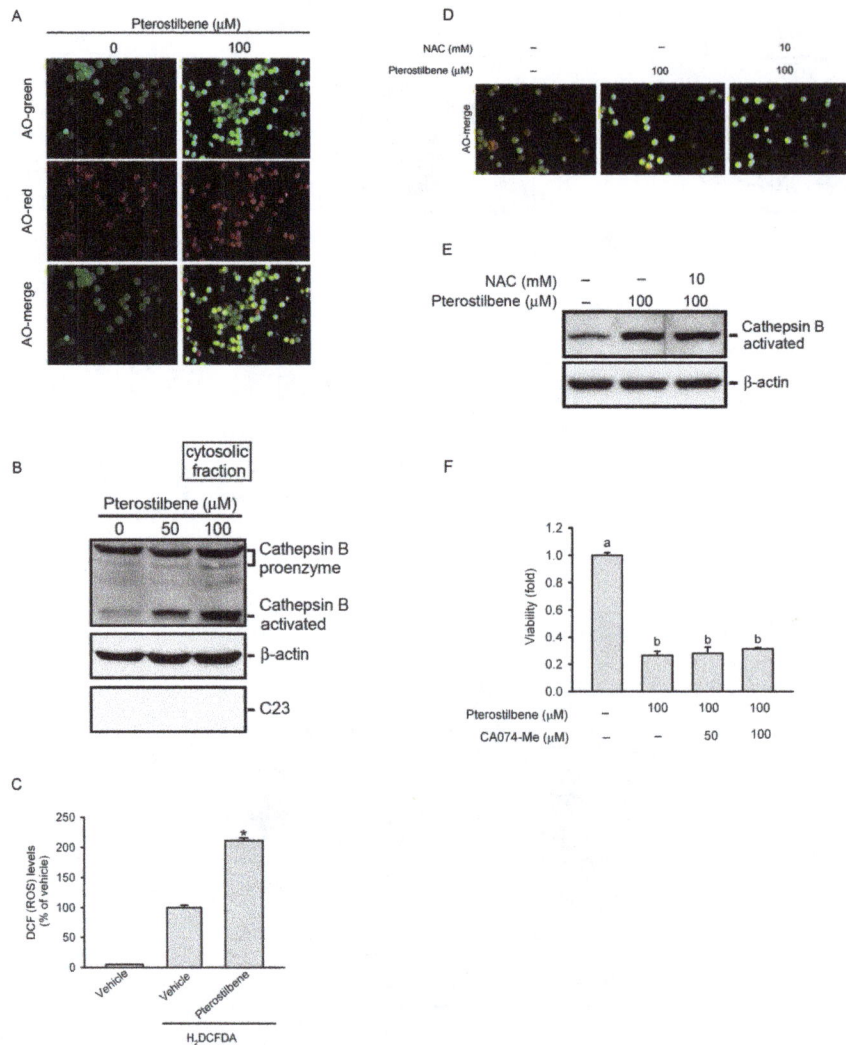

Figure 6. Effect of pterostilbene (PTER) on lysosomal membrane alterations in HL-60 cells. (A) PTER enhanced lysosome permeability. HL-60 cells were treated with 100 μM PTER for 12 h, then stained with acridine orange (5 μg/ml) for 15 min, and examined under a fluorescence microscope (×200 magnification). Representative images of three independent experiments are shown. (B) PTER concentration-dependently induced translocation of cathepsin B from lysosomes to the cytosol. Cytosolic cathepsin B levels were assessed by a Western blot analysis after treatment with various concentrations of PTER (0~100 μM) for 24 h. Protein levels of both the 37-kDa pro-cathepsin and 25-kDa activated cathepsin B are shown. β-actin and C23 were respectively used as positive and negative cytosolic internal controls. (C) HL-60 cells were treated with 100 μM PTER for 1 h and stained with H₂DCFDA; then total ROS level was analyzed by FACS, and data are presented as the mean multiples of increase in fluorescence compared to the control ± SE. *$p<0.05$, compared to the control. (D and E) The reactive oxygen species (ROS) scavenger, N-acetyl cysteine (NAC; 10 mM) was added 1 h prior to the addition of 100 μM PTER. Lysosome permeability (D) and cathepsin B cytosolic translocation (E) were analyzed 24 h later. (F) The cathepsin B inhibitor, CA074-Me (50 and 100 μM), was added 1 h prior to the addition of 100 μM PTER. Cell proliferation was determined by an MTS assay. Values are presented as the mean ± SE of three independent experiments. Data were analyzed using a one-way ANOVA with Tukey's post-hoc tests at 95% confidence intervals; Different letters represent significantly different, $p<0.05$.

Anticancer mechanisms elicited by natural polyphenols have been extensively studied for many years. RESV, one of the most studied polyphenols, has powerful growth-inhibitory and apoptosis-inducing effects on cancer cells [10,11]. Although potent anticancer effects were shown in cultured cells, potential inhibition of cancer growth by RESV in vivo is strongly limited due to its low bioavailability [12]. Therefore, it is important to consider other chemical structures, which may preserve the anticancer properties while possessing higher bioavailability.

PTER, a natural dimethylated analog of RESV with a longer half-life [16], represents an attractive option. Indeed, many in vitro and in vivo studies indicated that PTER may be a promising chemotherapeutic agent [15,17–20]. In this study, we

tested whether PTER treatment could be a new possibility for treating human AML and examined the mechanisms of the anticancer effect of PTER in human AML cells.

Our studies demonstrated that PTER concentration-dependently inhibited cell proliferation in five human AML cell lines, THP-1, U937, HL-60, OCI, and MV4-11. Cell proliferation is governed by the cell cycle, which is a complex and stepwise process, and uncontrolled cell proliferation is a hallmark of cancer [32]. The activity of CDKs is controlled by cyclin regulatory subunits. These form a complex with their catalytic subunit of CDKs and are regulated at a specific phase of the cell cycle [33]. In many cells, a transition through the G₁ phase of the cell cycle and entry into the S phase require activation of cyclin/CDK

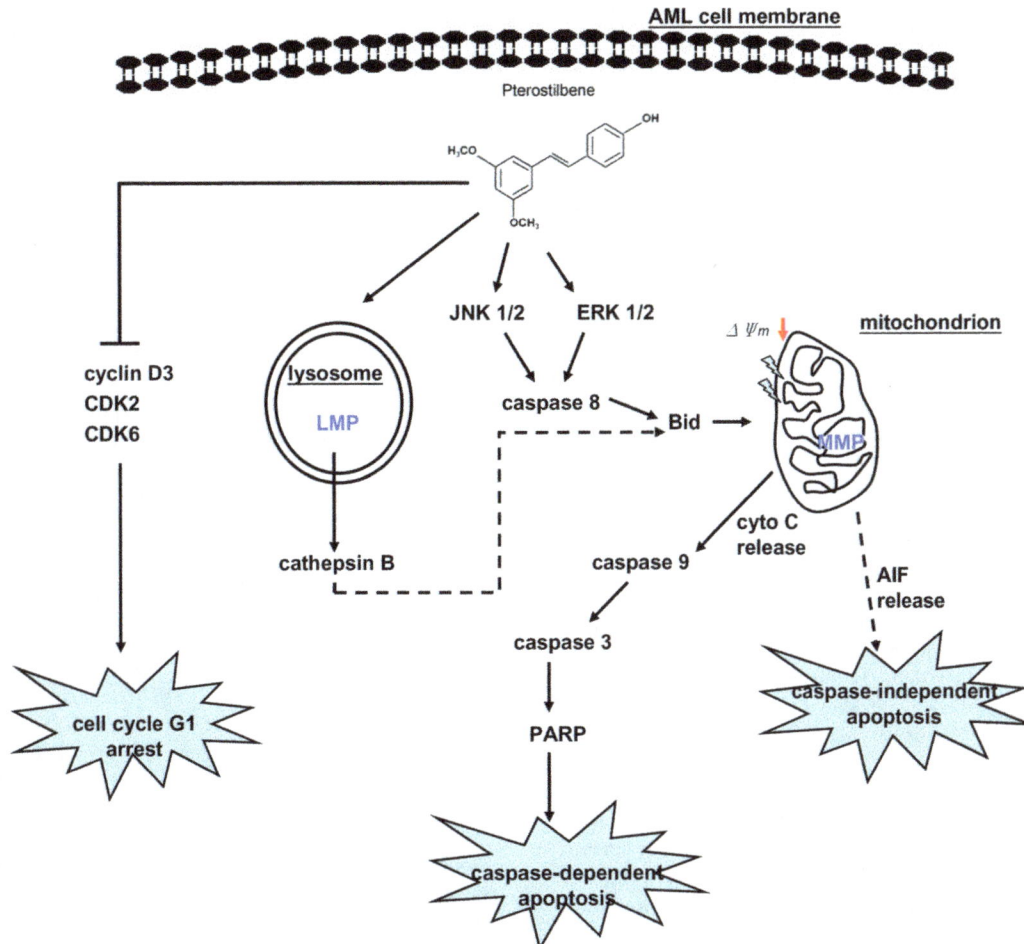

Figure 7. Proposed signal transduction pathways by which pterostilbene (PTER) inhibits the growth of HL-60 cells. 'Bold solid lines' indicate pathways affected by PTER. 'Bold dashed lines' indicate hypothetical pathways which might be affected by PTER. LMP, lysosomal membrane permeabilization; MMP, mitochondrial membrane permeabilization; cyto C, cytochrome C.

complexes, mainly cyclin D/CDK6 and cyclin E/CDK2 [32]. The kinase activity of these CDK-cyclin complexes is inhibited by two classes of CKIs [34]. Members of the INK4 family (p16 INK4A and p15 INK4B) inhibit only CDK4 and CDK6, while members of the cip family (p21 Cip1 and p27 Kip1) inhibit all CDKs [35]. In HL-60 cells, PTER treatment resulted in an accumulation of cells in the G_0/G_1 phase of the cell cycle. PTER-induced G_0/G_1 cell cycle arrest was also observed in AGS human gastric cancer cells [18], in MOLT4 human lymphoblastic leukemia cells [22], and in LNCaP human androgen-responsive prostate cancer cells [19]. Moreover, treatment of HL-60 cells with PTER decreased protein levels of cyclin D3, CDK2, and CDK6 but not p15INK4B, p21 Cip1, or p27 Kip1 indicating that changes in cyclin D3, CDK2, and CDK6 protein levels seem to make a major contribution to PTER-induced G_0/G_1 arrest in HL-60 cells.

Apoptosis is genetically programmed cell death that plays crucial roles in both the development and maintenance of tissue homeostasis. Chemical compounds that affect apoptotic pathways and eliminate cancer cells are considered promising anticancer drugs [36]. Recently, the targeted elimination of AML cells by inducing apoptosis has emerged as a valuable strategy for combating AML [37,38]. In this study, several hallmarks of apoptosis such as significant increases in chromatin condensation,

the sub-G_1 content, and Annexin-V-positive cells, were observed in HL-60 cells after PTER treatment. These results indicate that PTER can induce changes in phosphatidylserine externalization which belongs to apoptotic events and increases apoptotic DNA cleavage.

Mitochondria are emerging as promising targets for intervention and treatment of cancer [39]. Pan et al. [40] used transcript profiling techniques to identify cellular pathways targeted by PTER and found that it upregulated expressions of genes involved in mitochondrial functions. Caspases-8, -9, and -3 are believed to play crucial roles in mediating mitochondrion-mediated apoptosis pathways. Active caspase-8 can activate Bid, which then triggers the mitochondrial pathway to further activate caspase-9 and in turn activates the executioner, caspase-3, thus committing a cell to apoptosis [41]. Our present results showed that PTER activated the mitochondrial caspase-dependent apoptotic pathway in a concentration-dependent manner in HL-60 cells, and PTER-induced cell death was partly prevented by pretreatment with the caspase-3 inhibitor, Z-DEVE-FMK. Similar to our results, mitochondrial depolarization was also detected in PTER-treated human breast cancer cells [42] and lymphoblastic leukemia cells [22]. MAPKs are composed of several subfamilies, including ERK1/2, JNKs, and p38. These subfamilies regulate a variety of cellular responses, such as cell proliferation, differentiation, and apoptosis [43,44]. Previous reports found that MAPKs are involved in the effects of RESV in tumor cells [45], but the role of MAPKs in PTER-induced apoptosis of tumor cells was not investigated. In this study, we further investigated activation of MAPK family proteins in PTER-treated HL-60 cells and found that only ERK and JNK were activated after PTER treatment, and the ERK-specific inhibitor, U0126, and JNK-specific inhibitor, SP600125, respectively reversed activation of caspases-8, -9, and -3 induced by PTER. Taken together, these results suggest that activation of ERK and JNK plays important roles in PTER-induced apoptosis of HL-60 cells via regulation of caspase-8, -9, and -3 activities. Moreover, PTER-induced cell death might also occur via a caspase-independent mechanism.

LMP is an alternative mechanism for inducing cell death. Depending on the lethal stimulus, the extent of LMP, the amount and type of cathepsins released into the cytoplasm, and the abundance of cathepsin inhibitors, LMP can trigger the classical MMP-caspase pathway, as well as MMP-dependent but caspase-independent apoptosis [25]. Our results showed that PTER can dramatically induce LMP and an increase of activated cathepsin B release into the cytoplasm, indicating that PTER-induced cell apoptosis might occur through an LMP-triggered MMP-caspase pathway or an LMP-triggered caspase-independent pathway. A previous report indicated that cathepsin B-dependent Bid cleavage, a prominent MMP inducer, emerged as a key connection between LMP and MMP [25]. The correlation between Bid and cathepsin B in PTER-treated leukemia cells should be further confirmed in future work. Moreover, PTER was shown to induce oxidative stress by increasing ROS levels in breast cancer cells [42], and ROS are principal inducers of LMP. ROS-dependent LMP often initiates a cell death pathway that involves sequential cathepsin translocation and MMP with cytochrome c release and caspase-dependent apoptosis [25]. In this study, we also found that PTER also can induce ROS production in HL-60 cells. To further investigate the role of ROS in PTER-induced LMP in HL-60 cells, the antioxidant, NAC, was used. Results showed that inhibition of ROS by NAC did not prevent PTER-induced LMP or cathepsin B cytosolic translocation, indicating that ROS were not involved in PTER-mediated LMP.

Several reports indicated that LMP can also initiate a caspase-independent cell death pathway. For example, microtubule-stabilizing agents such as epothilone B, discodermolide, and paclitaxel reportedly induce cathepsin B-dependent and caspase-independent cell death, as evidenced by the significant cytoprotection conferred by the cathepsin B inhibitor, CA074-Me (but not the broad-spectrum caspase inhibitor, Z-VAD-FMK) [46]. Because cathepsin B is one of the most abundant lysosomal proteases released from lysosome to induce cell death after LMP [25]. Moreover, cathepsin B has also been implicated as an inducer of LMP. For example, hepatocytes from cathepsin B$^{-/-}$ mice display less LMP after exposure to TNF-α, which may reflect the direct induction of LMP by cathepsin B [47]. According to these observations, an amplification loop may exist through LMP induces cathepsin B activation, and cathepsin B then further triggers LMP. In our study, we used CA074-Me, the cathepsin B-specific inhibitor, as the blocker of LMP-mediated cell death.

Surprisingly, pretreatment of HL-60 cells with CA074-Me did not prevent cell death induced by PTER in our study. This might have been because the cytotoxic effect induced by the release of lysosomal hydrolases not only involves cathepsin B but also includes other cathepsins (e.g., cathepsin D, E, L, and H), and only blocking the activity of cathepsin B cannot sufficiently reverse the toxic effect of PTER. A previous report indicated that downregulation of heat shock protein (HSP) 70, which protects lysosomal membranes from LMP-inducing stimuli, induces caspase-independent cell death in breast cancer cells [48]. Moreover, PTER has also been reported to induce LMP-mediated cell death which depends on HSP70 levels in several solid tumor cell lines. This report indicated that endogenous HSP70 levels were found to be higher in cells with lower PTER susceptibility (HT29 and MCF-7 cells) than cells with higher PTER susceptibility (A375 and A549 cells) and knockdown of HSP70 in HT29 or MCF-7 cells can increase the PTER-induced cell death [49]. However, in our preliminary study, the endogenous HSP70 levels did not correlate with their susceptibility for PTER-mediated cell death in AML cell lines (Figure S6 in File S1). In addition to HSP70, the apoptosis-inducing factor (AIF) was shown to be an important effector of caspase-independent cell death induced by LMP [25]. The exact roles of HSP70 and AIF in PTER-induced apoptosis of leukemic cells must be further investigated in future work.

In summary, the present study demonstrated that PTER possesses an antileukemic effect on AML cells, and its anticancer activity was attributed to its induction of cell cycle arrest and apoptosis. The schematic mechanism is illustrated in Figure 7 and indicates that AML cell apoptosis elicited by PTER is mediated through MAPKs/caspases/MMP-dependent pathway, the disruption of LMP might also play a role in PTER-mediated apoptosis. The cell cycle arrest induced by PTER is mediated through downregulation of cyclin D3, CDK2 and CDK6 expressions. Our findings have elucidated the underlying mechanisms of the antileukemic effects of PTER and revealed that PTER may be a useful candidate as a chemotherapeutic agent for AML therapy.

Supporting Information

File S1 Figure S1, Effect of pterostilbene on U937 cell apoptosis as well as caspases activation. Figure S2, Effect of pterostilbene (PTER) on mitochondrial membrane permeability. Figure S3, Effects of ERK and JNK specific inhibitors on pterostilbene-induced activation of ERK and JNK. Figure S4, Effect of JNK specific inhibitor, JNK-IN-8 on pterostilbene-induced activation of caspases. Figure S5, Effect of pterostilbene on the ERK and JNK activation. Figure S6, The endogenous HSP70 levels in five AML cells.
(DOCX)

Author Contributions

Conceived and designed the experiments: PCH LML MHC. Performed the experiments: YEC MHC HYC. Analyzed the data: PT WJL SFY. Contributed reagents/materials/analysis tools: JMC CHL LML. Contributed to the writing of the manuscript: PCH LML MHC.

References

1. Bishop JF (1997) The treatment of adult acute myeloid leukemia. Semin Oncol 24: 57–69.
2. Tallman MS, Gilliland DG, Rowe JM (2005) Drug therapy for acute myeloid leukemia. Blood 106: 1154–1163.
3. Burns J, Yokota T, Ashihara H, Lean ME, Crozier A (2002) Plant foods and herbal sources of resveratrol. J Agric Food Chem 50: 3337–3340.
4. Jang M, Cai L, Udeani GO, Slowing KV, Thomas CF, et al. (1997) Cancer chemopreventive activity of resveratrol, a natural product derived from grapes. Science 275: 218–220.
5. Schneider Y, Vincent F, Duranton B, Badolo L, Gosse F, et al. (2000) Anti-proliferative effect of resveratrol, a natural component of grapes and wine, on human colonic cancer cells. Cancer Lett 158: 85–91.

6. Mgbonyebi OP, Russo J, Russo IH (1998) Antiproliferative effect of synthetic resveratrol on human breast epithelial cells. Int J Oncol 12: 865–869.

7. Sheth S, Jajoo S, Kaur T, Mukherjea D, Sheehan K, et al. (2012) Resveratrol reduces prostate cancer growth and metastasis by inhibiting the Akt/MicroRNA-21 pathway. PLoS One 7: e51655.

8. Garcia-Zepeda SP, Garcia-Villa E, Diaz-Chavez J, Hernandez-Pando R, Gariglio P (2013) Resveratrol induces cell death in cervical cancer cells through apoptosis and autophagy. Eur J Cancer Prev.

9. Liu P, Liang H, Xia Q, Li P, Kong H, et al. (2013) Resveratrol induces apoptosis of pancreatic cancers cells by inhibiting miR-21 regulation of BCL-2 expression. Clin Transl Oncol.

10. Tsan MF, White JE, Maheshwari JG, Bremner TA, Sacco J (2000) Resveratrol induces Fas signalling-independent apoptosis in THP-1 human monocytic leukaemia cells. Br J Haematol 109: 405–412.

11. Gautam SC, Xu YX, Dumaguin M, Janakiraman N, Chapman RA (2000) Resveratrol selectively inhibits leukemia cells: a prospective agent for ex vivo bone marrow purging. Bone Marrow Transplant 25: 639–645.

12. Aggarwal BB, Bhardwaj A, Aggarwal RS, Seeram NP, Shishodia S, et al. (2004) Role of resveratrol in prevention and therapy of cancer: preclinical and clinical studies. Anticancer Res 24: 2783–2840.

13. McCormack D, McFadden D (2012) Pterostilbene and cancer: current review. J Surg Res 173: e53–61.

14. Cichocki M, Paluszczak J, Szaefer H, Piechowiak A, Rimando AM, et al. (2008) Pterostilbene is equally potent as resveratrol in inhibiting 12-O-tetradecanoyl-phorbol-13-acetate activated NFkappaB, AP-1, COX-2, and iNOS in mouse epidermis. Mol Nutr Food Res 52 Suppl 1: S62–70.

15. Nutakul W, Sobers HS, Qiu P, Dong P, Decker EA, et al. (2011) Inhibitory effects of resveratrol and pterostilbene on human colon cancer cells: a side-by-side comparison. J Agric Food Chem 59: 10964–10970.

16. Kapetanovic IM, Muzzio M, Huang Z, Thompson TN, McCormick DL (2011) Pharmacokinetics, oral bioavailability, and metabolic profile of resveratrol and its dimethylether analog, pterostilbene, in rats. Cancer Chemother Pharmacol 68: 593–601.

17. Schneider JG, Alosi JA, McDonald DE, McFadden DW (2010) Pterostilbene inhibits lung cancer through induction of apoptosis. J Surg Res 161: 18–22.

18. Pan MH, Chang YH, Badmaev V, Nagabhushanam K, Ho CT (2007) Pterostilbene induces apoptosis and cell cycle arrest in human gastric carcinoma cells. J Agric Food Chem 55: 7777–7785.

19. Wang TT, Schoene NW, Kim YS, Mizuno CS, Rimando AM (2010) Differential effects of resveratrol and its naturally occurring methylether analogs on cell cycle and apoptosis in human androgen-responsive LNCaP cancer cells. Mol Nutr Food Res 54: 335–344.

20. Wang Y, Ding L, Wang X, Zhang J, Han W, et al. (2012) Pterostilbene simultaneously induces apoptosis, cell cycle arrest and cyto-protective autophagy in breast cancer cells. Am J Transl Res 4: 44–51.

21. Roslie H, Chan KM, Rajab NF, Velu SS, Kadir SA, et al. (2012) 3,5-dibenzyloxy-4′-hydroxystilbene induces early caspase-9 activation during apoptosis in human K562 chronic myelogenous leukemia cells. J Toxicol Sci 37: 13–21.

22. Siedlecka-Kroplewska K, Jozwik A, Kaszubowska L, Kowalczyk A, Boguslawski W (2012) Pterostilbene induces cell cycle arrest and apoptosis in MOLT4 human leukemia cells. Folia Histochem Cytobiol 50: 574–580.

23. Hwang JM, Kao SH, Hsieh YH, Li KL, Wang PH, et al. (2009) Reduction of anion exchanger 2 expression induces apoptosis of human hepatocellular carcinoma cells. Mol Cell Biochem 327: 135–144.

24. Chien MH, Ku CC, Johansson G, Chen MW, Hsiao M, et al. (2009) Vascular endothelial growth factor-C (VEGF-C) promotes angiogenesis by induction of COX-2 in leukemic cells via the VEGF-R3/JNK/AP-1 pathway. Carcinogenesis 30: 2005–2013.

25. Boya P, Kroemer G (2008) Lysosomal membrane permeabilization in cell death. Oncogene 27: 6434–6451.

26. Khan N, Afaq F, Mukhtar H (2007) Apoptosis by dietary factors: the suicide solution for delaying cancer growth. Carcinogenesis 28: 233–239.

27. Kim R, Emi M, Tanabe K (2006) Role of mitochondria as the gardens of cell death. Cancer Chemother Pharmacol 57: 545–553.

28. Chen T, Wong YS (2008) Selenocystine induces S-phase arrest and apoptosis in human breast adenocarcinoma MCF-7 cells by modulating ERK and Akt phosphorylation. J Agric Food Chem 56: 10574–10581.

29. Rammer P, Groth-Pedersen L, Kirkegaard T, Daugaard M, Rytter A, et al. (2010) BAMLET activates a lysosomal cell death program in cancer cells. Mol Cancer Ther 9: 24–32.

30. Groth-Pedersen L, Ostenfeld MS, Hoyer-Hansen M, Nylandsted J, Jaattela M (2007) Vincristine induces dramatic lysosomal changes and sensitizes cancer cells to lysosome-destabilizing siramesine. Cancer Res 67: 2217–2225.

31. Wang L, Liu L, Shi Y, Cao H, Chaturvedi R, et al. (2012) Berberine induces caspase-independent cell death in colon tumor cells through activation of apoptosis-inducing factor. PLoS One 7: e36418.

32. Sherr CJ (1996) Cancer cell cycles. Science 274: 1672–1677.

33. Jacks T, Weinberg RA (1996) Cell-cycle control and its watchman. Nature 381: 643–644.

34. Sherr CJ, Roberts JM (1999) CDK inhibitors: positive and negative regulators of G1-phase progression. Genes Dev 13: 1501–1512.

35. Ortega S, Malumbres M, Barbacid M (2002) Cyclin D-dependent kinases, INK4 inhibitors and cancer. Biochim Biophys Acta 1602: 73–87.

36. Chinkwo KA (2005) Sutherlandia frutescens extracts can induce apoptosis in cultured carcinoma cells. J Ethnopharmacol 98: 163–170.

37. Carter BZ, Mak DH, Shi Y, Fidler JM, Chen R, et al. (2012) MRx102, a triptolide derivative, has potent antileukemic activity in vitro and in a murine model of AML. Leukemia 26: 443–450.

38. Zhang S, Zhang Y, Zhuang Y, Wang J, Ye J, et al. (2012) Matrine induces apoptosis in human acute myeloid leukemia cells via the mitochondrial pathway and Akt inactivation. PLoS One 7: e46853.

39. Ralph SJ, Neuzil J (2009) Mitochondria as targets for cancer therapy. Mol Nutr Food Res 53: 9–28.

40. Pan Z, Agarwal AK, Xu T, Feng Q, Baerson SR, et al. (2008) Identification of molecular pathways affected by pterostilbene, a natural dimethylether analog of resveratrol. BMC Med Genomics 1: 7.

41. Elmore S (2007) Apoptosis: a review of programmed cell death. Toxicol Pathol 35: 495–516.

42. Alosi JA, McDonald DE, Schneider JS, Privette AR, McFadden DW (2010) Pterostilbene inhibits breast cancer in vitro through mitochondrial depolarization and induction of caspase-dependent apoptosis. J Surg Res 161: 195–201.

43. Matsukawa J, Matsuzawa A, Takeda K, Ichijo H (2004) The ASK1-MAP kinase cascades in mammalian stress response. J Biochem 136: 261–265.

44. Cobb MH (1999) MAP kinase pathways. Prog Biophys Mol Biol 71: 479–500.

45. Bai Y, Mao QQ, Qin J, Zheng XY, Wang YB, et al. (2010) Resveratrol induces apoptosis and cell cycle arrest of human T24 bladder cancer cells in vitro and inhibits tumor growth in vivo. Cancer Sci 101: 488–493.

46. Broker LE, Huisman C, Span SW, Rodriguez JA, Kruyt FA, et al. (2004) Cathepsin B mediates caspase-independent cell death induced by microtubule stabilizing agents in non-small cell lung cancer cells. Cancer Res 64: 27–30.

47. Werneburg NW, Guicciardi ME, Bronk SF, Gores GJ (2002) Tumor necrosis factor-alpha-associated lysosomal permeabilization is cathepsin B dependent. Am J Physiol Gastrointest Liver Physiol 283: G947–G956.

48. Nylandsted J, Rohde M, Brand K, Bastholm L, Elling F, et al. (2000) Selective depletion of heat shock protein 70 (Hsp70) activates a tumor-specific death program that is independent of caspases and bypasses Bcl-2. Proc Natl Acad Sci U S A 97: 7871–7876.

49. Mena S, Rodriguez ML, Ponsoda X, Estrela JM, Jaattela M, et al. (2012) Pterostilbene-induced tumor cytotoxicity: a lysosomal membrane permeabilization-dependent mechanism. PLoS One 7: e44524.

13

Evaluation and Structure-Activity Relationship Analysis of a New Series of *Arylnaphthalene lignans* as Potential Anti-Tumor Agents

Jiaoyang Luo, Yichen Hu, Weijun Kong, Meihua Yang*

Institute of Medicinal Plant Development, Chinese Academy of Medical Sciences and Peking Union Medical College, Beijing, P.R. China

Abstract

Arylnaphthalene lignan lactones have attracted considerable interest because of their anti-tumor and anti-hyperlipidimic activities. However, to our knowledge, few studies have explored the effects of these compounds on human leukemia cell lines. In this study, five arylnaphthalene lignans including 6′-hydroxy justicidin A (HJA), 6′-hydroxy justicidin B (HJB), justicidin B (JB), chinensinaphthol methyl ether (CME) and Taiwanin E methyl ether (TEME) were isolated from *Justicia procumbens* and their effects on the proliferation and apoptosis of the human leukemia K562 cell line were investigated then used to assess structure-activity relationships. To achieve these aims, cytotoxicity was assayed using the MTT assay, while intracellular SOD activity was detected using the SOD Activity Assay kit. Apoptosis was measured by both the using a cycle TEST PLUS DNA reagent kit as well as the FITC Annexin V apoptosis detection kit in combination with flow cytometry. Activation of caspase-mediated apoptosis was evaluated using a FITC active Caspase-3 apoptosis kit and flow cytometry. The results indicated that HJB, HJA and JB significantly inhibited the growth of K562 cells by decreasing both proliferation and SOD activity and inducing apoptosis. The sequence of anti-proliferative activity induced by the five tested arylnaphthalenes by decreasing strength was HJB > HJA > JB > CME > TEME. HJB, HJA and JB also decreased SOD activity and induced apoptosis in a dose-dependent manner. Activation of caspase-3 further indicated that HJB, HJA and JB induced caspase-dependent intrinsic and/or extrinsic apoptosis pathways. Together, these assays suggest that arylnaphthalene lignans derived from *Justicia procumbens* induce apoptosis to varying degrees, through a caspase-dependent pathway in human leukemia K562 cells. Furthermore, analysis of structure-activity relationships suggest that hydroxyl substitution at C-1 and C-6′ significantly increased the antiproliferative activity of arylnaphthalene lignans while a methoxyl at C-1 significantly decreased the effect.

Editor: Aditya Bhushan Pant, Indian Institute of Toxicology Research, India

Funding: This work received financial support from the Beijing Natural Science Foundation of China (7112092), the Program for PUMC Innovative Foundation and Specialized Research Fund for the Doctoral Program of Higher Education (20111106110034). The funders had no role in study design, data collection and analysis, decision to publish, or preparation of the manuscript.

Competing Interests: The authors have declared that no competing interests exist.

* E-mail: yangmeihua15@hotmail.com

Introduction

Lignans are a large group of dimeric phenylpropanoids that are widely distributed in higher plants. Like many other secondary metabolites, lignans represent a means of protection against herbivores for the plants that synthesize them. There is a growing interest in exploiting lignans, and their synthetic derivatives, as potential anti-cancer agents [1,2]. Indeed, some cytotoxic lignan derivatives have reached phase I and II clinical trials as anti-tumor agents including GP-11 [3], NK-611 [4,5], TOP-53 [6], NPF [7], GL-331 [8–12]. More recently, the lignan F11782 was shown to be a novel catalytic inhibitor of topoisomerases I and II, key promoters of DNA replication [13].

The majority of natural arylnaphthalene lignans are lactones [14]. These have attracted considerable interest because of their anti-tumor and anti-hyperlipidemic activities [15]. Cytotoxicity as well as anti-cancer activity has been reported for arylnapthalene lignan isolated from several genus including *Phyllantus*, *Cleistanthus*, and *Justicia* [1,16,17].

Justicia procumbens (*J. procumbens*) is an herb which can be used to prepare a traditional remedy for the treatment of fever, pain, and cancer [18]. The bioactive justicins isolated from *J. procumbens* include diphyllin, 6′-hydroxy justicidin A (HJA) and chinensi-naphthol methyl ether (CME), which share a similar chemical structure with that of podophyllotoxin (POD). Previous reports have demonstrated that these extracts promote cytotoxicity [19–23], antimicrobial [24], antiviral [25], and anti-platelet [26] activities. Indeed, the cytotoxicity of these arylnaphthalene lignans has been demonstrated in liver cancer HepG2, breast cancer MCF-7, lymphocytic leukemia P338 tumor cell lines, as well as human bladder cancer EJ cells. [18–20,27].

We have also previously shown that the extract of *J. procumbens* displays broad-spectrum anti-tumor activity, especially in the human leukemia K562 cell line. In addition, we have isolated five arylnaphthalene lignans from *J. procumbens* including HJA, 6′-hydroxy justicidin B (HJB), justicidin B (JB), CME and Taiwanin E methyl ether (TEME) [28,29] and demonstrated that these are the main arylnaphthalene lignans in *J. procumbens* [30]. Notably, these compounds share the same parent nucleus but harbor different substituent groups at the 1, 3′, 4′ and 6′ positions. However, the anti-cancer activity of these *J. procumbens*-derived compounds and their underlying mechanisms of action, especially the analysis of structure-activity relationships, have not been fully elucidated.

Mitochondria play a central role in various pathophysiological processes of cancer cells, in particular apoptosis. Most anti-tumor drugs can induce apoptosis in different types of tumor cells. There are two major apoptotic pathways, the intrinsic pathway and the extrinsic pathway, which both result in activation of effector caspases. The intrinsic apoptotic pathway involves an increase in mitochondrial membrane permeability and the subsequent increased release of cytochrome c into the cytoplasm, which in turn activates caspase-9 and caspase-3. These in turn mediate apoptotic damage [31,32]. The extrinsic pathway is initiated by the activation of death receptors involves the formation of a death-inducing signaling complex (DISC). DISC formation results in the activation of caspase-8, which activates caspase-3 [33]. In addition, reactive oxygen species (ROS), a by-product of mitochondrial oxidative metabolism, have been reported to exert a pathogenic role in different degenerative diseases as well as cancer [34,35].

In the present study, we investigated whether, and to what degree, arylnaphthalene lignans affect the survival of the human leukemia K562 cell line by measuring viability and apoptosis after exposure to the five compounds (Figure 1). We then used these results to clarify the structure-activity relationship between arylnaphthalene lignans and their anti-cancer activity.

Results

Effect of arylnaphthalene lignans on leukemia K562 cell survival

To test the cytotoxicity of different doses of HJA, HJB, JB, CME and TEME on human leukemia K562 cells, MTT assay were performed. As shown in Figure 2, arylnaphthalene lignans inhibited the viability of K562 cells to different degree in a dose-dependent manner. After treatment for 48 h, the average 50% inhibition concentrations (IC_{50}) of HJB, HJA, JB and CME were 20, 43.9, 45.4 and 106.2 μM, respectively. The IC_{50} of TEME, POD and etoposide (ETO) could not be calculated within the tested concentrations. We also investigated the cytotoxicity of the five arylnaphthalene lignans on HL-60, L1210 and P388D1 cell lines. The results showed that HJB exhibited the most cytotoxicity within these cell lines, with an average IC_{50} ranging from 3.9 to 26.2 μM (see Figure S1–S3). The sequence of the strength of cytotoxicity of the arylnaphthalene lignans was thus deduced to be HJB > HJA > JB > CME > TEME.

To further evaluate the structure-activity relationship, the cytotoxicity of another 10 lignans, derived from *J. procumbens*, was investigated in human colon cancer HCT-8 and human hepatocellular carcinoma Bel-7402 cell lines (Table S1 and Figure S4). Similar to the results obtained with the K562 cell line, HJB and HJA were again found to exhibit the most cytotoxicity, while CME and TEME were only mildly cytotoxic, when each was compared to a vehicle-treated control.

Arylnaphthalene lignans inhibit SOD activity of leukemia K562 cells

To test whether arylnaphthalene lignans altered redox system homeostasis in leukemia K562 cells, superoxide dismutase (SOD) activity, which is involved in the removal of ROS, was measured. Compared with the vehicle-treated control, the activity of SOD in leukemia K562 cells decreased significantly in response to increasing dose of either HJB or JB (Figure 3) while for CME

and TEME, only high doses showed inhibitory activity. The sequence of SOD activity inhibition by decreasing strength was HJB > JB > HJA > CME > TEME. Specifically, the SOD activity of cells treated with HJB decreased 59.1, 66.9 and 74.9% at dose of 12.5, 25 and 100 μM, respectively; while with JB it decreased 46.4, 52.6 and 84.3% at 3, 11.9 and 47.6 μM, respectively.

HJB, HJA and JB increase the proportion of subG0 phase K562 cells

Next, the effects of the five arylnaphthalene lignan lactones on the cell cycle were analyzed by flow cytometry. It has previously been demonstrated that POD arrests cell development at metaphases. In agreement with this data, K562 cells treated with 28.5 μM POD were arrested at metaphase. Indeed, the percentage of cells in metaphase significantly increased up to 94.1% compared with 6.99% in the vehicle-treated control group (Table 1, Figure 4A). In contrast, treatment of K562 with HJA, HJB, JB and ETO for 48 h dose-dependently increased the proportion of cells in the subG0 phase of the cell cycle while cells in the G2/M phase were barely detected. CME and TEME, however, did not significantly affect the subG0 phase K562 cells ($P>0.05$). Specifically, the percentages of apoptotic K562 cells following exposure to 12.5, 25 and 100 μM HJB were 9.2, 13.6 and 30.5%, respectively, while those of K562 cells exposed to 67.6 μM JB and 100 μM HJB were 14.6 and 30.5%, respectively.

Effect of arylnaphthalene lignans on apoptosis in K562 cells

The externalization of phosphatidylserine (PS) precedes the loss of membrane integrity which accompanies later stages of cell death induced by either apoptosis or necrosis. Staining with FITC Annexin V, with detects PS, is typically used in conjunction with a vital dye such as propidium iodide (PI) and subsequent analysis by flow cytometry to assess apoptosis. Viable cells with intact membranes exclude PI, whereas the membranes of dead and damaged cells are permeable to PI. As a result, viable cells are negative for both FITC Annexin V and PI; early apoptotic cells are FITC Annexin V positive and PI negative; and late apoptotic or dead cells are both FITC Annexin V and PI positive.

Using this approach, we clearly showed a dose-dependent apoptotic effect of arylnaphthalene lignans in K562 cells (Figure 4B). Indeed, treatment of cells with HJA, HJB, JB and CME at different doses for 48 h resulted in a shift from a population of largely live cells in the vehicle-treated control to populations with increasing proportions of early and late apoptotic cells with little change in the dead cell population (Figure 4B). More specifically, the positive control, ETO, induced apoptosis at a concentration of 22.7 μM (the viable cell population was 72.9%) but it did not increase when its dose was increased to 90.6 μM (the viable cell population was 70.6%). Meanwhile, the apoptotic percentages of K562 cells exposed to HJA, HJB, JB and CME increased in a dose-dependent manner. For example, the early apoptotic percentages of K562 cells exposed to 12.5, 25, and 100 μM HJB were 6.8, 12.4 and 19.8%, respectively; while the viable cell population was 86.7, 77.3 and 59.9%, respectively. The late apoptotic percentages of K562 cells exposed to 8.4, 16.9, and 67.6 μM JB were 6.2, 8.1 and 13.8%, respectively; while the viable cell population was 84.4, 77.7 and 76.2%, respectively.

Caspase-3 activity assay

The caspase family of cysteine proteases plays a key role in apoptosis and inflammation. Caspase-3 is a key protease that is

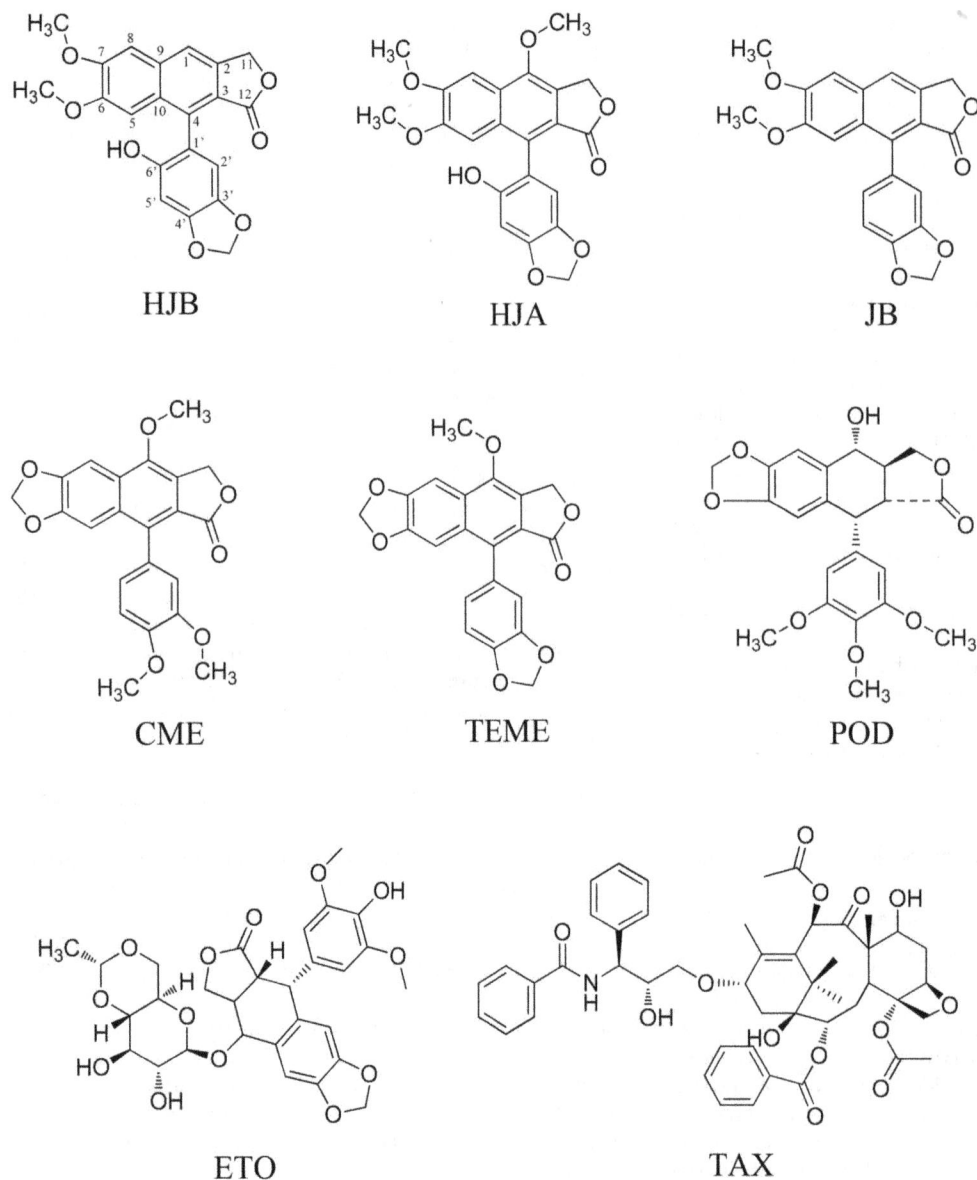

Figure 1. Chemical structures of 6′-hydroxy justicidin B (HJB), 6′-hydroxy justicidin A (HJA), justicidin B (JB), chinensinaphthol methyl ether (CME), Taiwanin E methyl ether (TEME), etoposide (ETO), paclitaxel (TAX) and podophyllotoxin (POD).

activated during the early stages of apoptosis and, like other members of the caspase family, is synthesized as an inactive pro-enzyme that is processed in cells undergoing apoptosis by self-proteolysis and/or cleavage by another protease [36]. Active caspase-3, a marker for cells undergoing apoptosis, consists of a heterodimer of 17 and 12 kDa subunits which is derived from the 32 kDa pro-enzyme. Active caspase-3 proteolytically cleaves and activates other caspases, as well as relevant targets in the cytoplasm, e.g., D4-GDI and Bcl-2, and in the nucleus (e.g. PARP). This antibody has been reported to specifically recognize the active form of caspase-3 in human and mouse cells.

As shown in Figure 5, among the tested compounds, HJA, HJB, JB and CME treatment induced caspase-3 activation in K562 cells in a dose-dependent manner. For example, while untreated cells were primarily negative (1.3%) for active caspase-3, treatment with 12.5, 25 and 100 μM HJB increased the percentages of active caspase-3 positive cells to 9.5, 12.4 and 20.6%, respectively.

Similarly, the percentages of active caspase-3-positive cells were increased 11.2, 13. 9 and 19.1% when treated with 8.4, 16.9 and 67.6 μM JB, respectively.

Discussion

Few studies have explored the effects of arylnaphthalene lignans on the human leukemia K562 cell line. Vasilev *et al.* first studied the cytotoxicity and apoptotic effects of JB on K562 cell line [37]. Later, Ionkova *et al.* reported a rare medicinal plant *Linum narbonense* that showed good cytotoxicity in tumor cells and provided a tool for the biotechnological production of JB [38]. However, the detailed effects of other arylnaphthalene lignans such as HJB, CME and TEME, on the leukemia K562 cell line have not been investigated. Moreover, the apoptosis pathways exploited as well as analysis of structure-activity relationships have not yet been illustrated.

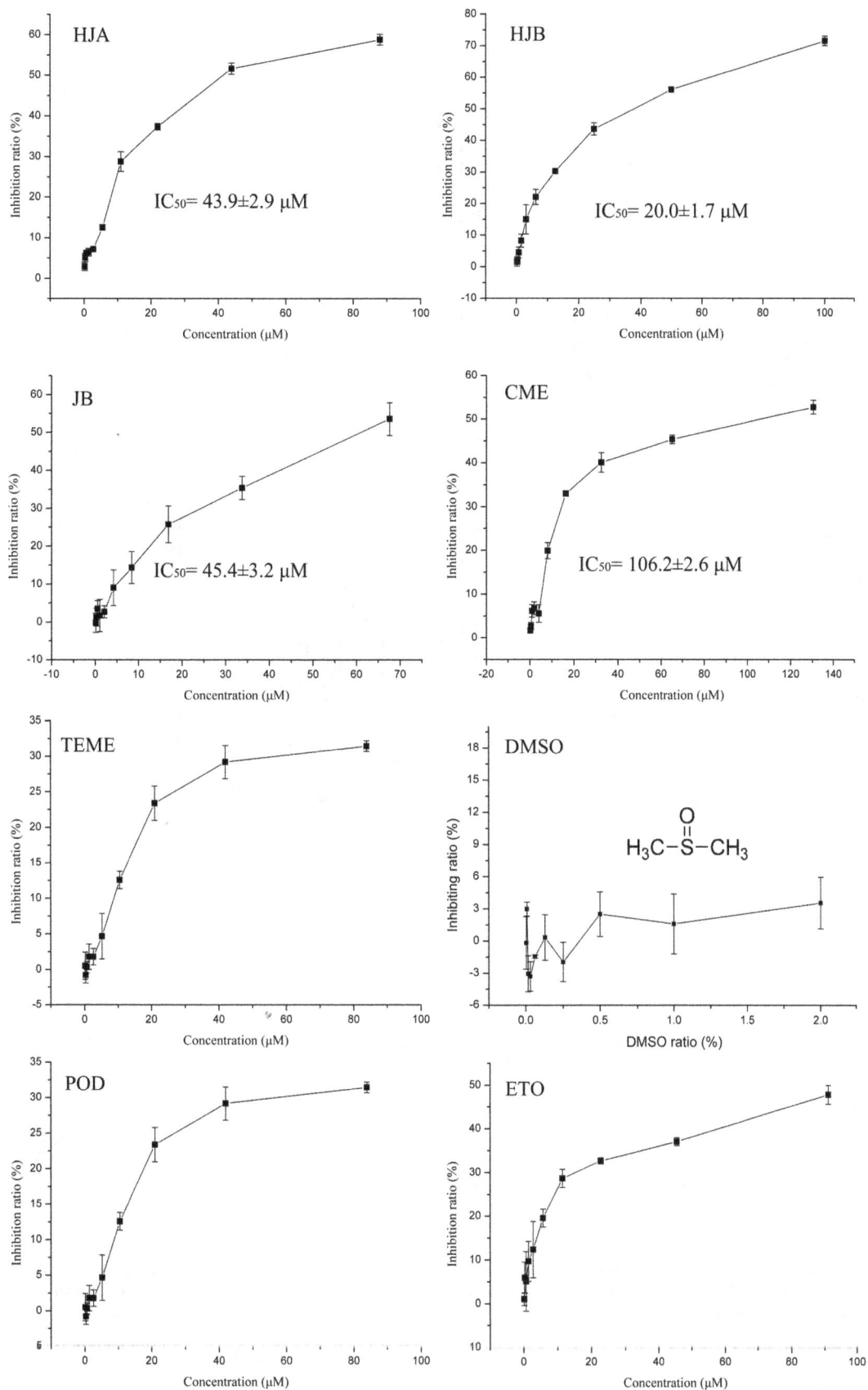

Figure 2. Effect of HJB, HJA, JB, CME, TEME, POD and ETO on K562 cell proliferation. Cells were exposed to the indicated concentrations of arylnaphthalene lignans and incubated for 48 h, MTT assays were then performed. Data represented the mean ± SD of three independent experiments, where each sample was tested in at least triplicate.

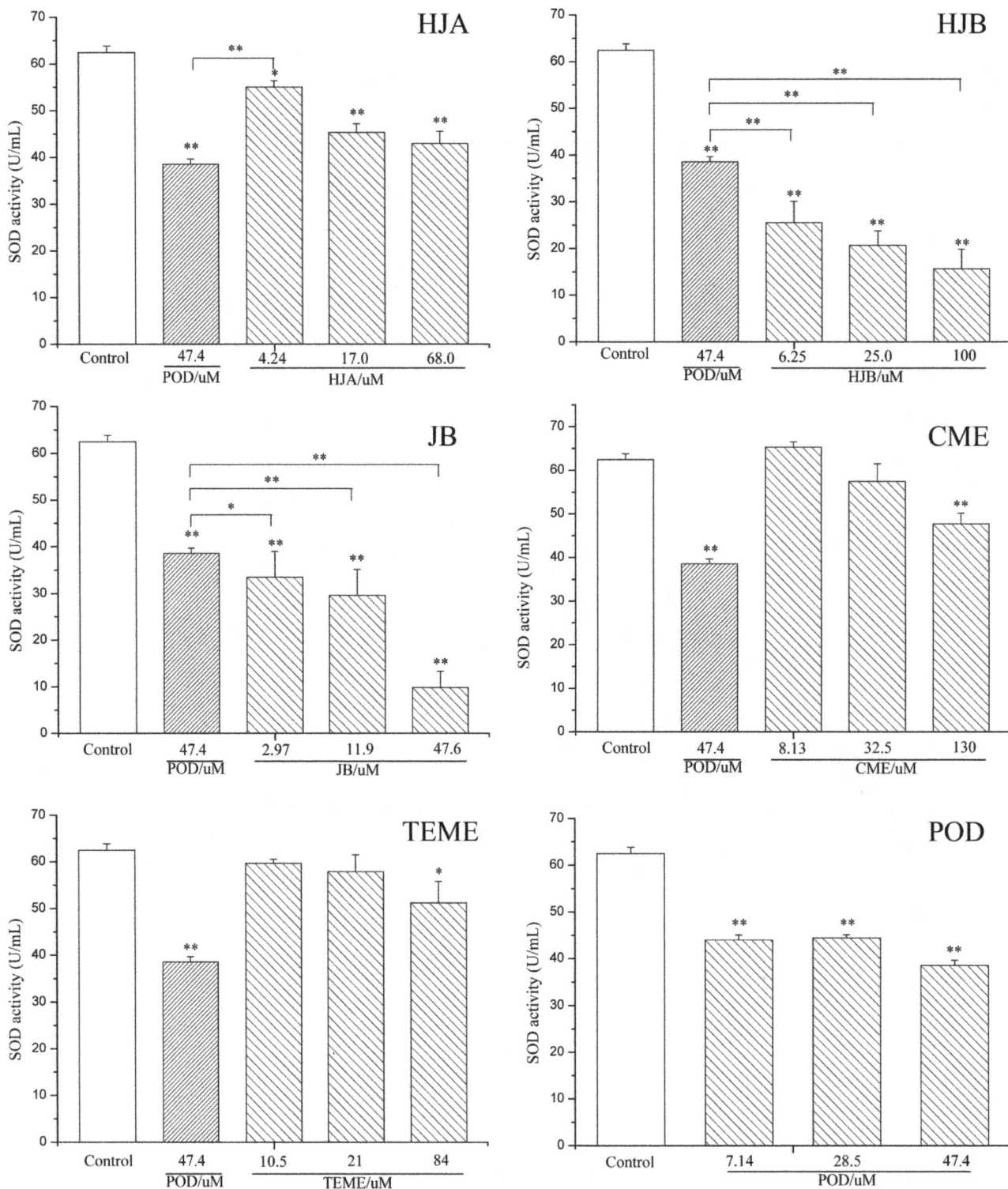

Figure 3. Effect of arylnaphthalene lignans on SOD activity in K562 cells. K562 cells were treated with of the indicated concentrations of HJA, HJB, JB, CME, TEME and POD for 48 h then the SOD activity assay was performed. Values are expressed as mean ± SD of five independent experiments; **$P<0.01$ compared with control group.

In this study, the cytotoxicity of new arylnaphthalene lignans extracted from *J. procumbens*, HJA, HJB, JB, CME and TEME, were tested on the tumor cell lines K562, HL-60, L1210 and P388D1. Of note, these compounds share the same parent nucleus but harbor different substituent groups at the 1, 3′, 4′ and 6′ positions that we hypothesized could underlie variances in activity. We found that the IC_{50} values of HJB in K562, HL-60 and P388D1 cell lines were lower than those of HJA and JB, as

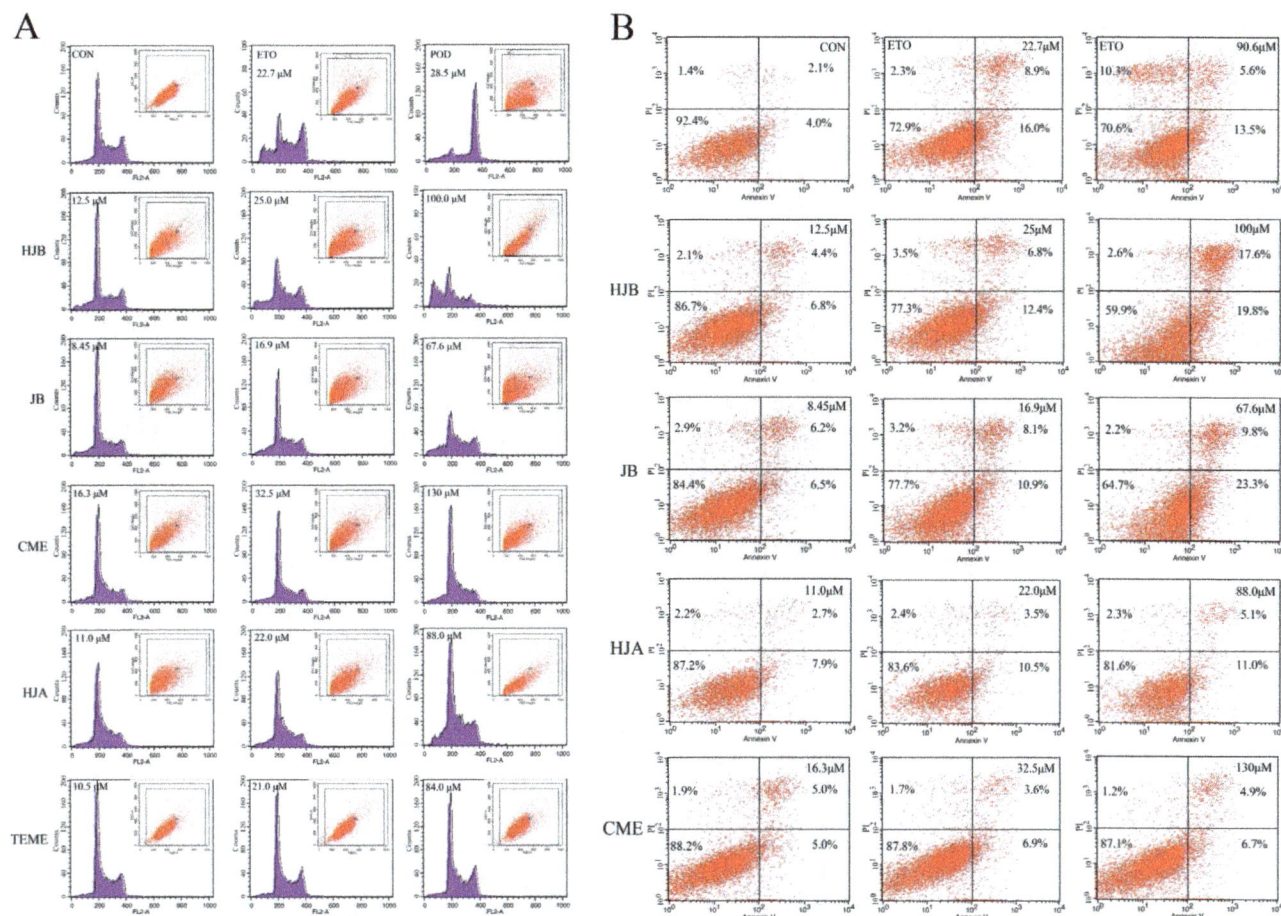

Figure 4. Effect of arylnaphthalene lignans on apoptosis in K562 cells. (A) The apoptosis rate and changes in the cell cycle of K562 cells treated with arylnaphthalene lignans at the indicated doses for 24 h were analyzed by PI staining and subsequent flow cytometry. Representative data are shown. (B) Apoptosis was further analyzed by annexin V/PI staining and flow cytometry of K562 cells treated with the indicated concentrations of HJA, HJB, JB, CME and ETO for 48 h. Representative FACS scatter-grams are shown. All results are representative of three independent experiments.

determined by MTT assay, indicating that HJB may be a stronger antiproliferative agent than the other tested arylnaphthalene lignans. This result was further validated by the SOD activity assay, cell-cycle analysis and Annexin V/PI staining. In agreement with these findings, we have previously reported that the oral absolute bioavailability of HJB is better than that of HJA (36.0 ± 13.4%) [39] and CME (3.2 ± 0.2%) [40]. Indeed, the sequence of the bioavailability was HJB > JB > HJC > HJA > CME.

ETO, a topoisomerase II inhibitor, is extensively used in the treatment of leukemia. However, K562 cells are known to be less sensitive to ETO than other cell lines [41]. Jiang et al used flow cytometry to measure the apoptosis rate induced by continuous exposure to ETO (10 μM) in K562 cells and found that apoptosis was barely detected 24 h after exposure to ETO [42]. In this study, The IC_{50} of TEME, POD and ETO were not determined within the tested concentrations. Moreover, the cytotoxicity of either POD or ETO on SOD activity was not significant when the concentration was less than 20 μM. In addition, the percentages of cells in both early and late apoptosis when the concentration of ETO was 90.6 μM were lower than those of cells treated with 100 μM HJB. In contrast, HJB, HJA and JB consistently showed greater cytotoxicity, including strong anti-proliferative and pro-apoptotic effects at low doses, suggesting that these compounds might be more effective than ETO in the treatment of leukemia.

In addition to the dose-dependent induction of apoptosis, HJB and JB also impaired SOD activity. SOD is the first line of defense against mitochondria-produced ROS which can protect cells from peroxidation injury induced by transferring one radical (O_2^-) to the next (H_2O_2) [43]. In this study, the activity of SOD decreased significantly in K562 cells after treatment with different concentrations of HJB and JB, suggesting that these compounds might elicit their cytotoxicity through the impairment of ROS removal.

Caspase-3 is a key effecter molecule of both extrinsic and intrinsic apoptosis. It cleaves a number of cellular proteins, leading to apoptosis [44]. Our study showed that HJB and JB significantly raised the enzymatic activity of caspase-3 in a dose-dependent manner suggesting that these compounds induced apoptosis in K562 cells. Notably, the activity of 100 μM HJB was equal to that of 48 μM paclitaxel (TAX) and 90.6 μM ETO. We thus concluded that arylnaphthalene-induced apoptosis in K562 cells occurred via a caspase-dependent pathway.

Taken together, the sequence of anti-proliferative activity was HJB > HJA > JB > CME > TEME. To explain the differences in anti-proliferative potency of the compounds, structure-activity relationships were examined. First, we found that the substituent at C-1 of the parent nucleus can affect its therapeutic effects. Specifically, a hydroxyl correlated with significantly increased anti-tumor activity while a methoxyl correlated with its decrease.

Table 1. The apoptosis rate and cell cycle analysis of K562 cells treated with arylnaphthalene lignans for 24 h.

Group	Concentration (μM)	Apoptosis (%)	G0/G1 (%)	S (%)	G2/M (%)
CON	---	2.9±0.2	35.5±2.59	57.5±4.8	7.0±0.3
ETO	22.7	15.3±1.5	19.5±2.0	72.5±5.2	8.0±0.4
POD	28.5	7.9±0.9	5.8±0.8	0.2±0.0	94.1±5.8
HJB	12.5	9.2±1.1	47.6±3.7	44.4±3.7	8.0±0.4
HJB	25.0	13.6±1.5	31.3±3.1	60.6±4.4	8.0±0.4
HJB	100	30.5±2.4	24.1±2.7	75.9±5.3	0.1±0.0
JB	8.4	7.5±0.8	48.5±3.7	47.2±3.9	4.3±0.2
JB	16.9	9.9±1.1	42.3±3.3	53.1±3.7	4.6±0.2
JB	67.6	14.6±1.3	27.4±2.6	64.6±4.1	8.0±0.2
CME	16.3	5.2±1.1	46.2±3.6	52.1±3.7	1.7±0.1
CME	32.5	5.8±0.6	48.5±3.0	45.8±3.3	5.7±0.1
CME	130	7.0±0.9	45.6±3.5	54.4±3.6	0.1±0.0
HJA	11.0	6.0±0.5	44.3±3.6	55.7±3.4	0.1±0.0
HJA	22.0	7.4±0.5	40.9±4.0	59.1±4.5	0.0±0.0
HJA	88.0	8.7±0.5	35.3±2.9	63.6±4.3	1.1±0.0
TEME	10.5	2.8±0.3	40.4±3.5	57.5±3.3	2.1±0.1
TEME	21.0	2.9±0.4	38.7±3.8	54.7±3.5	6.5±0.0
TEME	84.0	3.4±0.4	36.7±2.7	55.3±3.5	8.0±0.1

These data are representative of three independent experiments.

Second, a hydroxyl substituent at C-6′ also correlated with increased anti-tumor activity of the parent nucleus. Third, methylenedioxy between C-3′ and C-4′ correlated with deceased anti-tumor activity compared with methoxyl at the two positions. Of note, it has previously been reported in a structure-activity relationship study that di- and tetrahydronaphthalenes with a trans-lactone and a β-hydroxyl at C-4 have high therapeutic indices in tests for anti-neoplastic and anti-viral effects [45]. Together with our new data, this information could be used to select for arylnaphthalenes with likely high anti-tumor activity based on their structure.

Furthermore, diphyllin, a typical arylnaphthalene lignan isolated from the plant *J. procumbens* (*Acanthaceae*), has been found to have a wide spectrum of biological effects, such as cytotoxicity [19,20], antimicrobial [24] and antiviral [25] activities. As shown in Figure 1, the structure of HJB is similar to that of diphyllin. The only one difference is the substituted position of hydroxyl, i.e., the hydroxyl substituted at C-1 (diphyllin) translated to position C-6′ (HJB). Therefore diphyllin and HJB, and compounds that bare similar structure, could be good lead compounds for anti-cancer drug design and development.

Conclusion

This study systematically investigated the anti-tumor activity of five arylnaphthalene lignans isolated from *J. procumbens*. We found that HJB, HJA and JB significantly induced apoptosis in K562 cells via the activation of a caspase-dependent pathway. Structure-activity relationship analysis indicated that hydroxyl substitution at C-1 and C-6′ significantly increase the anti-tumor activity of arylnaphthalene lignans while a methoxyl at C-1 results in a significant decrease. Structure-activity differences could be used to select for arynaphthalenes with superior anti-cancer function for further testing and eventual drug development.

Materials and Methods

Materials

Reference standards of POD, ETO and TAX were purchased from Sigma (St. Louis, MO, USA). HJA, HJB, JB, CME, TEME, neojusticidin A, isodiphyllin, Taiwanin C, neesiinoside C, 6′-hydroxy azizin, 4′-demethylchinensinaphthol methyl ether, Diphyllin-1-O-β-D-apiofuranoside, ciliatoside C, Justicidinoside C and Justicidinoside B were isolated from *J. procumbens* and identified by UV, IR, ESI-MS, ^{1}H and ^{13}C-NMR [28,29]. The purity of the chemicals was greater than 95% as determined by normalization of the peak areas detected by HPLC-UV. The Cycle TEST PLUS DNA Reagent kit, FITC Active Caspase-3 Apoptosis Kit and FITC Annexin V Apoptosis Detection Kit were purchased from BD Pharmingen (San Diego, CA, USA). The SOD Activity Assay Kit was purchased from Nanjing Jiancheng Bioengineering Institute (Nanjing, China). Other reagents were purchased from Sigma (St. Louis, MO, USA).

Cell cultures

Human leukemia K562, human promyelocytic leukemia HL-60, mouse lymphocytic leukemia L1210, P388D1 mouse macrophage, human colon cancer HCT-8 and human hepatocellular carcinoma Bel-7402 cell lines were obtained from the Cancer Institute & Hospital, Chinese Academy of Medical Sciences, and the original commercial source was the American Type Culture Collection (ATCC, Manassas, VA, USA). The cell lines were cultured in RPMI-1640 (GIBCO BRL, Grand Island, NY, USA) containing 10% heat-inactivated fetal bovine serum, 100 U/ml penicillin, and 100 U/ml streptomycin. Cells were maintained at 37°C in an atmosphere of 5% carbon dioxide/95% air.

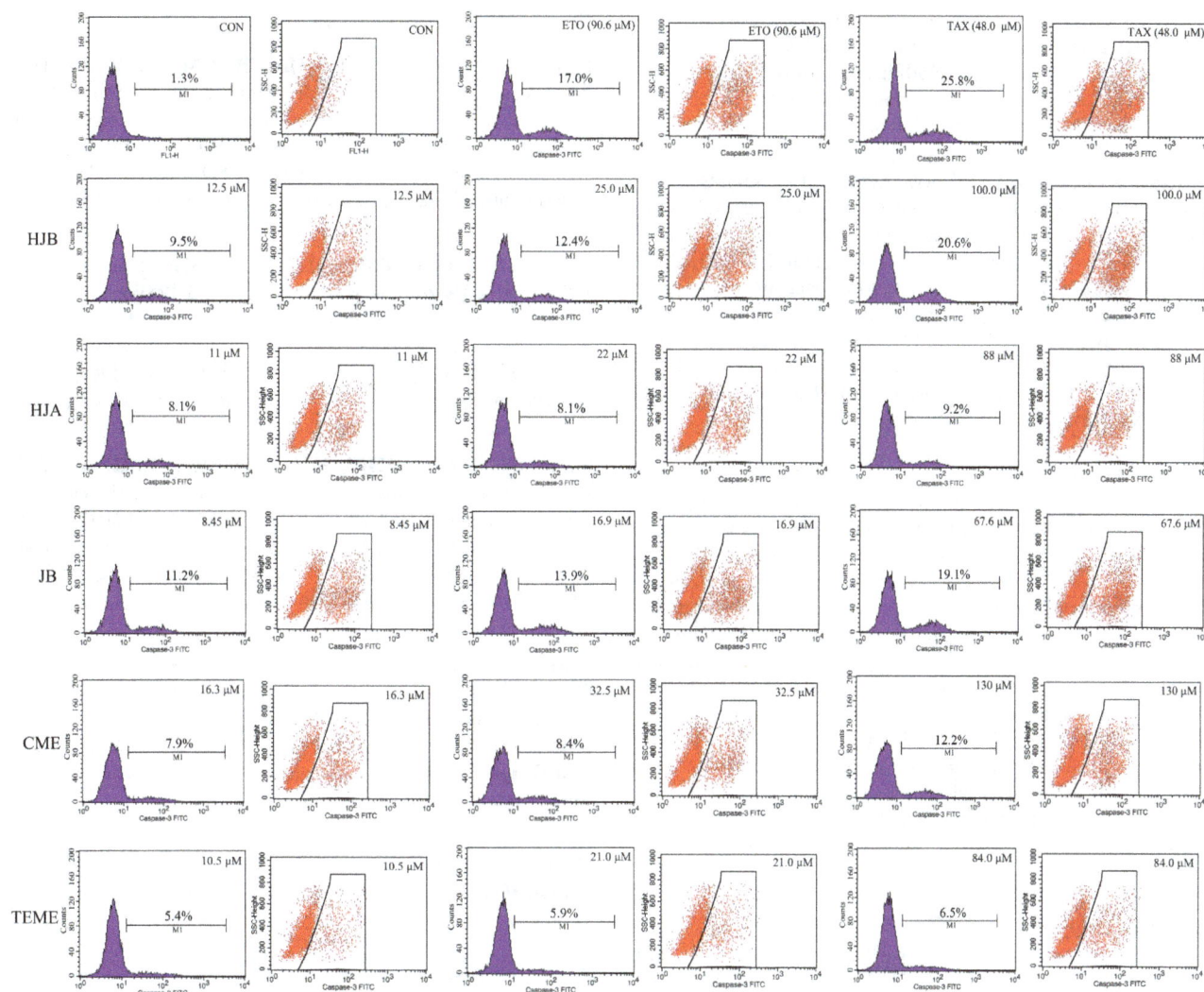

Figure 5. Effects of arylnaphthalene lignans on caspase-3 activity in K562 cells. Active caspase-3 expression was detected by flow cytometry in K562 cells after treatment with the indicated concentrations of HJA, HJB, JB, CME, TEME, ETO and TAX for 48 h. The results are representative of three independent experiments.

Cell viability assay

Cytotoxicity was determined using a modified MTT colorimetric assay [2]. HJA, HJB, JB, CME and TEME were dissolved in dimethylsulfoxide (DMSO; final concentration 0.1% (v/v)). DMSO (0.1%) was used as the control. Briefly, cells were seeded in 96-well plates (Nunc, Roskilde, Denmark) at 1×10^5 cells/ml and treated for 48 h with different concentrations of the test agent, as indicated. Next, 20 µl MTT (5 mg/ml) was added to each well and cells were incubated at $37°C$ for a further 4 h. Then, 100 µl 10% SDS-5% isopropanol-0.012 M HCl was added and cells were incubated overnight at $37°C$. The absorbance of each well was measured at 570 nm in a Multiscan photometer (BioTek, µQuant, USA). The IC_{50} was calculated by the following equation: $IC_{50} = Log^{-1}(Xm-I(\sum p-(3-Pm-Pn)/4))$, whereas Xm represents the logarithm of the maximum concentration, I represents the dilution factor, Pm represents the maximum inhibition rate, and Pn represents the minimum inhibition rate.

Measurement of SOD activity

The activity of SOD was detected by its ability to reduce cytochrome c, which causes an increase in absorbance at 550 nm. To do this, K562 cells were plated in 96-well plates at 1×10^5 cells/ml and allowed to attach for 24 h. Cells were then treated with different doses of the indicated arylnaphthalene or vehicle control. After 48 h, K562 cells were thawed three times at a temperature of $-80°C$. The supernatant was collected and used to measure intracellular SOD activity at 550 nm by using an automatic microplate reader.

Cell-cycle analysis

K562 cells were seeded at a density of 1×10^5 cells/ml in 12-well plates and incubated with different concentrations of the indicated arylnaphthalene for 48 h. After exposure, 10^6 cells were harvested, washed twice with ice-cold PBS, then centrifuged to recover the cell pellet which was subsequently resuspended and fixed with 70% ethanol overnight at $4°C$. The suspension was then washed and resuspended in 100 µl PBS containing 100 µg/ml RNase at RT for 10 min followed by staining with 200 µl of 100 µg/ml PI for 20 min in darkness. PI-stained cells were assayed using FACS Canto Becton Dickinson Flow Cytometry and cell cycle distributions were analyzed with the ModFit program (BD, San Diego, CA, USA). All samples were assayed in triplicate, and the fraction of each cell cycle phase was calculated.

Annexin V/PI staining and flow cytometry analysis

K562 cells were plated in 12-well plates at a density of 5×10^5 cells/well. The cells were treated with varying concentrations of the indicated arylnaphthalenes or the vehicle (0.1% DMSO) in complete medium for 48 h. At the end of each treatment, cells were collected and the quantitative apoptotic death assay was performed by Annexin V and PI staining (Molecular Probes) following the manufacturer's protocol. Staining was then analyzed immediately by flow cytometry using the FACS (BD, San Diego, CA, USA).

Caspase-3 activity assay

Caspase 3 enzymatic activity was measured using the caspase 3 activity assay kits (BioVision, USA) according to the manufacturer's instructions. In brief, cells were seeded at a density of 5×10^5 cells/ml in 12-well slides. After treatment with varying concentrations of the indicated Arylnaphthalene or the vehicle (0.1% DMSO) for 12 h, cells were collected and washed twice with ice-cold PBS, then resuspended in Cytofix/Cytoperm solution at a concentration of 1×10^5 cells/50 μl. The cells were incubated for 20 min on ice and then washed twice with Perm/Wash buffer at a volume of 0.5 ml buffer/1×10^6 cells at RT. The cells were then incubated with 20 μl FITC anti-active caspase-3/1×10^6 cells for 30 min at RT. After that, each sample was washed in 1 ml Perm/Wash buffer, and then resuspended in 0.5 ml Perm/Wash buffer and analyzed by flow cytometry using the FACS (BD, San Diego, CA, USA).

Statistical analysis

All experimental data are shown as means ± S.D. and accompanied by the number of experiments. Analysis was performed using one-way ANOVA followed by Dunnetts post-hoc test, and the values for significant difference were set at *$p <$ 0.05 and **$p < 0.01$.

References

1. Ramesh C, Ravindranath N, Ram TS, Das B (2003) Arylnaphthalide lignans from Cleistanthus collinus. Chem Pharm Bull (Tokyo) 51: 1299–1300.
2. Wu SJ, Wu TS (2006) Cytotoxic arylnaphthalene lignans from *Phyllanthus oligospermus*. Chem Pharm Bull (Tokyo) 54: 1223–1225.
3. Wang JZ, Tian X, Tsumura H, Shimura K, Ito H (1993) Antitumor activity of a new low immunosuppressive derivative of podophyllotoxin (GP-11) and its mechanisms. Anticancer Drug Des 8: 193–202.
4. Daley L, Guminski Y, Demerseman P, Kruczynski A, Etievant C, et al. (1998) Synthesis and antitumor activity of new glycosides of epipodophyllotoxin, analogues of etoposide, and NK 611. J Med Chem 41: 4475–4485.
5. Rassmann I, Thodtmann R, Mross M, Huttmann A, Berdel WE, et al. (1998) Phase I clinical and pharmacokinetic trial of the podophyllotoxin derivative NK611 administered as intravenous short infusion. Invest New Drugs 16: 319–324.
6. Utsugi T, Shibata J, Sugimoto Y, Aoyagi K, Wierzba K, et al. (1996) Antitumor activity of a novel podophyllotoxin derivative (TOP-53) against lung cancer and lung metastatic cancer. Cancer Res 56: 2809–2814.
7. Daley L, Meresse P, Bertounesque E, Monneret C (1997) A one-pot, efficient synthesis of the potent cytotoxic podophyllotoxin derivative NPF. Tetrahedron Lett 38: 2673–2676.
8. Van Vliet DS, Lee KH (1990) A high yield preparation of 2-fluoropodophyllo-toxin. Tetrahedron Lett 40: 2259–2262.
9. Huang TS, Lee CC, Chao Y, Shu CH, Chen LT, et al. (1999) A novel podophyllotoxin-derived compound GL331 is more potent than its congener VP-16 in killing refractory cancer cells. Pharmaceut Res 16: 997–1002.
10. Huang TS, Shu CH, Lee CC, Chen LT, Whang-Peng J (2000) *In vitro* evaluation of GL331's cancer cell killing and apoptosis-inducing activity in combination with other chemotherapeutic agents. Apoptosis 5: 79–85.
11. Lee CC, Huang TS (2001) A novel topoisomerase II poison GL331 preferentially induces DNA cleavage at (C/G) T sites and can cause telomere DNA damage. Pharm Res 18: 846–851.
12. Lin SK, Huang HC, Chen LL, Lee CC, Huang TS (2001) GL331 induces down-regulation of cyclin D1 expression via enhanced proteolysis and repressed transcription. Mol Pharmacol 60: 768–775.
13. Barret JM, Etievant C, Baudouin C, Skov K, Charveron M, et al. (2002) F 11782, a novel catalytic inhibitor of topoisomerases I and II, induces atypical, yet cytotoxic DNA double-strand breaks in CHO-K1 cells. Anticancer Res 22: 187–192.
14. Bringmann G, Walter R, Weirich R (1990) The Directed Synthesis of Biaryl Compounds: Modern Concepts and Strategies. Angew Chem 29: 977–991.
15. Kimura M, Suzuki J, Yamada T, Yoshizaki M, Kikuchi T, et al. (1985) Anti-inflammatory effect of neolignans newly isolated from the crude drug "Shin-I" (*Flos Magnoliae*). Planta Med 51: 291–293.
16. Nitiss JL (2009) Targeting DNA topoisomerase II in cancer chemotherapy. Nat Rev Cancer 9: 338–350.
17. Susplugas S, Hung NV, Bignon J, Thoison O, Kruczynski A, et al. (2005) Cytotoxic arylnaphthalene lignans from a Vietnamese Acanthaceae, *Justicia patentiflora*. J Nat Prod 68: 734–738.
18. Su CL, Huang LL, Huang LM, Lee JC, Lin CN, et al. (2006) Caspase-8 acts as a key upstream executor of mitochondria during justicidin A-induced apoptosis in human hepatoma cells. FEBS Lett 580: 3185–3191.
19. Day SH, Lin YC, Tsai ML, Tsao LT, Ko HH, et al. (2002) Potent cytotoxic lignans from *Justicia procumbens* and their effects on nitric oxide and tumor necrosis factor-alpha production in mouse macrophages. J Nat Prod 65: 379–381.

Supporting Information

Figure S1 Effect of HJB, HJA, JB, CME, TEME, POD, ETO and TAX on the proliferation of HL-60 cells. HL-60 cells were exposed to the indicated concentrations of arylnaphthalene lignans and incubated for 48 h, MTT assays were then performed. Data represent the mean ± SD of three independent experiments, where each sample was tested in at least triplicate.

Figure S2 Effect of HJB, HJA, JB, CME, TEME, POD, ETO and TAX on the proliferation of L1210 cells. L1210 cells were exposed to the indicated concentrations of arylnaphthalene lignans and incubated for 48 h, MTT assays were then performed. Data represent the mean ± SD of three independent experiments, where each sample was tested in at least triplicate.

Figure S3 Effect of HJB, HJA, JB, CME, TEME and TAX on the proliferation of P388D1 cells. P388D1 cells were exposed to the indicated concentrations of arylnaphthalene lignans and incubated for 48 h, MTT assays were then performed. Data represent the mean ± SD from three independent experiments, where each sample was tested in at least triplicate.

Figure S4 Chemical structures of 10 lignans isolated from *J. procumbens*, including neojusticidin A, isodi-phyllin, Taiwanin C, neesiinoside C, 6′-hydroxy azizin, 4′-demethylchinensinaphthol methyl ether, Diphyllin-1-O-β-D-apiofuranoside, ciliatoside C, Justicidinoside C and Justicidinoside B.

Table S1 Cytotoxicity of 14 lignans derived from *J. procumbens* on the HCT-8 and Bel-7402 cell lines.

Author Contributions

Conceived and designed the experiments: MY JL. Performed the experiments: JL YH. Analyzed the data: WK JL. Contributed reagents/materials/analysis tools: JL WK YH. Wrote the paper: JL.

20. Fukamiya N, Lee KH (1986) Antitumor agents, 81. Justicidin-A and diphyllin, two cytotoxic principles from *Justicia procumbens*. J Nat Prod 49: 348–350.

21. Zhang P, Dong XZ, Zhou YT, Yang MH, Bi MG (2009) Mechanism of JR6 to induce human bladder cancer EJ cells apoptosis. Chin Pharmacol Bull 25: 173–174.

22. Zhang P, Zhou WQ, Dong XZ, Yang MH, Bi MG (2010) Effect of 6'-hydroxy justicidin A on cell proliferation and redox system in tumor cells. Chin J Pharmacol Toxicol 24: 207–213.

23. Deng JY, Yang MH, Bi MG (2009) *In vitro* anti-tumor mechanism of JR6 on human colon cancer cell HT-29. Chin Pharmacol Bull 25: 190–191.

24. Di Giorgio C, Delmas F, Akhmedjanova V, Ollivier E, Bessonova I, et al. (2005) *In vitro* antileishmanial activity of diphyllin isolated from *Haplophyllum bucharicum*. Planta Med 71: 366–369.

25. Asano J, Chiba K, Tada M, Yoshii T (1996) Antiviral activity of lignans and their glycosides from *Justicia procumbens*. Phytochemistry 42: 713–717.

26. Chen CC, Hsin WC, Ko FN, Huang YL, Ou JC, et al. (1996) Antiplatelet arylnaphthalide lignans from *Justicia procumbens*. J Nat Prod 59: 1149–1150.

27. He XL, Zhang P, Dong XZ, Yang MH, Chen SL, et al. (2012) JR6, a new compound isolated from *Justicia procumbens*, induces apoptosis in human bladder cancer EJ cells through caspase-dependent pathway. J Ethnopharmacol 144: 284–292.

28. Yang M, Wu J, Cheng F, Zhou Y (2006a) Complete assignments of ^{1}H and ^{13}C NMR data for seven arylnaphthalide lignans from *Justicia procumbens*. Magn Reson Chem 44: 727–730.

29. Yang M, Wu J, Xu X, Jin Y, Guo Y, et al. (2006b) A new lignan from the Jian-er syrup and its content determination by RP-HPLC. J Pharm Biomed Anal 41: 662–666.

30. Luo Z, Kong W, Qiu F, Yang M, Li Q, et al. (2013) Simultaneous determination of seven lignans in *Justicia procumbens* by high performance liquid chromatography-photodiode array detection using relative response factors. J Sep Sci 36: 699–705.

31. Green DR, Reed JC (1998) Mitochondria and apoptosis. Science 281: 1309–1312.

32. Hanahan D, Weinberg RA (2000) The hallmarks of cancer. Cell 100: 57–70.

33. Roth W, Reed JC (2002) Apoptosis and cancer: When BAX is TRAILing away. Nat Med 8: 216–218.

34. Droge W (2002) Free radicals in the physiological control of cell function. Physiol Rev 82: 47–95.

35. Azad MB, Chen Y, Gibson SB (2009) Regulation of autophagy by reactive oxygen species (ROS): implications for cancer progression and treatment. Antioxid Redox Signal 11: 777–790.

36. Nicholson DW, Ali A, Thornberry NA, Vaillancourt JP, Ding CK, et al. (1995) Identification and inhibition of the ICE/CED-3 protease necessary for mammalian apoptosis. Nature 376: 37–43.

37. Vasilev N, Elfahmi, Bos R, Kayser O, Momekov G, et al. (2006) Production of justicidin B, a cytotoxic arylnaphthalene lignan from genetically transformed root cultures of *Linum leonii*. J Nat Prod 69: 1014–1017.

38. Ionkova I, Sasheva P, Ionkov T, Momekov G (2013) *Linum narbonense*: A new valuable tool for biotechnological production of a potent anticancer lignan Justicidine B. Pharmacogn Mag 9: 39–44.

39. Qiu F, Zhou S, Fu S, Kong W, Yang S, et al. (2012) LC-ESI-MS/MS analysis and pharmacokinetics of 6'-hydroxy justicidin A, a potential antitumor active component isolated from *Justicia procumbens*, in rats. J Pharm Biomed Anal 70: 539–543.

40. Zhou S, Qiu F, Tong Z, Yang S, Yang M (2012) Application of a sensitive and specific LC-MS/MS method for determination of chinensinaphthol methyl ether in rat plasma for a bioavailability study. J Chromatogr B Analyt Technol Biomed Life Sci 903: 75–80.

41. McGahon A, Bissonnette R, Schmitt M, Cotter KM, Green DR, et al. (1994) BCR-ABL maintains resistance of chronic myelogenous leukemia cells to apoptotic cell death. Blood 83: 1179–1187.

42. Jiang H, Hou C, Zhang S, Xie H, Zhou W, et al. (2007) Matrine upregulates the cell cycle protein E2F-1 and triggers apoptosis via the mitochondrial pathway in K562 cells. Eur J Pharmacol 559: 98–108.

43. Bechtel W, Bauer G (2009) Modulation of intercellular ROS signaling of human tumor cells. Anticancer Res 29: 4559–4570.

44. Potokar M, Milisav I, Kreft M, Stenovec M, Zorec R (2003) Apoptosis triggered redistribution of caspase-9 from cytoplasm to mitochondria. FEBS Lett 544: 153–159.

45. Charlton JL (1998) Antiviral activity of lignans. J Nat Prod 61: 1447–1451.

14

Genetic Variation in DNA Repair Pathways and Risk of Non-Hodgkin's Lymphoma

Justin Rendleman[1], Yevgeniy Antipin[2], Boris Reva[2], Christina Adaniel[1], Jennifer A. Przybylo[2], Ana Dutra-Clarke[2], Nichole Hansen[2], Adriana Heguy[2], Kety Huberman[2], Laetitia Borsu[2], Ora Paltiel[3], Dina Ben-Yehuda[3], Jennifer R. Brown[4], Arnold S. Freedman[4], Chris Sander[2], Andrew Zelenetz[2], Robert J. Klein[2], Yongzhao Shao[1], Mortimer Lacher[2], Joseph Vijai[2], Kenneth Offit[2], Tomas Kirchhoff[1]*

1 NYU School of Medicine, New York University, New York, New York, United States of America, 2 Memorial Sloan-Kettering Cancer Center, New York, New York, United States of America, 3 Hadassah-Hebrew University Medical Center, Jerusalem, Israel, 4 Dana Farber Cancer Center, Harvard University, Boston, Massachusetts, United States of America

Abstract

Molecular and genetic evidence suggests that DNA repair pathways may contribute to lymphoma susceptibility. Several studies have examined the association of DNA repair genes with lymphoma risk, but the findings from these reports have been inconsistent. Here we provide the results of a focused analysis of genetic variation in DNA repair genes and their association with the risk of non-Hodgkin's lymphoma (NHL). With a population of 1,297 NHL cases and 1,946 controls, we have performed a two-stage case/control association analysis of 446 single nucleotide polymorphisms (SNPs) tagging the genetic variation in 81 DNA repair genes. We found the most significant association with NHL risk in the *ATM* locus for rs227060 (OR = 1.27, 95% CI: 1.13–1.43, $p = 6.77 \times 10^{-5}$), which remained significant after adjustment for multiple testing. In a subtype-specific analysis, associations were also observed for the *ATM* locus among both diffuse large B-cell lymphomas (DLBCL) and small lymphocytic lymphomas (SLL), however there was no association observed among follicular lymphomas (FL). In addition, our study provides suggestive evidence of an interaction between SNPs in *MRE11A* and *NBS1* associated with NHL risk (OR = 0.51, 95% CI: 0.34–0.77, p = 0.0002). Finally, an imputation analysis using the 1,000 Genomes Project data combined with a functional prediction analysis revealed the presence of biologically relevant variants that correlate with the observed association signals. While the findings generated here warrant independent validation, the results of our large study suggest that *ATM* may be a novel locus associated with the risk of multiple subtypes of NHL.

Editor: Riccardo Dolcetti, IRCCS National Cancer Institute, Italy

Funding: The study was funded by Translational Research Grant from Leukemia and Lymphoma Society (TRP 6202-09, awarded to Tomas Kirchhoff). Funding support was also provided by the Lymphoma Foundation and the Filomena M. D'Agostino Foundation (both to Kenneth Offit). Further support was also provided by the Okonow-Lipton Fund (Jennifer R. Brown) and the National Institutes of Health (K23 CA115682, Jennifer R. Brown). Jennifer R. Brown is a Scholar of the American Society of Hematology as well as a Scholar in Clinical Research of the Leukemia and Lymphoma Society. MSKCC Sequenom facility is supported by the Anbinder Fund. The funders had no role in study design, data collection and analysis, decision to publish, or preparation of the manuscript.

Competing Interests: The authors have declared that no competing interests exist.

* Email: Tomas.Kirchhoff@nyumc.org

Introduction

The incidence of non-Hodgkin's lymphoma (NHL) in the U.S. has doubled over the past two decades. While the etiology of the disease remains largely unknown [1], surmounting evidence suggests that genetic predisposition plays a role in NHL development [2–4]. Besides recently completed genome-wide association studies (GWAS) [5–13], the search for missing genetic susceptibility to lymphoma in the past decade also involved the association analyses of common genetic variants in candidate molecular pathways putatively involved in lymphoma development. In contrast to GWAS, candidate scans allow for the focused assessment of biologically relevant molecular pathways by testing larger sample populations and maintaining a higher statistical power for detecting association effects [14]. Among the candidate networks previously investigated for the association with NHL risk, DNA repair was frequently explored [15–25] due to its strong relevance to lymphomagenesis [26–28].

Associations between DNA repair genes and lymphoma risk have been reported previously [15–19], however the results in many of these studies either failed to reach the necessary level of statistical significance, or lacked independent validation. In the present study, we attempted to improve on these prior efforts by performing a two-stage case-control analysis of 1,297 NHL cases and 1,946 controls to identify associations between 446 SNPs tagging 81 DNA repair genes and NHL risk. The two-stage design, thorough selection of DNA repair genes, assessment of genetic interactions, and identification of putatively functional variants by using public genomic and expression data are among the major innovations in our study, which provides yet another focused exploration of the role of DNA repair pathways in genetic susceptibility to NHL.

Materials and Methods

Ethics Statement

All cases were ascertained through Memorial Sloan-Kettering Cancer Center (MSKCC) IRB-approved protocols, or a protocol approved by the IRB at the Dana Farber Cancer Institute (DFCI) or Hadassah-Hebrew University. These protocols required written informed consent either for identified use of specimens for research into the genetic basis of lymphoma, or research use of specimens permanently de-identified prior to genotyping. Controls were part of the New York Cancer Project (NYCP) and all subjects gave written consent for use of samples in genetic studies of any disease state.

Study population

In total, the study involved 1,297 non-Hodgkin's lymphoma (NHL) cases from the combined resources at MSKCC, DFCI and Hadassah-Hebrew University, Israel as well as 1,946 controls collected from the NYCP, a study of 18,000 New York City residents originally designed to assess the role of environment and genetics in cancer risk, and described previously elsewhere [29–31]. The NYCP data include age, gender, history of cancers (including lymphoma) and ethnicity. A subset of NHL cases (n = 222) were probands from families with a strong family history (FH) of NHL, described in detail recently [32]. The remaining fraction of NHL patients (n = 1,075), were unrelated and unselected for FH. All cases and controls were of white European ancestry, with a fraction of cases (n = 534, 41.2%) and controls (n = 1,043, 53.6%) of self reported Ashkenazi Jewish (AJ) ancestry. In this study we have employed a two-stage design; the discovery stage (stage 1) consisting of 650 cases and 965 controls, and the replication stage (stage 2) involving 647 cases and 981 controls. The detailed structure, demographic, and clinical information of case/control populations in both stage 1 and 2 is summarized in Table S1. A subset of the patient collection in this study was previously included in a GWAS on lymphoma susceptibility [9]. Of the 944 lymphoma cases that constituted the GWAS phase of that prior study, 515 cases (39.7%) overlap with the 1,297 patients included here. While 1,043 controls (53.6%) overlap between the current study and the validation stage of the prior GWAS, there was no control overlap between this study and the GWAS discovery stage.

Selection of genes and tagging SNPs (tSNPs)

The selection of candidate DNA repair genes was performed as summarized in Figure S1. The initial subset of genes (n = 34) has been identified for their known role in DNA repair processes and queried for their catalytic activities from Gene Ontology (GO) [33] and KEGG [34]. The key networks of DNA repair defined by the catalytic domains in the seed list were further passed to: 1) GO search for genes containing identified catalytic activities and 2) yeast proteome database [35] identifying yeast homologues with experimental evidence demonstrating their effect on UV sensitivity, radiation, and DNA damage response. The yeast genes were subsequently queried for human homologues. The targets from 1) and 2) were crossed for gene overlap and passed to an interactome analysis (GeneGO, Ingenuity) to query interacting partners (defined by at least two independent reports, and confirmed by at least two experimental methods). After merging, 87 DNA repair genes were identified for the study (Table S2). The SNPs tagging 87 selected genes were chosen using Haploview with a haplotype Pearson's correlation coefficient (r^2) threshold <0.6 across selected gene regions (including 5 kb from 3′ and 5′ UTR), and minor allele frequency (MAF) >0.05. The tagging SNP selection has

been performed using the CEU data (120 individuals) of HapMap Phase II, the most accurate resource available for this purpose at the time of the study design and still serves as the most validated reference for capturing the common genetic variation in European populations. In total, 531 tagging SNPs (tSNPs) were selected to tag the 87 DNA repair genes.

Genotyping

For stage 1, the genotyping of 531 tSNPs from 87 selected DNA repair genes on 698 lymphoma cases and 1,041 controls was conducted using Sequenom MassARRAY iPLEX (Sequenom Inc., CA), multiplexed into a 16-plex design as per manufacturer's protocol and as described previously [30]. For quality control (QC), duplicates (8 per each 384-well plate) showed >99% concordance and non-template controls (2 per plate) revealed no evidence of cross-contamination. Thirty-four SNPs were excluded due to low genotyping rate across samples (<85%), poor clustering, or significant departure from Hardy-Weinberg Equilibrium (p<0.001 in control population); an additional 51 SNPs were dropped due to low MAF (<0.05) in our study population. Forty-eight cases and 76 controls were dropped due to low genotyping rate (<85%). After QC, in total 446 SNPs, tagging 81 DNA repair genes and n = 650 cases and n = 965 controls remained for the association analysis in stage 1. Twenty-eight SNPs associated with NHL (p<0.05) from stage 1 were passed to the validation analysis in stage 2 on an additional 684 cases and 1,042 controls. In order to perform downstream haplotype and imputation analyses, in stage 2 we also included 81 additional SNPs tagging the genes captured by the 28 significant loci in stage 1. A total of 109 SNPs were passed to the replication analysis in stage 2 using a re-plexed Sequenom design (iPLEX). While all 109 SNPs passed the QC in stage 2, 37 cases and 61 controls were dropped due to low genotyping rates across SNPs (<85%), resulting in the genotyping data on 109 SNPs in 647 cases and 981 controls. Data can be made available to other researchers: please contact the authors for details.

Statistical association analyses

Single SNP associations with NHL risk were tested using a logistic regression model under a per-allele test, calculating odds ratios (OR) and 95% confidence intervals (95% CI), adjusted for age, gender and AJ status. The associations were analyzed for stage 1, stage 2, and the aggregate sample set including both stages. In the aggregate sample set we also used a per-allele logistic regression model to test fifteen SNP associations within the three most common NHL subtypes in our dataset: diffuse large B-cell lymphoma (DLBCL), follicular lymphoma (FL) and small lymphocytic lymphoma/chronic lymphocytic leukemia (SLL/CLL). Quantile/quantile (Q/Q) plots were produced using ggplot2 in R, and inflation factors (λ) were calculated based on 90% of least significant SNPs. Statistical analyses were performed using PLINK [36]. The main analysis examining single SNP associations with NHL risk and the associations among subtypes were controlled for multiple testing using Bonferroni adjustment. The Bonferroni level of significance was defined as p<0.000154, accounting for 247 independent SNPs in stage 1, 33 independent SNPs in stage 2, and 15 SNPs tested among three NHL subtypes (number of tests = 247+33+(15*3) = 325; p = 0.05/325 – 0.000154). Independent SNPs were defined under Pearson's correlation coefficient (r-square) <0.5 calculated among our sample population.

Haplotypes were visualized by Haploview and haplotype associations were performed by logistic regression analysis adjusted for age, gender, and AJ status. We have also tested the homogeneity of the odds ratios between these three major subtypes by calculating the Breslow-Day statistics for each SNP.

In order to explore possible epistatic interactions associated with NHL risk, logistic regressions were modeled by adding an interaction term between the genotypes of each SNP pair. First, pairwise comparisons were performed between each SNP from the list of fifteen associations with NHL (105 tests), followed by pairwise comparisons of fifteen SNPs with the additional 94 SNPs included in the aggregate analysis (1,410 tests, Bonferroni adjusted p-value: $0.05/(105+1410) = 3.3 \times 10^{-5}$). This analysis was performed using PLINK [36]. For the targeted analysis of the MRN complex (MRE11A, NBS1), the multiplicative two-way gene-gene interactions were estimated using multiple logistic regression models. For each SNP pair, a logistic regression model was built to test case/control association based on the indicator variables (sex, age and AJ status) and the 2-SNP variable, for a total of 5 variables and an intercept. The 2-SNP variable was defined separately under three genetic models, based on the number of risk alleles in individual subjects.

For the assessment of SNP-gene association by incorporating expression information (expressed quantitative trait loci – eQTL) we used Genevar [37]. The eQTL associations were calculated by Spearman's rank correlation tests.

Imputation and functional prediction

The imputation of genotypes from 1,297 NHL cases and 1,946 controls was performed using IMPUTE2 [38] with a reference panel consisting of the 1,000 Genomes Project (1KG) data freeze from November 2010 for low-coverage genomes, May 2011 for high-coverage exomes, and the phased haplotypes released March 2012 (n = 1,092 individuals). Imputed loci were filtered based on the quality metric score (info score) >0.7 [39], chosen based on inflation estimates from a Q/Q analysis; the imputed SNPs with info score <0.7 showed significant inflations in our data (Figure S2). The functional annotation of the associated tagging SNPs and their correlated imputed SNPs was performed by ANNOVAR [40], focusing on 8 functional categories: coding regions, conserved transcription factor (TF) binding sites, TF binding sites based on ChIP-Seq data (using ENCODE database), enhancer sites based on H3K4me1 chromatin marks (using ENCODE database), DNase I hypersensitivity clusters (using ENCODE database), known CNVs, and 3′ UTR, and 5′ UTR.

Results

Sample population

The demographic and clinical composition of our sample population is summarized in Table S1. No significant difference was observed in the distribution of demographic variables or lymphoma subtypes between stage 1 and stage 2. Also, no significant difference between demographic characteristics or subtype distribution has been noted between cases with FH and NHL cases unselected for FH. However, there was a difference in the proportion of age, AJ ancestry and gender between the NHL cases and controls. Hence, age, AJ status and gender were used as covariates in all subsequent statistical analyses.

Single SNP associations with NHL risk

In this study we applied a two-stage design: in stage 1 we performed the association analysis on 446 SNPs tagging 81 DNA repair genes in the population of 650 cases and 965 controls. There was no significant inflation in observed versus expected associations ($\lambda = 1.07$), indicating no detectable genotyping arti-

facts or population substructures impacting our findings (Figure S3).

We first tested the association of DNA repair variants with NHL cases (all subtypes pooled). The association analysis of NHL cases in stage 1 identified 28 SNPs associated with NHL risk (p<0.05). The strongest associations in stage 1 were found for 3 SNPs in the ATM locus: rs611646, rs419716 and rs227060, the latter showing the strongest effect (OR = 1.27, 95% CI: 1.07–1.49, p = 0.005). Other associations in stage 1 included tSNPs in MRE11A (rs625245, OR = 0.78, 95% CI: 0.65–0.93, p = 0.006), GTF2H1 (rs4150606, OR = 0.82, 95% CI: 0.69–0.97, p = 0.02), and MSH2 (rs4952887, OR = 0.66, 95% CI: 0.47–0.91, p = 0.01).

The twenty-eight most significant SNPs from stage 1 and an additional 81 SNPs, as described in Materials and Methods (total 109 SNPs) were passed to stage 2, which involved 647 NHL cases and 981 controls. The associations were replicated for rs227060 and rs611646 in ATM with a more pronounced effect than in stage 1; rs227060 again shows the strongest association in stage 2 (OR = 1.30, 95% CI: 1.10–1.54, p = 0.002). Other SNPs that replicated in stage 2 include GTF2H1 (rs4150606, OR = 0.81, 95% CI: 0.68–0.95, p = 0.01), MSH2 (rs4952887, OR = 0.76, 95% CI: 0.58–1.01, p = 0.05) and MRE11A (rs625245, OR = 0.84, 95% CI: 0.69–1.01, p = 0.05). See Table S3 for the complete association results.

In the aggregate analysis of stage 1 and 2, fifteen SNPs showed associations with NHL risk (Table 1). These included two SNPs in the ATM locus: rs227060 and rs611646 (OR = 1.27, 95% CI: 1.13–1.43, $p_{agg} = 0.00007$; OR = 1.26, 95% CI: 1.12–1.43, $p_{agg} = 0.00015$, respectively, where p_{agg} is a p-value from aggregate analysis). Importantly, the associations for both loci remained significant after Bonferroni correction, as detailed in Material and Methods ($p_{adj} = 0.022$; $p_{adj} = 0.049$, respectively, where p_{adj} is the Bonferroni corrected p-value for each SNP). The two SNPs show incomplete LD ($r^2 = 0.642$, Figure S4). In order to test whether the associations in ATM were independent we conditioned the analyses by the status of rs227060 and found rs611646 and rs419716 no longer significant (data not shown), suggesting the association signals observed for ATM SNPs are correlated. No other SNP associations in the aggregate analysis passed Bonferroni correction. To further explore the structure of associated loci, we also examined common haplotypes (MAF> 0.05) for association with NHL risk. The strongest risk effect has been observed for a haplotype in ATM. Other loci have also shown specific haplotypes associated with NHL risk, however none were more significant than the associations from single SNP analyses (Table S4). As our study population includes a large fraction of AJ ancestry, we have investigated potential association differences between AJ and non-AJ samples. The majority of the 109 SNPs (n = 94) in the aggregate analysis show no more than a 5% difference in minor allele frequency (MAFs) between AJ and non-AJ subsets (Figure S5). Three SNPs (rs4150606, rs7149962, rs7562048) that present with >5% difference in MAF also show association with NHL. The analysis stratified by AJ status indicated that most associations, including our two most significant ATM SNPs, appear to be largely driven by non-AJ subsets which are predominant in our case population (Table S5). However, for other SNP associations such as rs4150606 (GTF2H1), rs4952887 (MSH2), and rs702019 (POLQ), both AJ and non-AJ subsets contribute to the association signal. Therefore, all analyses in the study were also adjusted by AJ status.

The associations of DNA repair genes with NHL subtypes

We have further tested the associations identified in the NHL pooled analysis among NHL subtypes on fifteen SNPs that

Table 1. Association analysis of genetic variants in DNA repair genes with the risk of NHL.

Gene	Chr.	SNP	Minor Allele	Allele Freq.	Stage 1 (650 Cases/965 Controls) OR (95% CI)	P	Stage 2 (647 Cases/981 Controls) OR (95% CI)	P	Stage 1 & 2 [Aggregate] (1,297 Cases/1,946 Controls) OR (95% CI)	P
ATM	11	rs2227060	T	0.37	1.27 (1.07–1.49)	0.0057	1.30 (1.10–1.54)	0.0020	1.27 (1.13–1.43)	6.77×10^{-5}
ATM	11	rs611646	T	0.45	1.24 (1.04–1.49)	0.016	1.30 (1.10–1.54)	0.0020	1.26 (1.12–1.43)	1.52×10^{-4}
GTF2H1	11	rs4150606	A	0.50	0.82 (0.69–0.97)	0.021	0.81 (0.68–0.95)	0.013	0.81 (0.72–0.92)	6.68×10^{-4}
MSH2	2	rs4952887	T	0.07	0.66 (0.47–0.91)	0.012	0.76 (0.58–1.01)	0.055	0.71 (0.57–0.87)	0.00128
MRE11A	11	rs625245	C	0.32	0.78 (0.65–0.93)	0.0066	0.84 (0.69–1.01)	0.059	0.81 (0.71–0.93)	0.0018
ATM	11	rs419716	T	0.42	0.8 (0.67–0.96)	0.014	0.85 (0.71–1.01)	0.056	0.83 (0.73–0.94)	0.0025
POLQ	3	rs702019	G	0.23	0.77 (0.62–0.95)	0.013	0.90 (0.74–1.09)	0.271	0.84 (0.73–0.96)	0.013
TDP1	14	rs7149962	C	0.06	1.49 (1.07–2.08)	0.020	1.19 (0.85–1.65)	0.307	1.33 (1.05–1.68)	0.019
NBS1	8	rs1805812	C	0.06	0.87 (0.59–1.27)	0.466	0.65 (0.46–0.94)	0.021	0.75 (0.58–0.97)	0.028
CCNH	5	rs3093819	T	0.46	1.14 (0.96–1.34)	0.128	1.13 (0.96–1.34)	0.139	1.14 (1.01–1.28)	0.030
MRE11A	11	rs10831227	A	0.34	0.93 (0.79–1.1)	0.382	0.83 (0.70–0.99)	0.035	0.88 (0.78–0.99)	0.030
CHEK1	11	rs565416	A	0.32	0.79 (0.66–0.94)	0.0075	0.99 (0.84–1.17)	0.892	0.88 (0.78–0.99)	0.037
MSH6	2	rs7562048	G	0.44	0.79 (0.66–0.93)	0.0062	0.98 (0.82–1.16)	0.818	0.88 (0.78–0.99)	0.039
NBS1	8	rs14448	C	0.06	0.99 (0.70–1.40)	0.936	1.61 (1.16–2.23)	0.0043	1.28 (1.01–1.62)	0.041
ATR	3	rs10804682	A	0.20	1.24 (1.02–1.51)	0.031	1.09 (0.90–1.32)	0.375	1.15 (1.01–1.32)	0.042

OR = odds ratio; CI = confidence interval.

associated with overall NHL risk in the aggregate analysis. We focused on the three most common NHL subtypes in our study population in order to maintain analytical power: diffuse large B-cell lymphomas (DLBCL), follicular lymphomas (FL), and small lymphocytic lymphoma/chronic lymphocytic leukemia (SLL/CLL). As shown in Table 2, associations were identified for the three *ATM* tSNPs in DLBCL (n = 412), with the strongest effect for rs611646 (OR = 1.37, 95% CI 1.14–1.64, p = 0.0008). Associations for rs611646 and rs227060 were also observed in SLL/CLL (n = 164). No *ATM* tSNPs were associated with risk in the FL subset (n = 301). In contrast, the strongest effects in FL was observed for *CHEK1* (rs565416, OR = 0.71, 95% CI: 0.58–0.87, p = 0.001) and *TDP1* (rs7149962, OR = 1.64, 95% CI: 1.14–2.35, p = 0.007), which were not associated with DLBCL or SLL/CLL. In SLL/CLL, the strongest association effect was found for rs4150606 tagging *GTF2H1* (OR = 0.51, 95% CI: 0.39–0.69, p = 4.84×10^{-6}); this association was not seen in FL or DLBCL sub-analyses. The association of rs4150606 with SLL/CLL remains significant after Bonferroni correction for multiple testing ($p_{adj} = 0.0016$). The SNP/MAF plot between AJ and non-AJ (Figure S5) identified rs4150606 as an outlier. Despite the MAF difference it appears that both AJ and non-AJ ancestries contribute to the observed association risk effect of rs4150606 (Table S5).

We have also tested the association heterogeneity among the three major subtypes in our analysis of fifteen SNPs (Table 2). The Breslow-Day test results showed an association for rs227060 (p = 0.037), indicating heterogeneity in the odds ratios between the DLBCL, SLL/CLL, and FL. Heterogeneity has also been observed for an additional two SNPs with subtype-specific associations: rs4150606 (*GTF2H1*, p = 0.001) and rs565416 (*CHEK1*, p = 0.006).

The epistatic SNP-SNP interactions in DNA repair genes and NHL risk

Using the additive model in pairwise SNP-SNP interaction analysis, we found several associations with NHL risk among the top fifteen SNPs from the aggregate analysis. However, none of these associations survived the adjustment for multiple testing (Table S6). Nonetheless, we noted several interactions of variants in *MRE11A* with SNPs in *NBS1* associated with NHL risk. Interestingly, both genes biologically interact in the MRN complex, a centerpiece of double strand break repair machinery, which prompted us to examine these interactions more closely using different genetic models. While all interactions involve rs1805812 in *NBS1*, for *MRE11A* there are four different variants which contribute to these associations (rs10831227, rs625245, rs607974, rs557148). After examination of the four pairwise associations (rs1805812 in *NBS1* with each of the four *MRE11A* SNPs) using three genetic models (Models 1–3 detailed in Table S7), we focused on two pairwise interactions with the strongest effects, rs1805812 (*NBS1*) x rs625245 (*MRE11A*) and rs1805812 (*NBS1*) x rs607974 (*MRE11A*). As shown in Table 3, the strongest interaction association was observed for rs1805812 x rs607974 under Model 3, with the strongest effect for heterozygotes or homozygotes for the minor allele on both gene loci (*MRE11A*' *NBS1*). The association observed for rs1805812 x rs625245 also shows the strongest effect under Model 3 (Table 4). Interestingly, both of these interactions replicate independently in both stage 1 and 2.

Imputation and functional predictions using data from the 1,000 Genomes Project

In order to identify the SNPs with putative functional impact, we imputed all associated loci from the aggregate analysis using data from the 1,000 Genomes Project (1KG; described in Material and Methods). As seen in Figure 1, the association analysis of imputed data did not yield association effects that were stronger than those observed in the analysis of genotyped SNPs. The imputation, however, identified variants that correlate with genotyped SNPs and show an association effect comparable with single SNP analyses of aggregate data (Figure 1). To investigate possible biological implications of these associations we tested the imputed SNPs using ANNOVAR (Materials and Methods). While only one non-synonymous SNP was found among the imputed variants (rs1381057 in *POLQ*), other imputed SNPs map within high-impact regulatory regions. In the *ATM* locus we found numerous putatively functional variants strongly correlated with associated tSNPs (Table 5). Of these, rs228594 merits particular attention; it maps in a DNase I hypersensitivity cluster as well as within *junD* and *FOSL2* binding sites, providing a rationale for future molecular exploration. The detailed list of imputed SNPs with predicted functional impact is in Table S8.

eQTL analysis

Using Genevar [37] we investigated eQTL associations for the *ATM* region by examining publicly available data collected from lymphoblastoid cell lines (LCL), T-cell lines (TCL), and fibroblast cell lines (FCL) derived from 75 individuals of European ancestry [41]. Out of the three *ATM* SNPs associated with NHL risk in our data, the most significant eQTL effect was observed for rs227060 in LCL based on data from probe ILMN_1716231, showing that reduced expression correlates with the risk allele (genetic correlation coefficient rho = 0.284, p = 0.0136; Figure S6). Interestingly, for the probe ILMN_1716231, the association of rs227060 with *ATM* expression was the second most significant eQTL in the region (Figure 2).

Discussion

Extensive published data suggest that DNA repair pathways are associated with lymphoma susceptibility [26,27]. The rare syndromes attributed to inherited mutations in DNA repair genes, such as ataxia talangiectasia (A-T; mutations in *ATM*) or Nijmegen breakage syndrome (NBS; mutations in *NBS1*) manifest with early onset lymphomas of various histological subtypes [42,43]. DNA repair plays a central role in B-cell development in germinal centers of primary and secondary lymphoid organs via V(D)J recombination, which is regulated by the genes involved in double strand break repair, mainly in non-homologous end-joining (NHEJ) [26]. The mouse knockout models of different components of NHEJ have serious defects in the V(D)J recombination process and manifest with increased incidence of B-cell specific lymphomas [26,44,45]. Also, inherited immunodeficiency syndromes (e.g. SCID), which are often associated with early onset lymphomas [26] are due to germline mutations in NHEJ genes. This and other evidence points to the importance of DNA repair genes in lymphomagenesis and suggest that these pathways are putative candidates in the susceptibility to lymphoma. In this study we tested common genetic variation in DNA repair genes for its role in susceptibility to NHL. The two-stage design, the thorough computational selection of DNA repair targets, the examination of potential epistatic effects of the associated loci, and the suggested functional implication of associated variants are among the major enhancements of our study design compared to prior efforts.

Table 2. Association analysis of genetic variants in DNA repair genes with the risk of major NHL subtypes.

Gene	Chr.	SNP	Minor Allele	Allele Freq.	DLBCL (412 Cases/1,946 Controls) OR (95% CI)	P	FL (301 Cases/1,946 Controls) OR (95% CI)	P	SLL/CLL (164 Cases/1,946 Controls) OR (95% CI)	P	Breslow-Day P
ATM	11	rs611646	T	0.45	1.37 (1.14–1.64)	7.7×10^{-4}	1.19 (0.96–1.46)	0.108	1.41 (1.06–1.87)	0.017	0.132
ATM	11	rs227060	T	0.37	1.34 (1.13–1.58)	8.7×10^{-4}	1.10 (0.91–1.34)	0.334	1.58 (1.21–2.06)	6.7×10^{-4}	0.037
ATM	11	rs419716	T	0.42	0.75 (0.62–0.90)	0.0026	0.84 (0.68–1.04)	0.107	0.84 (0.63–1.11)	0.217	0.229
MRE11A	11	rs10831227	A	0.34	0.77 (0.65–0.93)	0.0050	0.91 (0.75–1.11)	0.361	0.97 (0.74–1.26)	0.803	0.479
ATR	3	rs10804682	A	0.20	1.27 (1.05–1.55)	0.016	1.09 (0.86–1.37)	0.480	1.17 (0.87–1.59)	0.296	0.152
POLQ	3	rs702019	G	0.23	0.79 (0.64–0.97)	0.025	0.81 (0.64–1.03)	0.082	0.98 (0.71–1.34)	0.876	0.362
NBS1	8	rs14448	C	0.06	1.39 (1.01–1.93)	0.047	1.11 (0.74–1.65)	0.625	0.87 (0.48–1.58)	0.654	0.320
MSH2	2	rs4952887	T	0.07	0.72 (0.52–1.00)	0.048	0.71 (0.49–1.03)	0.073	0.63 (0.38–1.06)	0.079	0.432
CCNH	5	rs3093819	T	0.46	1.15 (0.98–1.37)	0.095	1.29 (1.06–1.57)	0.012	1.14 (0.87–1.49)	0.341	0.773
MRE11A	11	rs625245	C	0.32	0.85 (0.71–1.03)	0.106	0.78 (0.63–0.97)	0.028	0.87 (0.65–1.16)	0.347	0.810
GTF2H1	11	rs4150606	A	0.50	0.88 (0.74–1.05)	0.144	0.84 (0.69–1.02)	0.083	0.52 (0.39–0.69)	4.8×10^{-6}	0.001
CHEK1	11	rs565416	A	0.32	0.97 (0.82–1.16)	0.749	0.71 (0.58–0.87)	0.0012	0.99 (0.76–1.28)	0.915	0.006
TDP1	14	rs7149962	C	0.06	1.06 (0.73–1.52)	0.773	1.64 (1.14–2.35)	0.0076	0.91 (0.52–1.60)	0.754	0.921
NBS1	8	rs1805812	C	0.06	0.68 (0.45–1.04)	0.073	0.72 (0.46–1.15)	0.168	1.05 (0.58–1.88)	0.877	0.831
MSH6	2	rs7562048	G	0.44	0.87 (0.73–1.05)	0.146	0.87 (0.71–1.06)	0.162	0.84 (0.64–1.09)	0.188	0.150

DLBCL = diffuse large B-cell lymphoma; FL = follicular lymphoma; SLL/CLL = small lymphocytic lymphoma/chronic lymphocytic leukemia; OR = odds ratio; CI = confidence interval.

Table 3. Association analysis of rs1805812 x rs607974 interactions between *MRE11A* and *NBS1* with the risk of NHL.

NBS1 (rs1805812)/ MRE11A (rs607974) genotype	Stage 1			Stage 2			Stage 1 & 2 [Aggregate]		
	Cases	Controls	OR (95% CI)	Cases	Controls	OR (95% CI)	Cases	Controls	OR (95% CI)
Model 1									
NBS1 TT/*MRE11A* GG	167	333	1.0 (Ref)	241	362	1.0 (Ref)	408	695	1.0 (Ref)
NBS1 TT/*MRE11A* AG,AA; *NBS1* CT,CC/*MRE11A* GG	213	347	1.22 (0.95–1.58)	208	336	0.93 (0.73–1.18)	421	683	1.05 (0.88–1.25)
NBS1 CT,CC/*MRE11A* AG,AA	9	38	0.47 (0.22–1.00)	12	42	0.43 (0.22–0.83)	21	80	0.45 (0.27–0.73)
P for interaction	0.8713			0.03153			0.07991		
Model 2									
NBS1 TT, CT/*MRE11A* GG, AG	354	656	1.0 (Ref)	435	697	1.0 (Ref)	789	1353	1.0 (Ref)
NBS1 CC/*MRE11A* GG,AG,AA; *NBS1* TT,CT/*MRE11A* AA	35	62	1.05 (0.68–1.61)	26	43	0.97 (0.59–1.6)	61	105	1 (0.72–1.38)
P for interaction	0.4434			0.6881			0.9218		
Model 3									
NBS1 TT,CT,CC/*MRE11A* GG; *NBS1* TT/*MRE11A* AG,AA	380	680	1.0 (Ref)	449	698	1.0 (Ref)	829	1378	1.0 (Ref)
NBS1 CT,CC/*MRE11A* AG,AA	9	38	0.42 (0.2–0.89)	12	42	0.44 (0.23–0.85)	21	80	0.44 (0.27–0.71)
P for interaction	0.002537			0.002361			0.0000209		

OR = odds ratio; CI = confidence interval.

Table 4. Association analysis of rs1805812 x rs625245 interactions between *MRE11A* and *NBS1* with the risk of NHL.

NBS1 (rs1805812)/ *MRE11A* (rs625245) genotype	Stage 1			Stage 2			Stage 1 & 2 [Aggregate]		
	Cases	Controls	OR (95% CI)	Cases	Controls	OR (95% CI)	Cases	Controls	OR (95% CI)
Model 1									
NBS1 TT/*MRE11A* AA	148	246	1.0 (Ref)	205	278	1.0 (Ref)	353	524	1.0 (Ref)
NBS1 TT/*MRE11A* CA,CC and *NBS1* CT,CC/*MRE11A* AA	236	334	1.17 (0.90–1.53)	222	354	0.85 (0.66–1.09)	458	688	0.99 (0.83–1.18)
NBS1 CT,CC/*MRE11A* CA,CC	13	46	0.47 (0.25–0.90)	19	48	0.53 (0.31–0.94)	32	94	0.51 (0.33–0.77)
P for interaction	0.4211			0.02209			0.03183		
Model 2									
NBS1 TT,CT/*MRE11A* AA,CA	367	556	1.0 (Ref)	415	628	1.0 (Ref)	782	1184	1.0 (Ref)
NBS1 CC/*MRE11A* AA,CA,CC and *NBS1* TT,CT/*MRE11A* CC	30	70	0.65 (0.42–1.02)	31	52	0.90 (0.57–1.43)	61	122	0.76 (0.55–1.04)
P for interaction	0.03877			0.2747			0.03051		
Model 3									
NBS1 TT,CT,CC/*MRE11A* AA and *NBS1* TT/*MRE11A* CA,CC	384	580	1.0 (Ref)	427	632	1.0 (Ref)	811	1212	1.0 (Ref)
NBS1 CT,CC/*MRE11A* CA,CC	13	46	0.43 (0.23–0.80)	19	48	0.59 (0.34–1.01)	32	94	0.51 (0.34–0.77)
P for interaction	0.00436			0.01478			0.0002523		

OR = odds ratio; CI = confidence interval.

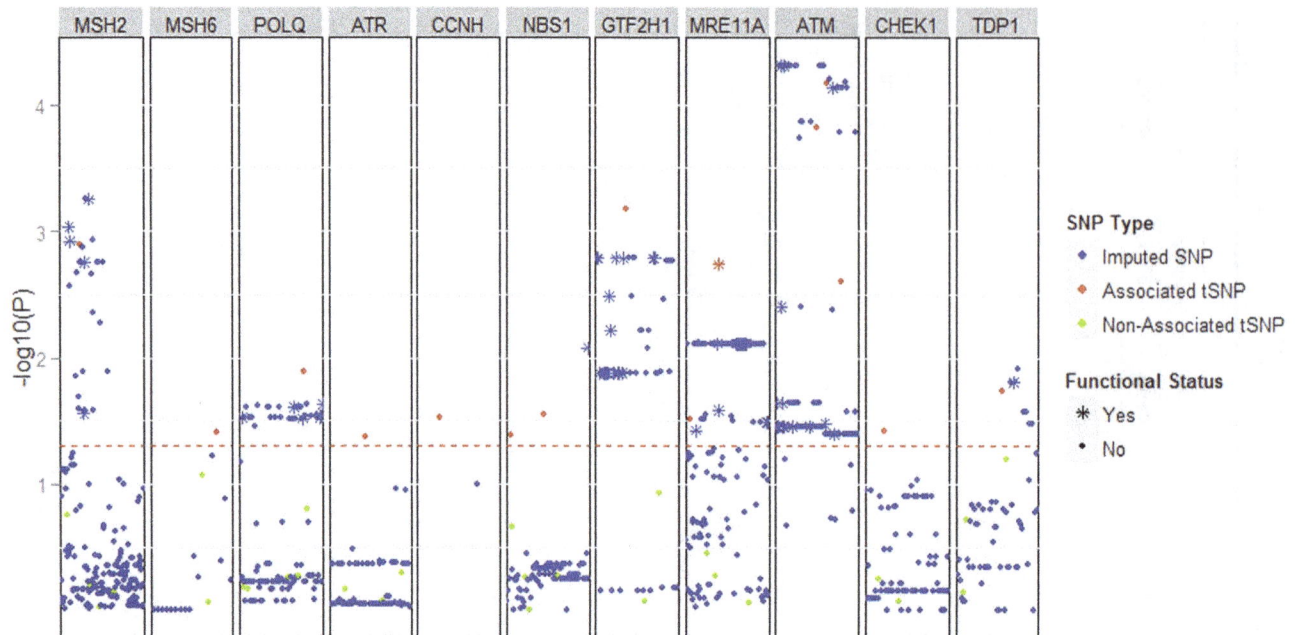

Figure 1. The results of association analysis, displayed as Manhattan plot, after imputation of 28 SNPs genotyped in both stage 1 and 2, which tag 11 DNA repair genes that showed association with NHL risk in our study. The SNPs and genes are ordered by chromosomal position (x-axis). The associations are displayed as $-\log_{10}$(p-value) for each SNP. Red dots represent fifteen tagging SNPs that were genotyped in our study and were associated with NHL risk. Green dots represent tagging SNPs that were genotyped in our study and that showed no association with NHL. Blue markers represent SNPs imputed by IMPUTE from 1KG. The red dotted line defines the threshold of p-value <0.05. * indicates an associated SNP with a putatively functional impact; non-synonymous coding change or SNP mapping in: transcription factor binding site, H3K4Me1 chromatin mark, DNaseI hypersensitivity cluster, 5′UTR, 3′UTR.

In this study, we report the most significant association with risk of NHL for two SNPs in the *ATM* locus, remaining significant after adjustment for multiple testing (Bonferroni). Although among FL patients there was no association observed, *ATM* SNPs did correlate with risk of DLBCL and SLL/CLL. While the FL subset was the second largest in the study (n = 301), many other subtypes were underrepresented (n<100) and hence it was not possible to assess risk among these smaller groups due to the limited power (although a suggestive, yet non-significant effect was observed among Mantle Cell lymphomas; rs611646, OR = 1.45, 95% CI: 1.03–2.05, p = 0.035). It is also important to note that the associations of *ATM* SNPs are stronger among the pooled NHL analysis (all subtypes) compared to separate associations with DLBCL or SLL/CLL. This evidence suggests for the first time that *ATM* is a putatively novel candidate NHL susceptibility locus.

In our study we have noted association differences in stratified analyses by AJ status (Table S5). This relates to the two most significant *ATM* SNPs, which show the significant risk effect only in non-AJ population. While the frequency of the risk allele of both SNPs appears to be similar among AJ and non-AJ cases (for rs227060 MAF = 40%, for rs611646 MAF = 48%), the MAF in AJ and non-AJ controls differs by approximately 4% (for rs227060 MAF = 37% and 33% respectively, for rs611646 MAF = 45% and MAF = 42% respectively). While there is a possibility of underlying genetic substructure [46,47], we believe reduced power of the AJ stratified sub-analysis is the most plausible explanation for the observed differences in the risk effects between AJ and non-AJ subsets, as AJ cases are underrepresented by ~43% compared to non-AJ cases in the study. It is likely that despite the differences in allele frequency of both SNPs in AJ, the risk would be detected by increasing the number of cases to a comparable size of the non-AJ subset. The issue of power reduction contributing to the observed

association differences between AJ and non-AJ is further supported by the same directionality of odds ratios in both AJ and non-AJ subsets and aggregate analysis. To explore both possibilities in detail, a larger validation analysis and possibly the detailed fine mapping of the *ATM* locus in AJ as well as non AJ populations will be needed.

Prior evidence linking *ATM* with lymphoid malignancies has been largely restricted to the somatic level; *ATM* somatic mutations were noted in particular lymphoma subtypes of DLBCL [48], CLL [49–52], and MCL [53,54], consistent with the results of the subtype-specific analysis in our data. Rare germline variants in *ATM* (MAF<0.05) have previously been associated with CLL susceptibility [25], however as the current study focused on common variants (MAF>0.05), these SNPs are not strongly correlated with tSNPs in our study (r^2<0.1). The study by Sipahimalani, *et al.* performed an extensive analysis exploring the association of six common genetic variants in *ATM* with lymphoma risk [55]. Notably, while the least significant *ATM* SNP associated with NHL risk in our data, rs419716, is strongly correlated with one of the SNPs from that prior study, rs664982 (r^2>0.9), no association was reported for rs664982 by Sipahimalani, *et al.* [55], although the directionality of the effects for both SNPs is similar. The smaller sample size (798 cases, 793 controls) of this prior report, together with a more heterogeneous population (>15% of Asian ancestry) likely explains the different association outcomes [55]. The different distribution of NHL subtypes in the study by Sipahimalani, *et al.* provides another possible explanation. While our strongest signals appear to be driven by associations of *ATM* SNPs in DLBCL and SLL/CLL, the study population from Sipahimalani, *et al.* had a much higher proportion of FL, for which we did not observe an association in our study. DLBCL specific GWAS studies have been previously

Table 5. Putatively functional SNPs imputed from the ATM locus associated with the risk of NHL.

SNP	r² with tSNP*	OR (95% CI)	P	phastCons 44-way	TFBS	H3K4me1 chromatin mark	DNase I Hypersensitivity cluster	UTR	Transcribed in GM12878
rs228594	0.991	0.71 (0.60–0.84)	4.85E-05	-	JunD, FOSL2	-	Yes	-	Yes
rs228599	0.991	0.71 (0.60–0.84)	4.85E-05	-	c-Jun	Yes	-	-	Yes
rs227070	0.997	0.71 (0.61–0.84)	7.32E-05	-	-	-	Yes	-	-
rs228595	1	1.16 (1.05–1.29)	0.003922	-	-	Yes	-	-	Yes
rs672655	0.994	0.89 (0.80–0.98)	0.02264	243	-	-	-	-	Yes
rs228596	0.994	0.89 (0.80–0.98)	0.02295	-	-	Yes	-	-	Yes
rs189037	0.994	0.89 (0.80–0.98)	0.02296	-	HEY1, TAF1, IRF4, PAX5-C20, POU2F2	-	-	5'	Yes
rs662578	0.994	0.90 (0.81–0.99)	0.03296	-	-	-	Yes	-	Yes
rs228590	0.994	0.90 (0.81–0.99)	0.03476	-	PAX5-C20	Yes	Yes	-	Yes
rs228598	0.994	0.90 (0.81–0.99)	0.03476	-	c-Jun	Yes	Yes	-	Yes
rs228591	0.994	0.90 (0.81–0.99)	0.03476	-	-	Yes	Yes	-	Yes
rs625120	0.994	0.90 (0.81–0.99)	0.03476	-	-	Yes	-	-	Yes
rs228597	0.994	0.90 (0.81–0.99)	0.03476	-	-	Yes	-	-	Yes
rs228592	0.994	0.90 (0.81–0.99)	0.03476	-	-	-	Yes	-	Yes
rs582157	0.994	0.90 (0.81–0.99)	0.03476	-	-	Yes	-	-	Yes
rs227072	0.998	0.90 (0.81–1.00)	0.04007	-	JunD	-	-	-	Yes
rs425061	0.998	0.90 (0.81–1.00)	0.04007	272	-	-	-	-	Yes
rs227092	0.998	0.90 (0.81–1.00)	0.04007	-	-	-	-	3'	Yes
rs227091	0.998	0.90 (0.81–1.00)	0.04007	-	-	-	-	3'	Yes
rs4585	0.998	0.90 (0.81–1.00)	0.04007	-	-	-	-	3'	Yes

OR = odds ratio; CI = confidence interval; TFBS = transcription factor binding site; UTR = untranslated region.
*Correlated tSNP for rs228595 is rs611646; all other SNPs are correlated with the tSNP rs419716.

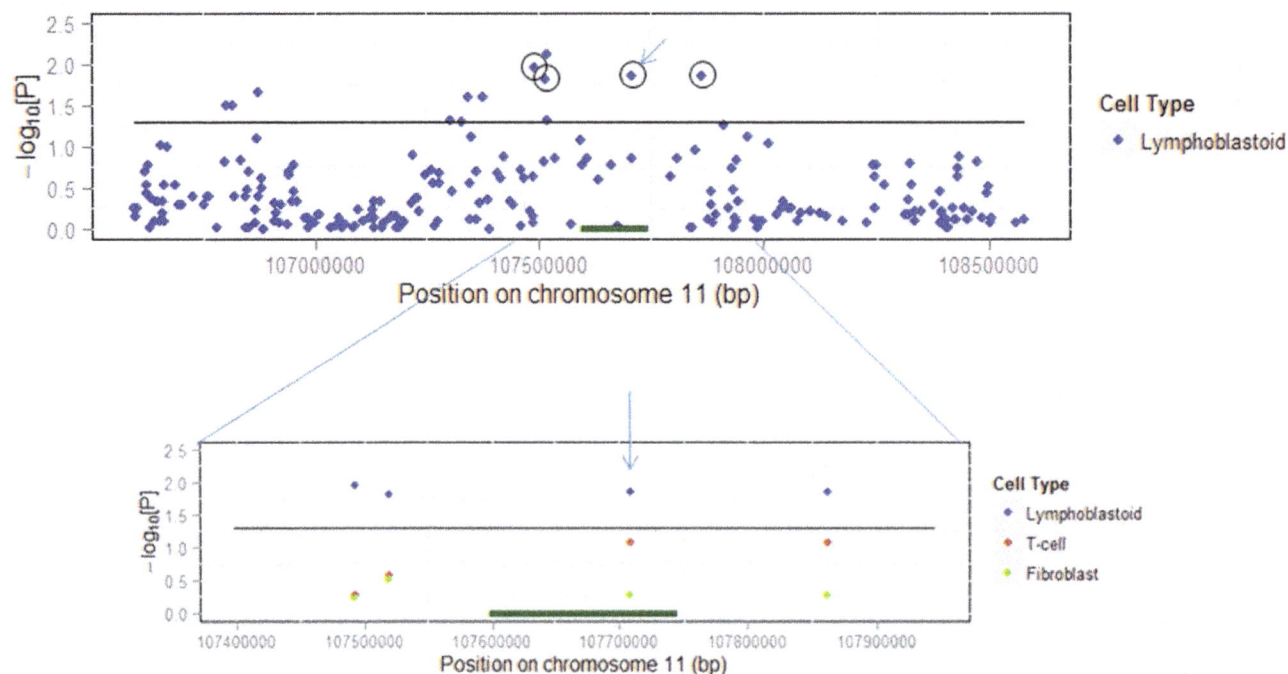

Figure 2. The distribution of eQTLs across the region of *ATM* determined by ILMN_1716231 probe from the data of lymphoblastoid cell lines from 75 individuals of European ancestry. The eQTLs were identified using Genevar. The eQTL association with rs227060 (arrow), the most significant SNP associated with NHL risk in our data, is the second strongest eQTL across *ATM* locus. The circles indicate all SNPs that correlate with rs227060. Zoom in shows eQTL associations of four correlated SNPs in lymphoblastoid cell line versus T-cell and fibroblastoid cell lines. The eQTL associations are displayed as −log$_{10}$(p-value) on y-axis.

reported [7,12], and most recently a large GWAS by international consortia has identified novel loci in apoptotic pathways associated with the risk of SLL/CLL [11]. While *ATM* was not among the reported associations in these prior studies, these reports focused only on the loci that passed the threshold of genome wide level of significance. For independent confirmation, a separate deeper analysis of this published data will be needed in the follow up study to validate the potential association effect of *ATM* with SLL/CLL and DLBCL in the large populations studied in these scans. Although the replication of our findings in NHL subtypes will be critical as part of the prior and upcoming GWAS studies from large consortia, it will also be very important to test the association effect of identified *ATM* variants in pooled NHL population, where we observed the most significant associations in our analysis. Such rationale is particularly relevant given the critical role of DNA repair pathways (with *ATM* as an important cell cycle checkpoint) in early development of progenitor B and T-cell lineages [56–59] via the process of V(D)J recombination producing diverse immune repertoire [60]. Because of the common origin of these precursor cell populations among different NHL subtypes, it is reasonable to hypothesize that variation in DNA repair networks in these progenitor cells could confer risk effects that are shared among multiple NHL subtypes, as we have suggested in our most recent GWAS scan [9] and as also discussed previously [7]. Additionally, double-stranded DNA break and non-homologous end joining repair mechanisms have been implicated in the occurrence of chromothripsis [61], which has recently been observed in both CLL and DLBCL [62–64] and proposed along with "chromoplexy" [65] to be involved in a punctuated cancer evolution. *ATM* is a critical checkpoint impacting both homologous recombination and non-homologous end joining [66]. It is possible that the inherited genetic variants in *ATM* may affect the

capacity of DSB repair in a way that would associate with the patterns of specific large-scale genomic alterations and rearrangements in a subset of cells in the tumor due to yet unknown genetic or microenvironment modifiers. Although in the context of this study it is highly speculative, given the associations with the *ATM* locus observed here, such a biological scenario is an attractive possibility and should be further investigated in detail on the somatic level of lymphomagenesis.

Numerous other studies have previously examined the germline variation in major DNA repair genes for their association with lymphoma risk [15–17,19]. However, mostly due to the limited selection of candidates, limited power or lack of independent validation, the results were of marginal significance. These borderline associations included the variants in nucleotide excision repair proteins, such as *XRCC1* and *XRCC2* [17], cell cycle protein *BLM* [19], and *MGMT*, a gene involved in DNA repair of alkylation damage [17]. We examined those previously associated loci, which had perfect proxies in our data and observed a borderline association in stage 1 for a proxy of rs1799782 in *XRCC1* [17], (rs3213344, OR = 1.44, 95% CI: 1.03–2.01, p = 0.03), however this SNP did not replicate in our stage 2. *MRE11A* and *NBS1*, which were associated with NHL risk in our study, were examined in a previous report on a small subset of NHL population [18]. Although some marginal associations with NHL risk were observed, the SNPs reported in that previous study were in weak correlation with the variants in *MRE11A* and *NBS1* associated with lymphoma risk in our analysis.

One novelty of our study design compared to prior efforts is the exploratory assessment of potential epistatic effects in DNA repair networks contributing to lymphoma risk. Our data suggest that the interactions between several genetic variants in *MRE11A* and *NBS1*, critical components of the MRN complex, associate with increased risk of NHL. Interestingly, these findings show that the carriers of at least one copy of the minor (protective) allele inherited in both *MRE11A* and *NBS1* are at more than a 2-fold reduced risk of developing NHL compared to the single SNP effect of each locus separately. While these findings are novel they are also exploratory, given the reduced power of this analysis and the fact that none of these observations reached the significance threshold adjusted for multiple testing. Importantly however, these epistatic interactions were observed in both stage 1 and 2 separately (Table 3 and Table 4) suggesting that the observed SNP-SNP associations merit further attention. Looking forward, the addition of other critical checkpoint DNA repair genes (such as *ATM* or *CHEK1/2*) to the MRN interaction model found in our study would be of interest. This analysis, along with the independent validation of epistatic and single SNP associations identified here, will need to be performed in a large consortium as part of the analyses following up on recent reports [11,67].

Our study provides a suggestive link between the associated SNPs and putatively functional variants to be pursued in subsequent molecular studies. By imputing our data from the public resources of 1KG we have identified several functional variants highly correlated with the SNPs associated with NHL risk in our study. Most notably, several of the variants in *ATM* were located within multiple functional regions, as annotated utilizing ENCODE data from lymphoblastoid cell lines. For example, rs228594, rs228599, and rs189037, which correlate with the associations observed in *ATM*, map within known transcription factor binding sites as well as chromatin marks, DNase I hypersensitivity clusters, and 5′ UTR, strongly supporting a possible impact on expression regulation.

The eQTL association with our top SNP, rs227060, was the second most significant eQTL association within the *ATM* region, and was detected in lymphoblastoid cell lines but not in fibroblast controls [41] (Figure 2). The observed eQTL effect shows the reduced expression of *ATM* correlating with the dosage of rs227060 risk allele. The reduction of *ATM* expression has been strongly linked with radiosensitivity and defective DNA damage-induced *ATM*-dependent signaling in various experimental studies, and was clearly shown to promote the tumor growth in lymphoma and other cancer models [68]. However, despite the potential biological implications of these associations, more detailed molecular investigations will be needed to link the imputed loci with lymphomagenesis. Nonetheless, the *in-silico* functional predictions as presented here can substantially improve subsequent fine mapping strategies of associated SNPs. At the same time this approach can reduce the need for a large scale re-sequencing by functional prioritizing the target variants for further molecular investigation.

Besides *ATM*, other loci also showed association effects in pooled NHL or subtype-specific analyses. As power limitations of our study may also be a concern, subsequent validation of these findings should be performed in large consortia. These future studies, with the concomitant collection of epidemiologic data and clinical characteristics, will also allow for a more in-depth analysis of potential gene-environment interactions attributed to DNA repair pathways. At the same time, the utilization of data from completed and ongoing lymphoma GWAS will be critical for the assessment of other interacting molecular pathways that may define the complex genetic susceptibility to NHL. For example, the HLA locus has been consistently replicated as a low-penetrant allele in recent NHL GWAS and follow-up meta-analyses [7,8,10,11,32,69]. It has been shown that the innate immunity

pathways are closely connected with particular DNA repair networks (e.g. B-cell maturation in germinal centers) [58,70], suggesting that detailed exploration of such interactions will be important. Our results strongly support the strategies for the pathway analysis of data from current and future GWAS on lymphoma susceptibility, using a deep validation of associations, considering the loci that did not reach genome-wide association thresholds, but may be biologically related. Our observations indicate that the genetic variants in key biological pathways, such as DNA repair, may account for an additional fraction of missing inherited susceptibility to lymphoid neoplasia. The associations observed here can also serve as the basis for further molecular investigations of the biological roles of the implicated loci on both a germline and somatic level. Such investigations will contribute not only to more efficient risk algorithms, but will lead to the improved understanding of lymphomagenesis for more effective targeting of therapy and prevention.

Supporting Information

Figure S1   Strategy schema for the selection of candidate DNA repair genes in the study.

Figure S2   Quantile/Quantile (Q/Q) plot comparing − $\log_{10}$(expected p-value) vs. − $\log_{10}$(observed p-value) under different quality metric scores (info). Based on imputation analysis of 109 genotyped SNPs using IMPUTE2. Q/Q analysis of imputed data was used to select quality score threshold with least inflation of significant SNPs, which we have set at 0.7.

Figure S3   Quantile/Quantile (Q/Q) plot of the association results from stage 1 SNPs genotyped in 650 NHL cases and 965 controls; − $\log_{10}$(expected p-value) vs. − $\log_{10}$(observed p-value). The blue dashded line indicates the inflation factor based on 90% of the least significant SNPs ($\lambda = 1.07$).

Figure S4   LD structure generated by Haploview shown for *ATM* gene region. The triangle plot displays correlation between the three tagging SNPs genotyped in the study (r^2 values). The associations of individual SNPs are displayed as − $\log_{10}$(p-value) for each SNP from the main effect aggregate analysis.

Figure S5   Minor allele frequency plot for non-AJ vs. AJ samples. Data based on allele frequencies in the aggregate analysis (for 109 SNPs with genotype information in stage 1 and stage 2). Blue dots indicate those SNPs associated with NHL in the aggregate analysis. Only 15 SNPs (14%) showed a difference in MAF >0.05. Indicated by arrows are NHL associated SNPs which did show a MAF difference >0.05 between non-AJ and AJ samples.

Figure S6   Genotype vs. expression (eQTL) results for rs227060 and four expression probes across the *ATM* locus. Data generated from lymphoblastoid cell lines (GenCord-L), T-cell lines (GenCord-T) and fibroblastoid cell lines (GenCord-F) established from 5 individuals of European ancestry. The most significant association for rs227060 in GenCord-L has been observed for ILMN-1716231. Data were generated using Genevar.

Table S1 Summary of the demographic characteristics of the case/control study population.

Table S2 List of DNA repair genes and tagging SNPs genotyped. Chromosome and base pair position are based on GRCh37/hg19 build. Allele frequencies calculated among our sample population.

Table S3 Results of single SNP associations analysis of tSNPs in DNA repair genes with the risk of NHL observed in our study, including 109 SNPs genotyped in stage 1 and stage 2.

Table S4 Full list of haplotype associations (p<0.05) for DNA repair genes associated with NHL in our study.

Table S5 Stratified AJ and non-AJ results for SNPs associated with NHL in the main effect aggregate analysis.

Table S6 Results from pairwise SNP-SNP interaction associations of tSNPs in DNA repair genes with NHL risk. A) Pairwise comparisons among the 15 tSNPs associated with NHL risk in the aggregate main effect analysis. B) Pairwise comparisons of 15 tSNPs with all additional SNPs genotyped in

both stage 1 and stage 2 (n = 94). Associations between *MRE11A* and *NBS1* are shaded in grey.

Table S7 Pairwise interaction results between *NBS1* (rs1805812) and *MRE11A* (rs607974, rs625245, rs557148, rs10831227) and NHL risk under three different genetic models. Each model was tested for a different SNP x SNP combination between rs1805812 and 4 SNPs tagging *MRE11A*. Indicated are the different combinations of genotypes used for each respective genetic model.

Table S8 Summary of tagging and imputed SNPs in DNA repair genes associated with NHL risk with high predicted functional impact. Functional information was annotated using ANNOVAR, and included data generated from the ENCODE project.

Acknowledgments

The authors thank Alex Lash for assistance with the study design and Vincent Devlin, Kimberly Phillips and Christine Thompson for excellent technical assistance.

Author Contributions

Conceived and designed the experiments: TK. Performed the experiments: JR JAP ADC AH KH LB. Analyzed the data: JR YA BR CS RJK YS TK. Contributed reagents/materials/analysis tools: AH OP DBY JRB ASF CS ML AZ KO TK. Wrote the paper: JR CA OP JRB RJK JV KO TK. Organized data and database construction: JR JP NH KH LB TK.

References

1. Skibola CF, Curry JD, Nieters A (2007) Genetic susceptibility to lymphoma. Haematologica 92: 960–969.
2. Chang ET, Smedby KE, Hjalgrim H, Porwit-MacDonald A, Roos G, et al. (2005) Family history of hematopoietic malignancy and risk of lymphoma. J Natl Cancer Inst 97: 1466–1474.
3. Wang SS, Slager SL, Brennan P, Holly EA, De Sanjose S, et al. (2007) Family history of hematopoietic malignancies and risk of non-Hodgkin lymphoma (NHL): a pooled analysis of 10 211 cases and 11 905 controls from the International Lymphoma Epidemiology Consortium (InterLymph). Blood 109: 3479–3488.
4. Siddiqui R, Onel K, Facio F, Offit K (2004) The genetics of familial lymphomas. Curr Oncol Rep 6: 380–387.
5. Slager SL, Rabe KG, Achenbach SJ, Vachon CM, Goldin LR, et al. (2011) Genome-wide association study identifies a novel susceptibility locus at 6p21.3 among familial CLL. Blood 117: 1911–1916.
6. Di Bernardo MC, Crowther-Swanepoel D, Broderick P, Webb E, Sellick G, et al. (2008) A genome-wide association study identifies six susceptibility loci for chronic lymphocytic leukemia. Nat Genet 40: 1204–1210.
7. Smedby KE, Foo JN, Skibola CF, Darabi H, Conde L, et al. (2011) GWAS of follicular lymphoma reveals allelic heterogeneity at 6p21.32 and suggests shared genetic susceptibility with diffuse large B-cell lymphoma. PLoS Genet 7: e1001378.
8. Conde L, Halperin E, Akers NK, Brown KM, Smedby KE, et al. (2010) Genome-wide association study of follicular lymphoma identifies a risk locus at 6p21.32. Nat Genet 42: 661–664.
9. Vijai J, Kirchhoff T, Schrader KA, Brown J, Dutra-Clarke AV, et al. (2013) Susceptibility loci associated with specific and shared subtypes of lymphoid malignancies. PLoS Genet 9: e1003220.
10. Skibola CF, Bracci PM, Halperin E, Conde L, Craig DW, et al. (2009) Genetic variants at 6p21.33 are associated with susceptibility to follicular lymphoma. Nat Genet 41: 873–875.
11. Berndt SI, Skibola CF, Joseph V, Camp NJ, Nieters A, et al. (2013) Genome-wide association study identifies multiple risk loci for chronic lymphocytic leukemia. Nat Genet.
12. Kumar V, Matsuo K, Takahashi A, Hosono N, Tsunoda T, et al. (2011) Common variants on 14q32 and 13q12 are associated with DLBCL susceptibility. J Hum Genet 56: 436–439.
13. Tan DE, Foo JN, Bei JX, Chang J, Peng R, et al. (2013) Genome-wide association study of B cell non-Hodgkin lymphoma identifies 3q27 as a susceptibility locus in the Chinese population. Nat Genet 45: 804–807.
14. Amos W, Driscoll E, Hoffman JI (2011) Candidate genes versus genome-wide associations: which are better for detecting genetic susceptibility to infectious disease? Proc Biol Sci 278: 1183–1188.
15. Smedby KE, Lindgren CM, Hjalgrim H, Humphreys K, Schollkopf C, et al. (2006) Variation in DNA repair genes ERCC2, XRCC1, and XRCC3 and risk of follicular lymphoma. Cancer Epidemiol Biomarkers Prev 15: 258–265.
16. Hill DA, Wang SS, Cerhan JR, Davis S, Cozen W, et al. (2006) Risk of non-Hodgkin lymphoma (NHL) in relation to germline variation in DNA repair and related genes. Blood 108: 3161–3167.
17. Shen M, Purdue MP, Kricker A, Lan Q, Grulich AE, et al. (2007) Polymorphisms in DNA repair genes and risk of non-Hodgkin's lymphoma in New South Wales, Australia. Haematologica 92: 1180–1185.
18. Schuetz JM, MaCarthur AC, Leach S, Lai AS, Gallagher RP, et al. (2009) Genetic variation in the NBS1, MRE11, RAD50 and BLM genes and susceptibility to non-Hodgkin lymphoma. BMC Med Genet 10: 117.
19. Shen M, Menashe I, Morton LM, Zhang Y, Armstrong B, et al. (2010) Polymorphisms in DNA repair genes and risk of non-Hodgkin lymphoma in a pooled analysis of three studies. Br J Haematol 151: 239–244.
20. Kim IS, Kim DC, Kim HG, Eom HS, Kong SY, et al. (2010) DNA repair gene XRCC1 polymorphisms and haplotypes in diffuse large B-cell lymphoma in a Korean population. Cancer Genet Cytogenet 196: 31–37.
21. Worrillow L, Roman E, Adamson PJ, Kane E, Allan JM, et al. (2009) Polymorphisms in the nucleotide excision repair gene ERCC2/XPD and risk of non-Hodgkin lymphoma. Cancer Epidemiol 33: 257–260.
22. Baris S, Celkan T, Batar B, Guven M, Ozdil M, et al. (2009) Association between genetic polymorphism in DNA repair genes and risk of B-cell lymphoma. Pediatr Hematol Oncol 26: 467–472.
23. Liu J, Song B, Wang Z, Song X, Shi Y, et al. (2009) DNA repair gene XRCC1 polymorphisms and non-Hodgkin lymphoma risk in a Chinese population. Cancer Genet Cytogenet 191: 67–72.
24. Shen M, Zheng T, Lan Q, Zhang Y, Zahm SH, et al. (2006) Polymorphisms in DNA repair genes and risk of non-Hodgkin lymphoma among women in Connecticut. Hum Genet 119: 659–668.
25. Rudd MF, Sellick GS, Webb EL, Catovsky D, Houlston RS (2006) Variants in the ATM-BRCA2-CHEK2 axis predispose to chronic lymphocytic leukemia. Blood 108: 638–644.
26. Bednarski JJ, Sleckman BP (2012) Lymphocyte development: integration of DNA damage response signaling. Adv Immunol 116: 175–204.

27. Economopoulou P, Pappa V, Papageorgiou S, Dervenoulas J, Economopoulos T (2011) Abnormalities of DNA repair mechanisms in common hematological malignancies. Leuk Lymphoma 52: 567–582.

28. de Miranda NF, Bjorkman A, Pan-Hammarstrom Q (2011) DNA repair: the link between primary immunodeficiency and cancer. Ann N Y Acad Sci 1246: 50–63.

29. Kirchhoff T, Chen ZQ, Gold B, Pal P, Gaudet MM, et al. (2009) The 6q22.33 locus and breast cancer susceptibility. Cancer Epidemiol Biomarkers Prev 18: 2468–2475.

30. Gallagher DJ, Vijai J, Cronin AM, Bhatia J, Vickers AJ, et al. (2010) Susceptibility loci associated with prostate cancer progression and mortality. Clin Cancer Res 16: 2819–2832.

31. Gold B, Kirchhoff T, Stefanov S, Lautenberger J, Viale A, et al. (2008) Genome-wide association study provides evidence for a breast cancer risk locus at 6q22.33. Proc Natl Acad Sci U S A 105: 4340–4345.

32. Vijai J, Kirchhoff T, Schrader KA, Brown J, Dutra-Clarke AV, et al. (2013) Susceptibility Loci associated with specific and shared subtypes of lymphoid malignancies. PLoS Genet 9: e1003220.

33. Ashburner M, Ball CA, Blake JA, Botstein D, Butler H, et al. (2000) Gene ontology: tool for the unification of biology. The Gene Ontology Consortium. Nat Genet 25: 25–29.

34. Kanehisa M (2000) Post-genome informatics. Oxford; New York: Oxford University Press. ix, 148 p. p.

35. Kals M, Natter K, Thallinger GG, Trajanoski Z, Kohlwein SD (2005) YPL.db2: the Yeast Protein Localization database, version 2.0. Yeast 22: 213–218.

36. Purcell S, Neale B, Todd-Brown K, Thomas L, Ferreira MA, et al. (2007) PLINK: a tool set for whole-genome association and population-based linkage analyses. Am J Hum Genet 81: 559–575.

37. Yang TP, Beazley C, Montgomery SB, Dimas AS, Gutierrez-Arcelus M, et al. (2010) Genevar: a database and Java application for the analysis and visualization of SNP-gene associations in eQTL studies. Bioinformatics 26: 2474–2476.

38. Howie BN, Donnelly P, Marchini J (2009) A flexible and accurate genotype imputation method for the next generation of genome-wide association studies. PLoS Genet 5: e1000529.

39. Marchini J, Howie B (2010) Genotype imputation for genome-wide association studies. Nat Rev Genet 11: 499–511.

40. Wang K, Li M, Hakonarson H (2010) ANNOVAR: functional annotation of genetic variants from high-throughput sequencing data. Nucleic Acids Res 38: e164.

41. Dimas AS, Deutsch S, Stranger BE, Montgomery SB, Borel C, et al. (2009) Common regulatory variation impacts gene expression in a cell type-dependent manner. Science 325: 1246–1250.

42. Kennedy RD, D'Andrea AD (2006) DNA repair pathways in clinical practice: lessons from pediatric cancer susceptibility syndromes. J Clin Oncol 24: 3799–3808.

43. Gumy-Pause F, Wacker P, Sappino AP (2004) ATM gene and lymphoid malignancies. Leukemia 18: 238–242.

44. Seymour R, Sundberg JP, Hogenesch H (2006) Abnormal lymphoid organ development in immunodeficient mutant mice. Vet Pathol 43: 401–423.

45. van der Burg M, Ijspeert H, Verkaik NS, Turul T, Wiegant WW, et al. (2009) A DNA-PKcs mutation in a radiosensitive T-B- SCID patient inhibits Artemis activation and nonhomologous end-joining. J Clin Invest 119: 91–98.

46. Olshen AB, Gold B, Lohmueller KE, Struewing JP, Satagopan J, et al. (2008) Analysis of genetic variation in Ashkenazi Jews by high density SNP genotyping. BMC Genet 9: 14.

47. Ostrer H, Skorecki K (2013) The population genetics of the Jewish people. Hum Genet 132: 119–127.

48. Gronbaek K, Worm J, Ralfkiaer E, Ahrenkiel V, Hokland P, et al. (2002) ATM mutations are associated with inactivation of the ARF-TP53 tumor suppressor pathway in diffuse large B-cell lymphoma. Blood 100: 1430–1437.

49. Stankovic T, Weber P, Stewart G, Bedenham T, Murray J, et al. (1999) Inactivation of ataxia telangiectasia mutated gene in B-cell chronic lymphocytic leukaemia. Lancet 353: 26–29.

50. Bullrich F, Rasio D, Kitada S, Starostik P, Kipps T, et al. (1999) ATM mutations in B-cell chronic lymphocytic leukemia. Cancer Res 59: 24–27.

51. Schaffner C, Stilgenbauer S, Rappold GA, Dohner H, Lichter P (1999) Somatic ATM mutations indicate a pathogenic role of ATM in B-cell chronic lymphocytic leukemia. Blood 94: 748–753.

52. Stankovic T, Stewart GS, Fegan C, Biggs P, Last J, et al. (2002) Ataxia telangiectasia mutated-deficient B-cell chronic lymphocytic leukemia occurs in pregerminal center cells and results in defective damage response and unrepaired chromosome damage. Blood 99: 300–309.

53. Schaffner C, Idler I, Stilgenbauer S, Dohner H, Lichter P (2000) Mantle cell lymphoma is characterized by inactivation of the ATM gene. Proc Natl Acad Sci U S A 97: 2773–2778.

54. Camacho E, Hernandez L, Hernandez S, Tort F, Bellosillo B, et al. (2002) ATM gene inactivation in mantle cell lymphoma mainly occurs by truncating mutations and missense mutations involving the phosphatidylinositol-3 kinase domain and is associated with increasing numbers of chromosomal imbalances. Blood 99: 238–244.

55. Sipahimalani P, Spinelli JJ, MacArthur AC, Lai A, Leach SR, et al. (2007) A systematic evaluation of the ataxia telangiectasia mutated gene does not show an association with non-Hodgkin lymphoma. Int J Cancer 121: 1967–1975.

56. Sherman MH, Bassing CH, Teitell MA (2011) Regulation of cell differentiation by the DNA damage response. Trends Cell Biol 21: 312–319.

57. Rossi DJ, Bryder D, Seita J, Nussenzweig A, Hoeijmakers J, et al. (2007) Deficiencies in DNA damage repair limit the function of haematopoietic stem cells with age. Nature 447: 725–729.

58. Alt FW, Zhang Y, Meng FL, Guo C, Schwer B (2013) Mechanisms of programmed DNA lesions and genomic instability in the immune system. Cell 152: 417–429.

59. Bredemeyer AL, Helmink BA, Innes CL, Calderon B, McGinnis LM, et al. (2008) DNA double-strand breaks activate a multi-functional genetic program in developing lymphocytes. Nature 456: 819–823.

60. Cobb RM, Oestreich KJ, Osipovich OA, Oltz EM (2006) Accessibility control of V(D)J recombination. Adv Immunol 91: 45–109.

61. Kloosterman WP, Tavakoli-Yaraki M, van Roosmalen MJ, van Binsbergen E, Renkens I, et al. (2012) Constitutional chromothripsis rearrangements involve clustered double-stranded DNA breaks and nonhomologous repair mechanisms. Cell Rep 1: 648–655.

62. Bassaganyas L, Bea S, Escaramis G, Tornador C, Salaverria I, et al. (2013) Sporadic and reversible chromothripsis in chronic lymphocytic leukemia revealed by longitudinal genomic analysis. Leukemia 27: 2376–2379.

63. Morin RD, Mungall K, Pleasance E, Mungall AJ, Goya R, et al. (2013) Mutational and structural analysis of diffuse large B-cell lymphoma using whole-genome sequencing. Blood 122: 1256–1265.

64. Stephens PJ, Greenman CD, Fu B, Yang F, Bignell GR, et al. (2011) Massive genomic rearrangement acquired in a single catastrophic event during cancer development. Cell 144: 27–40.

65. Baca SC, Prandi D, Lawrence MS, Mosquera JM, Romanel A, et al. (2013) Punctuated evolution of prostate cancer genomes. Cell 153: 666–677.

66. Giunta S, Belotserkovskaya R, Jackson SP (2010) DNA damage signaling in response to double-strand breaks during mitosis. J Cell Biol 190: 197–207.

67. Nieters A, Conde L, Slager SL, Brooks-Wilson A, Morton L, et al. (2012) PRRC2A and BCL2L11 gene variants influence risk of non-Hodgkin lymphoma: results from the InterLymph consortium. Blood 120: 4645–4648.

68. Williamson CT, Muzik H, Turhan AG, Zamo A, O'Connor MJ, et al. (2010) ATM deficiency sensitizes mantle cell lymphoma cells to poly(ADP-ribose) polymerase-1 inhibitors. Mol Cancer Ther 9: 347–357.

69. Foo JN, Smedby KE, Akers NK, Berglund M, Irwan ID, et al. (2013) Coding Variants at Hexa-allelic Amino Acid 13 of HLA-DRB1 Explain Independent SNP Associations with Follicular Lymphoma Risk. Am J Hum Genet 93: 167–172.

70. Gasser S, Orsulic S, Brown EJ, Raulet DH (2005) The DNA damage pathway regulates innate immune system ligands of the NKG2D receptor. Nature 436: 1186–1190.

15

Down-Regulation of CD9 by Methylation Decreased Bortezomib Sensitivity in Multiple Myeloma

Xiaotong Hu[1]*, Han Xuan[2], Huaping Du[2], Hao Jiang[2], Jinwen Huang[2]*

1 Biomedical Research Center, Sir Run Run Shaw Hospital, Zhejiang University and Key Laboratory of Biotherapy of Zhejiang Province, Hangzhou, China, **2** Department of Hematology, Sir Run Run Shaw Hospital, Zhejiang University, Hangzhou, China

Abstract

Bortezomib therapy has been proven successful for the treatment of relapsed and/or refractory multiple myeloma (MM). However, both intrinsic and acquired resistance has already been observed. In this study, we explored the relationship between CD9 expression and bortezomib sensitivity in MM. We found that down-regulation of CD9 by methylation decreased bortezomib sensitivity in multiple myeloma. CD9 expression obviously increased bortezomib sensitivity through inducing apoptosis, significantly inhibiting U266 cells' adhesion to HS-5 and primary bone marrow stromal cells, but increasing U266 cells' adhesion to fibronectin. CD9 expression also significantly inhibited U266 cell migration. The mechanisms may include: the endoplasmic reticulum stress pathway, cell adhesion related signaling pathway and osteoclast differentiation related signaling pathway. Combination therapy with de-methylation reagent 5-Aza-2-deoxycytidine may prove useful to the development of novel strategies for the treatment of bortezomib-resistant MM patients.

Editor: Irina U. Agoulnik, Florida International University, United States of America

Funding: This work was supported by grants from the Zhejiang Provincial Natural Science Foundation of China [No. R2100213], and the National Natural Science Foundation of China [No. 81372622] and Major Projects in Zhejiang Province [No. 2012C13014-1]. The funders had no role in study design, data collection and analysis, decision to publish, or preparation of the manuscript.

Competing Interests: The authors have declared that no competing interests exist.

* E-mail: hxt_hangzhou@sina.com (XH); huangjinwen@gmail.com (JH)

Introduction

Multiple myeloma (MM) is an incurable plasmatic neoplasm among the hematological malignancies. Despite great advances in understanding the molecular pathogenesis of MM and the development of promising new therapies, only 25–35% of patients respond to therapies in the relapsed and refractory setting. Bortezomib (PS-341; Velcade) therapy has proven successful for the treatment of relapsed and/or refractory multiple myeloma. However, both intrinsic and acquired resistance has already been observed in MM patients [1]. This prompts a growing interest in understanding its mechanisms of bortezomib treatment and resistance. Molecular studies have identified many potential therapeutic targets of bortezomib. Bortezomib can directly inhibits the proliferation of myeloma cells, induces their apoptosis, and abrogates paracrine tumor growth through alteration of interactions of myeloma and stromal cells. It is well established that the physical interaction between MM cells and the bone marrow (BM) microenvironment plays a crucial role in MM pathogenesis and drug resistance. Direct interaction between MM cells and BM cells activates pleiotropic signaling pathways that mediate growth, survival, migration of MM cells and drug resistance, as well as angiogenesis and BM osteoclastogenesis.

CD9, a member of tetraspanin family, was found to be down-regulated in relapsed MM cells after treatment with bortezomib (Li X *et al*, unpublished data). Tetraspanins span the membrane four times and accumulate in membrane microdomains, distinct from lipid rafts. More than 20 family members are reported for mammals, including CD9, CD63, CD81, CD82 and CD151.

They associate with other proteins in either a direct or indirect fashion. This entire complex of interactions has been termed the "tetraspanin web" [2–4]. CD9, one of the most characterized members of the tetraspanins, was initially reported to be expressed in pre-B cells and platelets [5,6], but further studies have revealed that it is expressed in a wide variety of hematopoietic and non-hematopoietic cells [7–10]. It interacts with other cell adhesion molecules and plays on the role of the organizer in tetraspanins net [11]. It has been implicated in various biological functions, including cell adhesion, motility, metastasis, growth, signal transduction, differentiation, and sperm-egg fusion [2,12,13].

The implication of CD9 in cancer has received much attention. An inverse correlation between its expression in primary tumors and the metastatic potential and patient survival rate has been established in various carcinomas [14–17]. For example, the expression of CD9 significantly decreased in metastatic breast cancer, colonic cancer and prostate cancer cells than in primary tumor cells, while the high expression of CD9 could weaken migration ability of various kinds of tumor cells [18,19]. For oral squamous cell carcinomas, the low expression of CD9 indicated the late stage of tumor development and the low survival rate [20]. Restore expression of CD9 in small cell lung cancer cells can significantly inhibit the proliferation and migration of tumor cells [21]. All of these results show that the down-regulation of CD9 plays an important role in the development of tumor.

In this study, we checked (1) the CD9 expression and their methylation control mechanism in MM cell lines and primary cases, (2) whether CD9 expression has a special relationship with bortezomib sensitivity in MM and (3) whether a combination of low dose de-methylation reagent 5-Aza-2-deoxycytidine (5-Aza) and bortezomib can overcome bortezomib resistance in MM.

Materials and Methods

Cell culture

The human multiple myeloma cell lines U266, NCI-H929, RPMI8226, MM.1S, OPM 2 and HS-5 were purchased from the American Type Culture Collection (ATCC, Manassas, VA, USA). The cells were maintained in RPMI 1640 medium supplemented with 15% fetal bovine serum, 100 units/mL penicillin, and 100 mg/mL streptomycin in a humidified atmosphere with 5% CO_2 at 37°C. Fresh bone marrow samples from newly diagnosed patients with MM without any treatment were obtained at the Sir Run Run Shaw Hospital, Zhejiang University. Written informed consent for the use of the tissues was obtained from all patients and the study was approved by the Institute Research Ethics Committee of Sir Run Run Shaw Hospital, Zhejiang University.

Isolation of primary myeloma and stromal cells from MM patients

Fresh CD138 positive MM cells were isolated from the mononuclear fraction using anti-human CD138 microbeads (Miltenyi Biotec, Auburn, CA) by AutoMACS according to manufacturer's instructions. Purity of plasma cells ranged between 60% and 90%, based on fluorescence-activated cell sorting (FACS) analysis of CD138 expression (FACSCaliber; BD Biosciences, San Jose, CA).

Bone marrow stromal cells (BMSC) were prepared by seeding the remaining mononuclear cells after CD138-positive selection. The cells were seeded in DMEM complete culture medium (10% fetal bovine serum, 100 units/ml penicillin, 100 mg/ml streptomycin, and 2 mM L-glutamin, Gibco). After 3 days of culture, non-adherent cells were removed, and the remaining cells were expanded and split after about 10 days.

Co-culture of MM cells with HS-5 or primary BMSC cells

HS-5 or primary BMSC cells were plated in 6-wells at 10^5 cells/well. Upon confluence, each group of U266 cells (0.5×10^6/well) were added. Drugs were added at the concentrations indicated. The cells were cultivated in a total volume of 200 ml/well.

Construction of the lentivirus-encoding CD9

To construct the lentivirus-encoding CD9 (lenti-CD9) plasmid (pLenO-DCE-Puro-CD9), the cDNA-encoding CD9 (NM_001769.3) was synthesized and cloned into the EcoRI and BamHI restriction endonuclease sites of the pLenO-DCE-Puro vector (Invabio, Shanghai, China), a mammalian expression vector containing green fluorescent protein (GFP) and puromycin resistance genes. The DH5a Escherichia coli strain was used for amplification of lenti-CD9. After the correct sequence was confirmed by sequencing, lenti-CD9 was introduced into 293T cells using four-plasmid co-transfection with pRSV-Rev (packaging helper plasmid), pMDLg/pRRE, pMD2G and pLenO-DCE-Puro-CD9 (transfer vector). A lentivirus containing the empty transfer vector pLenO-DCE-Puro (lenti-GFP) was also generated. At 48 h after infection, the number of GFP-positive cells was measured using FACS, and the titer was determined.

Generation of CD9 stably transfected U266 cells

Briefly, when the U266 cells reached 50-60% confluence, the medium was removed and washed twice with PBS. Polybrene was used to increase the infection rate, and the infection was performed with lenti-CD9 and lenti-GFP according to the manufacturer's instructions. At 2 days post-infection, the percentage of GFP-positive U266 cells was determined using a fluorescence microscope to evaluate the infectivity. GFP-positive cells were selected by flow cytometry.

RNA extraction, cDNA synthesis, and semi-quantitative RT-PCR

Total RNA was extracted from cell pellets by Trizol (Invitrogen, Carlsbad, CA, USA) and reverse transcribed into cDNA using MultiScribe Reverse Transcriptase (Applied Biosystems, Foster city, CA, USA) according to the manufacturer's instructions. The target gene expression was determined by semi-quantitative RT-PCR using specific primers of CD9 gene (Table S1). GAPDH was served as an internal control for total cDNA content. Samples were amplified using the ABI 7500 Real-Time PCR Systems (Applied Biosystems, Foster City, CA, USA).

5-Aza-2-deoxycytidine (5-Aza) treatment

Cells were treated with 10 μM de-methylating agent, 5-Aza (Sigma-Aldrich, St Louis, MO, USA) for 3 days. After treatment the cells were harvested for DNA and RNA extraction.

Bisulphite treatment and promoter methylation analysis

Bisulphite modification of DNA, Methylation Specific PCR (MSP) and Bisulphate Genome Sequencing (BGS) were carried out as described previously [22,23]. MSP and BGS primers are listed in Table S1.

Cell viability assay

Cells were seeded at 1×10^5 cells/100 ml/well in 96-well plates and exposed to various concentrations of bortezomib for 24 hours. Cell viability was quantified using the CellTiter 96 AQueous Non-Radioactive Cell Proliferation Assay (Promega, Madison, WI, USA). Each well was treated with MTS for 1 to 4 hours, after which absorbance at 490 nm was recorded using a 96-well plate reader. The quantity of formazan product as measured is directly proportional to the number of living cells. The results were derived from three independent experiments performed in triplicate. Calculation of the 50% inhibitory concentration (IC50) was done using SPSS 16.0 software.

Cell cycle analysis

Each group of cells were harvested, fixed with cold 70% ethanol, and suspended in 50 mg/ml PI (Sigma-Aldrich, St. Louis, MO, USA) with the addition of 0.1 mg/mL RNase A. After incubation at 37°C for 30 mins, cell cycle flow cytometry analysis was performed by means of fluorescence activated cell sorting (FACS).

Apoptotic assays

Each group of cells was harvested by pipetting, washed with phosphate buffered saline, and stained with PE-conjugated annexin-V (annexin-V/PE) (Beyotime, Nanjing, China). Cell apoptosis was judged by annexin-V reactivity in GFP positive populations using flow cytometer.

Cell adhesion assay

After 48-hour co-culture of U266 cells with primary BMSC, HS-5 cells or Fibronectin were performed, the cell adhesion assay was carried out using Vybrant@ Cell Adhesion Assay Kit (Invitrogen, Carlsbad, CA, USA) following the manufacturer's recommendations. We determined the percentage of adhesion by dividing the corrected (background subtracted) fluorescence of adherent cells by the total corrected fluorescence of cells added to each well.

Cell migration assay

Each group of U266 cells was serum starved overnight and then resuspended in 70 uL of RPMI1640 medium/0.5% fetal calf serum. Cell migration was conducted in 24-well, 6.5 mm internal diameter transwell cluster plates (Corning Costar; Cambridge, MA). Briefly, cells ($1 \times 10^5/250$ μl) were loaded onto polycarbonate membranes (8 μm pore size) separating 2 chambers of a transwell. Medium/0.1% FCS (500 μl) was added to the lower chamber of the transwell cluster plates. After 24 hours, cells migrating into the lower chamber were counted under a light microscope. The experiment was performed three times.

Methylcellulose colony formation assay

Methylcellulose media consisted of RPMI 1640 containing 1.1% methylcellulose (Aqua Solutions, Deer Park, TX), 30% fetal bovine serum, 100 units/ml penicillin, 100 mg/ml streptomycin, and puromycin at the appropriate concentration for each cell line. Cells were plated at a density of 500 cells/ml in 1 ml volume in humidified 24-well plates. Colonies were counted between 10 and 15 days after plating.

Western blot analysis

Proteins were separated from cell lysates by SDS-PAGE, transferred to nitrocellulose, and probed with FAK, P-397 FAK, P-925 FAK, P-576/577 FAK, TRB3, CHOP, PERK, Ero1 La, IRE1a, PDI, Calnexin antibodys (Cell Signaling Technology, Beverly, MA, USA). The blots were developed by enhanced chemiluminescence (ECL).

Microarray and data analysis

Total RNA from 6 sample (3 U266-CD9 and 3 U266-GFP) was quantified by the NanoDrop ND-1000 and RNA integrity was assessed by standard denaturing agarose gel electrophoresis and then used for labeling and array hybridization. The labeled cDNA samples were submitted to Roche NimbleGen and hybridized to Human 12×135K Gene Expression Arrays. The results were scanned using a Agilent Scanner G2505C and imported into NimbleScan software (version 2.5) for grid alignment and expression data analysis. Differentially expressed genes with statistical significance (Fold Change ≥ 2.0, P-value ≤ 0.05) were shown by Volcano Plot filtering (Figure S1). Pathway Analysis and GO analysis were applied to determine the roles of these differentially expressed genes played in these biological pathways or GO terms. The results obtained were submitted to Gene Expression Omnibus (GEO) database and the accession number is GSE55818.

Statistical analysis

Results are expressed as values of mean ± standard deviation (SD). Statistical analysis was performed using SPSS 16.0 for Windows (SPSS Inc., Chicago, IL, USA) and Student's t-test was used. p values less than 0.05 were considered statistically significant.

Results

During the study of MM cell lines resistant to bortezomib treatment, we found a most down-regulated gene was a tetraspanin family protein, CD9. CD9 expression was also found to be significantly higher in the patients sensitive to bortezomib

than in the patients resistant to bortezomib (Li X *et al*, unpublished data).

Then we evaluated the bortezomib IC50 in several myeloma cell lines. Our results suggested that in MM cells sensitive to bortezomib treatment, IC50 values being 5 nmol/L for RPMI-8226 cells and 6.2 nmol/L for MM.1S cells. However in MM cells resistant to bortezomib treatment, IC50 values were significantly higher, being 20.9 nmol/L for U266 cells and 18.5 nmol/L for NCI-H929 cells. Then we examined CD9 expression in these cell lines by semi-quantitative RT-PCR. CD9 expressed in bortezomib sensitive RPMI-8226 and MM.1S cells but silenced in bortezomib resistant U266 and NCI-H929 cells (Figure 1A).

Since CD9 gene has CpG island (CGI) in the promoter region, we designed methylation-specific PCR (MSP) primers to analyse its methylation status in these cell lines. The CD9 CGI was methylated in U266 and NCI-H929 cells with silenced CD9 expression (Figure 1A). Moreover, CD9 expression was significantly induced after 5-Aza treatment in these cells (Figure 1B). We further examined the detailed methylation profiles of CD9 CGI by bisulfite genomic sequencing (BGS) analysis of 37 CpG sites, including those CpG sites analysed by MSP (Figure 1C). Densely methylated CpG sites were detected in cells with no CD9 expression, representative results are shown in Figure 1D. Both MSP and BGS showed that the CD9 CGI was dramatically demethylated after 5-Aza treatment, showing a direct link between CGI methylation and CD9 silencing (Figure 1B and 1D). We also analysed CD9 methylation status in 16 primary MM cases. CD9 methylation was detectedin 37.5% (6/16) of tumors (Figure 1E).

By MTS analysis we also found that after pretreatment of 5-Aza, the sensitivity to bortezomib in U266 and NCI-H929 raised significantly while the bortezomib sentitive RPMI8226 raised a little bit (Figure 2), suggesting the synergistic interaction of 5-Aza and bortezomib inhibition in multiple myeloma may due to CD9 expression reversion.

In order to study the expression of CD9 and its corresponding cell behavior changes in myeloma cells and their microenvironment, we transfected CD9 in U266 cells and selected the stably transfected cells by flow sorting. CD9 expression was confirmed by RT-PCR and western blot analysis (Figure 3A).

Cell viability results showed that CD9 expression could obviously increase the drug sensitivity (Figure 3B). The main reason may be because the apoptosis ability had improved significantly (Figure 3C). We also tested the drug action on cell autophagy, there was no significant difference between groups of cells (data not shown).

In order to detect CD9's influence on the biological functions of cells in the bone marrow microenvironment, we mainly studied the effects of CD9 on U266 cell's clone formation ability, cell cycle arrest, cell adhesion and migration, which may be the possible mechanisms of bortezomib sensitivity in MM involving tetraspanins. CD9 did not affect the cell clone formation ability, cell cycle and the major cytokines (VEGF, IL-6 and IGF-1) secreted (data not shown). However, CD9 expression significantly affected the cell adhesion and migration ability. Ectopic expression of CD9 significantly inhibited U266 cells' adhesion to HS-5 (Figure 3D) and primary bone marrow stromal cells (Figure 3E), but CD9 expression increased U266 cells' adhesion to Fibronectin (Figure 3F). CD9 expression also significantly inhibited U266 cell migration (Figure 4G).

In order to study the molecular mechanisms of CD9's effects on bortezomib sensitivity in multiple myeloma, we did the genome-wide expression profile microarray to detect the differentially expressed genes and explore the molecular signaling pathways affected by CD9 expression. We found that CD9 expression

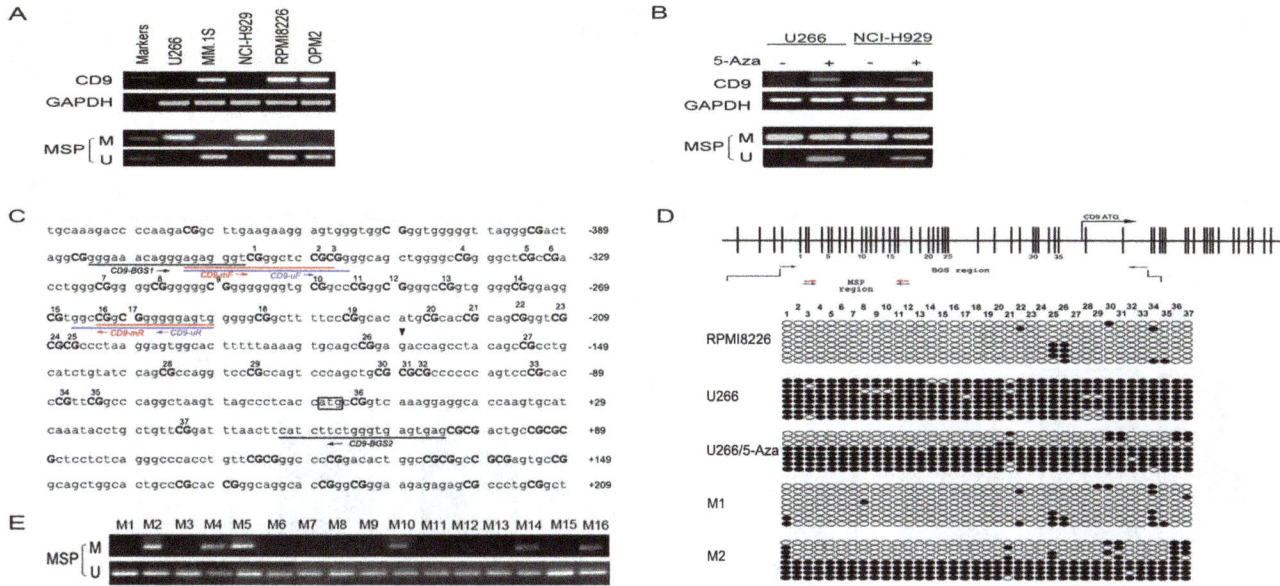

Figure 1. Analyses of methylation status of CD9 in multiple myeloma cell lines and cases. (A) Silencing of CD9 by promoter methylation in cell lines detected by semi-quantitative RT-PCR, with GAPDH as a control. M: methylated; U: unmethylated. (B) CD9 expression reserved with de-methylation reagent 5-Aza in U266 and NCI-H929. (C) Sequence of CD9 CGI with locations of the 37 CpG sites analysed and primers used. Methylation-specific PCR (MSP) and bisulfite genomic sequencing (BGS) regions are also shown. (D) Vertical lines indicate individual CpG sites. Cloned BGS-PCR products were sequenced and each clone was shown as an individual row, representing a single allele of the CGI. Filled circle, methylated; open circle, unmethylated. (E) Analysis of CD9 methylation in primary cases by MSP. M, methylated; U, unmethylated.

mainly affected the following three important signaling pathways respectively: the endoplasmic reticulum stress pathway, cell adhesion related signaling pathway and osteoclast differentiation related signaling pathway (Figure 4).

In addition to the differentially expressed genes shown by microarray, we futher checked protein expression level of several key genes involving ER stress pathway. The results showed that TRB3 and CHOP expressed higher in CD9 transfected U266 cells (Figure 5A).

Moreover, though FAK is not the differentially expressed gene detected by microarray, we checked some tyrosine-phosphorylated FAK protein expression using western blot. The results showed that only Phospho-FAK (Tyr925) expressed in cells and significantly increased in CD9 transfected U266 cells (Figure 5B).

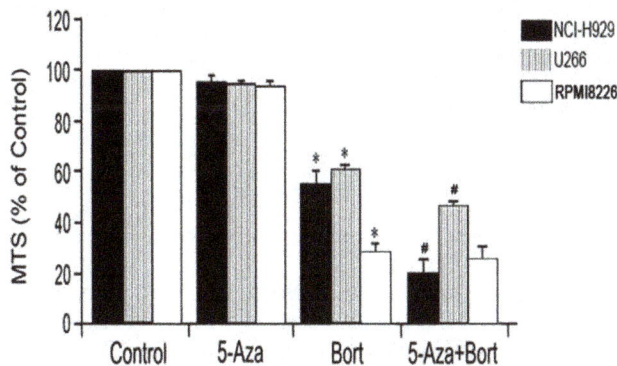

Figure 2. Synergy interaction of 5-Aza and bortezomib in MM cell lines. After pretreated with 5-Aza for 72 hours and then bortezomib, the sensitivity to bortezomib in U266 and NCI-H929 raised significantly while the bortezomib sentitive RPMI8226 raised a little bit.

Discussion

In this study, we identified that a tetraspanin family proteins, CD9 was significantly down-regulated and confered bortezomib resistance in MM. CD9 is constitutively expressed on a subpopulation of B cells [24,25]. Membranal tetraspanins are often inversely correlated with cancer prognosis and metastasis, however mutations were unidentified hitherto [26,27]. Their promoter characteristics and frequent down-regulation conform to transcriptional silencing by chromatin remodeling. We also found that down-regulation of CD9 due to promter hypermethylation in MM, consistant with previous studies [28–30]. Reverse expression of CD9 in the cell lines following de-methylation reagent 5-Aza treatment confirmed the mechanistic significance of methylation to its regulation. After pre-treatment of 5-Aza, the sensitivity to bortezomib in U266 and NCI-H929 raised significantly showed the synergistic interaction of 5-Aza and bortezomib inhibition in multiple myeloma. Moreover, CD9 transfected U266 cells had significantly increased bortezomib sensitivity suggested that one reason of the synergistic interaction of 5-Aza and bortezomib inhibition is CD9 expression.

From the CD9 functional study results, we found that CD9 expression did not affect the cell clone formation ability, cell cycle and the major cytokines (VEGF, IL-6 and IGF-1) secreted, but significantly affected the interaction beteen MM cells and their microenvironment. It significantly inhibited U266 cells' adhesion to HS-5 and also the primary bone marrow stromal cells, but CD9 expression increased U266 cells' adhesion to Fibronectin. MM cells localize within the BM through the interaction of adhesion receptors with their ligands on BM stromal cells and extracellular matrix proteins such as fibronectin [31]. It has been demonstrated that MM cells in the BM microenvironment are much less sensitive to chemotherapeutic agents [32,33]. This phenomenon is termed "cell adhesion-mediated drug resistance" (CAM-DR) and it is thought to be one of the major mechanisms by which MM

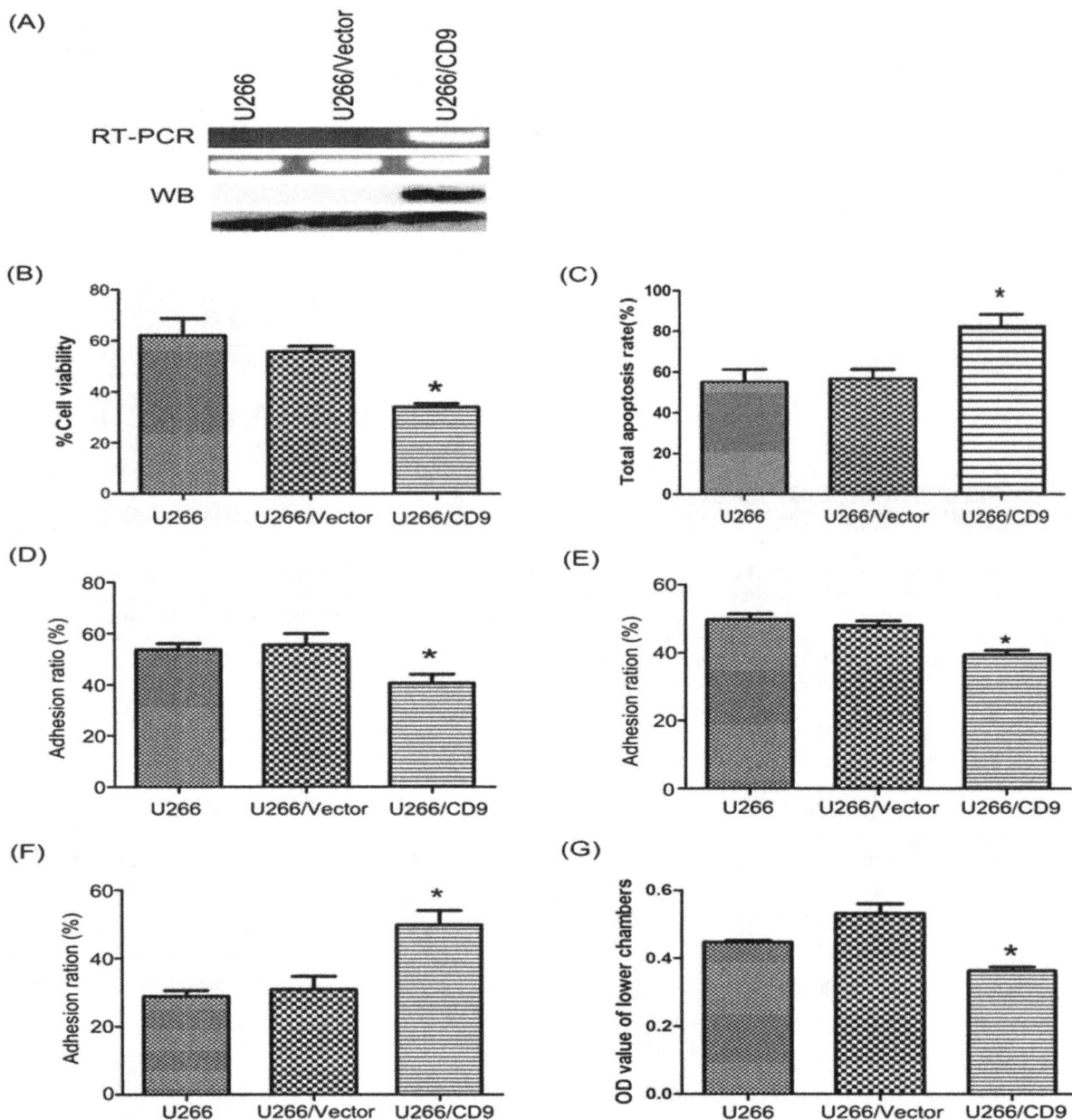

Figure 3. CD9 stablly transfected U266 cells construction and the effects of CD9 expression in U266 cell viability, apoptosis, adhesion and migration. (A) CD9 expression was confirmed by RT-PCR and western blot analysis. (B) CD9 expression obviously increased the bortezomib sensitivity compared to controls, *: p<0.05. (C) Bortezomib significantly promoted the apoptosis of U266/CD9 cells. *: p<0.05. (D) CD9 expression significantly inhibited U266 cells adhesion to bone marrow stromal cells HS-5. *: p<0.05. (E) CD9 expression significantly inhibited U266 cells' adhesion to the primary bone marrow stromal cells. *: p<0.05. (F) CD9 expression significantly increased U266 cells' adhesion to fibronectin. *: p<0.05. (G) CD9 expression significantly inhibited U266 cell migration. *: p<0.05.

cells escape the cytotoxic effects of therapeutic agents. However, until now, despite extensive investigations [34], the adhesion molecules critical for CAM-DR in MM is poorly understood. Here, we found that CD9 could overcome the CAM-DR of bortezomib through inhibiting MM cells' adherence to stromal cells but not fibronectin. This is consistent with Niranjan's report that fibronectin adherence did not protect MM cells from tipifarnib- or bortezomib-induced apoptosis. Stroma cell adhered MM cells were partially protected relative to suspension cells,

whereas fibronectin-adhered tumor cells seemed more sensitive to drug treatment [35].

Myeloma cell adhesion to BMSCs supports cell survival, proliferation, and cell adhesion-mediated drug resistance (CAM-DR) via signaling pathway activation, including the NF-kB (nuclear factor-kB), JAK/Stat3 (Janus kinase/signal transducer and activator of transcription-3), and MEK/MAPK (mitogen activated protein [MAP] kinase kinase/MAP kinase) pathways [36,37]. Our gene-expression profiling results suggested that CD9 expression mainly affected the following three important signaling

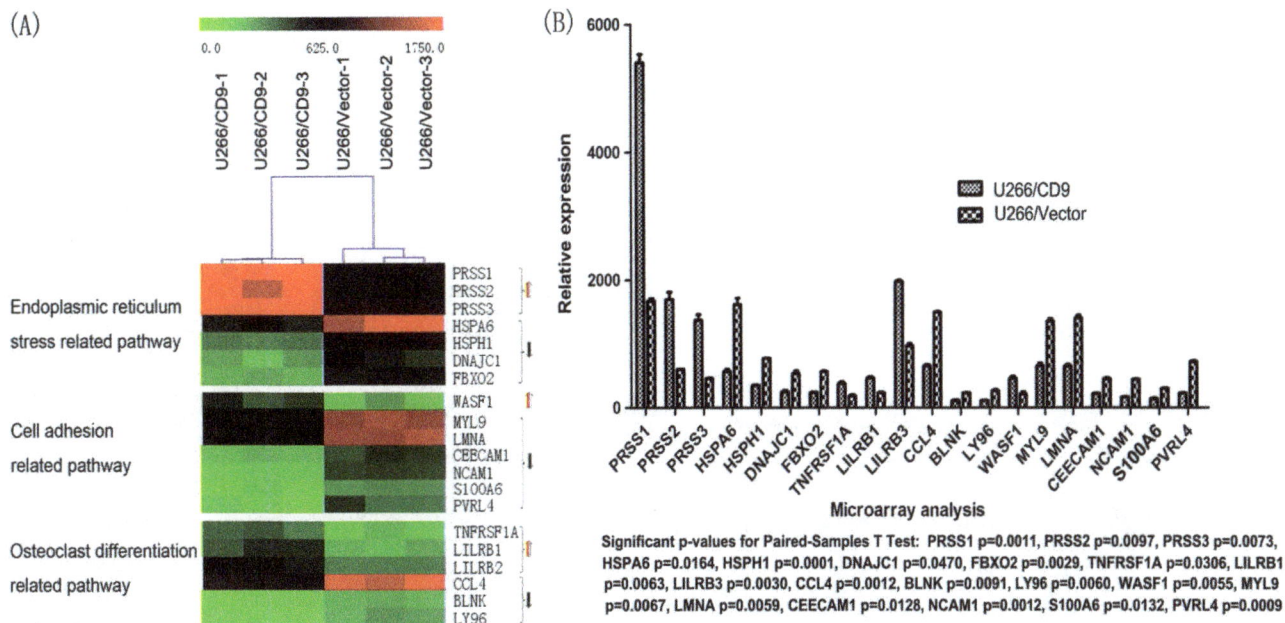

Figure 4. The differentially expressed genes in U266/CD9 and U266/Vector cells tested by genome-wide expression profile chip experiments and the analysis of related signaling pathways. CD9 expression mainly affected three important signaling pathways in MM. They are the endoplasmic reticulum stress pathway, cell adhesion related signaling pathways and osteoclast differentiation related signaling pathway, respectively (A). The degree of differentially expressed genes and p values were also analysed (B).

pathways respectively: the endoplasmic reticulum stress pathway, cell adhesion related signaling pathways and osteoclast differentiation related signaling pathway. The anti-cancer mechanisms of bortezomib elucidated by preclinical studies include induction of endoplasmic reticulum (ER) stress and pro-apoptotic Unfolded Protein Response (UPR) [38]. Activation of ER stress was further determined by checking several key proteins involving ER stress. CHOP and TRB3 expressed significantly higher in CD9

transfected U266 cells than in controls. During ER stress, the level of CHOP expression is elevated and CHOP functions to mediate programmed cell death [39]. TRB3 is also a stress-inducible nuclear protein, which has recently been shown to be involved in ER stress-induced apoptosis [40]. These data suggested that CD9 expression enhanced ER stress-mediated apoptosis by bortezomib in MM cells.

Our functional study results identified that CD9 really affected MM cells adhesion to the stromal cells and fibronectin. And this may be through cell adhesion related signaling pathways including upregulation of WASF1 and downregulation of MYL9, LMNA, CEECAM1, NCAM1, S100A6, PVRL4. Though mounting evidence has been shown that integrin-mediated cellular adhesion confers resistance to chemotherapy of multiple myeloma, our gene-expression profiling results didn't show that integrin as well as FAK expression changed. FAK is also an important mediator of focal adhesion formation and cell migration [41]. Then we checked some tyrosine-phosphorylated FAK protein expression using western blot. The results showed that only Phospho-FAK (Tyr925) expressed in cells and significantly increased in CD9 transfected U266 cells. Increased Phospho-FAK (Tyr925) was once reported to be correlated with loss of intercellular adhesion in breast cancer cells [42] and increased prostate cancer cell adhesion to fibronectin [43].

The gene-expression profiling results also show that CD9 expression may affect osteoclast differentiation in MM. Bone disease in patients with MM is characterized by increase in the numbers and activity of bone-resorbing osteoclasts and decrease in the number and function of bone-formation osteoblasts. CD9 may suppress osteoclastogenesis through up-regulation of TNFRSF1A, LILRB1, LILRB2 and down-regulation of CCL4, BLNK, LY96.

In conclusions (Figure 6), we found that down-regulation of CD9 by methylation decreased bortezomib sensitivity in multiple

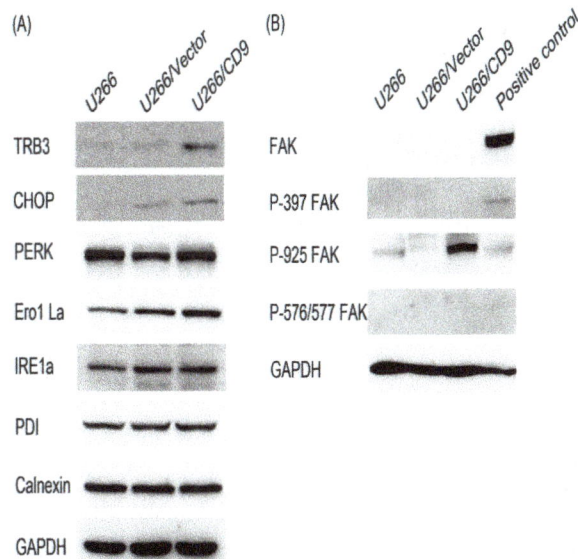

Figure 5. Several key ER Stress related protein and expression of FAK was analyzed by western blotting.

Promoter hypermethylation

↓

Down-regulation of CD9

↓

Ectopic expression of CD9

↓

| Endoplasmic reticulum Stress related pathway | Cell adhesion related pathway | Osteoclast differentiation related pathway |

↓ ↓ ↓

Pro-apoptosis | Inhibited adhesion to stromal cells ; Increased adhesion to Fibronectin | Inhibited Osteoclast differentiation

↓

increased bortezomib sensitivity in MM

↓

synergistic inhibition of 5-Aza and bortezomib in MM

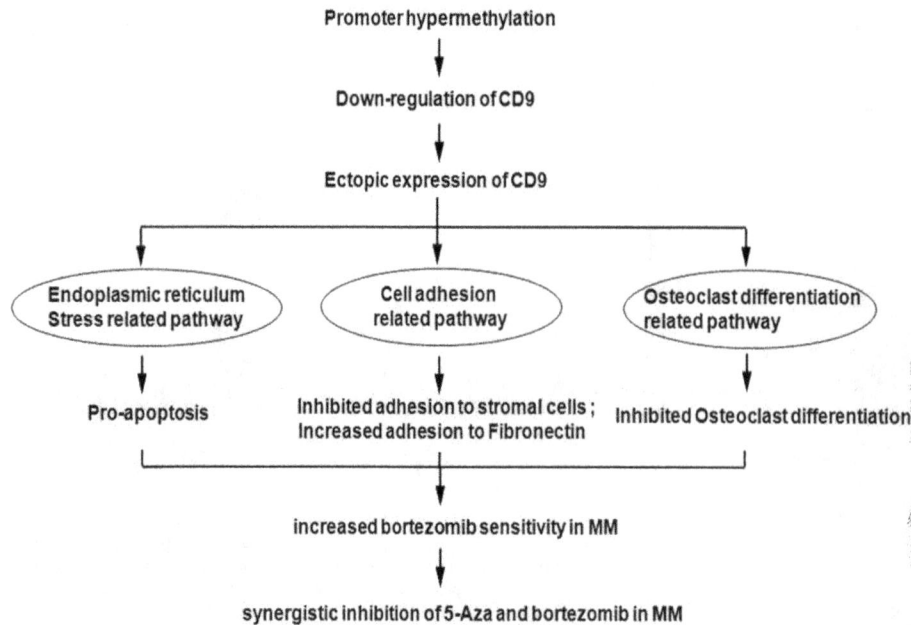

Figure 6. Diagram of the signaling pathways involved in CD9 expression's effect on bortezomib sensitivity in multiple myeloma.

myeloma. The mechanisms include three important signaling pathways: the endoplasmic reticulum stress pathway, cell adhesion related signaling pathway and osteoclast differentiation related signaling pathway. Combination therapy with de-methylation reagent 5-Aza may prove useful to the development of novel strategies for the treatment of bortezomib-resistant MM patients.

Supporting Information

Figure S1 Volcano Plot. Differentially expressed genes with statistical significance were shown by Volcano Plot. The vertical lines correspond to 2.0-fold up and down and the horizontal line

represents a P-value of 0.05. So the red point in the plot represents the differentially expressed mRNAs with statistical significance.

Table S1   PCR primers used in this study.

Author Contributions

Conceived and designed the experiments: XH JH. Performed the experiments: HX HD HJ. Analyzed the data: XH HX. Contributed reagents/materials/analysis tools: HD HJ JH. Wrote the paper: XH JH.

References

1. Anderson KC (2004) Bortezomib therapy for myeloma. Curr Hematol Rep 3: 65.
2. Hemler ME (2005) Tetraspanin functions and associated microdomains. Nat Rev Mol Cell Biol 6: 801–811.
3. Boucheix C, Rubinstein E (2001) Tetraspanins. Cell Mol Life Sci 58: 1189–1205.
4. Rubinstein E, Le Nour F, Lagaudriere-Gasbert C, Billard M, Conjeaud H, et al. (1996) CD9, CD63, CD61, CD81, and CD82 are components of a surface tetraspanin network connected to HLA-DR and VLA integrins. Eur J Immunol 26: 2657–2665.
5. Boucheix C, Soria C, Mirshahi M, Soria J, Perrot JY, et al. (1983) Characteristics of platelet aggregation induced by the monoclonal antibody ALB6 (acute lymphoblastic leukemia antigen p 24). Inhibition of aggregation by ALB6Fab. FEBS Lett 161: 289–295.
6. Kersey JH, LeBien TW, Abramson CS, Newman R, Sutherland R, et al. (1981) P-24: a human leukemia-associated and lymphohemopoietic progenitor cell surface structure identified with monoclonal antibody. J Exp Med 153: 726–731.
7. Boucheix C, Benoit P, Frachet P, Billard M, Worthington RE, et al. (1991) Molecular cloning of the CD9 antigen. A new family of cell surface proteins. J Biol Chem 266: 117–122.
8. Lanza F, Wolf D, Fox CF, Kieffer N, Seyer JM, et al. (1991) cDNA cloning and expression of platelet p24/CD9. Evidence for a new family of multiple membrane-spanning proteins. J Biol Chem 266: 10638–10645.
9. Iwamoto R, Senoh H, Okada Y, Uchida T, Mekada E (1991) An antibody that inhibits the binding of diphtheria toxin to cells revealed the association of a 27-kDa membrane protein with the diphtheria toxin receptor. J Biol Chem 266: 20463–20469.
10. Mitamura T, Iwamoto R, Umata T, Yomo T, Urabe I, et al. The 27-kD diphtheria toxin receptor-associated protein (DRAP27) from vero cells is the monkey homologue of human CD9 antigen: expression of DRAP27 elevates the number of diphtheria toxin receptors on toxin-sensitive cells. J Cell Biol 118: 1389–1399.
11. Fan J, Zhu GZ, Niles RM (2010) Expression and function of CD9 in melanoma cells. Mol Carcinog 49: 85–93.
12. Maecker HT, Todd SC, Levy S (1997) The tetraspanin superfamily: molecularfacilitators. FASEB J 11: 428–442.
13. Zoller M (2009) Tetraspanins: push and pull in suppressing and promoting metastasis. Nat Rev Cancer 9: 40–55.
14. Miyake M, Nakano K, Itoi SI, Koh T, Taki T (1996) Motility-related protein-1 (MRP-1/CD9) reduction as a factor of poor prognosis in breast cancer. Cancer Res 56: 1244–1249.
15. Higashiyama M, Doi O, Kodama K, Yokouchi H, Adachi M, et al. (1997) Immunohistochemically detected expression of motility-related protein-1 (MRP-1/CD9) in lung adenocarcinoma and its relation to prognosis. Int J Cancer 74: 205–211.
16. Huang CI, Kohno N, Ogawa E, Adachi M, Taki T, et al. (1998) Correlationof reduction in MRP-1/CD9 and KAI1/CD82 expression with recurrences in breast cancer patients. Am J Pathol 153: 973–983.
17. Mori M, Mimori K, Shiraishi T, Haraguchi M, Ueo H, et al. (1998) Motility related protein 1 (MRP1/CD9) expression in colon cancer. Clin Cancer Res 4: 1507–1510.
18. Hashida H, Takabayashi A, Tokuhara T, Hattori N, Taki T, et al. (2003) Clinical significance of transmembrane 4 superfamily in colon cancer. British Journal of Cancer 89: 158–167.
19. Sho M, Adachi M, Taki T, Hashida H, Konishi T, et al. (1998) Transmembrane 4 superfamily as a prognostic factor in pancreatic cancer. Int J Cancer 79: 509–516.
20. Buim ME, Lourenço SV, Carvalho KC, Cardim R, Pereira C. et al. (2010) Downregulation of CD9 protein expression is associated with aggressive behavior of oral squamous cell carcinoma. Oral Oncol 46: 166–171.

21. Zheng R, Yano S, Zhang H, Nakataki E, Tachibana I, et al. (2005) CD9 overexpression suppressed the liver metastasis and malignant ascites via inhibition of proliferation and motility of small-cell lung cancer cells in NK cell-depleted SCID mice. Oncology Research 15: 365–372.

22. Murray PG, Qiu GH, Fu L, Waites ER, Srivastava G, et al. (2004) Frequent epigenetic inactivation of the RASSF1A tumor suppressor gene in Hodgkin's lymphoma. Oncogene 23: 1326–1331.

23. Ying J, Li H, Seng TJ, Langford C, Srivastava G, et al. (2006) Functional epigenetics identifies a protocadherin PCDH10 as a candidate tumor suppressor for nasopharyngeal, esophageal and multiple other carcinomas with frequent methylation. Oncogene 25: 1070–1080.

24. Won WJ, Kearney JF. (2002) CD9 is a unique marker for marginal zone Bcells, B1 cells, and plasma cells in mice. J Immunol 168: 5605–5611.

25. Barrena S, Almeida J, Yunta M, López A, Fernández-Mosteirín N, et al. (2005) Aberrant expression of tetraspanin molecules in B-cell chronic lymphoproliferative disorders and its correlation with normal B-cell maturation. Leukemia 19: 1376–1383.

26. Wang HX, Li Q, Sharma C, Knoblich K, Hemler ME (2011) Tetraspanin protein contributions to cancer. Biochem Soc Trans 39: 547–552.

27. Richardson MM, Jennings LK, Zhang XA (2011) Tetraspanins and tumor progression. Clin Exp Metastasis 28: 261–270.

28. De Bruyne E, Bos TJ, Asosingh K, Vande Broek I, Menu E, et al. (2008) Epigenetic silencing of the tetraspanin CD9 during disease progression in multiple myeloma cells and correlation with survival. Clin Cancer Res 14: 2918–2926.

29. Heller G, Schmidt WM, Ziegler B, Holzer S, Müllauer L, et al. (2008) Genome-wide transcriptional response to 5-aza-2'-deoxycytidine and trichostatin a in multiple myeloma cells. Cancer Res 68: 44–54.

30. Drucker L, Tohami T, Tartakover-Matalon S, Zismanov V, Shapiro H, et al. (2006) Promoter hypermethylation of tetraspanin members contributes to their silencing in myeloma cell lines. Carcinogenesis 27: 197–204.

31. Hideshima T, Mitsiades C, Tonon G, Richardson PG, Anderson KC (2007) Understanding multiple myeloma pathogenesis in the bone marrow to identify new therapeutic targets. Nat Rev Cancer 7: 585–598.

32. Damiano JS, Cress AE, Hazlehurst LA, Shtil AA, Dalton WS (1999) Cell adhesion mediated drug resistance (CAM-DR): role of integrins and resistance to apoptosis in human myeloma cell lines. Blood 93: 1658–1667.

33. Nefedova Y, Landowski TH, Dalton WS (2003) Bone marrow stromal-derived soluble factors and direct cell contact contribute to de novo drug resistance of myeloma cells by distinct mechanisms. Leukemia 17: 1175–1182.

34. Neri P, Bahlis NJ (2012) Targeting of adhesion molecules as a therapeutic strategy in multiple myeloma. Curr Cancer Drug Targets 12: 776–796.

35. Yanamandra N, Colaco NM, Parquet NA, Buzzeo RW, Boulware D, et al. (2006) Tipifarnib and bortezomib are synergistic and overcome cell adhesion-mediated drug resistance in multiple myeloma and acute myeloid leukemia. Clin Cancer Res 12: 591–599.

36. Hazlehurst LA, Dalton WS (2001) Mechanisms associated with cell adhesion mediated drug resistance (CAM-DR) in hematopoietic malignancies. Cancer Metastasis Rev 20: 43–50.

37. Li ZW, Dalton WS (2006) Tumor microenvironment and drug resistance in hematologic malignancies. Blood Rev 20: 333–342.

38. Mujtaba T, Dou QP (2011) Advances in the understanding of mechanisms and therapeutic use of bortezomib. Discov Med 12: 471–480.

39. Zinszner H, Kuroda M, Wang X, Batchvarova N, Lightfoot RT, Remotti H, Stevens JL, Ron D. CHOP is implicated in programmed cell death in response to impaired function of the endoplasmic reticulum. Genes Dev. 1998 Apr 1;12(7):982–95.

40. Ohoka N, Yoshii S, Hattori T, Onozaki K, Hayashi H (2005) TRB3, a novel ER stress-inducible gene, is induced via ATF4-CHOP pathway and is involved in cell death. EMBO J 24: 1243–1255.

41. Pelletier AJ, Kunicki T, Ruggeri ZM, Quaranta V (1995) The activation state of the integrin alpha IIb beta 3 affects outside-in signals leading to cell spreading and focal adhesion kinase phosphorylation. J Biol Chem 270: 18133–18140.

42. Nagaharu K, Zhang X, Yoshida T, Katoh D, Hanamura N, et al. (2011) Tenascin C induces epithelial-mesenchymal transition-like change accompanied by SRC activation and focal adhesion kinase phosphorylation in human breast cancer cells. Am J Pathol 178: 754–763.

43. Su B, Gao L, Meng F, Guo LW, Rothschild J, et al. (2013) Adhesion-mediated cytoskeletal remodeling is controlled by the direct scaffolding of Src from FAK complexes to lipid rafts by SSeCKS/AKAP12. Oncogene 32: 2016–2026.

16

Dendritic Cells Pulsed with Leukemia Cell-Derived Exosomes More Efficiently Induce Antileukemic Immunities

Ye Yao[1][◐], **Chun Wang**[2][◐], **Wei Wei**[1], **Chang Shen**[2], **Xiaohui Deng**[1], **Linjun Chen**[1], **Liyuan Ma**, **Siguo Hao**[1]*

1 Department of Hematology, Xinhua Hospital Affiliated to Shanghai Jiaotong University School of Medicine, Shanghai, China, **2** Department of Hematology, The First People's Hospital of Shanghai Affiliated to Shanghai Jiaotong University, Shanghai, China

Abstract

Dendritic cells (DCs) and tumor cell-derived exosomes have been used to develop antitumor vaccines. However, the biological properties and antileukemic effects of leukemia cell-derived exosomes (LEXs) are not well described. In this study, the biological properties and induction of antileukemic immunity of LEXs were investigated using transmission electron microscopy, western blot analysis, cytotoxicity assays, and animal studies. Similar to other tumor cells, leukemia cells release exosomes. Exosomes derived from K562 leukemia cells (LEX$_{K562}$) are membrane-bound vesicles with diameters of approximately 50–100 μm and harbor adhesion molecules (*e.g.*, intercellular adhesion molecule-1) and immunologically associated molecules (*e.g.*, heat shock protein 70). In cytotoxicity assays and animal studies, LEXs-pulsed DCs induced an antileukemic cytotoxic T-lymphocyte immune response and antileukemic immunity more effectively than did LEXs and non-pulsed DCs ($P<0.05$). Therefore, LEXs may harbor antigens and immunological molecules associated with leukemia cells. As such, LEX-based vaccines may be a promising strategy for prolonging disease-free survival in patients with leukemia after chemotherapy or hematopoietic stem cell transplantation.

Editor: Gabriele Multhoff, Technische Universitaet Muenchen, Germany

Funding: This research was supported by the National Natural Science Foundation of China (grant No. 81070432). The funders had no role in study design, data collection and analysis, decision to publish, or preparation of the manuscript.

Competing Interests: The authors have declared that no competing interests exist.

* E-mail: haosghj88@hotmail.com

◐ These authors contributed equally to this work.

Introduction

In patients with leukemia, the presence of minimal residual leukemia cells (MRLs) after chemotherapy and hematopoietic stem cell transplantation (HSCT) is a major cause of disease recurrence [1]. At present, eradication of MRLs is achieved with high-dose chemotherapy and allogeneic HSCT (allo-HSCT). The graft-versus-leukemia effects of allogeneic lymphocytes contribute to the antileukemic effect of allo-HSCT. However, these antileukemic immunological effects are nonspecific; as such, they are inefficient and can cause serious graft-versus-host disease, which contributes to morbidity after allo-HSCT. Several clinical and pre-clinical studies have identified immunotherapy as an approach to eliminate MRLs after chemotherapy and transplantation in order to reduce and prevent leukemia relapse. Indeed, several clinical studies have demonstrated the effectiveness of leukemia immunotherapy [2–4]. However, immunotherapy is limited by the lack of reliable leukemia-associated antigens. Therefore, it is important to identify leukemia cell-associated antigens in order to develop immunotherapies for leukemia and other hematologic malignancies.

Exosomes (EXOs) are vesicles that harbor multiple cell-membrane molecules and other proteins secreted by eukaryotes [5,6]. EXOs are secreted by several cell types, particularly hematopoietic cells, including antigen-presenting cells such as dendritic cells (DCs), lymphocytes, mast cells, enterocytes, and tumor cells [2].

Recently, tumor cell-derived EXOs (TEXs) have attracted attention as a source of tumor antigens for use in vaccines [7–9]. TEXs harbor tumor-related antigens and can induce potent antitumor immune responses [5,10]. TEXs isolated from malignant effusions can transfer tumor antigens to DCs to induce specific cytotoxic T-lymphocyte (CTL) responses and antitumor immunity [11–14]. Therefore, TEXs may be a source of tumor antigens for antitumor immunotherapy. However, a previous study reported that TEXs can induce antigen-specific tolerance through T-cell apoptosis and suppression of T-cell receptor/CD3-zeta by Fas ligand-containing EXOs from ovarian tumors [15]. In contrast, ours and other studies have demonstrated that EXOs secreted by tumor peptide-pulsed DCs can induce a specific antitumor response. Specifically, DCs can take up TEXs and the antigens harbored within, thus inducing strong antitumor immunity [16,17]. These studies have demonstrated that TEXs and DCs can be implemented as cancer immunotherapy [4,5]. The K562 cell line is a human chronic myelogenous leukemia cell line that contains the *BCR:ABL* fusion gene [18]. In this study, we investigated the biological characteristics of EXOs derived from K562 leukemia cells (LEX$_{K562}$) and their ability to induce antileukemic immunity. Our results revealed that LEX$_{K562}$ harbor the BCR-ABL fusion protein, which is expressed in the original

K562 cell line. Furthermore, our results suggested that LEX can be taken up by DCs *in vitro* and that LEX-pulsed DCs induce a stronger antigen-specific antileukemic CTL immune response *in vivo*.

Materials and Methods

Reagents, cell lines, and animals

The research on "Dendritic cells pulsed with leukemia cell-derived exosomes induce more efficiently anti-leukemia immunities" will be carried out by Prof. Siguo Hao's research team, this research mainly focus on the biological properties and its anti-leukemia immunities of Dendritic cells pulsed with leukemia cell-derived exosomes. In this study, DBA/2 will be used as animal model and immunized with Dendritic cells pulsed with leukemia cell-derived exosomes and then mouse will be challenged with L1210 leukemia cells and the incidence of tumor growth will be monitored.

The Ethics Committee of Xinhua Hospital Affiliated to Shanghai Jiaotong University School of Medicine carried out a comprehensive assessment of the animals, including experimental purposes, the expected benefits and causing injury, death, etc.

The Ethics Committee concluded that this study was carried out in strict accordance with the recommendations in the Guide for the Care and Use of Laboratory Animals of the National Institutes of Health. The protocol was approved by the Committee on the Ethics of Animal Experiments of Xinhua Hospital Affiliated to Shanghai Jiaotong University (Permit Number: XHEC-E 2011-006). All surgery was performed under sodium pentobarbital anesthesia, and all efforts were made to minimize suffering.

RPMI-1640 cell culture medium, fetal bovine serum (FBS), and serum-free medium AIM-V were purchased from Invitrogen (Shanghai, China). Rabbit anti-human ABL and rat anti-human heat shock protein 70 (HSP70) antibodies were purchased from Santa Cruz Biotechnology (Shanghai, China). Recombinant mouse granulocyte-macrophage colony-stimulating factor (rmGM-CSF), recombinant human interleukin (rhIL)-4, and rhIL-2 were purchased from PeproTech (Shanghai, China). The CytoTox 96 non-radioactive cytotoxicity assay kit was purchased from Promega BioSciences (Shanghai, China). The K562 cell line was provided by the Shanghai Institute of Hematology. The L1210 cell line, an acute lymphoblastic leukemia cell line derived from DBA/2 mice, was purchased from the Shanghai Institute for Biological Science (Shanghai, China). Both cell lines were cultured in RPMI 1640 medium supplemented with 10% FBS. To prevent contamination with plasma EXOs, cells were transferred to serum-free medium (AIM V) and cultured for 24 h. This culture medium was then used as the source of EXOs. DBA/2 female mice were purchased from the Shanghai Laboratory Animal Center (Shanghai, China) and used at 6–14 weeks of age. Mice were allowed to adapt to their environment for 1 week before initiation of the experiments. During the course of the experiments, DBA/2 mice were maintained under standard environmental conditions with free access to food and water. DBA/2 mice were treated according to the guidelines of The Ethics Committee of Xinhua Hospital Affiliated to the Shanghai Jiaotong University School of Medicine.

Generation and purification of EXOs *from leukemia cells*

Generation and purification of EXOs from leukemia cells were performed as previously described [19]. Briefly, the culture supernatants of K562 and L1210 cells were subjected to 4 successive centrifugations: $300 \times g$ for 5 min to remove whole cells, $1,200 \times g$ for 20 min, $10,000 \times g$ for 30 min to remove debris, and $100,000 \times g$ for 1 h to pellet EXOs. The LEX pellets were washed twice in a large volume of phosphate-buffered saline (PBS) and recovered by centrifugation at $100,000 \times g$ for 1 h. LEXs were purified using sucrose density gradient centrifugation [19]. Briefly, EXOs were underlain with 1.5 mL of a 30% sucrose/D_2O density cushion (density 1.210 g/cm^3) followed by ultracentrifugation at $100,000 \times g$ at 4°C for 1 h. Approximately 2 mL of the cushion was collected from the bottom of the tube and diluted in 50 mL of PBS. Finally, the EXOs were concentrated to a volume of 10 mL by centrifugation for 60 min at $1000 \times g$ in a pre-rinsed 100-kDa molecular weight cut-off Amicon Ultra capsule filter (Millipore, Billerica, MA, USA). The amount of recovered exosomal proteins was measured using the Bradford assay (Bio-Rad, Richmond, CA). EXOs of K562 and L1210 cells were termed LEX$_{K562}$ and LEX$_{L1210}$, respectively.

Morphological characteristics of LEX$_{K562}$

LEX$_{K562}$ (10 μg) were washed in cacodylate buffer, fixed in 2.5% glutaraldehyde (Polysciences, Shanghai, China) in cacodylate buffer overnight at 4°C, dehydrated by graded alcohol processing, and flat embedded in LX-112 epoxy resin. Sections were cut with an ultramicrotome. Mounted sections were collected on copper grids, stained with a saturated solution of uranyl acetate, and submitted for observation and imaging under a Philips CM12 transmission electron microscope (TEM) [20].

Detection of expression of ABL and HSP70 in LEX$_{K562}$

The LEX$_{K562}$ suspension (20 μL) was added to 20 μL of a 2% paraformaldehyde solution and incubated at room temperature for 1 h. Next, 3–6 μL of fixed EXOs was dripped onto a nickel grid, allowed to dry completely, and stained with diluted rat anti-human HSP70 and ABL antibodies. Samples were first incubated at room temperature for 30 min and then overnight at 4°C. Next, 25 μL diluted scintillation proximity assay (SPA) suspension was dripped onto a clean and flat hydrophobic membrane to form liquid drops. The grid was gently placed on the SPA drops with the film facing down, incubated at room temperature for 2 h, and then rinsed with PBS. Then, 5% uranyl acetate staining solution was dripped onto the nickel grid for negative staining and incubated at room temperature for 10 min. A blank control was included in which the primary antibody was replaced with PBS. EXO staining was visualized under TEM [19]. EXOs containing black colloidal gold particles on the extramembrane and cavum of the vesicles were considered to be positive.

To further confirm the expression of BCR-ABL and HSP70 in LEX$_{K562}$, we performed western blotting as previously described [19]. Briefly, 10 μg of LEX$_{K562}$ and K562 cell extracts was resuspended in sodium dodecyl sulfate buffer and heated at 95°C for 5 min. Then, 0.13 M dithiothreitol was added to the samples, and they were subjected to 7.5% sodium dodecyl sulfate polyacrylamide gel electrophoresis. Following electrotransfer to nitrocellulose membranes, blocking was performed with 5% bovine serum albumin at room temperature for 2 h. Rabbit anti-human HSP70 and ABL antibodies were added separately, and the blots were incubated at room temperature for 1 h. Then, blots were incubated for 1 h with horseradish peroxidase-labeled secondary antibodies. Proteins were visualized by enhanced chemiluminescence substrate, and the blots were developed with the Pico West illumination kit (Promega, Shanghai, China).

Generation of DCs

DBA/2 murine bone marrow-derived DCs were generated from bone marrow cells cultured in the presence of GM-CSF and IL-4 as previously described [17]. Briefly, bone marrow cells from the femurs and tibias of mice were flushed with RPMI 1640 medium. Red blood cells were depleted with 0.84% ammonium chloride, and the cells were plated in DC culture medium containing 10% FBS, GM-CSF (10 ng/mL), and IL-4 (10 ng/mL). On day 3, non-adherent cells, including granulocytes and T- and B-lymphocytes, were gently removed, and fresh medium containing GM-CSF and IL-4 was added. Two days later, loosely adherent proliferating DC aggregates were dislodged and replated. On day 7, non-adherent DCs were harvested and matured by incubation with 1 μg/mL lipopolysaccharide (Sigma-Aldrich, Shanghai, China) for 6 h. DCs were then harvested for further use.

LEX uptake by DCs *in vitro*

Our previous study demonstrated that DC-derived EXOs are taken up by DCs *in vitro*. In the present study, we investigated whether LEXs are taken up by DCs *in vitro*. LEXs were stained with carboxyfluorescein succinimidyl ester (CFSE) and then co-cultured with DCs. CFSE-positive cells were visualized at different time points for up to 10 h by confocal microscopy. To investigate the rate of decay, DCs incubated with LEX_{K562} for 4 h were washed twice with PBS, further cultured in media, and then visualized by confocal microscopy at different time points for up to 72 h. DCs pulsed with LEX_{K562} and LEX_{L1210} were termed DC/LEX_{K562} and DC/LEX_{L1210}, respectively.

Animal study

To examine the ability of LEX_{L1210} and DC/LEX_{L1210} to induce protective antitumor immunity, DBA/2 mice were randomly divided into 4 groups (n = 8 per group). The animals were immunized subcutaneously (s.c.) on the inner side of their thighs with the following: PBS (control), LEX_{L1210} (30 μg), non-pulsed DCs (1×10^6/mouse), and different doses of DC/LEX_{L1210} ($1.0–4.0 \times 10^6$ cells/mouse). On days 7–10 after immunization, all mice were challenged with L1210 leukemia cells on the outer side of the same thighs (0.5×10^6 cells/mouse). To determine immune specificity, after immunization, a group of tumor-free mice were challenged s.c. with P388 cells, another DBA/2 mouse leukemia cell line (Shanghai Institute for Biological Science) (5×10^5 cells/mouse). Tumor growth was monitored daily for up to 4 weeks using a caliper. For ethical treatment of the animals, all mice were euthanized when the tumor diameter reached 1.5 cm.

To examine the therapeutic effect on established tumors, DBA/2 mice (n = 8 per group) were s.c. inoculated with L1210 cells (0.5×10^6 cells/mouse). After 5 d, when the tumors became palpable (~5 mm in diameter), mice were s.c. immunized with LEX_{L1210} and different doses of DC/LEX_{L1210} ($1.0–4.0 \times 10^6$ cells/mouse). Animal mortality and tumor growth or regression were monitored daily for up to 10 weeks; for ethical treatment of the animals, the mice were euthanized when the tumor diameter reached 1.5 cm.

Cytotoxicity assay

Cytotoxic responses were evaluated by lactate dehydrogenase (LDH) release using the CytoTox 96 cytotoxicity assay kit according to the manufacturer's instructions. Splenic T-cells from mice immunized intravenously with LEX_{L1210}, DC/LEX_{L1210}, and PBS (control) were harvested and purified over nylon wool. Cells were prepared at 1.5×10^6/mL in complete medium. They were then co-cultured with 1.5×10^5 irradiated L1210 cells in 100-mm Petri dishes containing 100 U/mL of rhIL-2 at 37°C for 6 d. On days 2 and 5, rhIL-2 was added. Cells were harvested at the end of the culture period, and viable T-cells were isolated using Ficoll-Paque centrifugation (Pharmacia Biotech, Shanghai, China). These cells were thereafter referred to as effector cells. The

LDH assay is an enzymatic method that colorimetrically quantifies LDH released from lysed target cells. L1210 and P388 cells served as controls and were mixed at different ratios with effector cells after incubation for 4 h at 37°C. The spontaneous/maximal release ratio was <20% in all experiments. Specific lysis (%) was calculated as follows: (experimental LDH release − effector cell spontaneous LDH release − target spontaneous LDH release)/(target maximum LDH release)×100.

Statistical analysis

For the mouse study, the Kaplan-Meier product-limit method was used to calculate survival rates. Differences between groups were determined using the generalized Log-rank test. Survival data are also presented as median survival time (MST), which is the time point at which half of the mice were alive. Data have been expressed as X±S; statistical analysis was performed using the Student's *t*-test. For all statistical analyses, $P<0.05$ was considered statistically significant.

Results

Leukemia cells secrete exosomes

We first assessed whether the K562 cell line releases EXOs similar to other tumor cell lines. When the K562 culture supernatant was differentially centrifuged up to $100,000 \times g$, the pellet was similar to previously reported EXOs, as determined by electron microscopy. The vesicles of these preparations were <100 nm in diameter and had the dimpled, cup-shaped morphologies characteristic of EXOs (Fig. 1a). In order to explore whether LEX_{K562} harbored specific proteins from its parental K562 cells, we analyzed the expression of BCR-ABL, a fusion protein in K562 cells, using anti-ABL antibodies in LEX_{K562}. More than 60% of LEX_{K562} were positively stained for ABL (Fig. 1c and 1e), indicating that LEXs harbor proteins of their parental leukemia cells. To further confirm this finding, we performed a western blot to analyze ABL expression in LEX_{K562}. Our data suggested that LEX_{K562} harbored BCR-ABL molecules expressed in K562 cells (Fig. 1d and 1e). In addition, LEX_{K562} expressed HSP70 (Fig. 1b and 1d), a chaperone protein involved in the induction of immunity. we also examined ER-residing protein Grp94 in exosomes derived from K562 leukemia cells by western blot and our data showed that ER-residing protein Grp94 was absent in LEX_{K562} (Figure S1). Acetylcholinesterase activity, a characteristic enzyme in reticulocyte-derived exosomes also were detectable in LEX_{K562} (data not shown). Taken together, these results indicated that vesicles obtained from cell-free supernatants of K562 leukemia cells exhibited biophysical properties of exosomes. and LEXs contain known leukemia cell associated antigens as well as HSP70, a molecule that facilitates antigen presentation and CTL induction. Together, these data indicate that LEXs are a potential source of leukemia cell-associated antigens.

LEXs are taken up by DCs

To determine whether LEX_{K562} are taken up by DCs and to understand the kinetics of DCs sensitized by LEX_{K562} *in vitro*, LEX_{K562} were labeled with CFSE and then co-cultured with DCs. CFSE expression in DCs was tested at different time points using flow cytometry and confocal fluorescence microscopy. CFSE-positive DCs (23%) were detectable as early as 1 h after incubation (Figure 2a and 2b). The number of CFSE-positive cells (86.5%) reached a plateau 3–4 h after incubation. To investigate the rate of decay of LEX_{K562} in DCs, DCs were incubated with CFSE-labeled LEX_{K562} for 4 h, washed twice with PBS, further cultured

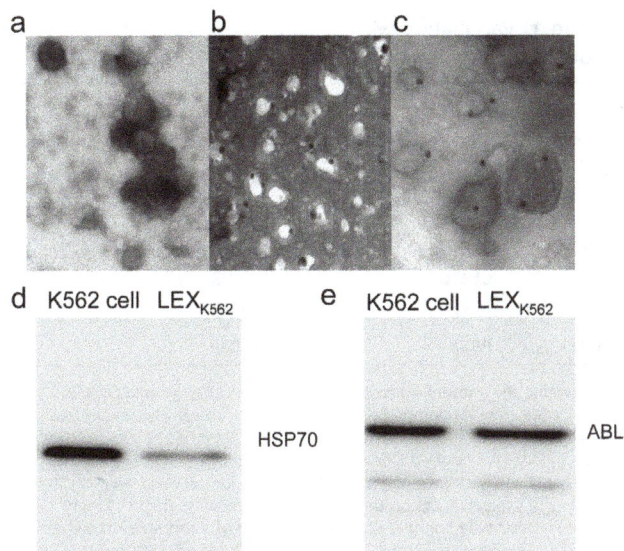

Figure 1. Morophology and expression of heat shock protein 70 and ABL in LEX$_{K562}$. (a) Transmission electron micrograph of K562 cell-secreted exosomes (×100K). (b and c) Electron micrograph of heat shock protein 70 (HSP70)- and ABL-labeled exosomes. (d) Western blot analysis demonstrating the presence of HSP70 and ABL molecules in K562 cells and K562-derived exosomes (LEX$_{K562}$).

in culture medium, and then examined at different time points for up to 72 h. The number of CFSE-positive DCs decreased over time (Fig. 2c). CFSE-positive DCs (18%) remained detectable at 72 h after culturing, indicating that the uptake of LEX$_{K562}$ by DCs is stable.

LEX-pulsed DCs induced a strong cytotoxic antileukemic immune response *ex vivo*

In order to examine whether LEXs induced an antileukemic CTL immune response, L1210 leukemia cells were implanted in DBA/2 mice as an animal model of tumor growth. Splenic T-cells

were isolated from mice immunized with PBS (control), non-pulsed DCs, LEX$_{L1210}$, and DC/LEX$_{L1210}$. T cells from mice immunized with PBS and non-pulsed DCs did not show killing activity against L1210 cells, whereas T cells from LEX$_{L1210}$-immunized mice showed weak killing activity against L1210 cells ($23.5\% \pm 3.21\%$; E:T ratio, 50:1) (Fig. 3). Interestingly, T-cells from DC/LEX$_{L1210}$-immunized mice showed significantly stronger killing activity ($57.15\% \pm 6.13\%$; E:T ratio, 50:1) than T-cells from LEX$_{L1210}$-immunized mice ($P < 0.01$). Thus, LEX-pulsed DCs induce a more potent antileukemic CTL response. Further, LEX$_{L1210}$- and LEX$_{L1210}$-pulsed DCs induce specific antileukemic effects against L1210 cells, as evidenced by the lack of killing activity in T-cells from DC/LEX$_{L1210}$-immunized mice against P388 leukemia cells (Fig. 3).

LEX-pulsed DCs induce strong protective immunity against leukemia cells

Because the strength of *ex vivo* CTL cell responses was comparable between mice immunized with LEX$_{L1210}$ and DC/LEX$_{L1210}$, we examined the immune protection conferred by these 2 vaccines *in vivo*. To do so, we evaluated the efficacy of vaccination with LEX$_{L1210}$ and DC/LEX$_{L1210}$ in preventing tumor growth. L1210 leukemia cells were implanted in DBA/2 mice as an animal model of tumor growth. DBA/2 mice were immunized s.c. with PBS (control), LEX$_{L1210}$, non-pulsed DCs, and different doses of DC/LEX$_{L1210}$. On days 7–10 after immunization, all mice were challenged with L1210 leukemia cells. All mice injected with PBS and non-pulsed DCs showed tumor growth (100%), while only half (50%) of mice injected with LEX$_{L1210}$ showed tumor growth (Table 1), indicating that LEXs induce protective immunity against leukemia cells. Interestingly, 87.5% (7/8) of DC/LEX$_{L1210}$-immunized mice were tumor-free, indicating that LEX-pulsed DCs induce stronger antileukemic immunity than LEX alone. In addition, our data demonstrated that LEX$_{L1210}$ and DC/LEX$_{L1210}$ induce specific antileukemic immunity, because no protective immunity was observed in mice challenged with P388 leukemia cells. Moreover, our data also showed that immunization with LEX$_{L1210}$ and DC/LEX$_{L1210}$ significantly improved survival (Fig. 4). Vaccination with non-pulsed DCs (MST, 20 d) did not significantly prolong survival as

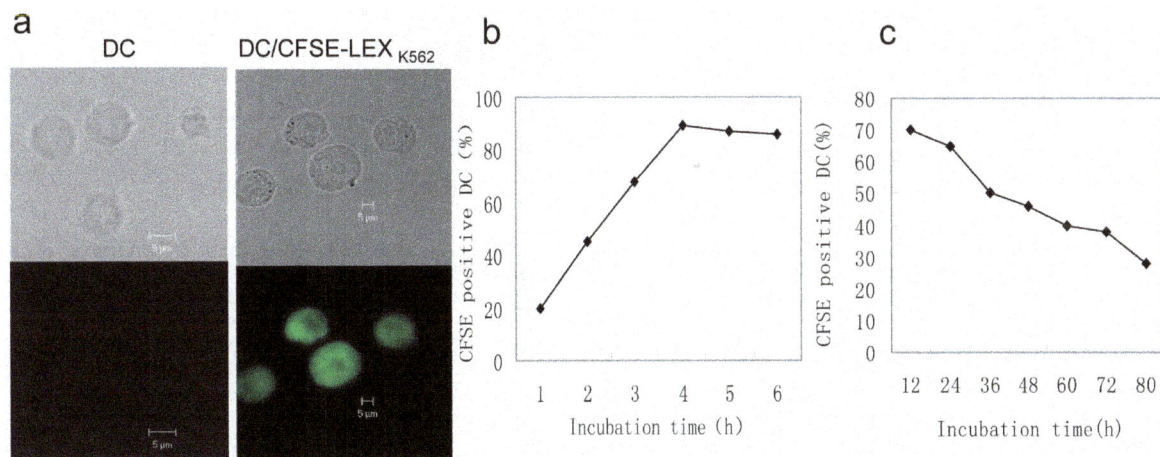

Figure 2. Exosome-uptaking by dendritic cells (a) Carboxyfluorescein succinimidyl ester (CFSE)-labeled exosomes were co-cultured *in vitro* with dendritic cells (DCs), and CFSE-positive DCs were detected using flow cytometry at different times during the culture. Confocal microscopy was used concurrently with flow cytometry to visualize the cultured DCs. (b) Phase changes of CFSE expression in DCs at different time points during the culture. (c) To investigate the rate of decay of exosomes (EXOs) in DCs, DCs were incubated with CFSE-labeled EXOs for 4 h, washed twice with phosphate-buffered saline, cultured in culture medium, and examined at different time points for up to 72 h.

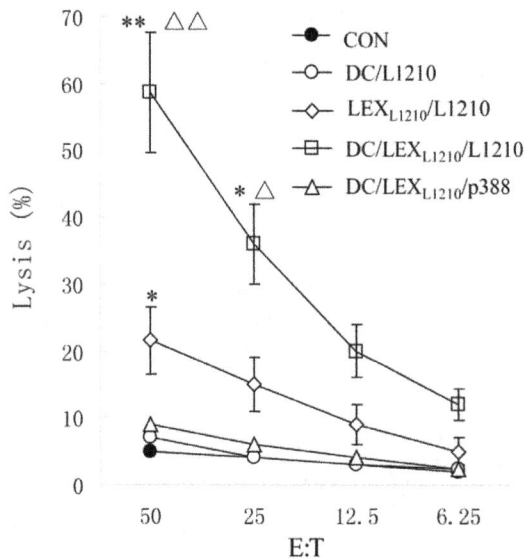

Figure 3. Cytotoxicity assay. Cytotoxic responses were evaluated by the lactate dehydrogenase (LDH)-releasing method. Splenic T-cells from mice immunized intravenously with L1210-derived exosomes (LEX$_{L1210}$) and dendritic cells (DCs) pulsed with LEX$_{L1210}$ or phosphate-buffered saline (PBS) as a control were harvested and co-cultured with irradiated L1210 cells. At the end of the culture period, viable T-cells were separated using Ficoll-Paque centrifugation and were thereafter referred to as effector cells. The LDH assay is an enzymatic method used to colorimetrically quantify LDH released from lysed target cells, including L1210 or P388 cells, which served as the control and were mixed at different ratios with effector cells after incubation for 4 h at 37°C. The spontaneous/maximal release ratio was <20% in all experiments. Specific lysis (%) was calculated as follows: (experimental LDH release − effector cell spontaneous LDH release − target spontaneous LDH release)/(target maximum LDH release)×100. * $P<0.05$ compared with the PBS, DC, and P388 groups; ** $P<0.01$ compared with the PBS control group; △ $P<0.05$ compared with the LEX$_{L1210}$ group; △△ $P<0.01$ compared with the LEX$_{L1210}$ group. Experiments were performed in triplicate. One representative experiment is shown.

compared to the non-vaccinated group (MST, 15 d), whereas LEX$_{L1210}$ vaccination (MST, 30 d) improved survival as compared to the non-vaccinated group ($P<0.05$). In contrast, mice receiving different doses of DC/LEX$_{L1210}$ (particularly $2×10^6$ and $4×10^6$) had a significantly improved survival as compared to non-vaccinated mice and LEX$_{L1210}$-vaccinated mice, ($P<0.0001$). The MST was >60 d in 50%, 70%, and 100% of mice vaccinated with 1, 2, and $4×10^6$ DC/LEX$_{L1210}$, respectively.

To further examine the therapeutic effect of LEX$_{L1210}$ and DC/LEX$_{L1210}$, mice bearing palpable tumors (~5 mm in diameter) were immunized with LEX$_{L1210}$ and DC/LEX$_{L1210}$. All mice in the control group died at approximately 18 d after immunization, and 5 of 8 mice in the LEX$_{L1210}$ group died (Fig. 5). However, immunization with DC/LEX$_{L1210}$ dose-dependently protected mice from established-tumor growth, because tumor retarded were observed in 5/8 (62.5%), 7/8 (87.5%), and 8/8 (100%) of tumor-bearing mice, which immunized with $1×10^6$, $2×10^6$, and $4×10^6$ DC/LEX$_{L1210}$, respectively. Taken together, these data indicate that LEX$_{L1210}$-pulsed DCs more efficiently induce protective antileukemic immunity than LEX$_{L1210}$ alone.

Table 1. Vaccination with LEXO and LEXO-targeted DC protects against tumor growth.

Vaccines	Tumor cell challenge	Incidence of tumor growth (%)
PBS	**L1210**	100% (8/8)
DC	**L1210**	100% (8/8)
LEX$_{L1210}$	**L1210**	50% (4/8)
DC/LEX$_{L1210}$	**L1210**	12.5% (1/8)
LEX$_{L1210}$	**P388**	100% (8/8)
DC/LEX$_{L1210}$	**P388**	100% (8/8)

To examine the antitumor immunity conferred by LEX$_{L1210}$ and DC/LEX$_{L1210}$, DBA/2 mice were randomly divided into 4 groups (n=8) and immunized s.c. with the following vaccines on the inner side of their thighs: PBS (control), LEX$_{L1210}$ (30 μg), unpulsed DCs ($1×10^6$ cells), and LEX$_{L1210}$-pulsed DCs (DC/LEX$_{L1210}$) ($1×10^6$ cells). On day 7 after immunization, all mice were challenged with L1210 leukemia cells on the outer side of the same thighs ($0.5×10^6$ cells/mice). To determine immune specificity, a group of tumor-free mice after immunization, were challenged s.c. with p388 cells ($5×10^5$ cells/mouse). Tumor growth was monitored daily for up to 4 weeks using a caliper. For ethical treatment of the animals, all mice were euthanized when the tumor diameter reached 1.5 cm. Three total experiments were performed. One representative experiment is shown.

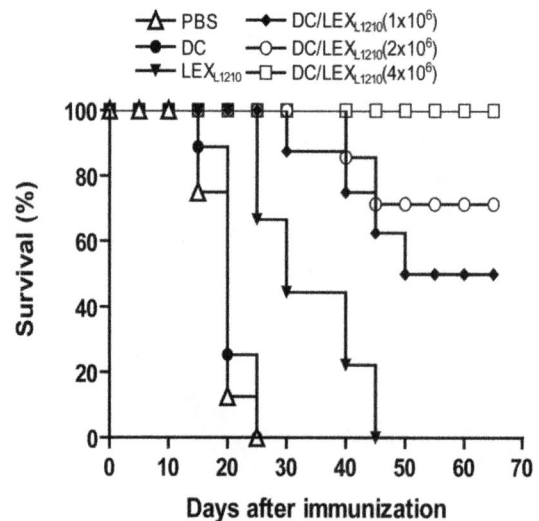

Figure 4. LEX$_{L1210}$ and LEX$_{L1210}$-pulsed DCs induce anti-leukemia protective immunity against L1210 leukemia cells. Survival of mice prophylactically immunized with different vaccines. DBA/2 mice (n=8 per group) were immunized with phosphate-buffered saline (PBS), L1210-derived exosomes (LEX$_{L1210}$), non-pulsed dendritic cells (DCs), and different doses of LEX$_{L1210}$-pulsed DCs (DC/LEX$_{L1210}$). On days 7–10 after immunization, all mice were challenged with L1210 leukemia cells. Vaccination with non-pulsed DCs (median survival time [MST], 20 d) did not significantly prolong the survival of mice as compared to the non-vaccinated PBS group (MST, 15 d), whereas LEX$_{L1210}$ vaccination (MST, 30 d) improved survival as compared to the control group of non-vaccinated mice ($P<0.05$). In contrast, mice receiving different doses of DC/LEX$_{L1210}$ (particularly $2×10^6$ and $4×10^6$) had significantly improved survival as compared to non-vaccinated mice ($P<0.0001$). Results were combined from 2 separate experiments.

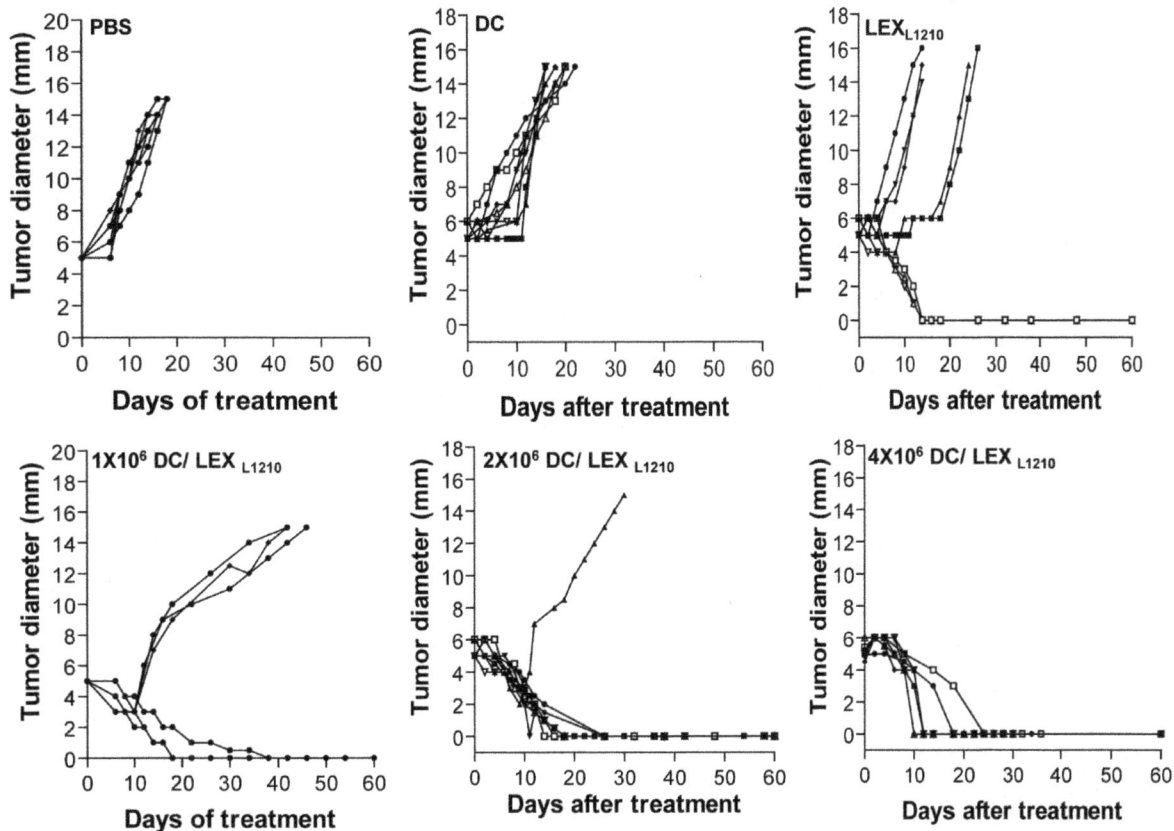

Figure 5. Therapeutic effect of LEX$_{L1210}$-pulsed DCs on established tumors. To examine the therapeutic effect on established tumors, DBA/2 mice (n = 8 per group) were subcutaneously (s.c.) inoculated with L1210 cells (0.5×10^6 cells/mouse). After 5 d, when tumors became palpable (~5 mm in diameter), mice were s.c. immunized with L1210-derived exosomes (LEX$_{L1210}$) and different doses of dendritic cells (DCs) pulsed with LEX$_{L1210}$ (DC/LEX$_{L1210}$) ($1.0–4.0 \times 10^6$ cells/mouse). Animal mortality and tumor growth or regression were monitored daily for up to 10 weeks. For ethical treatment of the animals, mice were euthanized when the tumor diameter reached 1.5 cm. Experiments were performed in triplicate. One representative experiment is shown.

Discussion

Recent studies have demonstrated that TEXs harbor tumor cell-associated antigens and can induce antitumor immunological effects [7,11]. Wolfers et al. [12] reported that the morphological characteristics and density of TEXs are similar to those of DEXs. TEXs can be isolated and purified from the supernatant of tumor cell cultures, blood, and malignant effusions [11,12,21]. TEXs also harbor major histocompatibility complex class I antigens (MHC-I), lysosome-associated membrane glycoprotein 1, HSP70, and other tumor-related antigens. They can induce immunological responses and antitumor immunological effects of T-cells that are restricted by tumor antigen-specific MHC-I. Therefore, TEXs may be a source of tumor antigens for tumor immunotherapy.

Leukemia cells, which originate from hematopoietic cells, also secrete EXOs. Although K562 chronic myelogenous leukemia cells [22,23] have been reported to produce EXOs, little is known about their role in the biology of chronic myelogenous leukemia. In this study, EXO$_{K562}$ were systemically characterized by electron microscopy, confocal microscopy, and flow cytometry. We demonstrated that EXO$_{K562}$ expressed membrane molecules derived from K562 cells but at significantly lower levels than expressed by K562 cells (data not shown). TEM analysis and western blotting indicated that EXO$_{K562}$ expressed HSP70 and ABL proteins. Two-dimensional protein electrophoresis revealed that EXO$_{K562}$ harbor most proteins expressed in K562 cells

although at lower levels. Interestingly, some proteins were expressed at higher levels in EXO$_{K562}$ than in K562 cells (unpublished data), suggesting that EXO$_{K562}$ preparation enriches for some proteins from the parental K562 cells. The specific proteins that are enriched remain to be determined using proteomic techniques, such as mass spectrometry.

Membrane transfer occurs in systems that do or do not require cell-to-cell contacts [24]. Knight et al. reported that DCs acquire antigens from cell-free DC supernatants [25]. In the present study, we demonstrated that EXOs are taken up by DCs.

Among antigen-presenting cells, DCs most potently initiate cellular immune responses through stimulating naive T-cells. The action of DCs mainly results from constitutive upregulated expression of adhesion molecules, MHC, and costimulatory molecules [26]. DCs play a central role in various immunotherapies by generating CTL. Accordingly, DC-based vaccines have been successfully used for cancer prophylaxis [27] and some murine tumor models [14,16], which has provided a basis for using DCs in human anticancer vaccinations. Several strategies have been investigated for DC loading with tumor cells [28,29], including transfecting DCs with RNA encoding TAA [30,31], acid-eluted tumor peptides [32,33], and TEXs [16,17,34,35].

EXO$_{K562}$ and K562 cell lysates induced CTL activity, but relatively weakly. Previous studies indicated that TEXs might depress the host's immunologic response [15], which may limit immunotherapy using TEX-based vaccines. Therefore, it is important to overcome these drawbacks of TEXs and enhance their antitumor effects in order to develop highly effective TEX-based tumor vaccines. In our previous study, we demonstrated that EXO-pulsed DCs induce stronger antitumor immunity than EXOs and DCs alone [17]. In the present study, we demonstrated that EXO_{K562}-pulsed DCs activate CTLs *in vitro*, which kill target cells more potently than CTLs induced by EXO_{K562} alone or by DCs pulsed with cell lysates. To further confirm whether EXO_{K562} and EXO_{K562}-pulsed DCs have an effect *in vivo*, we performed preliminary experiments in an animal model. Our data demonstrated that LEXs induce antileukemic immunity and that LEX-pulsed DCs had more potent antigen-specific antileukemic effects, because all mice injected with non-pulsed DCs developed tumors. Therefore, we conclude that LEXs are an important source of leukemia cell antigens and that LEX-pulsed DCs

represent a new, highly effective DC-based vaccine for the induction of antileukemic immunity.

Supporting Information

Figure S1 Detection of expression of Grp94 in K562-derived exosomes. Western blot analysis demonstrating the presence of ER-residing protein Grp94 in K562 cells and K562-derived exosomes (LEX_{K562}).

Author Contributions

Conceived and designed the experiments: SGH. Performed the experiments: YY CW WW CS XHD LJC. Analyzed the data: SGH YY LYM. Contributed reagents/materials/analysis tools: YY WW CW CS LYM. Wrote the paper: SGH CW.

References

1. San Miguel JF, Martinez A, Macedo A, Vidriales MB, Lopez-Berges C, et al. (1997) Immunophenotyping investigation of minimal residual disease is a useful approach for predicting relapse in acute myeloid leukemia patients. Blood 90: 2465–2470.
2. Oka Y, Tsuboi A, Taguchi T, Osaki T, Kyo T, et al. (2004) Induction of WT1 (Wilms' tumor gene)-specific cytotoxic T lymphocytes by WT1 peptide vaccine and the resultant cancer regression. Proc Natl Acad Sci U S A 101: 13885–13890.
3. Mailander V, Scheibenbogen C, Thiel E, Letsch A, Blau IW, et al. (2004) Complete remission in a patient with recurrent acute myeloid leukemia induced by vaccination with WT1 peptide in the absence of hematological or renal toxicity. Leukemia 18: 165–166.
4. Barrett AJ, Le Blanc K (2010) Immunotherapy prospects for acute myeloid leukaemia. Clin Exp Immunol 161: 223–232.
5. Denzer K, Kleijmeer MJ, Heijnen HF, Stoorvogel W, Geuze HJ (2000) Exosome: from internal vesicle of the multivesicular body to intercellular signaling device. J Cell Sci 113 Pt 19: 3365–3374.
6. Thery C, Zitvogel L, Amigorena S (2002) Exosomes: composition, biogenesis and function. Nat Rev Immunol 2: 569–579.
7. Andre F, Schartz NE, Chaput N, Flament C, Raposo G, et al. (2002) Tumor-derived exosomes: a new source of tumor rejection antigens. Vaccine 20 Suppl 4: A28–31.
8. Kim JV, Latouche JB, Riviere I, Sadelain M (2004) The ABCs of artificial antigen presentation. Nat Biotechnol 22: 403–410.
9. Chaput N, Schartz NE, Andre F, Zitvogel L (2003) Exosomes for immunotherapy of cancer. Adv Exp Med Biol 532: 215–221.
10. Thery C, Duban L, Segura E, Veron P, Lantz O, et al. (2002) Indirect activation of naive CD4+ T cells by dendritic cell-derived exosomes. Nat Immunol 3: 1156–1162.
11. Andre F, Schartz NE, Movassagh M, Flament C, Pautier P, et al. (2002) Malignant effusions and immunogenic tumour-derived exosomes. Lancet 360: 295–305.
12. Wolfers J, Lozier A, Raposo G, Regnault A, Thery C, et al. (2001) Tumor-derived exosomes are a source of shared tumor rejection antigens for CTL cross-priming. Nat Med 7: 297–303.
13. Altieri SL, Khan AN, Tomasi TB (2004) Exosomes from plasmacytoma cells as a tumor vaccine. J Immunother 27: 282–288.
14. Hao S, Bai O, Yuan J, Qureshi M, Xiang J (2006) Dendritic cell-derived exosomes stimulate stronger CD8+ CTL responses and antitumor immunity than tumor cell-derived exosomes. Cell Mol Immunol 3: 205–211.
15. Taylor DD, Gercel-Taylor C, Lyons KS, Stanson J, Whiteside TL (2003) T-cell apoptosis and suppression of T-cell receptor/CD3-zeta by Fas ligand-containing membrane vesicles shed from ovarian tumors. Clin Cancer Res 9: 5113–5119.
16. Zitvogel L, Regnault A, Lozier A, Wolfers J, Flament C, et al. (1998) Eradication of established murine tumors using a novel cell-free vaccine: dendritic cell-derived exosomes. Nat Med 4: 594–600.
17. Hao S, Bai O, Li F, Yuan J, Laferte S, et al. (2007) Mature dendritic cells pulsed with exosomes stimulate efficient cytotoxic T-lymphocyte responses and antitumour immunity. Immunology 120: 90–102.
18. Lozzio CB, Lozzio BB (1975) Human chronic myelogenous leukemia cell-line with positive Philadelphia chromosome. Blood 45: 321–334.
19. Shen C, Hao SG, Zhao CX, Zhu J, Wang C (2011) Antileukaemia immunity: effect of exosomes against NB4 acute promyelocytic leukaemia cells. J Int Med Res 39: 740–747.
20. Merchant ML, Powell DW, Wilkey DW, Cummins TD, Deegens JK, et al. (2010) Microfiltration isolation of human urinary exosomes for characterization by MS. Proteomics Clin Appl 4: 84–96.
21. Thery C, Amigorena S, Raposo G, Clayton A (2006) Isolation and characterization of exosomes from cell culture supernatants and biological fluids. Curr Protoc Cell Biol Chapter 3: Unit 3 22.
22. Savina A, Furlan M, Vidal M, Colombo MI (2003) Exosome release is regulated by a calcium-dependent mechanism in K562 cells. J Biol Chem 278: 20083–20090.
23. Abache T, Le Naour F, Planchon S, Harper F, Boucheix C, et al. (2007) The transferrin receptor and the tetraspanin web molecules CD9, CD81, and CD9P-1 are differentially sorted into exosomes after TPA treatment of K562 cells. J Cell Biochem 102: 650–664.
24. Akira S, Takeda K, Kaisho T (2001) Toll-like receptors: critical proteins linking innate and acquired immunity. Nat Immunol 2: 675–680.
25. Knight SC, Iqball S, Roberts MS, Macatonia S, Bedford PA (1998) Transfer of antigen between dendritic cells in the stimulation of primary T cell proliferation. Eur J Immunol 28: 1636–1644.
26. Bancherau J, Steinman RM (1998) Dendritic cells and the control of immunity. Nature 392: 245–252.
27. Prasad SJ, Farrand KJ, Matthews SA, Chang JH, McHugh RS, et al. (2005) Dendritic cells loaded with stressed tumor cells elicit long-lasting protective tumor immunity in mice depleted of CD4+CD25+ regulatory T cells. J Immunol 174: 90–98.
28. Parkhurst MR, DePan C, Riley JP, Rosenberg SA, Shu S (2003) Hybrids of dendritic cells and tumor cells generated by electrofusion simultaneously present immunodominant epitopes from multiple human tumor-associated antigens in the context of MHC class I and class II molecules. J Immunol 170: 5317–5325.
29. Avigan D, Vasir B, Gong J, Borges V, Wu Z, et al. (2004) Fusion cell vaccination of patients with metastatic breast and renal cancer induces immunological and clinical responses. Clin Cancer Res 10: 4699–4708.
30. Dorfel D, Appel S, Grunebach F, Weck MM, Muller MR, et al. (2005) Processing and presentation of HLA class I and II epitopes by dendritic cells after transfection with in vitro-transcribed MUC1 RNA. Blood 105: 3199–3205.
31. Fukui M, Nakano-Hashimoto T, Okano K, Maruta Y, Suehiro Y, et al. (2004) Therapeutic effect of dendritic cells loaded with a fusion mRNA encoding tyrosinase-related protein 2 and enhanced green fluorescence protein on B16 melanoma. Tumour Biol 25: 252–257.
32. Delluc S, Tourneur L, Michallet AS, Boix C, Varet B, et al. (2005) Autologous peptides eluted from acute myeloid leukemia cells can be used to generate specific antileukemic CD4 helper and CD8 cytotoxic T lymphocyte responses in vitro. Haematologica 90: 1050–1062.
33. Ostankovitch M, Buzyn A, Bonhomme D, Connan F, Bouscary D, et al. (1998) Antileukemic HLA-restricted T-cell clones generated with naturally processed peptides eluted from acute myeloblastic leukemia blasts. Blood 92: 19–24.
34. Chaput N, Schartz NE, Andre F, Taieb J, Novault S, et al. (2004) Exosomes as potent cell-free peptide-based vaccine. II. Exosomes in CpG adjuvants efficiently prime naive Tc1 lymphocytes leading to tumor rejection. J Immunol 172: 2137–2146.
35. Yao Y, Chen L, Wei W, Deng X, Ma L, et al. (2013) Tumor cell-derived exosome-targeted dendritic cells stimulate stronger CD8+ CTL responses and antitumor immunities. Biochem Biophys Res Commun 436: 60–65.

17

The MEC1 and MEC2 Lines Represent Two CLL Subclones in Different Stages of Progression towards Prolymphocytic Leukemia

Eahsan Rasul[1]*, Daniel Salamon[1], Noemi Nagy[1], Benjamin Leveau[1], Ferenc Banati[2], Kalman Szenthe[2], Anita Koroknai[3], Janos Minarovits[3,4], George Klein[1], Eva Klein[1]

1 Department of Microbiology, Tumor and Cell Biology (MTC), Karolinska Instititet, Stockholm, Sweden, 2 RT-Europe Nonprofit Research Ltd, Mosonmagyaróvár, Hungary, 3 Microbiological Research Group, National Center for Epidemiology, Budapest, Hungary, 4 University of Szeged, Faculty of Dentistry, Department of Oral Biology and Experimental Dental Research, Szeged, Hungary

Abstract

The EBV carrying lines MEC1 and MEC2 were established earlier from explants of blood derived cells of a chronic lymphocytic leukemia (CLL) patient at different stages of progression to prolymphocytoid transformation (PLL). This pair of lines is unique in several respects. Their common clonal origin was proven by the rearrangement of the immunoglobulin genes. The cells were driven to proliferation *in vitro* by the same indigenous EBV strain. They are phenotypically different and represent subsequent subclones emerging in the CLL population. Furthermore they reflect the clinical progression of the disease. We emphasize that the support for the expression of the EBV encoded growth program is an important differentiation marker of the CLL cells of origin that was shared by the two subclones. It can be surmised that proliferation of EBV carrying cells *in vitro*, but not *in vivo*, reflects the efficient surveillance that functions even in the severe leukemic condition. The MEC1 line arose before the aggressive clinical stage from an EBV carrying cell within the subclone that was in the early prolymphocytic transformation stage while the MEC2 line originated one year later, from the subsequent subclone with overt PLL characteristics. At this time the disease was disseminated and the blood lymphocyte count was considerably elevated. The EBV induced proliferation of the MEC cells belonging to the subclones with markers of PLL agrees with earlier reports in which cells of PLL disease were infected *in vitro* and immortalized to LCL. They prove also that the expression of EBV encoded set of proteins can be determined at the event of infection. This pair of lines is particularly important as they provide *in vitro* cells that represent the subclonal evolution of the CLL disease. Furthermore, the phenotype of the MEC1 cells shares several characteristics of ex vivo CLL cells.

Editor: Joseph S. Pagano, The University of North Carolina at Chapel Hill, United States of America

Funding: This work was supported by the Swedish Cancer Society and by the Cancer Research Institute (New York, NY)/Concern Foundation (Los Angeles, CA). The funders had no role in study design, data collection and analysis, decision to publish, or preparation of the manuscript.

Competing Interests: The authors declare no competing financial interests.

* Email: eahsan.rasul@ki.se

Introduction

Epstein-Barr virus can infect several human cell types. B lymphocytes are uniquely sensitive targets. Their differentiation marker CD21 serves as receptor for the virus. In the infected cells, interaction with cellular genes regulates the expression of viral genes. In a defined phase of differentiation a virally encoded growth program is expressed that induces proliferation. Practically all humans carry EBV. In health, the danger of proliferating EBV carrying B cells is constantly supervised and eliminated by immunological mechanisms [1].

Lymphoblastoid cell lines (LCLs) can be obtained by infecting B cells *in vitro*.[2] They can also emerge spontaneously from tissue explants that contain EBV genome carrying B lymphocytes when the *in vitro* condition modifies or eliminates the immunological cell mediated controls.[3] When the highly efficient control is compromised *in vivo* by immunosuppression, EBV positive B cell proliferations can occur such as in post transplant lymphoproliferative disease (PTLD) and AIDS associated lymphomas [4].

The viral growth program, latency Type III comprises nine EBV encoded proteins; EBNA1-6, LMP-1, -2A and -2B. Although their quantitative expression varies considerably, EBNA-2 and LMP-1 are essential for induction of proliferation. Presence of these two proteins is a marker for the proliferative EBV carrying B cell. Due to the requirement of specific transcription factors, the resident viral genes are expressed differently as the B cell proceeds in the differentiation path and it is also determined by the differentiation phase of B cell at the event of infection.[1,5,6,7] When the virus infects B cells that are outside the appropriate differentiation window, either EBNA-2 or LMP-1, or both are not expressed. These "restricted expressions" are denoted as latency Type 0, I, IIa, IIb. The fate of these cells differs considerably. Only the Type IIa cells proliferate and develop malignancy; generated by a complex interaction with microenvironment as in EBV positive Hodgkin's lymphoma, HL. In the autoregulatory circuit the cells with Type IIa latency elicit a granulomatous tissue reaction that produces growth factors [1,8].

In CLL disease, B lymphocyte clones proliferate. These originate from self-renewing hematopoietic stem cells, stimulated by autoantigens and by the stroma cells.[9,10] The clinical course of disease differs remarkably depending on the mutation status of immunoglobulin (IGHV) genes, expression of CD38 and zeta-chain-associated protein kinase 70 KDa and ZAP-70 [10].

Recently, attention was directed to the subclonal heterogeneity of the CLL populations with emerging dominant clones that lead to distinct periods in the progression of the disease.[11] In some patients progression to the aggressive prolymphocytic cell profile occurs in the terminal stage.[12] Rarely, progression is accompanied by phenotypical cellular changes resulting in HL, PLL or diffuse large B cell lymphoma, DLBCL-like diseases [13,14,15,16].

EBV is not involved in the pathogenesis of CLL. The CLL cells can be infected *in vitro* but only rare clones are induced to proliferate. The infected cells express a viral program that lacks LMP-1, we referred to it as latency Type IIb.[1] In contrast, *in vitro* infected PLL cells could express the complete growth program [17].

Cells of occasional CLL patients were transformed to LCLs, when infected *in vitro*.[18] In addition, LCLs could be established from explanted CLL cells even without experimental infection.[19] The origin of the MEC1 and MEC2 lines was similar. They grew from subsequent explants of the patient.[20] As reported in the original and in several subsequent publications, the phenotype and biological behavior of the 2 cell lines differ.[21,22,23] We extended the study of this unique pair of lines.

Acquisition of EBV by CLL cells in different stages of the disease provided these *in vitro* lines with features that reflected the clinical status of the patient at the time of their origin. Two features can be singled out from our analyses that are in line with the development of the disseminated final stage. MEC2 but not the MEC1 cells express CD38 that is a marker for progression in CLL and MEC1 express CXCR4 that is present on CLL cells, while it is conspicuously reduced in the MEC2 line. According to a recent report, the expression of the suppressor microRNAs, MiR-15/-16 differs in the two MEC lines. Their processing and maturation are impaired in the MEC2 cells.[21] This may provide an important property that contributes to the aggressive behavior of the cell of origin which with the contribution of EBV grew *in vitro* and established as the MEC2 line.

Materials and Methods

Cell culture

The two lines, MEC1 and MEC2 were established from the spontaneous outgrowth of explanted CLL cells on subsequent occasions with one year interval when the disease underwent marked prolymphocytoid transformation.[20] The characteristics of the ex vivo cells were described in the original publication. The disease was diagnosed as CLL though the cells were not typical in that they had strong surface immunoglobulin expression and lacked CD23. LCL derived from cord blood, CBM1-Ral-STO, and the Burkitt's lymphoma (BL) line, Daudi, were used as EBV positive and the Ramos line as EBV negative control.[24,25,26] The cells were cultured in RPMI 1640 supplemented with 10% heat-inactivated FBS, 100 units/ml penicillin, and 100 µg/ml streptomycin in humidified incubator at 37°C and 5% CO_2.

Immunoglobulin gene analysis

PCR amplification of IGH gene rearrangements was performed on genomic DNA using subgroup-specific framework 1 (FR1) primers, together with a consensus IGHJ primer as previously described.[27] Sequences were analyzed using the IMGT database and the IMGT/V-QUEST tool (http://www.imgt.org) [28,29].

Immunofluorescence staining

The details of the staining and imaging were described previously.[30] For single staining, mouse monoclonal antibody (mAb) specific for EBNA-2 (PE-2, culture supernatant prepared in our laboratory), for LMP-1, CS1-4, mixture of 4 mAb (Novocastra Laboratories Ltd, UK) or mAB S-12 (prepared in our laboratory) and for simultaneous detection, isotype specific anti LMP-1, S-12 (IgG_{2a}) and anti EBNA-2, PE-2 (IgG_1) were used. Alexa fluor 488 and 594 labeled isotype specific goat anti mouse IgG_1 and IgG_{2a}, accordingly (Life technologies, USA) were used as secondary antibodies.

Immunoblotting

The cells were lysed in sodium dodecyl sulfate (SDS) gel-loading buffer. Lysates corresponding to 1.5×10^5 cells were loaded from CBM1-Ral-STO and Ramos. 5×10^5 cells were loaded from MEC1 and MEC2. Immunoblotting was performed with the antibodies, PE-2 (EBNA-2), CS1-4 (LMP-1), and 3H2- E8 (Blimp-1, Novus Biologicals), as described previously.[31] As a control for protein loading, mAb specific for β-actin, clone AC-15 (Sigma–Aldrich, USA) was used.

Real Time Quantitative PCR

The primer sequences and PCR conditions used were described in our earlier publication and also shown in Table S1.[31] GAPDH served as endogenous control.

Control DNA sequencing

Genomic DNAs were amplified with PCR using the primers and PCR conditions listed in Table S1. Both strands of the PCR products were sequenced on a MegaBACE DNA sequencing system (GE healthcare) using dye-labeled ddNTPs, according to the manufacturer's instructions.

Automated genomic sequencing of sodium bisulfite-treated DNA

We used the method as described earlier.[32] Primers used for the amplification of Cp are shown in Table S1.

Terminal repeat fragment analysis

Genomic DNAs were digested with BamHI and the resulting fragments were separated on a 0.8% agarose gel, blotted to a Hybond N membrane and hybridized with a DIG-dUTP-labelled PCR product generated from the B95-8 prototype EBV genome with primers 5′-GTA TGC CTG CCT GTA ATT GTT G-3′ and 5′-ACG AAA GCC AGT AGC AGC AG-3′.

Flow Cytometry

The cells were washed in cold PBS containing 2% FCS and then stained with FITC-, or PE-, or PE-Cy5-conjugated mouse anti-human monoclonal antibodies. The following specificities were used: CD5, CD10, CD11c, CD19, CD20, CD21, CD23, CD25, CD27, CD38, CD45, CD54, IgM, HLA-ABC, HLA-DR and CD19 (Becton Dickinson, Ca). Antibodies detecting CXCR4, CXCR5, CCR7 and CCR10 (R & D Systems, MN) were also used. Ten thousand events were collected on a FACScan flow cytometer, and the results were analyzed using CELLQUEST (Becton Dickinson) software.

Exposure to IL-21 and to CD40L

IL-21: As described in our earlier publication, IL-21 (100 ng/ml, PeproTech EC, UK) was added to cultures containing 0.16×10^6 cells/ml.[31] The cultures were readjusted on third day to 0.16×10^6 cells/ml and IL-21 was re-added. The cells were harvested on the 6th day for analysis.

CD40 ligand, CD40L: 0.5×10^6 irradiated (15,000RAD) L or CD40L-L cells were plated in wells of a 24 well plate and used 24 hours later. Equal number of MEC1 and MEC2 cells were seeded on the monolayer and incubated for 3 days at 37°C and 5% CO_2 [33].

Results

Identity of the lines

We list the characteristics of the MEC1 and MEC2 cells used in the current study. The analysis includes features that correspond well with those described in the original publication [20].

The derivation of the cell lines from the patient's CLL cells was proven by the identity of the DNA rearrangement in the IgH loci in the ex vivo sample and in the lines. Both lines belonged to the VH4 family. The cell lines used in the present study carry IGHV4-59/IGHD2-21/IGHJ6 gene rearrangements with 94% identity to germline as it is described in the original publication [20].

The MEC2 cells are larger than the MEC1 cells. MEC1 cells are mainly solitary. They form few and small aggregates. The social behavior of MEC2 cells is different. The majority of the cells create large aggregates. Morphological and proliferation properties and the surface marker profiles of the cells corresponded at large to that reported originally [20].

The lines carry the same EBV strain but the infection events differed

Based on their sequence of the Cp region from 10480 to 11461 (European Nucleotide Archive accession numbers for MEC1 and MEC2 are HG380070 and HG380071 respectively), the two lines contained the same EBV strain, differing from the widely used prototype, B95-8 [34].

The cells carry predominantly latent episomal EBV genomes. The terminal repeat analysis showed single fragment with different size in the lines (Figure S1). Therefore we can conclude that the cells of origin were infected at different occasions.[35] This was in accordance with the difference in the promoter usage for EBNA-2 expression.

Expression and regulation of the EBV encoded latent proteins, EBNA-2 and LMP-1

All cells in the MEC1 and MEC2 lines express both EBNA-2 and LMP-1. Thus they correspond to Type III latency (Fig. 1A) (also see Figure S2). Two antibodies were used for LMP-1 detection, CS1-4 and S-12 and they localized mainly to the cell membrane. The pattern with CS1-4 was dotted while it was patchy with the S-12. The LMP-1 staining showed also that MEC2 cells are larger and analysis of the populations shows a shift to the larger sizes in the MEC2 culture (Figure S2). The immunoblots detected higher level of EBNA-2 in the MEC2 cells (Fig. 1B).

Analysis of the promoter activities confirmed the Type III latency with difference in the transcription program of EBNA-s (Fig. 2C). In MEC1 cells only the W promoter, Wp, while in the MEC2 cells Cp and Wp were active. Wp activity was twofold higher in MEC1 than in MEC2. Dual usage of Wp and Cp is regular in the Type III LCLs.[36] The LMP-1 mRNA was expressed in both lines but it was lower in the MEC1 cells. Q promoter, Qp was silent in both lines.

The difference in the lines with regard of EBNA-2 regulation does not seem to be determined by their methylation pattern since the genomic sequence of Cp region was unmethylated in both (Figure S3).

Similarly, it is unlikely that the B cell specific transcription factor ARID3A/Bright that is known to upregulate Cp activity accounts for this difference because the mRNA levels were similar in MEC1 and MEC2. It was about half in comparison to a regular LCL, CBM1-Ral-STO (Fig. 1C) [37].

Kelly et al. suggested that BL cells which use exclusively the Wp are particularly resistant to apoptosis because of Wp driven expression of the viral bcl2 homologue BHRF1.[38] The MEC lines do not show this correlation. Both MEC lines express low level of BHRF1, though in MEC1 the Wp activity is twofold higher (Fig. 1C). In MEC1 the BHRF1 level was similar to the Cp user LCL, CBM1-Ral-STO and it was even lower in the MEC2 cells that use both Wp and Cp.

Phenotypic differences determined by surface marker expression

Expression of surface markers by the MEC lines reported in the original publication as well as additional markers is summarized in Table S2. Selected FACS profiles are shown in Fig. 1D. The B cell markers, CD19, CD20 and HLA-ABC, HLA-DR, CD30, CD54/ICAM-1 and CCR7 were detected with similar profiles on both lines, while they differed in the expression of CD38, CD27, CD23, CD21, IL-21R, FMC7, CXCR4, and CXCR10. We discuss here the markers that may be relevant to the biological behavior of the cells.

CD38 is a marker for poor prognosis as it indicates activation and recent proliferative history of the CLL cells. CD38 positive cells in the blood are assumed to be recent emigrants from the proliferation centers; lymph nodes and bone marrow.[39] CD38 was expressed by the majority (64%) of MEC2 while it was absent on the MEC1 cells. The difference indicates that the lines arose from different subclones and it is in accordance with the clinical status of the patient; the disease being more extended at the time of the derivation of the MEC2 line.

CD27, the memory B cell marker is expressed by CLL cells.[40,41] It is present on a significant proportion of MEC1 cells (23%) but not on MEC2 cells (2%).

CD23 is a B cell activation marker. It is expressed by LCLs.[42] CLL cells also express CD23 and has positive correlation with CD38.[43,44,45] In accordance, it was detected on lower proportion on MEC1 cells (51%) than on MEC2 cells (83%).

CD21, the complement receptor, is expressed by CLL cells.[19] It serves as receptor for EBV. Its expression was higher on MEC1 (91%) than on MEC2 (56%) cells. This difference is in good correlation with its expression on CLL and PLL. It was reported to be lower on PLL than on CLL cells [46,47].

IL-21R was shown to be inversely correlated with CD38 expression in CLL cells.[48] Similar tendency was observed on the MEC lines. The CD38 negative MEC1 line had higher (51%) expression than the CD38 positive MEC2 line (28%).

FMC7 is strongly expressed by CLL cells when they proceed to prolymphocytoid transformation.[44] Although a major proportion of (81%) the CLL cells in the ex vivo sample was FMC7 positive, the established MEC1 line contained only 8% positive cells.[20] In our present analysis, the majority of the MEC1 cells

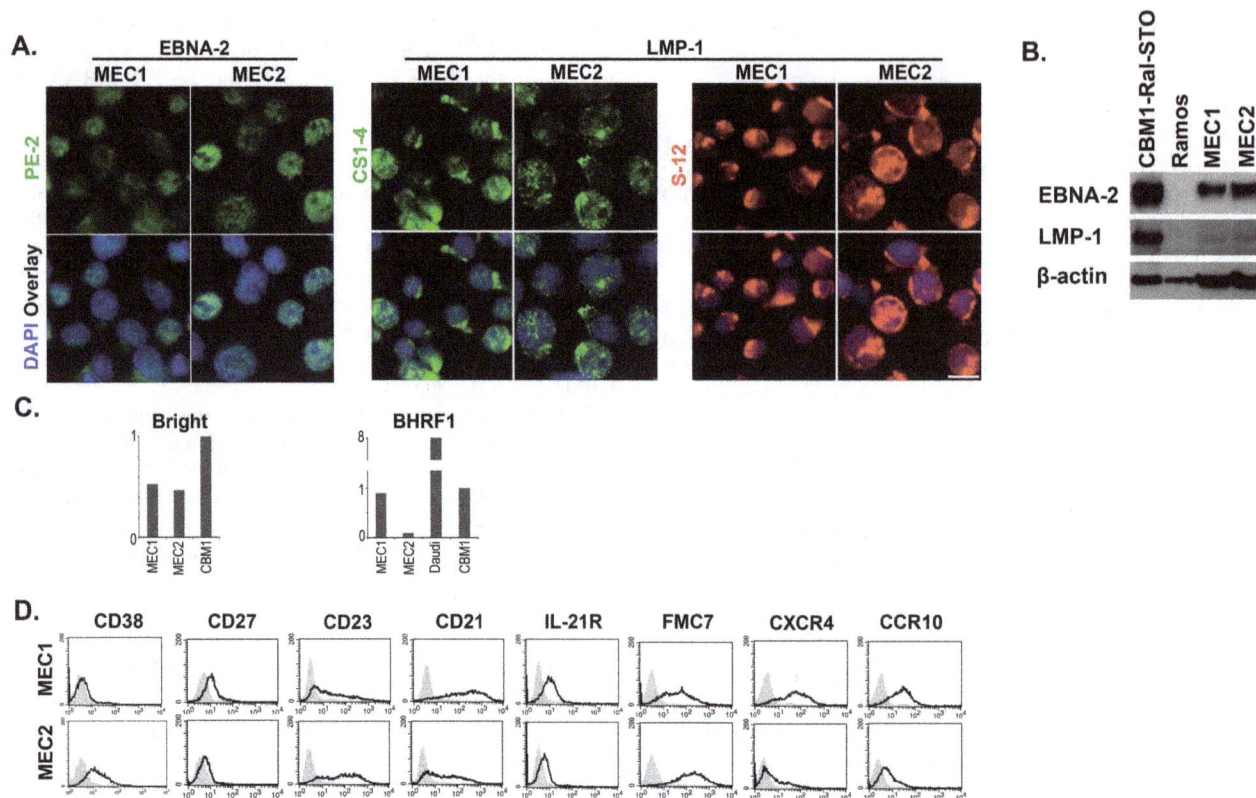

Figure 1. Comparison of the MEC1 and MEC2 cells. (A) Expression of EBV encoded proteins EBNA-2 and LMP-1 by immunofluorescence; magnification (×100), scale bar 25 μm. Note: the MEC2 cells are larger. (B) Expression of EBNA-2 and LMP-1 by immunoblotting; positive control: CBM1-Ral-STO, negative control: Ramos. 1.5×10^5 cells were loaded in control lanes and 5×10^5 were loaded in MEC1 and MEC2 lanes. Note MEC2 expresses higher amount of EBNA-2. (C) Expression of Bright and BARF1 by Q-PCR. (D) FACS analysis of surface markers that are differently expressed in the 2 lines.

expressed FMC7 (74%) and all MEC2 cells expressed this marker. The patient's CLL cell that generated the MEC1 line may have been in an early transition towards the PLL stage and progressed further *in vitro*.

Chemokine receptors and adhesion molecules guide the migration of CLL cells between the tissues and the circulation.[49,50] Resting B cells in the blood have high expression of CXCR4 and CCR7 and low expression of CCR10. On EBV immortalized LCL cells, CXCR4 and CCR10 are expressed reciprocally, low CXCR4 and high CCR10 [51].

CXCR4 was shown to be present on resting CLL cells in the blood. The recently emigrated cells from the proliferation centers have low levels.[11,52] The majority of MEC1 (84%) cells but only a small proportion of MEC2 (26%) cells express CXCR4. This can be related to the aggressive clinical stage of the disease, when high cell numbers are discharged from the proliferation centers. Expression of this marker is similar in the MEC2 and LCL cells.

CCR10 expression was higher on MEC1 (75%) than on MEC2 (26%) cells. Neither the CXCR4 nor the CCR10 markers conform with the phenotypic relationship with LCL cells and with EBV positive B cells localized at the periphery of tonsil in infectious mononucleosis [51].

CCR7 is similarly expressed by MEC cells and LCL cells.[51] The relationship between the MEC lines and LCLs with regard to the chemokine receptor doesn't provide any clue to their biological behavior.

The surface marker profile of the MEC1 line has many similarities with CLL cells. At the time of its establishment, the patient's clinical condition did not progress yet and as published earlier, similar to CLL cells, MEC1 could grow in immunosuppressed mice while the MEC2 cell did not.[22,23] Some of the markers, such as the high Ig expression, the transformation to Type III cells by EBV infection, indicate that at the time of establishment of MEC1, the disease already entered progression to PLL. Subsequently, cells in further stage of transformation dominated and lead to the aggressive clinical stage.

Influence of IL-21 and CD40 Ligand on the expression of EBV encoded proteins

Soluble factors produced by activated CD4[+] T cell was shown to influence the expression of EBV encoded proteins and thus change the EBV latency type.[53] IL-21 is known to induce plasmacytoid differentiatioin of LCLs, and plasma cells do not support Type III expression.[31,54] Treatment of LCL with IL-21 downregulated EBNA-2 expression thus it changed the latency from Type III to Type IIa. Concomitantly, the cells ceased to proliferate. IL-21 also upregulated LMP-1 protein expression. Similar changes were induced in the MEC lines (Fig. 2A, & B). The IL-21 induced plasmocytoid differentiation was substantiated by expression of Blimp-1 (Fig. 2B).

The changes were confirmed by the corresponding promoter activities (Fig. 2C). Wp activity decreased in MEC1 cells and both Wp and Cp activity decreased in the MEC2 cells and the LMP-1 mRNA level was elevated in both lines.

Similar to earlier report, co-culture of LCL with CD40 ligand (CD40L) expressing L cells reduced EBNA-2 and LMP-1

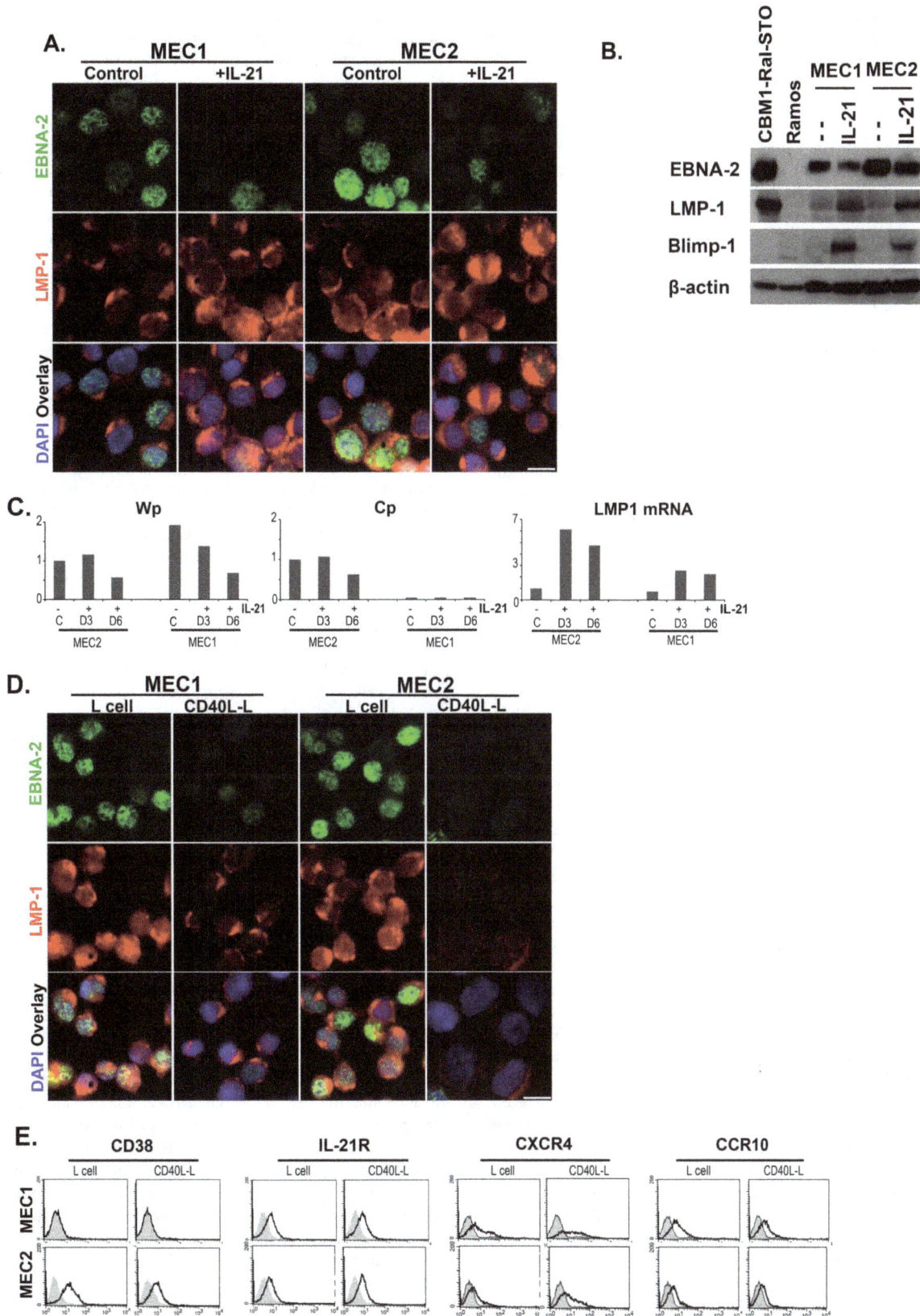

Figure 2. The effect of IL-21 and CD40L exposure on MEC1 and MEC2 cells. Expression of EBNA-2 and LMP-1 in IL-21 treated cells (A, B). (A) Simultaneous immunofluorescence staining of EBNA-2 (Green) and LMP-1 (Red); magnification (×100), scale bar 25 μm. Note the downregulation of EBNA-2 and upregultion of LMP-1 after IL-21 treatment. (B) Expression of EBNA-2, LMP-1 and Blimp-1 by immunoblotting; positive control: CBM1-Ral-STO, negative control: Ramos. 1.5×10^5 cells were loaded in the control lanes and 5×10^5 were loaded in both untreated and IL-21 treated MEC1 and MEC2 lanes. Note low expression of EBNA-2 and high expression of LMP-1 after IL-21 treatment and induction of Blimp-1 after IL-21 treatment. (C)

Activity of the W and C promoters that regulate EBNA-2 expression and LMP-1 mRNA expression by Q-PCR. Note the difference in EBNA-2 regulation; the MEC2 cell uses both Wp and Cp while in MEC1 only Wp is active. (D) Expression of EBNA-2 and LMP-1 in cells exposed to CD40L. Simultaneous immunofluorescence staining; for details see (A). Note: EBNA-2 and LMP-1 are downregulated by CD40L in both lines. (E) CD40L induced modulation of surface marker by FACS analysis.

expression, in the MEC lines (Fig. 2D).[33] On the basis of the known effects of CD40L on the differentiation of B cells, both normal and LCLs, it is likely that alteration of the EBV encoded protein expression is a consequence of change of differentiation towards germinal center and memory B cells.[33,55] Co-cultivation with L cells (without CD40L) elevated also the LMP-1 expression on the MEC cells, though to a lesser degree (Fig. 2D). For base line LMP-1 expression see Fig. 2A.

CD40L induced modulation of CD38 and chemokine receptors, CXCR4 and CCR10

CD40L exposure resulted in upregulation of CXCR4 in the MEC lines (Fig. 2E). This upregulation of CXCR4 might be due to CD40L induced downregulation of EBNA-2 and LMP-1.[51] Similar to CLL cells, slight upregulation of IL-21R and downregulation of CD38 was noted in MEC2 cells in response to CD40L.[48] CD40L induced no significant change in IL-21R and CD38 expression in MEC1. However, CCR10 was down-regulated following CD40L exposure in both lines. CD40L induced change of differentiation is reflected by the change of surface marker phenotypes in MEC cells.

Discussion

EBV is not involved in the pathogenesis of CLL. Presently it is emphasized that subclonal variation and selection lead to the evolution of the disease with alteration of the biological behavior, activation state and proliferation of the cells.[9,10,11] In some cases EBV carrying subclones have been detected by their capacity to proliferate in vitro; giving rise to LCLs with proven CLL origin.[56,57] In vitro infected CLL cells exhibit an unusual viral latency, Type IIb; the cells express EBNA-2 but not LMP-1 and they do not proliferate. EBV positive B cells with Type IIb program were detected in tissues of PTLD, IM and in EBV infected humanized mice.[1] We detected rare cells with Type IIb latency in in vitro infected cord blood derived lymphocyte population.[30] In contrast to the CLL cells, EBV can induce in vitro proliferation of PLL cells.[17] It is important to note that even when EBV positive subclones were detected in the CLL population, these cells did not lead to development of EBV positive disease.[19] This indicates that the proliferation of EBV carrying B cell can be efficiently controlled even in the severe leukemia condition. This is in contrast with the development of EBV positive B cell proliferation in PTLD, when the immune response is compromised due to the immunosuppressive treatment [4].

EBV carrying lines have been established from CLL cells in a few experiments.[20,58] Similar to the MEC1 and MEC2, cell lines with somewhat differing properties were established earlier from explanted lymphocyte samples of a CLL patient.[19] During the 5 final years of the case history, lines were established from cultures to which the anti-viral agent phosphonoformate and virus-neutralizing antibodies were added. These prevented virus release and infection of B cells in vitro. One group of lines was the descendants of one clonal CLL cell that carried the virus in vivo. It was estimated that these cells represented 0.1% of the CLL cell population. On the last occasion of sampling, 8 lines were established. 4 of these belonged to the same clone that provided the earlier lines, 4 other lines grew from another clone that was

infected in vivo with a different EBV sub-strain. The detection of EBV encoded proteins indicated that these cells were Type I or IIa cells. Because they seemed to lack EBNA-2. It seems therefore that the CLL cells that acquired the virus in vivo expressed the growth program in vitro, probably because they were released from the immunological control.

In the ex vivo sample that gave rise to the MEC lines, DNA encoding EBNA-2 was not detected.[20] Therefore the authors favored the possibility that infection of the CLL cells occurred in vitro by virus released from normal B cells in the culture. It cannot be ruled out however that the viral EBNA-2 code present in very few cells in the ex vivo sample evaded detection. Though we have no direct evidence for presence of the EBV infected cells in the CLL population, we like to consider this for discussion.

The analysis of the EBV terminal repeat and the EBNA-2 promoter expression in the lines indicated that the cells of origin were infected in vivo and at different occasions. The following scenario can be proposed. The CLL cell which was the origin of the line entered into a differentiation state that allowed the expression of the EBV encoded growth program but T cell derived factors, suppressed one or both proteins pivotal for proliferation (EBNA-2 and LMP-1). The cell then followed its own EBV independent proliferation dynamic in vivo. However, since CLL cells do not proliferate in vitro, upon explantation the rare EBV carrying cells were selected in the culture. This assumption may be justified by the cessation of proliferation and deregulation of the viral growth program when the cells were treated with IL-21 or with CD40L. In vitro experiments and the emergence of EBV positive proliferating B cell malignancies in immunosuppressive conditions indicate that the EBV carrying B cells can be controlled by immunological mechanisms [4].

The important massage of this work is that the viral gene harboring lines reflect the characteristics of their cell of origin. The phenotypic difference between the two MEC lines represents two considerably different phases of the CLL to PLL transition. Analysis of the MEC1 cell population showed already conspicuous change for some of the markers. For others, the population was still heterogeneous. MEC2 was established when the lymphocyte count was very high and the PLL character was evident.

The unusual phenotype of the MEC1 line deserves attention. While it expresses the growth program, Type III, CD23 is expressed by a smaller proportion of cells and it does not express the activation marker CD38. The MEC1 line provides an eminent example for the differential assortment of markers related to the EBV induced biological behavior. The properties of the two lines exemplify the complexity of EBV and the target interaction regulated by the differentiation of the B cell. Based on phenotypic marker expression, the MEC1 line would be a mixture of virus carrying cells in different phases of CLL progression towards PLL, while MEC2 would represent the fully developed PLL.

The two MEC lines were utilized in several studies for different objectives.[21,22,23,59,60] A noteworthy difference related to the characteristics of the disease conditions was found when the cells were inoculated to Rag2$-/-\gamma$c$-/-$ mice. MEC1 cells were detected in bone marrow, blood, lymph node and peritoneum.[22] The engrafted MEC2 cells did not grow.[23] In this respect the MEC lines conformed with CLL versus LCLs established from normal B cells. MEC1 has been stated to behave like CLL cells while MEC2 similar to LCLs do not establish as tumors in immunocompromised mice [61].

We emphasize 3 aspects of the characteristics of the MEC lines. 1. The EBV encoded growth program was expressed by both lines but the cells differed in phenotype and the MEC1 line retained some features of CLL cells. These are so prominent that the line was used in several studies as representative for CLL cells. Thus the expression of EBV in the MEC1 line did not override the B phenotype. 2. The expression of the incoming EBV gene can be determined by the event of infection. 3. The EBV carrying CLL cells do not express the Type III growth program *in vivo* even in a serious state of the disease indicating the immunological control is still in function.

Supporting Information

Figure S1   Terminal repeat analysis of MEC1 and MEC2 cell line.

Figure S2   Staining with secondary antibody and comparison of cell size by FSC.

Figure S3   Nucleic acid sequences of Cp after bisulfite-modification. Overlapping raw sequencing data of bisulfite-modified DNAs of the MEC1 and MEC2 lines, from nucleotide

10664 to 11341, according to the prototype B95-8 sequence.[34] Boxes indicate the positions of the CBF1 and CBF2 binding sites. Green line: adenine; blue line: cytosine; black line: guanine; red line: thymine.

Table S1   Primers used in PCR.

Table S2   Phenotypic analysis of MEC1 and MEC2.

Acknowledgments

We thank Dr Kenneth Nilsson, Department of Immunology, Genetics & Pathology, Uppsala University for providing us MEC1 and MEC2 cell lines. We thank also Dr Nicola Cahill, and Dr Richard Rosenquist, Department of Immunology, Genetics & Pathology, Uppsala University for Immunoglobulin gene sequencing and analysis.

Author Contributions

Conceived and designed the experiments: ER EK DS NN. Performed the experiments: ER DS NN BL FB KS AK. Analyzed the data: ER DS NN JM GK EK. Contributed reagents/materials/analysis tools: ER DS NN BL FB KS AK JM EK. Contributed to the writing of the manuscript: ER DS NN BL FB KS AK JM GK EK.

References

1. Klein E, Nagy N, Rasul AE (2013) EBV genome carrying B lymphocytes that express the nuclear protein EBNA-2 but not LMP-1: Type IIb latency. Oncoimmunology 2: e23035.
2. Pope JH, Horne MK, Scott W (1968) Transformation of foetal human leukocytes in vitro by filtrates of a human leukaemic cell line containing herpes-like virus. Int J Cancer 3: 857–866.
3. Bird AG, McLachlan SM, Britton S (1981) Cyclosporin A promotes spontaneous outgrowth in vitro of Epstein-Barr virus-induced B-cell lines. Nature 289: 300–301.
4. Brink AA, Dukers DF, van den Brule AJ, Oudejans JJ, Middeldorp JM, et al. (1997) Presence of Epstein-Barr virus latency type III at the single cell level in post-transplantation lymphoproliferative disorders and AIDS related lymphomas. J Clin Pathol 50: 911–918.
5. Thorley-Lawson DA, Allday MJ (2008) The curious case of the tumour virus: 50 years of Burkitt's lymphoma. Nature Reviews Microbiology 6: 913–924.
6. Kurth J, Hansmann ML, Rajewsky K, Kuppers R (2003) Epstein-Barr virus-infected B cells expanding in germinal centers of infectious mononucleosis patients do not participate in the germinal center reaction. Proc Natl Acad Sci U S A 100: 4730–4735.
7. Babcock GJ, Hochberg D, Thorley-Lawson AD (2000) The expression pattern of Epstein-Barr virus latent genes in vivo is dependent upon the differentiation stage of the infected B cell. Immunity 13: 497–506.
8. Kuppers R (2009) The biology of Hodgkin's lymphoma. Nat Rev Cancer 9: 15–27.
9. Rosen A, Murray F, Evaldsson C, Rosenquist R (2010) Antigens in chronic lymphocytic leukemia–implications for cell origin and leukemogenesis. Semin Cancer Biol 20: 400–409.
10. Chiorazzi N, Rai KR, Ferrarini M (2005) Chronic lymphocytic leukemia. N Engl J Med 352: 804–815.
11. Calissano C, Damle RN, Hayes G, Murphy EJ, Hellerstein MK, et al. (2009) In vivo intraclonal and interclonal kinetic heterogeneity in B-cell chronic lymphocytic leukemia. Blood 114: 4832–4842.
12. Matutes E, Attygalle A, Wotherspoon A, Catovsky D (2010) Diagnostic issues in chronic lymphocytic leukaemia (CLL). Best Pract Res Clin Haematol 23: 3–20.
13. Reiniger L, Bodor C, Bognar A, Balogh Z, Csomor J, et al. (2006) Richter's and prolymphocytic transformation of chronic lymphocytic leukemia are associated with high mRNA expression of activation-induced cytidine deaminase and aberrant somatic hypermutation. Leukemia 20: 1089–1095.
14. Tsimberidou AM, O'Brien S, Kantarjian HM, Koller C, Hagemeister FB, et al. (2006) Hodgkin transformation of chronic lymphocytic leukemia: the M. D. Anderson Cancer Center experience. Cancer 107: 1294–1302.
15. Tsimberidou AM, Keating MJ, Bueso-Ramos CE, Kurzrock R (2006) Epstein-Barr virus in patients with chronic lymphocytic leukemia: a pilot study. Leuk Lymphoma 47: 827–836.
16. Ansell SM, Li CY, Lloyd RV, Phyliky RL (1999) Epstein-Barr virus infection in Richter's transformation. Am J Hematol 60: 99–104.

17. Walls EV, Doyle MG, Patel KK, Allday MJ, Catovsky D, et al. (1989) Activation and immortalization of leukaemic B cells by Epstein-Barr virus. Int J Cancer 44: 846–853.
18. Rosen A, Bergh AC, Gogok P, Evaldsson C, Myhrinder AL, et al. (2012) Lymphoblastoid cell line with B1 cell characteristics established from a chronic lymphocytic leukemia clone by in vitro EBV infection. Oncoimmunology 1: 18–27.
19. Lewin N, Avila-Carino J, Minarovits J, Lennette E, Brautbar C, et al. (1995) Detection of two Epstein-Barr-virus (EBV)-carrying leukemic cell clones in a patient with chronic lymphocytic leukemia (CLL). Int J Cancer 61: 159–164.
20. Stacchini A, Aragno M, Vallario A, Alfarano A, Circosta P, et al. (1999) MEC1 and MEC2: two new cell lines derived from B-chronic lymphocytic leukaemia in prolymphocytoid transformation. Leuk Res 23: 127–136.
21. Allegra D, Bilan V, Garding A, Dohner H, Stilgenbauer S, et al. (2014) Defective DROSHA processing contributes to downregulation of MiR-15/-16 in chronic lymphocytic leukemia. Leukemia 28: 98–107.
22. Bertilaccio MT, Scielzo C, Simonetti G, Ponzoni M, Apollonio B, et al. (2010) A novel Rag2−/−gammac−/−xenograft model of human CLL. Blood 115: 1605–1609.
23. Loisel S, Ster KL, Quintin-Roue I, Pers JO, Bordron A, et al. (2005) Establishment of a novel human B-CLL-like xenograft model in nude mouse. Leuk Res 29: 1347–1352.
24. Ernberg I, Falk K, Minarovits J, Busson P, Tursz T, et al. (1989) The role of methylation in the phenotype-dependent modulation of Epstein-Barr nuclear antigen 2 and latent membrane protein genes in cells latently infected with Epstein-Barr virus. J Gen Virol 70 (Pt 11): 2989–3002.
25. Klein E, Klein G, Nadkarni JS, Nadkarni JJ, Wigzell H, et al. (1968) Surface IgM-kappa specificity on a Burkitt lymphoma cell in vivo and in derived culture lines. Cancer Res 28: 1300–1310.
26. Klein G, Lindahl T, Jondal M, Leibold W, Menezes J, et al. (1974) Continuous lymphoid cell lines with characteristics of B cells (bone-marrow-derived), lacking the Epstein-Barr virus genome and derived from three human lymphomas. Proc Natl Acad Sci U S A 71: 3283–3286.
27. Ghia P, Stamatopoulos K, Belessi C, Moreno C, Stilgenbauer S, et al. (2007) ERIC recommendations on IGHV gene mutational status analysis in chronic lymphocytic leukemia. Leukemia 21: 1–3.
28. Brochet X, Lefranc MP, Giudicelli V (2008) IMGT/V-QUEST: the highly customized and integrated system for IG and TR standardized V-J and V-D-J sequence analysis. Nucleic Acids Res 36: W503–508.
29. Lefranc MP, Giudicelli V, Ginestoux C, Jabado-Michaloud J, Folch G, et al. (2009) IMGT, the international ImMunoGeneTics information system. Nucleic Acids Res 37: D1006–1012.
30. Rasul AE, Nagy N, Sohlberg E, Adori M, Claesson HE, et al. (2012) Simultaneous detection of the two main proliferation driving EBV encoded proteins, EBNA-2 and LMP-1 in single B cells. J Immunol Methods 385: 60–70.
31. Kis LL, Salamon D, Persson EK, Nagy N, Scheeren FA, et al. (2010) IL-21 imposes a type II EBV gene expression on type III and type I B cells by the

repression of C- and activation of LMP-1-promoter. Proc Natl Acad Sci U S A 107: 872–877.

32. Salamon D, Banati F, Koroknai A, Ravasz M, Szenthe K, et al. (2009) Binding of CCCTC-binding factor in vivo to the region located between Rep* and the C promoter of Epstein-Barr virus is unaffected by CpG methylation and does not correlate with Cp activity. J Gen Virol 90: 1183–1189.

33. Pokrovskaja K, Ehlin-Henriksson B, Kiss C, Challa A, Gordon J, et al. (2002) CD40 ligation downregulates EBNA-2 and LMP-1 expression in EBV-transformed lymphoblastoid cell lines. Int J Cancer 99: 705–712.

34. Baer R, Bankier AT, Biggin MD, Deininger PL, Farrell PJ, et al. (1984) DNA sequence and expression of the B95-8 Epstein-Barr virus genome. Nature 310: 207–211.

35. Raab-Traub N, Flynn K (1986) The structure of the termini of the Epstein-Barr virus as a marker of clonal cellular proliferation. Cell 47: 883–889.

36. Elliott J, Goodhew EB, Krug LT, Shakhnovsky N, Yoo L, et al. (2004) Variable methylation of the Epstein-Barr virus Wp EBNA gene promoter in B-lymphoblastoid cell lines. J Virol 78: 14062–14065.

37. Borestrom C, Forsman A, Ruetschi U, Rymo L (2012) E2F1, ARID3A/Bright and Oct-2 factors bind to the Epstein-Barr virus C promoter, EBNA1 and oriP, participating in long-distance promoter-enhancer interactions. J Gen Virol 93: 1065–1075.

38. Kelly GL, Long HM, Stylianou J, Thomas WA, Leese A, et al. (2009) An Epstein-Barr virus anti-apoptotic protein constitutively expressed in transformed cells and implicated in burkitt lymphomagenesis: the Wp/BHRF1 link. PLoS Pathog 5: e1000341.

39. Malavasi F, Deaglio S, Damle R, Cutrona G, Ferrarini M, et al. (2011) CD38 and chronic lymphocytic leukemia: a decade later. Blood 118: 3470–3478.

40. Damle RN, Calissano C, Chiorazzi N (2010) Chronic lymphocytic leukaemia: a disease of activated monoclonal B cells. Best Pract Res Clin Haematol 23: 33–45.

41. Ranheim EA, Cantwell MJ, Kipps TJ (1995) Expression of CD27 and its ligand, CD70, on chronic lymphocytic leukemia B cells. Blood 85: 3556–3565.

42. Wang F, Gregory CD, Rowe M, Rickinson AB, Wang D, et al. (1987) Epstein-Barr virus nuclear antigen 2 specifically induces expression of the B-cell activation antigen CD23. Proc Natl Acad Sci U S A 84: 3452–3456.

43. Matutes E, Polliack A (2000) Morphological and immunophenotypic features of chronic lymphocytic leukemia. Rev Clin Exp Hematol 4: 22–47.

44. Dungarwalla M, Matutes E, Dearden CE (2008) Prolymphocytic leukaemia of B- and T-cell subtype: a state-of-the-art paper. Eur J Haematol 80: 469–476.

45. Damle RN, Temburni S, Calissano C, Yancopoulos S, Banapour T, et al. (2007) CD38 expression labels an activated subset within chronic lymphocytic leukemia clones enriched in proliferating B cells. Blood 110: 3352–3359.

46. Berrebi A, Bassous-Guedj L, Vorst E, Dagan S, Shtalrid M, et al. (1990) Further characterization of prolymphocytic leukemia cells as a tumor of activated B cells. Am J Hematol 34: 181–185.

47. Takeuchi H, Katayama I (1993) Surface phenotype and adhesion activity of B-cell chronic lymphoid leukemias. Leuk Lymphoma 10: 209–216.

48. de Totero D, Meazza R, Zupo S, Cutrona G, Matis S, et al. (2006) Interleukin-21 receptor (IL-21R) is up-regulated by CD40 triggering and mediates proapoptotic signals in chronic lymphocytic leukemia B cells. Blood 107: 3708–3715.

49. Davids MS, Burger JA (2012) Cell Trafficking in Chronic Lymphocytic Leukemia. Open J Hematol 3.

50. Burger JA (2012) Targeting the microenvironment in chronic lymphocytic leukemia is changing the therapeutic landscape. Curr Opin Oncol 24: 643–649.

51. Nakayama T, Fujisawa R, Izawa D, Hieshima K, Takada K, et al. (2002) Human B cells immortalized with Epstein-Barr virus upregulate CCR6 and CCR10 and downregulate CXCR4 and CXCR5. J Virol 76: 3072–3077.

52. Calissano C, Damle RN, Marsilio S, Yan XJ, Yancopoulos S, et al. (2011) Intraclonal complexity in chronic lymphocytic leukemia: fractions enriched in recently born/divided and older/quiescent cells. Mol Med 17: 1374–1382.

53. Nagy N, Adori M, Rasul A, Heuts F, Salamon D, et al. (2012) Soluble factors produced by activated CD4+ T cells modulate EBV latency. Proc Natl Acad Sci U S A 109: 1512–1517.

54. Anastasiadou E, Vaeth S, Cuomo L, Boccellato F, Vincenti S, et al. (2009) Epstein-Barr virus infection leads to partial phenotypic reversion of terminally differentiated malignant B cells. Cancer Lett 284: 165–174.

55. Arpin C, Dechanet J, Van Kooten C, Merville P, Grouard G, et al. (1995) Generation of memory B cells and plasma cells in vitro. Science 268: 720–722.

56. Lewin N, Minarovits J, Weber G, Ehlin-Henriksson B, Wen T, et al. (1991) Clonality and methylation status of the Epstein-Barr virus (EBV) genomes in in vivo-infected EBV-carrying chronic lymphocytic leukemia (CLL) cell lines. Int J Cancer 48: 62–66.

57. Lewin N, Aman P, Mellstedt H, Zech L, Klein G (1988) Direct outgrowth of in vivo Epstein-Barr virus (EBV)-infected chronic lymphocytic leukemia (CLL) cells into permanent lines. Int J Cancer 41: 892–895.

58. Lanemo Myhrinder A, Hellqvist E, Bergh AC, Jansson M, Nilsson K, et al. (2013) Molecular characterization of neoplastic and normal "sister" lymphoblastoid B-cell lines from chronic lymphocytic leukemia. Leuk Lymphoma.

59. Voltan R, di Iasio MG, Bosco R, Valeri N, Pekarski Y, et al. (2011) Nutlin-3 downregulates the expression of the oncogene TCL1 in primary B chronic lymphocytic leukemic cells. Clin Cancer Res 17: 5649–5655.

60. Zauli G, Voltan R, Bosco R, Melloni E, Marmiroli S, et al. (2011) Dasatinib plus Nutlin-3 shows synergistic antileukemic activity in both p53 wild-type and p53 mutated B chronic lymphocytic leukemias by inhibiting the Akt pathway. Clin Cancer Res 17: 762–770.

61. Nilsson K, Giovanella BC, Stehlin JS, Klein G (1977) Tumorigenicity of human hematopoietic cell lines in athymic nude mice. Int J Cancer 19: 337–344.

18

Less Graft-Versus-Host Disease after Rabbit Antithymocyte Globulin Conditioning in Unrelated Bone Marrow Transplantation for Leukemia and Myelodysplasia: Comparison with Matched Related Bone Marrow Transplantation

Elias Hallack Atta[1]*, **Danielli Cristina Muniz de Oliveira**[1], **Luis Fernando Bouzas**[1], **Márcio Nucci**[2], **Eliana Abdelhay**[1]

1 CEMO, Instituto Nacional de Câncer, Rio de Janeiro, Brazil, **2** University Hospital, Universidade Federal do Rio de Janeiro, Rio de Janeiro, Brazil

Abstract

One of the major drawbacks for unrelated donor (UD) bone marrow transplantation (BMT) is graft-versus-host disease (GVHD). Despite results from randomized trials, antithymocyte globulin (ATG) is not routinely included for GVHD prophylaxis in UD BMT by many centers. One of ways to demonstrate the usefulness of rabbit ATG in UD BMT is to evaluate how its results approximate to those observed in matched related (MRD) BMT. Therefore, we compared the outcomes between UD BMT with rabbit ATG (Thymoglobulin) for GVHD prophylaxis (n = 25) and MRD BMT (n = 91) for leukemia and myelodysplasia. All but one patient received a myeloablative conditioning regimen. Grades II–IV acute GVHD were similar (39.5% vs. 36%, p = 0.83); however, MRD BMT recipients developed more moderate-severe chronic GVHD (36.5% vs. 8.6%, p = 0.01) and GVHD-related deaths (32.5% vs. 5.6%, p = 0.04). UD BMT independently protected against chronic GVHD (hazard ratio 0.23, p = 0.04). The 6-month transplant-related mortality, 1-year relapse incidence, and 5-year survival rates were similar between patients with non-advanced disease in the MRD and UD BMT groups, 13.8% vs. 16.6% (p = 0.50), 20.8% vs. 16.6% (p = 0.37), and 57% vs. 50% (p = 0.67), respectively. Stable full donor chimerism was equally achieved (71.3% vs. 71.4%, p = 1). Incorporation of rabbit ATG in UD BMT promotes less GVHD, without jeopardizing chimerism evolution, and may attain similar survival outcomes as MRD BMT for leukemia and myelodysplasia especially in patients without advanced disease.

Editor: Vassiliki A. Boussiotis, Beth Israel Deaconess Medical Center, Harvard Medical School, United States of America

Funding: The authors have no support or funding to report.

Competing Interests: The authors have declared that no competing interests exist.

* Email: elias.atta@inca.gov.br

Introduction

Allogeneic hematopoietic stem cell transplantation (HSCT) is the treatment of choice for patients with high-risk hematologic malignancies. However, only 30% of patients have an HLA-matched related donor (MRD) [1]. Unrelated donor (UD) transplantation is an alternative for these patients, particularly with the increasing availability of registered volunteer donors and the regular use of high-resolution HLA typing techniques [2,3]. However, one of the major drawbacks to UD HSCT is graft-versus-host disease (GVHD), with reported incidences as high as 28% for grades III–IV acute GVHD and 44% for chronic GVHD in patients submitted to an 8/8 allele-level matched UD HSCT [3]. In addition to HLA compatibility, other donor-recipient non-HLA antigen mismatches such as cytokine polymorphisms may also play a role in the development of GVHD [4].

Many approaches have been evaluated to reduce GVHD complications after UD HSCT, especially methods designed to deplete donor alloreactive T cells in the graft [5,6]. Of particular interest is the administration of antithymocyte globulin (ATG) during the conditioning regimen to promote *in vivo* T cell depletion of the graft [7–9]. The use of rabbit ATG as a GVHD prophylaxis agent is more compelling than horse ATG, because of its stronger lymphocytotoxicity secondary to its longer half-life and higher lymphocyte affinity [10,11]. Three randomized trials demonstrated the efficacy of rabbit ATG in reducing GVHD after UD myeloablative HSCT in patients with hematologic malignancies: two with Thymoglobulin and one with ATG-Fresenius [12–14]. Although Thymoglobulin and ATG-Fresenius are rabbit-derived preparations, they differ in the antigen used to elicit the immune response and probably have different biological and clinical properties in HSCT [15,16].

Only 57% of the European centers routinely include ATG in the prophylaxis for recipients of a graft from an UD, as demonstrated in a survey conducted with 79 out of the 372 centers which perform allogeneic HSCT in Europe [17]. Data from the Center for International Blood and Marrow Transplant Research (CIBMTR) display a similar picture, only 37% of patients with hematologic malignancies submitted to an UD HSCT in 2009 received ATG for GVHD prophylaxis [18]. Therefore, the regular use of ATG in UD HSCT is still controversial, mainly because this approach has not conferred any survival advantage in the randomized trials [19].

One of the ways to assess the role of rabbit ATG in UD HSCT is to evaluate how its outcomes approximate to those observed in MRD HSCT. In the current study, we compared GVHD incidences between MRD bone marrow transplant (BMT) and UD BMT after rabbit ATG (Thymoglobulin) in patients with leukemia and myelodysplasia. Infectious complications and chimerism evolution were also analyzed, since these outcomes might be influenced by the T cell depletion promoted by rabbit ATG in UD BMT. Additionally, survival outcomes were compared to determine whether UD BMT after rabbit ATG achieves similar results as those seen in MRD BMT.

Patients and Methods

Eligibility

This study included all consecutive patients submitted to MRD and UD BMT between January 2005 and September 2011 at the Brazilian National Cancer Institute with the following hematologic malignancies: acute lymphoblastic leukemia, acute myelogenous leukemia (AML), chronic myelogenous leukemia, and myelodysplasia. Only patients who received bone marrow as graft were included. This study was approved by the Ethics Committee of the Brazilian National Cancer Institute and was in accordance with the Brazilian legislation and the Declaration of Helsinki. Informed consent was not obtained since the retrospective nature of this study did not affect the healthcare of the included individuals.

Moreover, confidentiality was preserved: patient records and data were anonymized and de-identified prior to analysis.

Conditioning regimens, GVHD prophylaxis, and GVHD treatment

All but one patient underwent a myeloablative conditioning regimen based on either busulfan or total body irradiation (TBI). TBI-based regimens were used mainly in patients with acute lymphoblastic leukemia, and busulfan-based regimens in those with myeloid malignancies. The following regimens were employed: oral busulfan 16 mg/kg and cyclophosphamide 120 mg/kg (n = 63), oral busulfan 16 mg/kg and melphalan 140 mg/m^2 (n = 2), hyperfractionated TBI 1320 cGy and cyclophosphamide 120 mg/kg (n = 49), hyperfractionated TBI 1320 cGy and melphalan 140 mg/m^2 (n = 1), or fludarabine 125 mg/m^2 and melphalan 140 mg/m^2 (n = 1).

All patients received cyclosporine and methotrexate as GVHD prophylaxis. UD BMT recipients also received rabbit ATG (Thymoglobulin, Sanofi-Aventis); total dose was 8 mg/kg (n = 22), 10 mg/kg (n = 2), or 15 mg/kg (n = 1), beginning on day -4 with its end on day -1. Cyclosporine was adjusted to target a serum level between 200 and 400 ng/mL. Cyclosporine was discontinued after BMT as soon as possible in both the MRD and UD groups, particularly in patients who were GVHD free.

Corticosteroids were used as first-line treatment for grades II–IV acute GVHD, with second-line therapies (extracorporeal photopheresis, anti-tumor necrosis factor antibody, and mycophenolate mofetil) individually or sequentially employed in patients with steroid-refractory acute GVHD. Moderate-severe chronic GVHD was treated with prednisone with the introduction of other agents to unresponsive patients.

Table 1. Comparison of baseline characteristics between matched related and unrelated BMT.

	Matched related BMT (n = 91)	Unrelated BMT (n = 25)	p value
Age (years), median (range)	31 (3–64)	17 (4–55)	0.11
Male gender, n (%)	59 (64.8%)	15 (60%)	0.65
Diagnosis, n (%)			
ALL	26 (28.6%)	12 (48%)	0.09
AML	31 (34.1%)	5 (20%)	0.22
MDS	13 (14.3%)	5 (20%)	0.53
CML	21 (23%)	3 (12%)	0.27
Advanced disease at the time of BMT, n (%)	19 (20.9%)	13 (52%)	0.004
Previous HSCT, n (%)	5 (5.5%)	2 (8%)	0.64
Pre-BMT positive CMV serology, n (%)	84 (92.3%)	22 (88%)	0.44
Serum ferritin before BMT (mg/dL), median (range)	881 (8.5–7496)	1367 (18.9–10474)	0.16
Donor-recipient gender mismatch, n (%)	39 (42.9%)	15 (60%)	0.17
ABO match	68 (74.7%)	8 (32%)	0.0002
TBI-based preparative regimen, n (%)	31 (34.1%)	19 (76%)	0.0002
Busulfan-based preparative regimen, n (%)	59 (64.8%)	6 (24%)	0.0005
Rabbit ATG dose (mg/kg), median (range)	0	8 (8–15)	<0.0001
Nucleated cell dose (x10^8/Kg), median (range)	2.39 (1.01–6.04)	2.92 (1.22–8.50)	0.50
G-CSF before day +15, n (%)	5 (5.5%)	2 (8%)	0.64

Abbreviations: ALL, acute lymphoblastic leukemia; AML, acute myelogenous leukemia; ATG, antithymocyte globulin; BMT, bone marrow transplantation; CML, chronic myelogenous leukemia; CMV, cytomegalovirus; G-CSF, granulocyte colony-stimulating factor; HSCT, hematopoietic stem cell transplantation; MDS, myelodysplastic syndrome; TBI, total body irradiation.

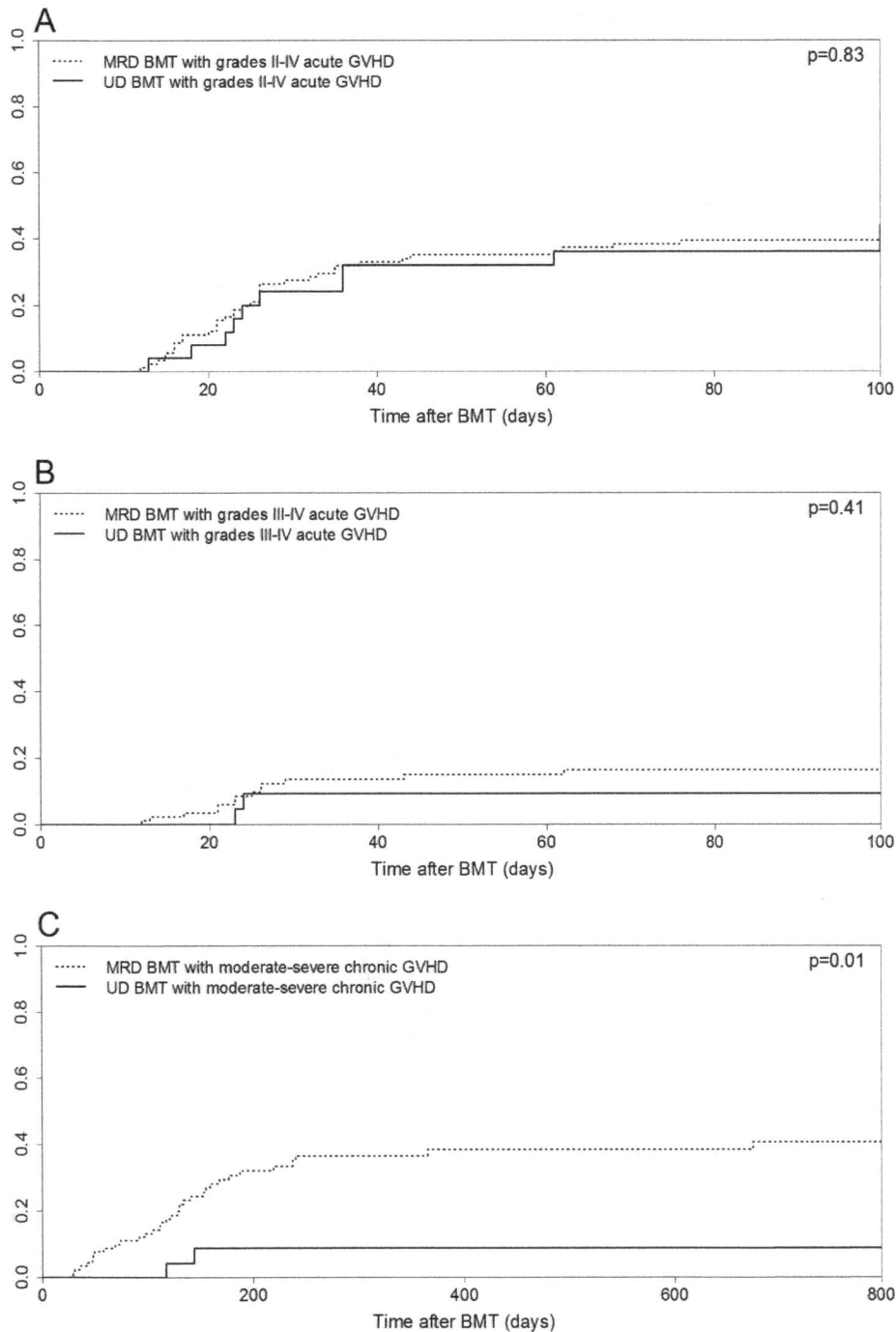

Figure 1. Cumulative incidence curves for matched related donor (MRD) and unrelated donor (UD) bone marrow transplantation (BMT). (A) Cumulative incidences for grades II–IV acute graft-versus-host disease (GVHD). (B) Cumulative incidences for grades III–IV acute GVHD. (C) Cumulative incidences for moderate-severe chronic GVHD.

Donor characteristics

All related BMTs were performed with a genotypically identical donor. The UD search process was performed by the Brazilian National Register of Bone Marrow Recipients (REREME). All UDs were matched to the recipient by low/intermediate-resolution technique for HLA-A and HLA-B, and by a high-resolution technique for HLA-DRB1. However, donor-recipient matching with high-resolution techniques for HLA-A, HLA-B, HLA-C, HLA-DQB1, and HLA-DRB1 were also performed in 17

pairs (68% of UD BMT) with only three pairs mismatched at two or more alleles (12% of UD BMT).

Supportive care and infection prophylaxis

Transplants were performed in single rooms with HEPA filters and positive air pressure. Acyclovir was begun during conditioning and continued until one year post-BMT. Weekly cytomegalovirus (CMV) pp65 antigenemia assays were performed from neutrophil engraftment until day +100 or beyond in cases with extended

Table 2. Cox regression analysis of variables predictive for moderate-severe chronic GVHD.

	Univariate analysis		Multivariate analysis	
	p value	Hazard ratio (95% CI)	p value	Hazard ratio (95% CI)
Age	0.03	1.02 (1.00–1.03)	0.05	–
ALL	0.45	0.75 (0.36–1.58)	–	–
AML	0.81	1.09 (0.52–2.27)	–	–
MDS	0.13	0.40 (0.12–1.33)	–	–
CML	0.03	2.09 (1.03–4.20)	0.06	–
Advanced disease at BMT	0.22	0.55 (0.21–1.43)	–	–
Pre-BMT serum ferritin	0.73	1.00 (1.00–1.00)	–	–
Donor-recipient gender mismatch	0.12	1.69 (0.87–3.29)	–	–
Busulfan-based conditioning	0.35	1.38 (0.69–2.75)	–	–
TBI-based conditioning	0.35	0.72 (0.36–1.43)	–	–
Unrelated BMT	0.04	0.23 (0.05–0.95)	0.04	0.23 (0.05–0.95)
Total nucleated cell dose	0.13	0.78 (0.57–1.07)	–	–

Abbreviations: ALL, acute lymphoblastic leukemia; AML, acute myelogenous leukemia; BMT, bone marrow transplantation; CML, chronic myelogenous leukemia; CI, confidence interval; GVHD, graft-versus-host disease; MDS, myelodysplastic syndrome; TBI, total body irradiation.

systemic immunosuppression. Ganciclovir was used for preemptive therapy in patients who developed positive antigenemia. Epstein-Barr virus polymerase chain reaction (PCR) was not routinely performed. Antifungal prophylaxis was prescribed on a case-by-case basis at the discretion of the attending clinician, with the following agents employed: fluconazole (n = 102), voriconazole (n = 12), or lipid-based amphotericin B (n = 2). Granulocyte-colony-stimulating factor (G-CSF) was administered only to patients with life-threatening infections during neutropenia.

End-points and definitions

The variables analyzed included acute and chronic GVHD, CMV reactivation, CMV disease, invasive fungal disease (IFD), transplant-related mortality (TRM), relapse, overall survival (OS), and chimerism evolution. Infectious complications were analyzed up to day +100, in order to evaluate the impact of rabbit ATG on these outcomes. Acute and chronic GVHD were diagnosed and classified according to the 1994 Consensus Conference and the National Institutes of Health Consensus, respectively [20,21]. CMV reactivation was defined as the presence of one or more positive cells in a CMV pp65 antigenemia assay, and CMV disease as the combination of symptoms or signs secondary to tissue lesion along with virus detection [22]. Diagnosis of IFD was based on criteria previously established [23]. Chimerism was monitored with PCR-based analysis of variable number of tandem repeats, and more recently with PCR-based analysis of short tandem repeats. Full donor chimerism (FDC) was defined as the establishment of more than 95% donor hematopoietic cells.

Patients were classified into two groups regarding the status of the hematologic malignancy at the time of BMT: advanced disease (acute leukemia beyond second remission or active at BMT, chronic myelogenous leukemia in blast crisis, or myelodysplastic syndrome with excess of blasts) and non-advanced disease (remaining patients).

Statistical analyses

Baseline characteristics were compared using Chi-square or Fisher's exact test for categorical variables and Mann-Whitney nonparametric test for continuous variables. Acute and chronic

GVHD, IFD, and CMV reactivation were analyzed as time-to-event outcomes with death by other causes treated as a competing event. Patients who did not develop IFD or CMV reactivation until day +100 were censored at that point in time for these outcomes. Patients submitted to donor lymphocyte infusion were also censored at this time for analysis of both acute and chronic GVHD incidences. TRM was measured from BMT until death without previous relapse or progression. Relapse was analyzed as the time from BMT to relapse, with death in remission treated as a competing event. Acute and chronic GVHD, IFD, CMV reactivation, TRM, and relapse were analyzed as cumulative incidence rates with the Fine and Gray's proportional hazards model to compare outcomes in the presence of competing risks [24]. OS was measured from BMT to death or last follow-up, analyzed with the Kaplan-Meier method, and compared with the log-rank test. Patients submitted to a second HSCT were censored at that time for all outcomes, except for survival analysis. Univariate Cox regression analyses were performed to identify the variables associated with chronic GVHD, variables with a p-value<0.10 were entered in the multivariate model. All p-values were two-sided, with p<0.05 indicating statistical significance. Registration and analysis of data were carried out using IBM SPSS version 15 software. Cumulative incidences, the Fine and Gray's test, and graphs were generated using R Statistical Software (R-project version 3.0.1, http://www.r-project.org/).

Results

Comparison of baseline characteristics

During the study period, 91 MRD and 25 UD BMT were identified and analyzed. Baseline characteristics were similar between the groups, except that the UD BMT group was more likely to have advanced disease at BMT, receive a graft with donor-recipient ABO mismatch, and be submitted to a TBI-based conditioning regimen than the MRD BMT group (Table 1).

Graft-versus-host disease

The cumulative incidence of grades II–IV acute GVHD at day +100 was 39.5% (95% confidence interval [CI] 29.4–49.4%) and

36% (95% CI 17.7–54.6%) in patients submitted to MRD and UD BMT, respectively (p = 0.83, Figure 1A). Grades III–IV acute GVHD incidences at day +100 were also similar: 16.2% (95% CI 9–25.2%) for MRD and 9.1% (95% CI 1.4–25.6%) for UD BMT (p = 0.41, Figure 1B). Steroid-refractory acute GVHD was observed in 31.4% (11 out of 35) and 20% (two out of 10) of patients who developed acute GVHD in the MRD and UD BMT groups, respectively (p = 0.69).

The 1-year incidence of moderate-severe chronic GVHD was higher in MRD than in UD BMT recipients: 36.5% (95% CI 26.1–46.9%) vs. 8.6% (95% CI 1.3–24.6%, p = 0.01, Figure 1C). Multivariate analysis indicated that UD BMT remained independently associated with moderate-severe chronic GVHD, displaying a protective effect (hazard ratio [HR] 0.23, 95% CI 0.05–0.95, p = 0.04, Table 2).

Infectious complications

The cumulative incidences of proven or probable IFD on day + 100 were 8.7% (95% CI 4–15.7%) and 16% (95% CI 4.8–33%) in MRD and UD BMT recipients (p = 0.34, Figure 2A). Eight cases of proven/probable IFD developed in MRD BMT patients: invasive aspergillosis (n = 4) and invasive candidiasis (n = 4); whereas the UD BMT group registered four cases: invasive aspergillosis (n = 2), disseminated fusariosis (n = 1), and cryptococcosis (n = 1).

CMV reactivation incidence at day +100 was higher in UD than in MRD BMT: 76% (95% CI 52–89.1%) vs. 57.1% (95% CI 46.2–66.6%, p = 0.003, Figure 2B). However, only 6.6% of the MRD (six out of 91) and 8% of the UD BMT (two out of 25) patients developed CMV disease (p = 0.68).

Transplant-related mortality, relapse, and survival

The median follow-up for all patients was 592.5 days (range, 12–2948 days). Since there were more patients with advanced disease in the UD BMT group, the results regarding TRM, relapse, and OS were classified into two categories: non-advanced and advanced disease.

In patients with non-advanced disease at the time of BMT, the 6-month TRM was similar between the two groups, 13.8% (95% CI 7–22.9%) in MRD and 16.6% in UD BMT (95% CI 2.3–42.5%, p = 0.50, Figure 3A). However, in patients with advanced disease, the 6-month TRM was higher in UD BMT: 30.7% (95% CI 8.4–56.9%) vs. 15.7% (95% CI 3.6–35.7%, p = 0.06, Figure 3B). The high mortality observed in patients with advanced disease receiving UD BMT was mainly attributable to infectious complications: CMV disease (n = 2), disseminated fusariosis (n = 1), neurotoxoplasmosis (n = 1), and *Pseudomonas aeruginosa* bacteremia (n = 1).

The 1-year relapse incidences were similar between the MRD and UD BMT groups both among patients with non-advanced disease (20.8% [95% CI 12.3–30.9%] and 16.6% [95% CI 22.9–42.7%], respectively, p = 0.37, Figure 3C) and advanced disease (42.1% [95% CI 19.5–63.2%] and 53.8% [95% CI 21.7–77.8%], respectively, p = 0.49, Figure 3D).

No difference was found in the 5-year OS between patients with non-advanced disease submitted to MRD and UD BMT: 57% and 50%, respectively (p = 0.67, Figure 4A). However, the 5-year OS was higher in MRD BMT patients with advanced disease: 35.1% vs. 7.7% (p – 0.008, Figure 4B).

Relapse of the hematologic malignancy was the most common cause of death in the population analyzed (Table 3). However, GVHD-related deaths were more common in MRD than in UD BMT recipients, 32.5% (14 out of 43) vs. 5.6% (one out of 18), p = 0.04. On the contrary, infection-related deaths were less common in MRD than in UD BMT recipients, 4.7% (two out of 43) vs. 33.3% (six out of 18), p = 0.006.

Chimerism data

Chimerism assessment was available in 88.9% (80 out of 90) and 95.5% (21 out of 22) of patients surviving beyond day +30 in the MRD and UD BMT groups, respectively (p = 0.68). The proportion of patients who achieved stable FDC was similar between the groups, 71.3% in MRD and 71.4% in UD BMT recipients (p = 1).

Discussion

Our results suggest that the incorporation of rabbit ATG in UD BMT protects against GVHD-related complications, with less chronic GVHD and fewer GVHD-related deaths in UD compared to MRD BMT. In addition, UD BMT after rabbit ATG was independently associated with protection against chronic GVHD. Despite the observed efficacy of rabbit ATG for GVHD prophylaxis in UD BMT, achievement of stable FDC was not impaired. TRM, relapse, and OS were similar between MRD and UD BMT in patients with leukemia and myelodysplasia without advanced disease at the time of BMT, in the setting where most patients received a myeloablative conditioning regimen.

The incidence of grades II–IV acute GVHD in our UD BMT recipients was 40.9%, with only 10% developing grades III–IV acute GVHD. These incidences are lower than those reported in two randomized trials conducted by Bacigalupo *et al*, in which grades II–IV acute GVHD developed in 72% and 79% of patients and grades III–IV developed in 36% and 50% of patients in the UD BMT arms without rabbit ATG (Thymoglobulin) [12]. In another study with the National Marrow Donor Program data, the incidences of grades III–IV acute GVHD were 28%, 37%, and 44% in patients undergoing an 8/8 (n = 1,840), 7/8 (n = 985), and 6/8 (n = 633) allele-matched UD HSCT, respectively; incidences substantially higher than that observed in our study [3]. Therefore, rabbit ATG protected our UD BMT recipients against acute GVHD; reducing its incidence to that observed in MRD BMT. Moreover, a smaller proportion of the UD BMT recipients developed severe (grades III–IV) and steroid-refractory acute GVHD; however, these differences were not statistically significant possibly due to the small number of cases. In our study, moderate-severe chronic GVHD was considerably more common after MRD than after UD BMT. In addition, UD BMT with rabbit ATG was independently associated with protection against chronic GVHD by multivariate analysis. This protective effect was observed despite some patients who were not matched by high-resolution techniques for HLA class I antigens or not completely HLA allele-matched with their UD. Previous studies have also observed an inferior incidence of chronic GVHD in recipients of UD HSCT conditioned with rabbit ATG (Thymoglobulin, total dose ≥6 mg/kg) compared to MRD HSCT, without differences in acute GVHD incidences [25,26]. However, differently from these studies, our population was uniform with respect to stem cell source, since all patients received bone marrow as graft [25,26]. Another important finding from our study was that, despite protecting against GVHD, conditioning with rabbit ATG did not jeopardized the achievement of stable FDC in UD BMT recipients. To our knowledge, the current study is the first to demonstrate that, at least in the setting where most patients received a myeloablative regimen, MRD and UD BMT after rabbit ATG (Thymoglobulin) display a similar chimerism profile.

Infection-related deaths were the main cause of non-relapse mortality in UD BMT recipients, especially in those with

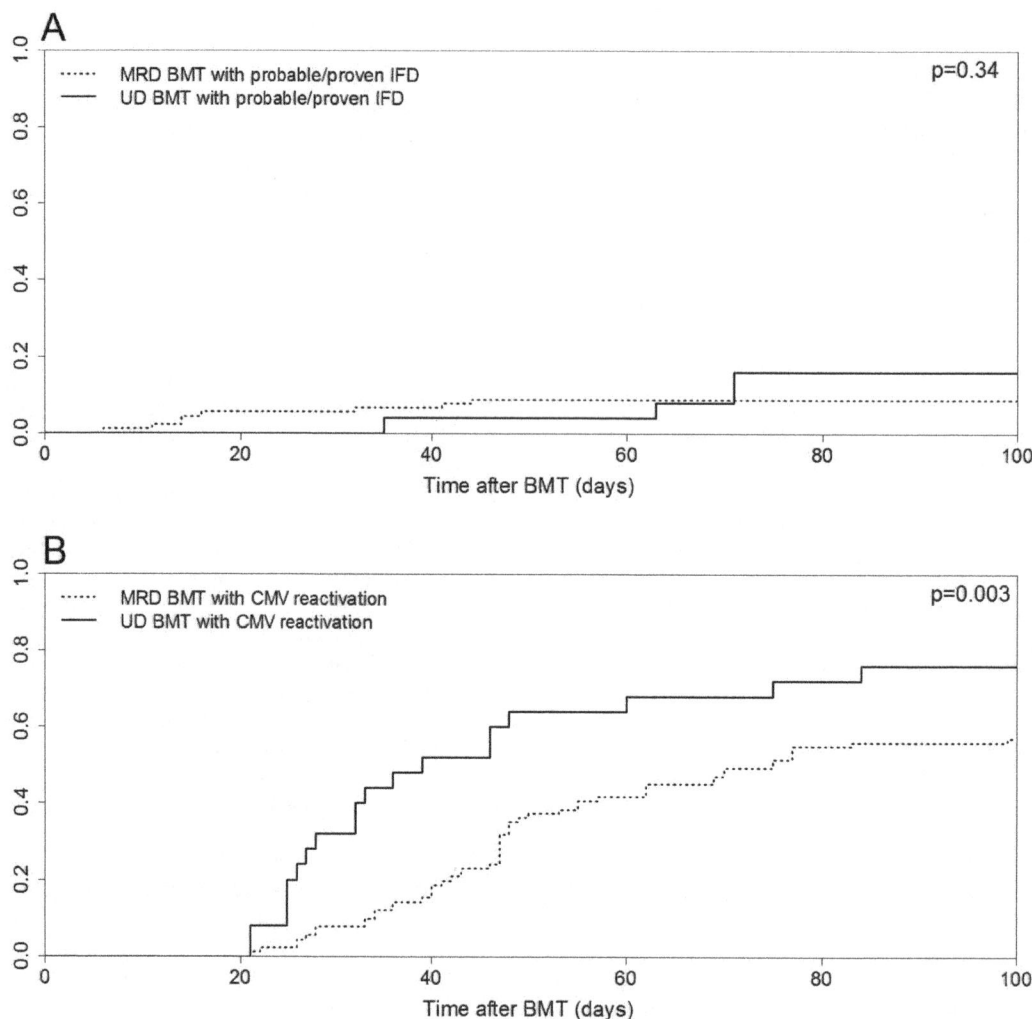

Figure 2. Cumulative incidence curves for matched related donor (MRD) and unrelated donor (UD) bone marrow transplantation (BMT). (A) Day +100 probability for proven or probable invasive fungal disease (IFD). (B) Day +100 probability for cytomegalovirus (CMV) reactivation.

advanced disease. Infectious complications were manageable in UD BMT patients without advanced disease, owing to adequate prophylaxis and treatment. Despite a higher incidence of CMV reactivation in UD BMT, this was not translated to more cases of CMV disease, highlighting the efficacy of the preemptive approach adopted. IFD incidence was slightly higher in the UD BMT group, although this difference was not statistically significant. No case of post-transplant lymphoproliferative disorder was observed; however, our UD BMT population was not large, and the regular monitoring of Epstein-Barr virus DNA levels after rabbit ATG conditioning is recommended to allow preemptive treatment. Most of our UD BMT patients received rabbit ATG (Thymoglobulin) at a total dose of 8 mg/kg, a dose which probably allows a balance between protection against GVHD and an increase in the risk of infectious complications [27,28]. A study conducted by Remberger *et al* found that the ideal dose of Thymoglobulin for GVHD prophylaxis in UD myeloablative HSCT is 6–8 mg/kg, since lower doses (4 mg/kg) increased the risk of severe acute GVHD, whereas higher doses (10 mg/kg) promoted more infectious death [28]. In reduced-intensity HSCT, the optimal dose of Thymoglobulin was 6 mg/kg, since an 8 mg/kg dose was associated with an inferior relapse-free survival particularly in patients with high-risk disease [29].

Patients with non-advanced disease undergoing UD BMT experienced similar TRM, relapse, and OS compared with MRD BMT recipients. However, TRM was higher in UD BMT recipients with advanced disease, promoting poor survival in this subgroup. This higher TRM was probably secondary to the use of fully myeloablative regimens in patients with low functional reserve after multiple lines of chemotherapy to control disease progression during the UD search. Previous studies in patients with hematologic malignancies also found similar TRM, relapse, and OS between UD myeloablative HSCT after rabbit ATG (Thymoglobulin) and MRD HSCT [25,26,30]. However, a recent retrospective analysis with data from the Center for International Blood and Marrow Transplant Research (CIBMTR) found that ATG conditioning in reduced-intensity HSCT increased the likelihood of relapse, which negatively influenced disease-free survival in patients with hematologic malignancies [31]. Therefore, immune modulation with ATG in the reduced-intensity setting might abrogate the graft-versus-leukemia effect that is responsible for the elimination of residual malignant cells that persist after a less intensive preparative regimen.

Our study has various limitations. First, data was retrospectively collected; however, information was easily retrieved with minimal loss. Second, some baseline characteristics were different between

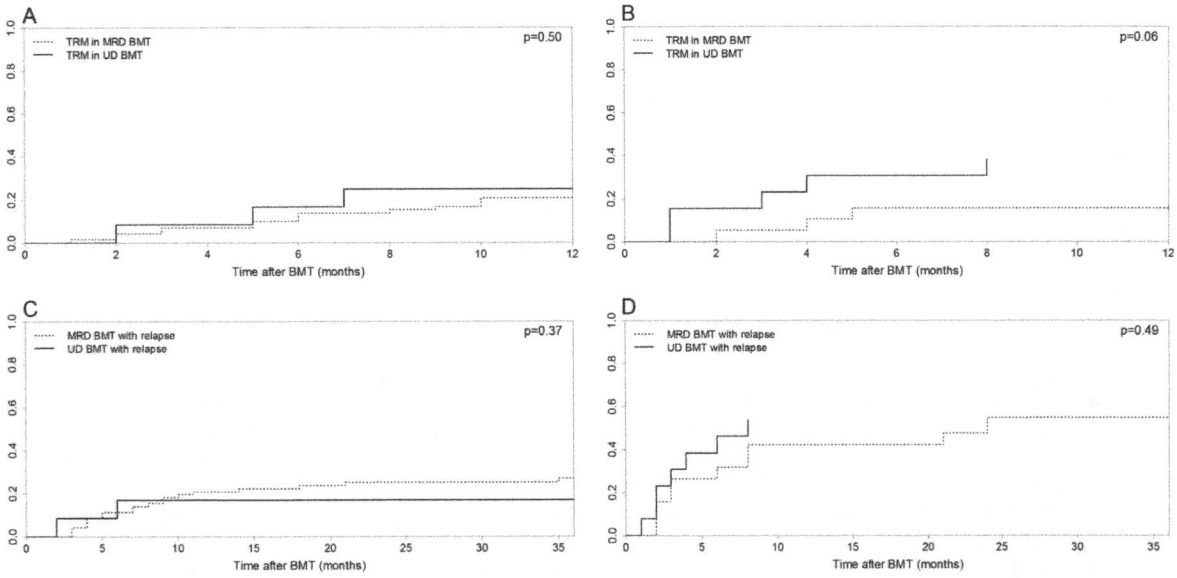

Figure 3. Cumulative incidence curves for matched related donor (MRD) and unrelated donor (UD) bone marrow transplantation (BMT). (A) Transplant-related mortality (TRM) in patients with non-advanced disease at the time of BMT. (B) TRM in patients with advanced disease at the time of BMT. (C) Relapse incidences in patients with non-advanced disease at the time of BMT. (D) Relapse incidences in patients with advanced disease at the time of BMT.

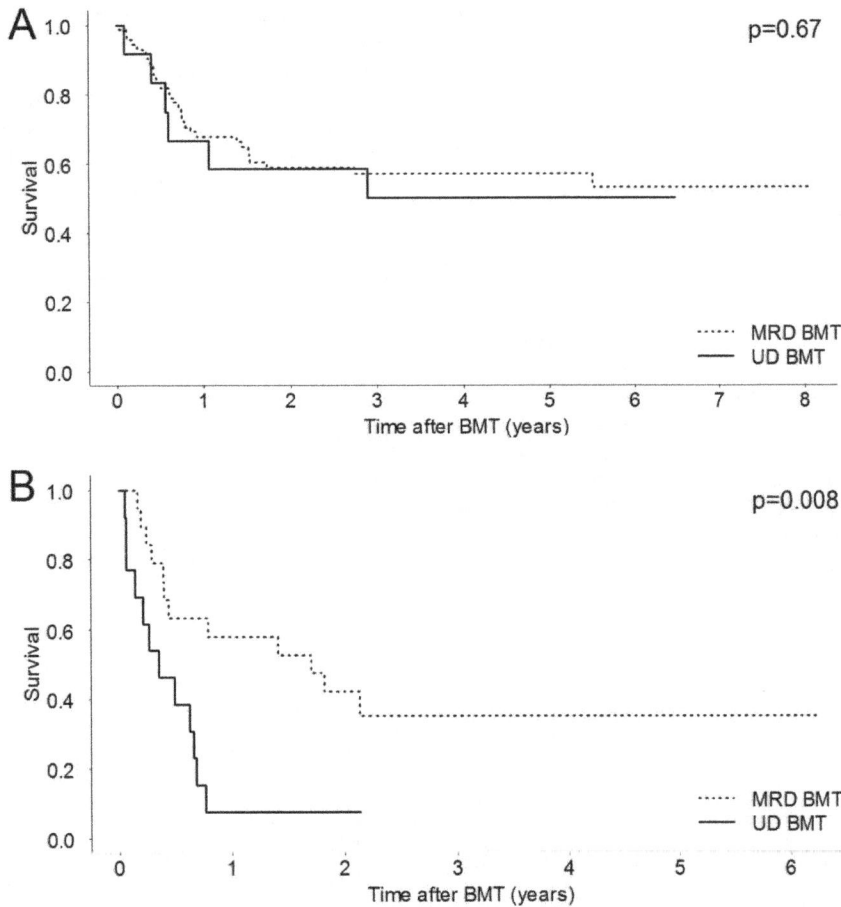

Figure 4. Kaplan-Meier curves for matched related donor (MRD) and unrelated donor (UD) bone marrow transplantation (BMT). (A) Overall survival in patients with non-advanced disease at the time of BMT. (B) Overall survival in patients with advanced disease at the time of BMT.

Table 3. Comparison of death causes between related and unrelated BMT.

Death causes	Related BMT (n = 91)	Unrelated BMT (n = 25)	p value
Relapse, n (%)	23 (53.4%)	8 (44.4%)	0.58
Infection, n (%)	2 (4.7%)	6 (33.3%)	0.006
Toxicity, n (%)	2 (4.7%)	2 (11.1%)	0.57
GVHD, n (%)	14 (32.5%)	1 (5.6%)	0.04
Other, n (%)	2 (4.7%)	1 (5.6%)	1.00

Abbreviations: BMT, bone marrow transplantation; GVHD, graft-versus-host disease.

the groups and this could be associated with the observed outcomes. For instance, the UD group was younger and composed mainly by patients with acute lymphoblastic leukemia. However, by multivariate analysis, we were able to identify the variables independently associated with chronic GVHD. Another limitation is the small and heterogeneous patient population, particularly in the UD BMT group. The small sample size probably precluded the detection of other clinically significant differences between the groups and also hampered multivariate Cox regression analyses regarding outcomes such as relapse and OS. Finally, to counteract the higher mortality observed in the UD BMT group, chronic GVHD cumulative incidence was estimated using death without this event as a competing risk.

Notwithstanding these limitations, the current study has implications for both the research and clinical settings as several outstanding questions remain. In the translational research setting, more research is needed to understand the exact mechanisms by which rabbit ATG prevents GVHD: Which specific cells from the allograft are depleted and what are rabbit ATG's effects on the recipient [32,33]. From a clinical standpoint, our study suggests that UD HSCT after myeloablative conditioning with rabbit ATG offers less GVHD with similar survival outcomes as MRD HSCT for leukemia and myelodysplasia, especially in patients without advanced disease at BMT. These results are particularly important because they differ from the current transplant strategy adopted by many centers as demonstrated in two recent studies with CIBMTR data which also compared UD and MRD HSCT for AML (8/8 UD, n = 1193; MRD, n = 624) and myelodysplasia (8/8 UD, n = 413; MRD, n = 176) [34,35]. Despite similar survival rates, B–D acute GVHD was more common after 8/8 allele-matched UD than MRD HSCT both for AML (51% vs. 33%, p< 0.001) and myelodysplasia (54% vs. 42%, p = 0.006). Also, the 1-year probability of chronic GVHD was higher in AML patients submitted to an 8/8 allele-matched UD HSCT (45% vs. 39%, p = 0.008). In the previously cited studies, the higher incidence of

GVHD was mainly because most patients were not conditioned with ATG and received peripheral blood as graft. However, ATG conditioning might also counteract the increased risk of GVHD after peripheral blood HSCT [36]. The burden of GVHD should be taken into account in UD HSCT, because it might increase TRM, worsen quality of life, prolong immunosuppressive therapy, and increase health care costs [13,36,37]. Both acute and chronic GVHD are associated with worse quality of life in many aspects: physical functioning, role functioning, social functioning, mental health, and general health [38]. Therefore, although UD HSCT might be the only option for patients without a MRD, physicians may offer improved quality of life through GVHD reduction [39]. Finally, our results were obtained after rabbit ATG (Thymoglobulin) conditioning; therefore, comparative studies are necessary to characterize the differences among ATG brands and other *in vivo* T-cell depleting agents in UD HSCT.

In summary, our results demonstrate the protective effect of rabbit ATG against GVHD in UD BMT, overcoming donor-recipient HLA and non-HLA disparities. Incorporation of rabbit ATG in the preparative regimen of UD BMT promotes less GVHD compared to MRD BMT, without jeopardizing the achievement of stable FDC, and may attain similar TRM, relapse, and survival in patients with leukemia and myelodysplasia especially in those without advanced disease at BMT. Prospective randomized trials in the era of high-resolution HLA typing techniques and better supportive care are needed to define the exact role of rabbit ATG in UD HSCT.

Author Contributions

Conceived and designed the experiments: EHA DCMDO LFB MN EA. Performed the experiments: EHA DCMDO LFB MN EA. Analyzed the data: EHA DCMDO LFB MN EA. Contributed to the writing of the manuscript: EHA DCMDO LFB MN EA.

References

1. Beatty PG, Hansen JA, Longton GM, Thomas ED, Sanders JE, et al. (1991) Marrow transplantation from HLA-matched unrelated donors for treatment of hematologic malignancies. Transplantation 51: 443–447.
2. Walker T, Milford E, Chell J, Maiers M, Confer D (2011) The National Marrow Donor Program: improving access to hematopoietic cell transplantation. Clin Transpl: 55–62.
3. Lee SJ, Klein J, Haagenson M, Baxter-Lowe LA, Confer DL, et al. (2007) High-resolution donor-recipient HLA matching contributes to the success of unrelated donor marrow transplantation. Blood 110: 4576–4583.
4. Mullighan C, Heatley S, Doherty K, Szabo F, Grigg A, et al. (2004) Non-HLA immunogenetic polymorphisms and the risk of complications after allogeneic hemopoietic stem-cell transplantation. Transplantation 77: 587–596.
5. Spencer A, Szydlo RM, Brookes PA, Kaminski E, Rule S, et al. (1995) Bone marrow transplantation for chronic myeloid leukemia with volunteer unrelated donors using ex vivo or in vivo T-cell depletion: major prognostic impact of HLA class I identity between donor and recipient. Blood 86: 3590–3597.
6. Champlin RE, Passweg JR, Zhang MJ, Rowlings PA, Pelz CJ, et al. (2000) T-cell depletion of bone marrow transplants for leukemia from donors other than HLA-identical siblings: advantage of T-cell antibodies with narrow specificities. Blood 95: 3996–4003.
7. Zander AR, Zabelina T, Kroger N, Renges H, Kruger W, et al. (1999) Use of a five-agent GVHD prevention regimen in recipients of unrelated donor marrow. Bone Marrow Transplant 23: 889–893.
8. Byrne JL, Stainer C, Cull G, Haynes AP, Bessell EM, et al. (2000) The effect of the serotherapy regimen used and the marrow cell dose received on rejection, graft-versus-host disease and outcome following unrelated donor bone marrow transplantation for leukaemia. Bone Marrow Transplant 25: 411–417.
9. Finke J, Bertz H, Schmoor C, Veelken H, Behringer D, et al. (2000) Allogeneic bone marrow transplantation from unrelated donors using in vivo anti-T-cell globulin. Br J Haematol 111: 303–313.

10. Thomas FT, Griesedieck C, Thomas J, Carver M, Whitley T, et al. (1984) Differential effects of horse ATG and rabbit ATG on T cell and T cell subset levels measured by monoclonal antibodies. Transplant Proc 16: 1561–1563.

11. Scheinberg P, Fischer SH, Li L, Nunez O, Wu CO, et al. (2007) Distinct EBV and CMV reactivation patterns following antibody-based immunosuppressive regimens in patients with severe aplastic anemia. Blood 109: 3219–3224.

12. Bacigalupo A, Lamparelli T, Bruzzi P, Guidi S, Alessandrino PE, et al. (2001) Antithymocyte globulin for graft-versus-host disease prophylaxis in transplants from unrelated donors: 2 randomized studies from Gruppo Italiano Trapianti Midollo Osseo (GITMO). Blood 98: 2942–2947.

13. Bacigalupo A, Lamparelli T, Barisione G, Bruzzi P, Guidi S, et al. (2006) Thymoglobulin prevents chronic graft-versus-host disease, chronic lung dysfunction, and late transplant-related mortality: long-term follow-up of a randomized trial in patients undergoing unrelated donor transplantation. Biol Blood Marrow Transplant 12: 560–565.

14. Finke J, Bethge WA, Schmoor C, Ottinger HD, Stelljes M, et al. (2009) Standard graft-versus-host disease prophylaxis with or without anti-T-cell globulin in haematopoietic cell transplantation: a randomised, open-label, multicentre phase 3 trial. Lancet Oncol 10: 855–864.

15. Basara N, Baurmann H, Kolbe K, Yaman A, Labopin M, et al. (2005) Antithymocyte globulin for the prevention of graft-versus-host disease after unrelated hematopoietic stem cell transplantation for acute myeloid leukemia: results from the multicenter German cooperative study group. Bone Marrow Transplant 35: 1011–1018.

16. Terasako K, Sato K, Sato M, Kimura S, Nakasone H, et al. (2010) The effect of different ATG preparations on immune recovery after allogeneic hematopoietic stem cell transplantation for severe aplastic anemia. Hematology 15: 165–169.

17. Ruutu T, van BA, Hertenstein B, Henseler A, Garderet L, et al. (2012) Prophylaxis and treatment of GVHD after allogeneic haematopoietic SCT: a survey of centre strategies by the European Group for Blood and Marrow Transplantation. Bone Marrow Transplant 47: 1459–1464.

18. Pidala J, Tomblyn M, Nishihori T, Ayala E, Field T, et al. (2011) ATG prevents severe acute graft-versus-host disease in mismatched unrelated donor hematopoietic cell transplantation. Biol Blood Marrow Transplant 17: 1237–1244.

19. Appelbaum FR, Bacigalupo A, Soiffer R (2012) Anti-T cell antibodies as part of the preparative regimen in hematopoietic cell transplantation–a debate. Biol Blood Marrow Transplant 18: S111–S115.

20. Przepiorka D, Weisdorf D, Martin P, Klingemann HG, Beatty P, et al. (1995) 1994 Consensus Conference on Acute GVHD Grading. Bone Marrow Transplant 15: 825–828.

21. Filipovich AH, Weisdorf D, Pavletic S, Socie G, Wingard JR, et al. (2005) National Institutes of Health consensus development project on criteria for clinical trials in chronic graft-versus-host disease: I. Diagnosis and staging working group report. Biol Blood Marrow Transplant 11: 945–956.

22. Ljungman P, Griffiths P, Paya C (2002) Definitions of cytomegalovirus infection and disease in transplant recipients. Clin Infect Dis 34: 1094–1097.

23. De PB, Walsh TJ, Donnelly JP, Stevens DA, Edwards JE, et al. (2008) Revised definitions of invasive fungal disease from the European Organization for Research and Treatment of Cancer/Invasive Fungal Infections Cooperative Group and the National Institute of Allergy and Infectious Diseases Mycoses Study Group (EORTC/MSG) Consensus Group. Clin Infect Dis 46: 1813–1821.

24. Scrucca L, Santucci A, Aversa F (2007) Competing risk analysis using R: an easy guide for clinicians. Bone Marrow Transplant 40: 381–387.

25. Remberger M, Mattsson J, Hausenberger D, Schaffer M, Svahn BM, et al. (2008) Genomic tissue typing and optimal antithymocyte globuline dose using

26. Portier DA, Sabo RT, Roberts CH, Fletcher DS, Meier J, et al. (2012) Antithymocyte globulin for conditioning in matched unrelated donor hematopoietic cell transplantation provides comparable outcomes to matched related donor recipients. Bone Marrow Transplant 47: 1513–1519.

27. Meijer E, Cornelissen JJ, Lowenberg B, Verdonck LF (2003) Antithymocyte globulin as prophylaxis of graft failure and graft-versus-host disease in recipients of partially T-cell-depleted grafts from matched unrelated donors: a dose-finding study. Exp Hematol 31: 1026–1030.

28. Remberger M, Svahn BM, Mattsson J, Ringden O (2004) Dose study of thymoglobulin during conditioning for unrelated donor allogeneic stem-cell transplantation. Transplantation 78: 122–127.

29. Remberger M, Ringden O, Hagglund H, Svahn BM, Ljungman P, et al. (2013) A high antithymocyte globulin dose increases the risk of relapse after reduced intensity conditioning HSCT with unrelated donors. Clin Transplant 27: E368–374.

30. Duggan P, Booth K, Chaudhry A, Stewart D, Ruether JD, et al. (2002) Unrelated donor BMT recipients given pretransplant low-dose antithymocyte globulin have outcomes equivalent to matched sibling BMT: a matched pair analysis. Bone Marrow Transplant 30: 681–686.

31. Soiffer RJ, Lerademacher J, Ho V, Kan F, Artz A, et al. (2011) Impact of immune modulation with anti-T-cell antibodies on the outcome of reduced-intensity allogeneic hematopoietic stem cell transplantation for hematologic malignancies. Blood 117: 6963–6970.

32. Na IK, Wittenbecher F, Dziubianau M, Herholz A, Mensen A, et al. (2013) Rabbit antithymocyte globulin (Thymoglobulin(R)) impairs the thymic output of both conventional and regulatory CD4+ T cells after allogeneic hematopoietic stem cell transplantation in adult patients. Haematologica 98: 23–30.

33. Hoegh-Petersen M, Amin MA, Liu Y, Ugarte-Torres A, Williamson TS, et al. (2013) Anti-thymocyte globulins capable of binding to T and B cells reduce graft-vs-host disease without increasing relapse. Bone Marrow Transplant 48: 105–114.

34. Saber W, Opie S, Rizzo JD, Zhang MJ, Horowitz MM, et al. (2012) Outcomes after matched unrelated donor versus identical sibling hematopoietic cell transplantation in adults with acute myelogenous leukemia. Blood 119: 3908–3916.

35. Saber W, Cutler CS, Nakamura R, Zhang MJ, Atallah E, et al. (2013) Impact of donor source on hematopoietic cell transplantation outcomes for patients with myelodysplastic syndromes (MDS). Blood 122: 1974–1982.

36. Socie G, Schmoor C, Bethge WA, Ottinger HD, Stelljes M, et al. (2011) Chronic graft-versus-host disease: long-term results from a randomized trial on graft-versus-host disease prophylaxis with or without anti-T-cell globulin ATG-Fresenius. Blood 117: 6375–6382.

37. Svahn BM, Ringden O, Remberger M (2006) Treatment costs and survival in patients with grades III–IV acute graft-versus-host disease after allogenic hematopoietic stem cell transplantation during three decades. Transplantation 81: 1600–1603.

38. Pidala J, Anasetti C, Jim H (2009) Quality of life after allogeneic hematopoietic cell transplantation. Blood 114: 7–19.

39. Yu ZP, Ding JH, Wu F, Liu J, Wang J, et al. (2012) Quality of life of patients after allogeneic hematopoietic stem cell transplantation with antihuman thymocyte globulin. Biol Blood Marrow Transplant 18: 593–599.

19

Outcome of Central Nervous System Relapses In Childhood Acute Lymphoblastic Leukaemia – Prospective Open Cohort Analyses of the ALLR3 Trial

Ashish Narayan Masurekar[1🌑], Catriona A. Parker[1🌑], Milensu Shanyinde[2], Anthony V. Moorman[3], Jeremy P. Hancock[4], Rosemary Sutton[5], Philip J. Ancliff[6], Mary Morgan[7], Nicholas J. Goulden[6], Chris Fraser[8], Peter M. Hoogerbrugge[9], Tamas Revesz[10], Philip J. Darbyshire[11], Shekhar Krishnan[12], Sharon B. Love[2], Vaskar Saha[12]*

1 Children's Cancer Group, Centre for Paediatric, Teenage and Young Adult Cancer, Institute of Cancer, Manchester Academic Health Science Centre, Central Manchester University Hospitals Foundation Trust, The University of Manchester, Manchester, United Kingdom, 2 Centre for Statistics in Medicine, University of Oxford, Oxford, United Kingdom, 3 Leukaemia Research Cytogenetics Group, Northern Institute for Cancer Research, Newcastle University, Newcastle upon Tyne, United Kingdom, 4 Bristol Genetics Laboratory, Southmead Hospital, Bristol, United Kingdom, 5 Children's Cancer Institute Australia, Lowy Cancer Research Centre, University of New South Wales, Sydney, Australia, 6 Great Ormond Street Hospital, London, United Kingdom, 7 Child Oncology and Haematology Centre, Southampton General Hospital, Southampton, United Kingdom, 8 Queensland Children's Cancer Centre, Brisbane, Australia, 9 Childrens Hospital, Radboud University Nijmegen Medical Centre, Nijmegen, The Netherlands Dutch Childhood Oncology Group, The Hague, The Netherlands, 10 Department of Haematology-Oncology, SA Pathology at Women's and Children's Hospital and University of Adelaide, Adelaide, Australia, 11 Department of Haematology, Birmingham Children's Hospital, Birmingham, United Kingdom, 12 Paediatric Oncology, Tata Translational Cancer Research Centre, Kolkata, India

Abstract

The outcomes of Central Nervous System (CNS) relapses in children with acute lymphoblastic leukaemia (ALL) treated in the ALL R3 trial, between January 2003 and March 2011 were analysed. Patients were risk stratified, to receive a matched donor allogeneic transplant or fractionated cranial irradiation with continued treatment for two years. A randomisation of Idarubicin with Mitoxantrone closed in December 2007 in favour of Mitoxantrone. The estimated 3-year progression free survival for combined and isolated CNS disease were 40.6% (25·1, 55·6) and 38.0% (26.2, 49.7) respectively. Univariate analysis showed a significantly better survival for age <10 years, progenitor-B cell disease, good-risk cytogenetics and those receiving Mitoxantrone. Adjusting for these variables (age, time to relapse, cytogenetics, treatment drug and gender) a multivariate analysis, showed a poorer outcome for those with combined CNS relapse (HR 2·64, 95% CI 1·32, 5·31, p = 0·006 for OS). ALL R3 showed an improvement in outcome for CNS relapses treated with Mitoxantrone compared to Idarubicin; a potential benefit for matched donor transplant for those with very early and early isolated-CNS relapses.

Editor: Maria R. Baer, University of Maryland, United States of America

Funding: This study was funded in part by a programme grant from Cancer Research UK [http://www.cancerresearchuk.org/] (VS - programme grant C8230); grants from Leukaemia Lymphoma Research [http://leukaemialymphomaresearch.org.uk/] funded the Leukaemia Research Cytogenetics Group (AVM - programme grant 11004). The Cancer Council NSW (PG11-06) [http://www.cancercouncil.com.au/], Sporting Chance Cancer Foundation Cancer Fund 2011 [http://sportingchance.com.au/] and NH&MRC grant (1024232) [http://www.nhmrc.gov.au/] funded analysis of minimal residual disease at CCIA (RS). Hospira provided a non-conditional educational grant for ANZCHOG data management (TR). The authors confirm the funders had no role in this study. The funders had no role in study design, data collection and analysis, decision to publish, or preparation of the manuscript.

Competing Interests: Hospira provided help for the data entry for the Australian and New Zealand patients by providing a non-conditional educational grant for ANZCHOG.

* Email: vaskar.saha@manchester.ac.uk

🌑 These authors contributed equally to this work.

Introduction

Acute lymphoblastic leukaemia (ALL) of childhood is a systemic disease with a propensity for post-therapeutic recurrence in the central nervous system (CNS) [1]. Modern chemotherapeutic regimens have significantly decreased the incidence of all types of relapses [2–9], primarily by intensification of systemic rather than CNS directed therapy (cranial irradiation and intrathecal therapy)

[10,11]. Nevertheless, 20–40% of relapses continue to occur in the CNS as either isolated (i-CNS) or combined (c-CNS) disease [10]. Management of these relapses remains problematic. In general, early and combined relapses have a poorer prognosis when compared with late and isolated CNS disease [12–15]. A combination of 6–12 months systemic therapy with intrathecal methotrexate, followed by cranial irradiation has yielded good results [16–21]. Other approaches used have either focused on

intensifying CNS directed therapy, such as craniospinal irradiation [20], or intensifying systemic therapy with autologous [18] and allogeneic stem cell transplantation (allo-SCT) [16,17,21].

As a significant proportion of patients relapsing off UK frontline trials had CNS disease [10], we designed CNS directed therapy into the ALL R3 relapse trial [22]. Drugs reported to cross the blood brain barrier e.g. dexamethasone, high dose methotrexate and high dose cytarabine were used in systemic chemotherapy along with intrathecal methotrexate. At the end of three blocks of chemotherapy, lasting 13 weeks, patients were either eligible for cranial radiotherapy with continuing chemotherapy or allo-SCT without cranial radiotherapy, based on risk stratification and minimal residual disease (MRD) levels at the end of induction. Patients with late isolated CNS relapses (more than 6 months after stopping therapy) were not eligible for the allo-SCT option, based on previous observations showing that the majority are cured with chemotherapy and CNS directed radiotherapy [14,15]. All other patients were treated on an uniform strategy for relapsed disease. Very early CNS relapses (within 18 months from first diagnosis) and early (more than 18 months from first diagnosis but within 6 months of stopping therapy) or late c-CNS relapses with high MRD were eligible for allo-SCT. In patients with early or late c-CNS disease where MRD results were not available, based on our previous reported experience [14], allo-SCT was offered to all those in whom relapse had occurred within 24 months of stopping therapy. Relapses occurring 24 months after stopping therapy were not eligible for an allo-SCT. Using these criteria, all early i-CNS relapses were eligible for an allo-SCT. In ALL R3, a randomisation of Mitoxantrone and Idarubicin was performed. The Idarubicin metabolite idarubicinol is thought to cross the blood brain barrier and Mitoxantrone to be active against quiescent cells. Thus the former could be more active in CNS disease and the latter in systemic relapses. We recently reported on the premature closure of the randomisation due to overall benefits of Mitoxantrone in all categories of relapsed ALL [22]. What remained unclear, in the light of the different properties of the drugs, whether this extended to those with CNS relapse? Though the randomisation is now closed, the trial continues to recruit to answer secondary objectives.

We now report on a prospective cohort analysis of the subgroup of patients with CNS relapses treated on the ALL R3 trial. The analysis thus includes patients recruited in both the randomised and non-randomised phases of the trial.

Materials and Methods

The protocol for this trial and supporting CONSORT checklist are available as supportive information; see Checklist S1 and Protocol S1.

Patients

Patients aged 1–18 years with a first relapse of ALL, who had not received an allo-SCT in first complete remission (CR1), were eligible for the trial and were recruited from centres of the Children's Cancer and Leukaemia Group in UK and Ireland; Australian and New Zealand Children's Haematology and Oncology Group and the Dutch Children's Oncology Group. This reports includes patients recruited between 1st January 2003 and 31st March 2011, with a median follow up of 46 months. The trial was registered (ISRCTN 45724312 http://www.controlled-trials.com/ISRCTN45724312/ALLR3) on 1st October 2003, after recruitment started. At the time of trial start, it was recommended that trials be registered but not necessarily prior to subject recruitment, hence the short delay in ISRCTN

registration. The authors confirm that all ongoing and related trials for this drug/intervention are registered.

Ethics Statement

Ethics approval obtained from Research Ethics Committee for Wales in the UK, Research Ethics Committee, Our Lady's Children's Hospital in Ireland, Committee for Human Research (Arnhem – Nimegen Region) in the Netherlands and the Multi-Region Ethics Committee in New Zealand. The following Institutional Review Boards approved the study in Australia: Ethics Committee, The Children's Hospital at Westmead; Children, Youth and Women's Health Service Research Ethics Committee, Government of South Australia; Ethics in Human Research Committee, The Royal Children's Hospital, Melbourne; Royal Children's Hospital and Health Service District Ethics Committee, Queensland Government; Human Research Ethics Committee C, Southern Health; Hunter New England Human Research Ethics Committee, New South Wales Health; Mater Health Services in Human Research Ethics Committee, Brisbane. Written informed consent was obtained from patients or from parents or legal guardians.

Definitions

i-CNS disease was defined as more than 5 or more white blood cells per µl of CSF with morphological evidence of blasts or biopsy proven recurrence in the eye or brain with no morphological bone marrow involvement. A c-CNS relapse was defined as presence of CNS disease with $\geq 5\%$ blasts in a concomitant bone marrow aspirate. An isolated bone marrow (i-BM) relapse was defined as the presence of $\geq 25\%$ blasts in the bone marrow. Patients were defined as having achieved a second complete remission (CR2) if they had $<5\%$ blasts in the marrow; no blasts in the CSF or regression of extramedullary disease including ocular infiltration at the end of induction. Time to relapse was defined as, very early, within 18 months from first diagnosis; early, after 18 months of first diagnosis but within 6 months after end of therapy and late if more than 6 months after end of therapy. Progression Free Survival (PFS) was defined as time from registration date to the first of induction failure ($\geq 5\%$ blasts in the bone marrow or persistence of CSF blasts at the end of induction), relapse, death from any cause or a second malignancy. Overall Survival (OS) was defined as time from registration to date of death from any cause. For risk stratification at first diagnosis, the presence of $<25\%$ blasts in the marrow after 8 days (4-drug induction, NCI High Risk) or 15 days (3-drug induction, NCI Standard Risk) were defined as a rapid early response; $\geq 25\%$ blasts in the same categories was defined as a slow early response.

MRD

MRD was measured from marrow samples obtained at relapse for those with c-CNS at the end of induction using clonotypic markers for Ig/TCR rearrangements, by quantitative PCR as previously described [22]. MRD^{lo} was defined as fewer than 10^{-4} cells with two sensitive markers (quantitative range 10^{-4}) and MRD^{hi} as at least one marker of 10^{-4} cells or more at the end of induction. End of induction MRD analysis was not possible in patients with i-CNS [23].

Cytogenetics

Cytogenetic analysis was done in local laboratories and reviewed centrally by the Leukaemia Research Cytogenetic Group at the Northern Institute for Cancer Research, University of Newcastle. Diagnostic and relapse karyotypes were used to classify

Table 1. Characteristics of those with isolated (i-CNS) or combined (c-CNS) CNS relapses compared with those with an isolated bone marrow relapse (i-BM).

	c-CNS	i-CNS	i-BM
N	43	80	207
Age at relapse in years			
median (25th–75th)	8·7 (6·8–13·7)	8·4 (6·1–11·5)	9·75 (7–13·4)
Range	2·5–18·8	2·0–17·9	1·1–18·8
Gender			
Male:Female	27:16	61:19	104:103
Ratio	1·7:1	3·2:1	1:1
Time to Relapse in months			
median (25th–75th)	37 (23–47)	27 (21–34·3)	44 (33–61)
Range	6–92	5–90	5–155
Late	20 (47%)	12 (15%)	142 (69%)
Early	16 (37%)	55 (69%)	48 (23%)
Very Early	7 (16%)	13 (16%)	17 (8%)
Risk category (%)			
Standard	-	12 (15%)	-
Intermediate	20 (47%)	68 (85%)	135 (65%)
High	23 (53%)	-	72 (35%)
Immunophenotype			
B:T	36:7	61:19	189:18
Ratio	5:1	3:1	11:1
CSF blast count			
median (range)	97 (14–188)	97 (27–392)	NA
Bone Marrow Blast %			
median (range)	83·5 (48·5–95)	NA	90 (78–95)
Cytogenetics (%)			
progenitor B			
Good	15 (35)	28 (35)	77 (37)
Intermediate	11 (25)	18 (23)	63 (30)
Poor	5 (12)	6 (8)	34 (16)
Unknown	5 (12)	9 (11)	15 (7)
T-cell	7 (16)	19 (24)	18 (9)

Relapses within 18 months of first diagnosis were termed as Very Early; after 18 months but within 6 months of stopping therapy as Early and after 6 months of stopping therapy as Late. B = progenitor B cell; T = T-cell; CSF = cerebrospinal fluid. CSF blast count is presented as cells/μl of CSF. Risk stratification and cytogenetic classification have previously been described.

patients with progenitor B-cell into good, intermediate and poor risk cytogenetic subgroups based on the presence of specific chromosomal abnormalities and characterised by their relapse risk [24]. T-cell patients were characterised separately.

Treatment

The therapeutic protocol has been published [22] and available at http://www.medicine.manchester.ac.uk/images/cancer/PAYAC/documents/pdf/R3Protocolv4_31Aug2007.pdf. As per the trial design, all very early relapses and early and late c-CNS relapses with MRD levels $\geq 10^{-4}$ (MRD^{hi}) at the end of induction were eligible for allo-SCT as were early i-CNS relapses where an end of induction MRD assessment is uninformative. Where MRD was unavailable for technical reasons in patients with early or late c-CNS relapse, allo-SCT was recommended if disease recurrence was within 24 months of stopping therapy. Early and late c-CNS

relapses with MRD $<10^{-4}$ (MRD^{lo}) and late isolated CNS relapses were not eligible for transplantation, received 24 Gy as fractionated cranial irradiation prior to week 14 and continued on chemotherapy for a total of 104 weeks with no further intrathecal methotrexate. Transplanted patients were conditioned with cyclophosphamide and total body irradiation, There was a day 1 randomisation of Mitoxantrone versus Idarubicin. As previously reported, this randomisation closed in December 2007 after 212 patients had been recruited and all subsequent patients registered on the trial have received Mitoxantrone. Thus the patients analysed represent those in the randomised cohort as well as those enrolled post randomisation.

Statistical Analyses

This is a cohort analysis of those with CNS relapse from the ALL R3 trial. PFS and OS, time was calculated in months and the

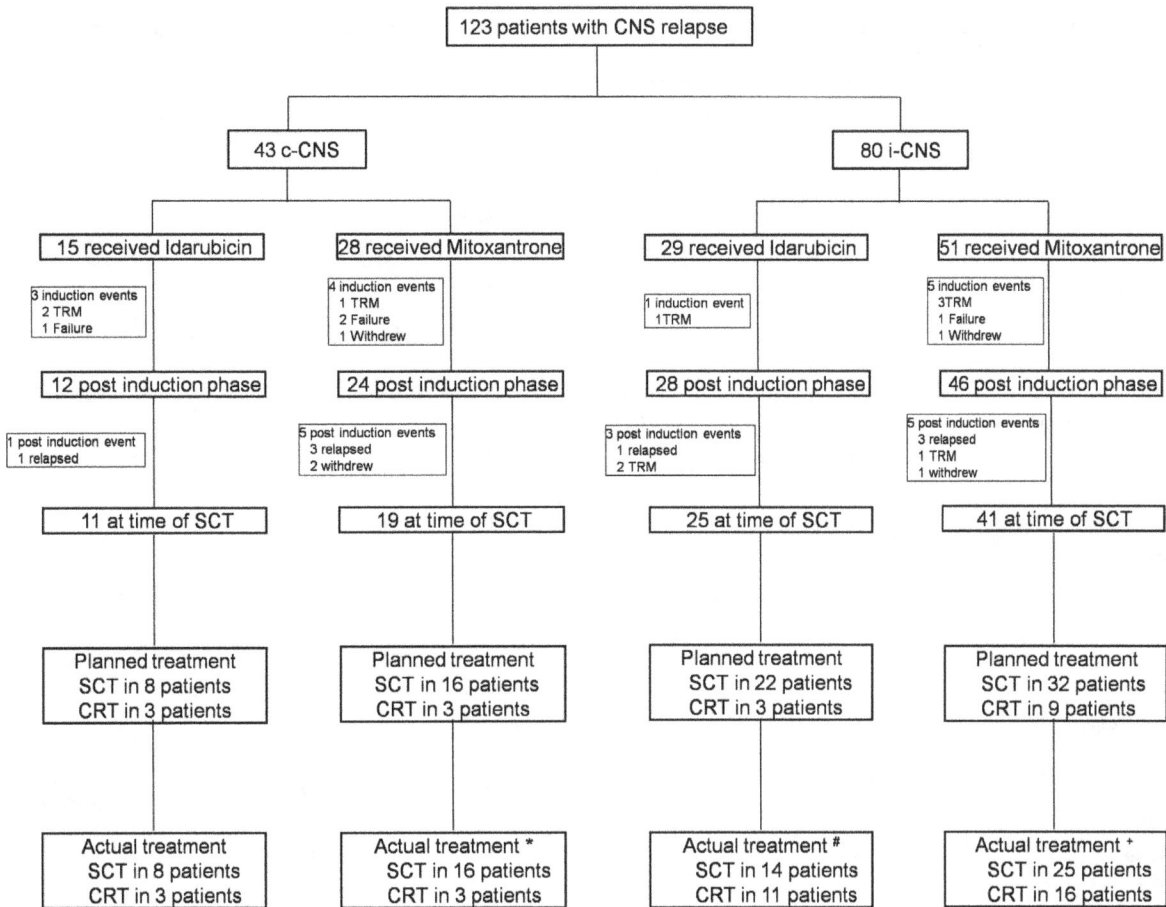

Figure 1. Consort diagram. Showing the details of patients with central nervous system (CNS) relapse. c-CNS = combined bone marrow and CNS relapse; i-CNS = isolated CNS relapse; TRM = treatment related mortality; SCT = allogenic bone marrow transplant; CRT = chemo-radiotherapy. *1 patient planned for SCT received CRT and vice-versa; #9 patients planned for SCT received CRT; +9 patients planned for SCT received CRT and 2 patients planned for CRT got SCT. No patients with i-CNS had detectable MRD in the marrow at the end of induction. Twenty four patients with c-CNS has detectable marrow disease at week 5; 13 MRD positive and 9 MRD negative.

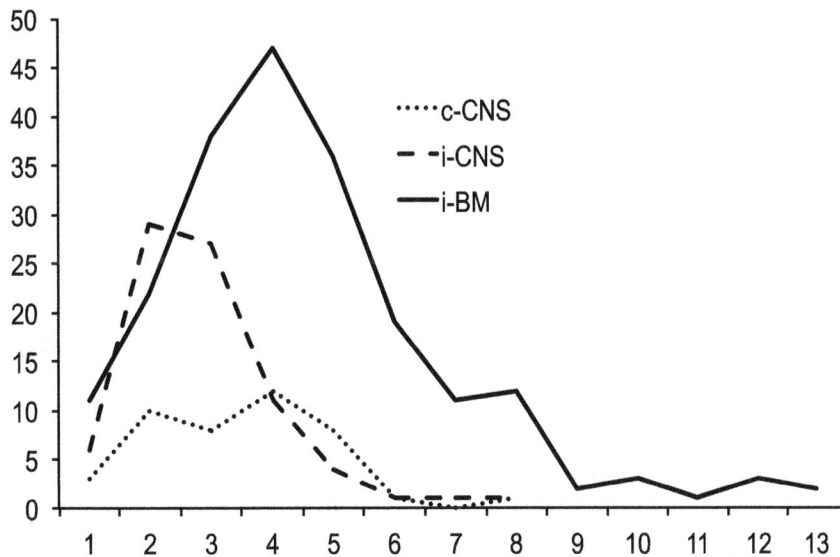

Figure 2. Temporal pattern of relapses. Isolated (iCNS) and combined (c-CNS) relapses occur significantly earlier than those with isolated bone marrow (iBM) relapses (Log rank p = <0.001). Figures in parenthesis show mean duration of remission in months for each group with ± standard deviation.

Table 2. Differences in outcome in patients with CNS relapse, allocated either transplantation or chemoradiotherapy according to whether they received Idarubicin or Mitoxantrone.

	c-CNS		i-CNS	
n	**43**		**80**	
	Ida	Mito	Ida	Mito
Induction				
n	**15**	**28**	**29**	**51**
TRM	2	1	1	3
Failure	1	2	0	1
Withdrawn	0	1	0	1
Allocated Treatment*				
n	**12**	**24**	**28**	**46**
SCT	9	21	25	36
No SCT	3	3	3	10
Post Induction				
n	**12**	**24**	**28**	**46**
TRM	0	0	2	2
Relapse	1	3	2	1
Withdrawn	0	2	0	2
SCT Time point				
Not Reached	0	0	0	3
Reached	11	19	24	38
Outcome				
SCT Group	8	16	21	30
Actual SCT	8	15	13	21
CR2	3	12	5	16
TRM	3	1	1	2
Relapse	2	2	6	3
Accidental Death	0	0	1	0
No-SCT	0	1	8	9
CR2	0	0	0	4
TRM	0	1	0	0
Relapse	0	0	8	5
Non-SCT Group	3	3	3	8
Actual non-SCT	3	2	3	6
CR2	1	1	3	5
TRM	1	0	0	0
Relapse	1	1	0	1
SCT	0	1	0	2
CR2	0	1	0	1
Second Malignancy	0	0	0	1

c-CNS = combined CNS relapse; i-CNS = isolated CNS relapse; TRM = Therapy related mortality; SCT = allogeneic transplantation; CR2 = second remission; Ida = Idarubicin; Mito = Mitoxantrone. *Patients allocated SCT were, all those with very early relapse; early i-CNS relapses and early and late c-CNS relapses with MRD $\geq 10^{-4}$ at the end of induction. Where MRD was not evaluable, decision to transplant was based on duration of CR1. All other patients were allocated chemoradiotherapy.

primary hypothesis generating analysis was performed using the Kaplan Meier method and log rank test. Cox regression analysis was done to assess the effect of type of CNS relapse after adjusting for pre-specified prognostic covariates; age group (<10, ≥ 10 years), immunophenotype (B-cell, T-cell), time to relapse (very early, early and late), cytogenetics (poor, intermediate, good, failed/unknown and T-cell), treatment drug (Idarubicin, Mitoxantrone) and sex. The Cox model for PFS was used to separately assess interactions of the treatment drug with the following variables; time to relapse, relapse site, immunophenotype and actual SCT. Interactions with the type of CNS relapse were assessed using the following covariates; time to relapse, immunophenotype and CSF blast count (≤ 50, 51–99, ≥ 100). For MRD at day 35, only intermediate risk patients were included. The proportional hazards assumption was assessed using Schoenfeld

Table 3. Endpoint of PFS and OS in patients with CNS relapse grouped by treatment allocation, and according to drug received Idarubicin vs Mitoxantrone.

	n	3 yr PFS (95% CI)	p-value	3 yr OS (95% CI)	p-value
Intended SCT	91				
Idarubicin	34	22·2% (9·9, 37·4)		34·0 (18·7, 49·9)	
Mitoxantrone	57	55·0% (39·4, 68·1)	0·02	63·0% (46·7, 75·5)	0·02
Intended No SCT	19				
Idarubicin	6	66·7% (19·5, 90·4)		66·7% (19·5, 90·4)	
Mitoxantrone	13	61·5% (26·6, 83·7)	0·90	68·6% (21·3, 91·2)	0·81
Actual SCT	60				
Idarubicin	21	36·4% (16·6, 56·6)		35·7% (16·1, 56·0)	
Mitoxantrone	39	72·2% (52·8, 84·7)	0·02	76·0% (55·6, 87·9)	0·01
Actual No SCT	32				
Idarubicin	14	28·6% (8·8, 52·4)		50·0% (22·9, 72·2)	
Mitoxantrone	18	50·4% (22·6, 72·9)	0·20	59·2% (17·6, 85·4)	0·39

residuals and was found to be acceptable in all cases. This analysis was performed using STATA version 11.

The cumulative distribution function was used to describe potential differences between age groups by treatment related events, defined as post induction failure and toxic-related deaths. For censored patients, time from registration to date last known alive or date of death if the patient did not have a disease related event was used. For toxic deaths, time to event was defined as time from date of registration to date of death if cause of death was due to toxicity.

Results

Three hundred and thirty children were recruited to the trial between January 1, 2003 and March 31, 2011. Of these, 207 had i-BM; 43 c-CNS and 80 i-CNS relapses (Table 1 and Figure 1). Comparing the two groups, CNS recurrence, in particular i-CNS was significantly higher for males (p = <0·001). Of the 44 T-cell relapses, 26 (59%) had recurrence in the CNS compared to 97 (34%) of 286 progenitor B-cell relapses (p = 0·001). The temporal patterns of CNS relapses were similar and peaked before i-BM disease (p = <0.001) (Figure 2). The median follow up was 46·1 (39·8–52·7) months for all patients (95% CI, reverse Kaplan-Meier method). The estimated 3-year PFS and OS of the whole group (n = 330) were 51·2% (45·3, 56·9) and 58·3% (52·3, 63·9) respectively. Further analyses with respect to this report are restricted to the outcome of those with a CNS relapse (n = 123). The estimated 3-year PFS for those with c-CNS and i-CNS were 40·6% (25·1, 55·6) and 38·0% (26·2, 49·7) p = 0.876 respectively. The estimated 3-year OS for those with c-CNS and i-CNS were 40·9% (24·9, 56·3), 50·8% (37·5, 62·6) p = 0·303 respectively.

A schema of the risk stratified treatment approach, based on duration of first remission, immunophenotype and site of relapse, for those with CNS disease is shown in Table S1 in File S1, along with the numbers of patients in each risk group and the allocation for allo-SCT or chemoradiotherapy. Table 2 shows the progression with therapy. 30/43 (70%) and 62/77 (81%) evaluable c-CNS and i-CNS patients completed 3 blocks of intensive therapy to reach the time to transplant (chi-squared test, p = 0.182). Excluding the 13 patients who were withdrawn or had an event during induction, as per the stratification adopted in the trial, 91 patients were eligible for allo-SCT and 19 for chemoradiotherapy.

We have previously reported a better outcome for 87 of the 123 patients with CNS relapse who received Mitoxantrone [22]. This continues to the case in this extended cohort with a significant (log rank p = 0.042) increase in disease recurrence in patients who received Idarubicin (Figure S1 in File S1). Mitoxantrone was associated with a significant PFS and OS 3-year survival rates advantage in patients eligible for/or who received an allo-SCT when compared to those patients eligible for/who received Idarubicin (Table 3 and Figure S2 in File S1).

Fifty one i-CNS patients, with very early or early relapse and eligible for allo-SCT reached the time point for transplantation (week 13). In the Idarubicin group, 3 of 4 very early and 10 of 17 early relapses were transplanted. In the Mitoxantrone group, all 5 very early and 16 of 25 early relapses were transplanted. The 3-year PFS and OS for 21 i-CNS patients treated with Idarubicin was 21.2 [11.9, 30.5] and 35.6 [24.9, 46.3]; and for 30 patients treated with Mitoxantrone were 60.7 [50.8, 70.6] and 70.8 [61.4, 80.2] respectively (p = 0.027 for PFS and p = 0.032 for OS). Of those eligible for but not transplanted, 13/17 have relapsed. In contrast, there has been only 1 relapse in the 11 patients with late i-CNS relapses not eligible for allo-SCT. For those with c-CNS relapses, the numbers are small, but 15 of 24 patients eligible for allo-SCT are in CR2 (3-year PFS 62.2 [51.4, 73], 3-year OS 65.5 [54.6, 76.4]).

Table 4 shows the 3-year PFS, OS and the univariate unadjusted hazard ratio (HR) for PFS and OS for various factors contributing to outcome. From the analysed risk factors at original diagnosis, presenting age, but not white cell count or early response to therapy were predictive of outcome at CNS relapse. At relapse, late recurrence, age less than 10 years, progenitor B-cell disease, standard and intermediate risk groups, good risk cytogenetics and those who received Mitoxantrone had a better prognosis. As the randomisation was terminated early there was an imbalance in patients receiving Mitoxantrone. Adjusting for the variables (age at relapse, time to relapse, cytogenetics, treatment drug and gender) in a multivariate analysis, showed a poorer outcome for those with c-CNS relapse (HR 1·82, 95% CI 0·98, 3·40, p = 0·059 c-index = 0.70 95% CI 0.64,0.75 for PFS and HR 2·64, 95% CI 1·32, 5·31, p = 0·006 c-index = 0.72 95% CI 0.66,0.78 for OS).

Table 4. Outcome of those with a CNS relapses in ALL R3 by risk parameters defined at first diagnosis, and at relapse.

	N	%PFS	%OS	Univariate Analysis			
				PFS		OS	
				Hazard ratio	p-value	Hazard ratio	p-value
At Original Diagnosis							
Presenting WC							
WC <50×10⁹/l	73	53·8 (40·2, 65·6)	46·6 (34·1,58·1)	1		1	
WC ≥50×10⁹/l	35	42·9 (25·0, 59·6)	31·6 (16·0-48·3)	1·37 (0·81, 2·32)	0·246	1·19 (0·67, 2·13)	0·549
Unknown	15	-	-				
Age at Diagnosis							
<10 years	97	54·8 (43·1, 65·1)	46·0 (34·8, 56·4)	1		1	
≥10 years	26	15·5 (2·9, 37·3)	9·9 (0·9,31·9)	3·03 (1·79, 5·12)	<0·001	2·76 (1·57, 4·87)	<0·001
Early Response							
Rapid Early Response	67	47·5 (33·7, 60·0)	39·6 (27·1, 51·8)	1		1	
Slow Early Response	29	42·1 (23·5, 59·7)	35·8 (18·6, 53·4)	1·40 (0·79, 2·46)	0·245	1·41 (0·77, 2·58)	0·261
Unknown	27	-	-				
At Relapse							
Age at relapse							
<10 years	78	48·2 (36·6, 59·8)	55·4 (42·1, 66·7)	1		1	
≥10 years	45	22·9 (10·7, 37·9)	33·1 (17·9, 49·0)	2·11 (1·31, 3·40)	0·002	1·94 (1·15, 3·24)	0·012
Gender							
Female	35	44·5 (26·1, 61·4)	42·3 (23·9, 59·5)	1		1	
Male	88	36·5 (25·6, 47·6)	49·1 (36·8, 60·3)	1·30 (0·75, 2·50)	0·354	0·98 (0·56, 1·72)	0·94
Immunophenotype							
B-cell	97	41·9 (31·1, 52·3)	51·7 (39·9, 62·2)	1		1	
T-cell	26	33·9 (16·7, 52·0)	33·3 (14·8, 53·1)	1·95 (1·12, 3·41)	0·019	2·09 (1·16, 3·76)	0·014
Time to Relapse							
Late	32	64·0 (44·2, 78·3)	69·1 (48·7, 82·7)	1		1	
Early	71	27·1 (15·8, 39·8)	36·2 (22·9, 49·7)	2·45 (1·29, 4·70)		2·56 (1·26, 5·17)	
Very Early	20	32·0 (12·3, 53·8)	41·9 (19·5, 63·0)	2·95 (1·34, 6·52)	0·012	2·53 (1·07, 5·98)	0·029
Site of Relapse							
i-CNS	80	38·0 (26·2, 49·7)	50·8 (37·5, 62·6)	1		1	
c-CNS	43	40·6 (25·1, 55·6)	40·9 (24·9, 56·3)	1·04 (0·634, 1·704)	0·876	1·32 (0·78, 2·22)	0·304
CNS Blast Count (/µl)							
<50	42	35·9 (20·0, 52·0)	39·3 (22·4, 55·9)	1		1	
50-99	13	-	16·2 (1·1, 48·1)	1·59 (0·75, 3·36)		1·31 (0·57, 2·97)	
≥100	54	39·4 (25·1, 53·4)	52·8 (36·6, 66·7)	0·93 (0·54, 1·60)	0·335	0·69 (0·38, 1·25)	0·238

Table 4. Cont.

| | N | %PFS | %OS | Univariate Analysis | | | | |
| | | | | PFS | | OS | | |
				Hazard ratio	p-value	Hazard ratio	p-value
Unknown	14	-	-				
Risk category							
Standard	12	64·8 (31·0, 85·2)	80·2 (40·3, 94·8)	1		1	
Intermediate	88	41·4 (30·0, 52·3)	50·5 (38·3, 61·5)	1·87 (0·67, 5·21)		3·29 (0·79, 13·63)	
High	23	15·5 (3·0, 37·2)	11·6 (1·0, 36·9)	3·99 (1·34, 11·94)	0·008	7·85 (1·79, 34·43)	0·002
Cytogenetics							
progenitor B							
Good	43	54·8 (38·1, 68·8)	63·5 (45·0, 77·3)	1		1	
Intermediate	29	32·8 (16·0, 50·8)	41·8 (22·7, 59·9)	1·71 (0·89,3·27)		1·96 (0·95, 4·01)	
Poor	11	10·2 (1·0,36·4)	35·1 (8·4, 64·1)	4·38 (1·95,9·82)		3·55 (1·43, 8·82)	
Unknown	14	43·5 (8·3, 75·7)	43·5 (8·3, 75·7)	1·21 (0·45,3·25)		1·95 (0·70, 5·43)	
T-cell	26	33·9 (16·7, 52·0)	33·3 (14·8, 53·1)	2·85 (1·46,5·54)	0·0018	3·31 (1·60, 6·84)	0·0126
Therapy							
Idarubicin	44	26·5 (14·4, 40·1)	35·5 (21·7,49·5)	1		1	
Mitoxantrone	79	48·9 (36·0, 60·6)	56·9 (42·9,68·7)	0·65 (0·40,1·04)	0·075	0·57 (0·34, 0·97)	0·036

Rapid early response = <25% blasts in the marrow aspirate on day 8/15 of induction; Slow early response = ≥25% blasts in the marrow aspirate on day 8/15 of induction.

Table 5. Characteristics of patients aged younger than 10, or 10 and older with CNS relapses.

Age at Relapse (years)	<10	≥10
n	**78**	**45**
CNS relapse (%)		
Isolated	53 (68)	27 (60)
Combined	25 (32)	18 (40)
Gender		
Male: Female	51:27	37:8
Time to Relapse (%)		
median in months (range)	29 (5–92)	33 (6–90)
Late	18 (23)	14 (31)
Early	48 (62)	23 (51)
Very Early	12 (15)	8 (18)
Risk category		
Standard	4 (5)	8 (18)
Intermediate	63 (81)	25 (55)
High	11 (14)	12 (27)
Immunophenotype		
B:T	66:12	31:14
Cytogenetics (%)		
progenitor-B cell		
Good	32 (41)	11 (24)
Intermediate	18 (23)	11 (24)
Poor	5 (6)	6 (13)
Unknown	11 (14)	3 (7)
T-cell	12 (15)	14 (22)

The late isolated relapses in the i-CNS group have the best outcome (10 of 11 patients are in CR2) and a better salvage rate, so a difference in the adjusted outcome is to be expected. Additionally for PFS multivariate analyses separate assessments of interaction of the treatment drug with time to relapse, relapse site, immunophenotype and actual SCT were not statistically significant. Similarly, the interaction of type of CNS with time to relapse, immunophenotype and CSF blast count were not statistically significant. Exploratory multivariate analysis using pre-specified subgroups showed that age at relapse ≥10 years had an unfavourable outcome (HR 1.91, 95% CI 1.11, 3.28, p = 0.018 for PFS and HR 1.90, 95% CI 1.07, 3.35, p = 0.027 for OS). We tested the effect of potential imbalances of prognostic factors in the two age groups. There were proportionately more c-CNS, males, standard risk, T-cell immunophenotype and fewer good risk cytogenetic patients in the ≥10 year age group (Table 5). Figure 3, shows the risk ratios for PFS, for age at relapse according to the different characteristics. Patients age ≥10 years had a significantly worse outcome in all categories except in those who had good risk cytogenetics. To investigate whether differences seen between the two age groups was due to disease progression and/or side effects of treatment we examined the cumulative percentage of events. As shown in Figure 4 although disease related events are similar between the two groups 24/77 (31%) and 13/44 (30%) for age groups <10 and > = 10 respectively (p = 0.852), older patients relapsed earlier. Overall treatment related mortality was higher in older patients in all phases of

therapy 10/77 (13%) and 13/44 (30%) for age groups <10 and > = 10 respectively (p = 0.026).

Of the 36 second relapses, five (14%) (Four with i-CNS and one with c-CNS) have subsequently achieved CR3 (Table S2 in File S1). Of the 28 patients who relapsed after either receiving a transplant or cranial radiotherapy, there were 19 CNS (17 i-CNS and 2 c-CNS) and 9 i-BM relapses. Thirteen of the 19 CNS relapses were patients who had not been transplanted but had received cranial irradiation. Six of the nine post transplant relapses in the i-CNS group occurred in those with a very early relapse. Thus, salvage after a CNS relapse remains low with a high frequency of disease recurrence in those who received cranial irradiation.

Discussion

The survival rates of patients treated with mitoxantrone reported here are better than we have previously reported for c-CNS and comparable for those with i-CNS [14]. All relapses described here are of children treated on protocols in existence from 2000 onwards. In the UK these are primarily ALL97 [25] and ALL2003 [26]. This analysis suggests that there has been a change in pattern of CNS relapses in the post 2000 era. While we previously reported i-CNS to c-CNS ratio of 1·1 [10], in this report it is 1·9. There also appears to be a temporal change in the pattern of i-CNS relapses with a decrease in very early from 42% to 16% and a proportionate increase in early to 69% from 45%. Thus with

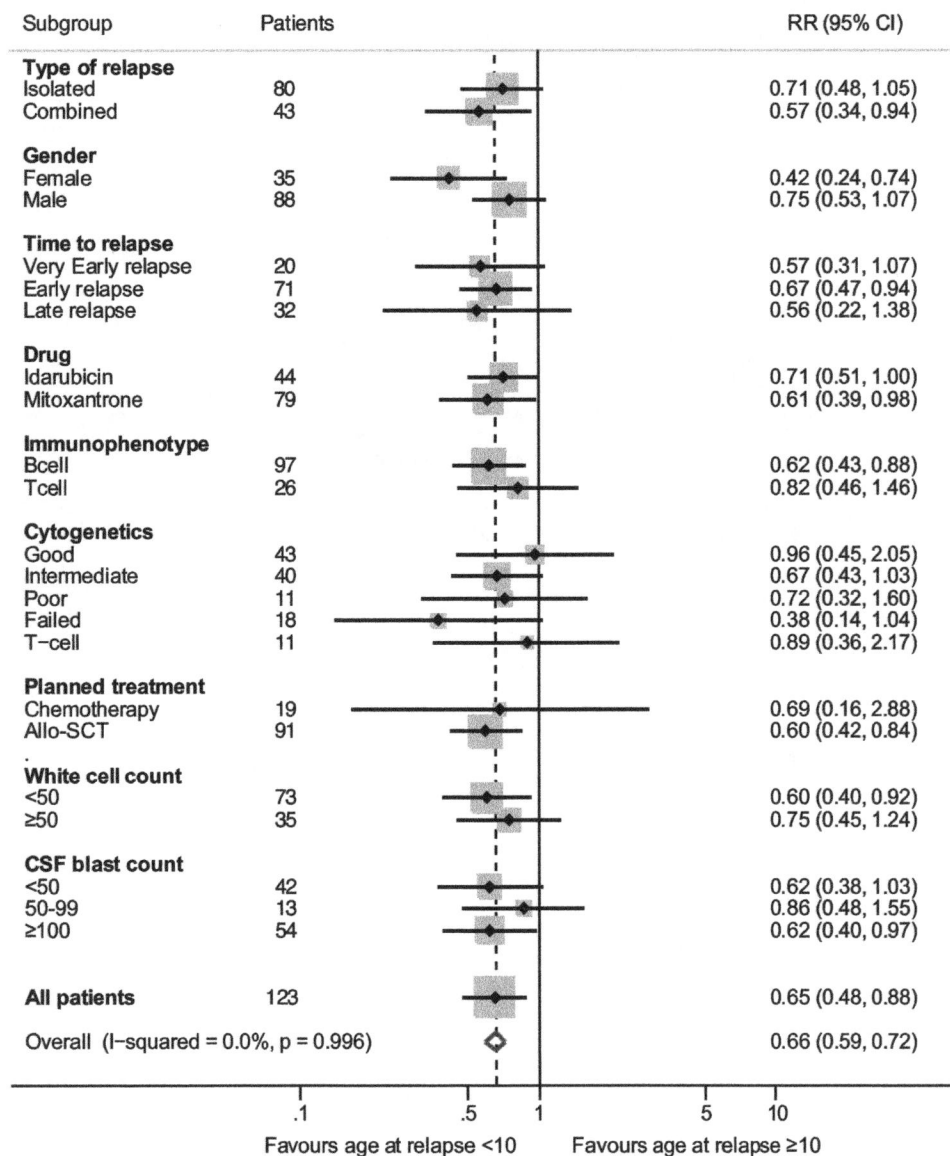

Figure 3. Age at relapse (<10 or ≥10 years) effect on progression-free survival by patient characteristics, from Cox models with interactions. White cell count is the presenting count ($\times 10^9$/L) at first diagnosis. Relative risk ratios indicate that all subgroups show a poorer outcome in those ≥10 years, except good risk cytogenetics.

time there is an apparent shift towards earlier and c-CNS relapses both of which are associated with an inferior outcome.

The rarity of relapse makes subgroup analyses problematical. However relapsed ALL remains the leading cause of death in children with cancer and our observations may help physicians managing such patients. The key findings of this study are the benefits of, Mitoxantrone for all patients and allo-SCT for early and very early i-CNS relapses. We have previously suggested that the benefit of Mitoxantrone may be related to its toxic effect on the microenvironment [22]. Allogeneic transplantation may have a similar effect, though this study is not designed to answer this question. What is evidenced is that after intensive systemic therapy, consolidation of remission with allo-SCT offers a better curative approach over targeted CNS directed therapy for very early and early CNS relapses. In those with early and very early i-CNS disease, 71% of those allocated allo-SCT but not transplanted (receiving chemoradiotherapy) suffered a second

relapse, while recurrence rates were 21% in those transplanted. Late i-CNS relapses occurring off modern intensive chemotherapy regimens continue to be curable with chemo-radiotherapy. There were only a few patients with c-CNS disease not eligible for transplantation. Of the 5 not transplanted, 2 are in CR2. Of the 23 transplanted, 15 are in CR2. Given the poor salvage rate after a second relapse, a more simple approach would be to offer an allo-SCT to all CNS relapses except those with a late i-CNS recurrence.

The poorer outcome of adolescent patients with CNS relapse has been previously reported in a retrospective analysis. Therapy was not uniform and other potential contributing factors to the worse outcome were not examined [9]. In our study, a uniform therapeutic approach, stratified for risk, was taken for all patients, with good results in those aged under 10 but not for older children. The older age group had proportionately more patients with T-cell disease and less with good-risk cytogenetics. The inferior

A

B

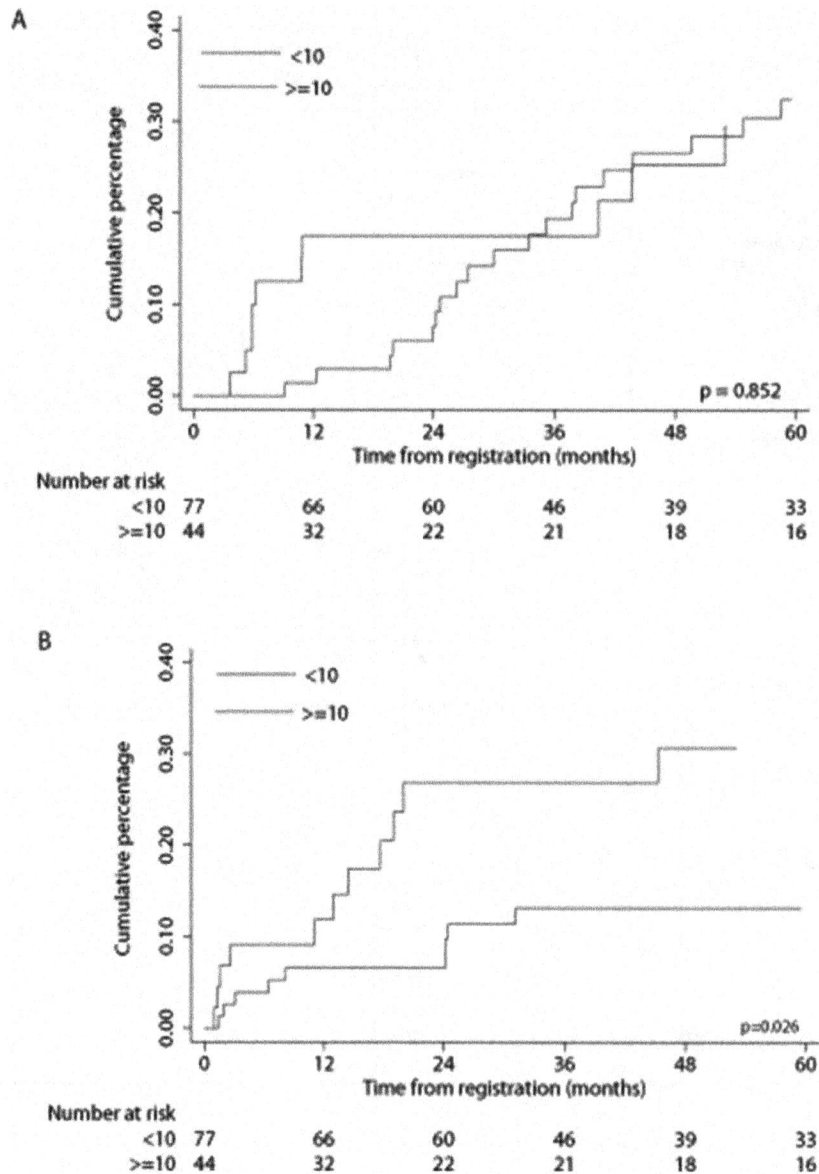

Figure 4. Cumulative percentage of events, in those aged <10 and ≥10 years at first relapse. (A) Therapeutic failure, which includes both induction failures and second relapses. (B) Treatment related deaths.

survival of very early and T-cell relapses has been a consistent theme [13–15] and in this study, T-cell relapses occurred earlier and in older patients. Good-risk cytogenetics are associated with late relapses [24] and a better prognosis in older patients [27]. Thus both immunophenotype and cytogenetics contributed to the earlier relapse pattern observed in those ≥10 years of age.

The worse outcomes for the ≥10 year age group in this trial were primarily related to toxicity. Paediatric type protocols have considerably improved the outcome of adolescents and young adults newly diagnosed with ALL [28,29]. This improvement comes at a price of increased toxicity, primarily that of sepsis, osteonecrosis and thrombosis [29,30]. In ALL R3 we shortened the duration of steroid exposure and used a pegylated derivative to decrease the dose of asparaginase. Neither thrombosis nor osteonecrosis have been of significance though sepsis in older children remains a problem. As older patients tend to relapse early further cytotoxic intensification is not possible. The successor trial

for ALLR3, IntReALL 2010 [31] will use the non-toxic targeted drug Epratuzamab in conjunction with post induction therapy patients with late and early CNS relapses. Though Epratuzamab does not cross the blood-brain, our data suggests that systemic therapy is key to maintaining remission in those with a CNS relapse. Thus IntReALL will evaluate if a non-toxic intervention is able to improve the outcome of older patients with relapses in the CNS.

The pathogenesis of CNS disease in ALL remains enigmatic, hindering the development of more targeted less toxic strategies. Recent evidence suggests that leukemic blasts circulate in the blood to the CNS, where they transgress blood-brain and blood-CSF barriers by diapedesis rather than by haemorrhage [32]. The subarachnoid tissue may then provide a chemoprotective microenvironment for lymphoblasts [33] giving rise to recurrence once therapy is discontinued. This supports the use of systemic therapy to prevent and treat CNS recurrence. As illustrated by this report, while the management of relapsed CNS disease using intensive systemic approaches has met with some success, it remains less than satisfactory. We need new agents and novel approaches, based on a better understanding of the disease process. A good proportion of patients eligible for early phase trials are in the older age group. Thus when evaluating new agents, we will also need to allow for age related variations in the therapeutic response, both with regards to efficacy and toxicity, lest we come to inexact conclusions.

Supporting Information

File S1 Additional information on survival and further relapse rates by drug (Idarubicin & Mitoxantrone). Details of risk stratification and treatment allocation and also outcome following second relapse.

Checklist S1 CONSORT checklist.

Protocol S1 Trial Protocol.

Acknowledgments

The Central Manchester University Hospitals NHS Trust is the current sponsor of the trial. We thank the participating children and their families and the physicians who enrolled their patients into the study and members of the CRUK IS team who maintain the trial database. We acknowledge the members of the Data Monitoring Committee, Mike Stevens, Moira Stewart and Rob Edwards for their role.

Author Contributions

Conceived and designed the experiments: VS SL. Performed the experiments: JH NG RS AVM. Analyzed the data: AM CP VS SL MS. Contributed reagents/materials/analysis tools: JH NG RS AVM. Wrote the paper: AM CP SL MS VS. Trial coordinators: VS PD CF TR MM PA PH.

References

1. Pui CH, Thiel E (2009) Central nervous system disease in hematologic malignancies: historical perspective and practical applications. Seminars in Oncology 36: S2–S16.
2. Conter V, Arico M, Basso G, Biondi A, Barisone E, et al. (2010) Long-term results of the Italian Association of Pediatric Hematology and Oncology (AIEOP) Studies 82, 87, 88, 91 and 95 for childhood acute lymphoblastic leukemia. Leukemia 24: 255–264.
3. Gaynon PS, Angiolillo AL, Carroll WL, Nachman JB, Trigg ME, et al. (2010) Long-term results of the children's cancer group studies for childhood acute lymphoblastic leukemia 1983–2002: a Children's Oncology Group Report. Leukemia 24: 285–297.
4. Kamps WA, van der Pal-de Bruin KM, Veerman AJ, Fiocco M, Bierings M, et al. (2010) Long-term results of Dutch Childhood Oncology Group studies for children with acute lymphoblastic leukemia from 1984 to 2004. Leukemia 24: 309–319.
5. Mitchell C, Richards S, Harrison CJ, Eden T (2010) Long-term follow-up of the United Kingdom medical research council protocols for childhood acute lymphoblastic leukaemia, 1980–2001. Leukemia 24: 406–418.
6. Moricke A, Zimmermann M, Reiter A, Henze G, Schrauder A, et al. (2010) Long-term results of five consecutive trials in childhood acute lymphoblastic leukemia performed by the ALL-BFM study group from 1981 to 2000. Leukemia 24: 265–284.
7. Schmiegelow K, Forestier E, Hellebostad M, Heyman M, Kristinsson J, et al. (2010) Long-term results of NOPHO ALL-92 and ALL-2000 studies of childhood acute lymphoblastic leukemia. Leukemia 24: 345–354.
8. Silverman LB, Stevenson KE, O'Brien JE, Asselin BL, Barr RD, et al. (2010) Long-term results of Dana-Farber Cancer Institute ALL Consortium protocols for children with newly diagnosed acute lymphoblastic leukemia (1985–2000). Leukemia 24: 320–334.
9. Tsurusawa M, Shimomura Y, Asami K, Kikuta A, Watanabe A, et al. (2010) Long-term results of the Japanese Childhood Cancer and Leukemia Study Group studies 811, 841, 874 and 911 on childhood acute lymphoblastic leukemia. Leukemia 24: 335–344.
10. Krishnan S, Wade R, Moorman AV, Mitchell C, Kinsey SE, et al. (2010) Temporal changes in the incidence and pattern of central nervous system relapses in children with acute lymphoblastic leukaemia treated on four consecutive Medical Research Council trials, 1985–2001. Leukemia 24: 450–459.
11. Pui CH, Campana D, Pei D, Bowman WP, Sandlund JT, et al. (2009) Treating childhood acute lymphoblastic leukemia without cranial irradiation. N Engl J Med 360: 2730–2741.
12. Gaynon PS, Qu RP, Chappell RJ, Willoughby ML, Tubergen DG, et al. (1998) Survival after relapse in childhood acute lymphoblastic leukemia: impact of site and time to first relapse–the Children's Cancer Group Experience. Cancer 82: 1387–1395.
13. Nguyen K, Devidas M, Cheng SC, La M, Raetz EA, et al. (2008) Factors influencing survival after relapse from acute lymphoblastic leukaemia: a Children's Oncology Group study. Leukemia 22: 2142–2150.
14. Roy A, Cargill A, Love S, Moorman AV, Stoneham S, et al. (2005) Outcome after first relapse in childhood acute lymphoblastic leukaemia - lessons from the United Kingdom R2 trial. British Journal of Haematology 130: 67–75.
15. Tallen G, Ratei R, Mann G, Kaspers G, Niggli F, et al. (2010) Long-Term Outcome in Children With Relapsed Acute Lymphoblastic Leukemia After Time-Point and Site-of-Relapse Stratification and Intensified Short-Course Multidrug Chemotherapy: Results of Trial ALL-REZ BFM 90. Journal of

clinical oncology : official journal of the American Society of Clinical Oncology: 10.1200/JCO.2009.1225.1983
16. Eapen M, Zhang MJ, Devidas M, Raetz E, Barredo JC, et al. (2008) Outcomes after HLA-matched sibling transplantation or chemotherapy in children with acute lymphoblastic leukemia in a second remission after an isolated central nervous system relapse: a collaborative study of the Children's Oncology Group and the Center for International Blood and Marrow Transplant Research. Leukemia 22: 281–286.
17. Harker-Murray PD, Thomas AJ, Wagner JE, Weisdorf D, Luo X, et al. (2008) Allogeneic hematopoietic cell transplantation in children with relapsed acute lymphoblastic leukemia isolated to the central nervous system. Biology of Blood and Marrow Transplantation 14: 685–692.
18. Messina C, Valsecchi MG, Arico M, Locatelli F, Rossetti F, et al. (1998) Autologous bone marrow transplantation for treatment of isolated central nervous system relapse of childhood acute lymphoblastic leukemia. AIEOP/FONOP-TMO group. Associazione Italiana Emato-Oncologia Pediatrica. Bone marrow transplantation 21: 9–14.
19. Ribeiro RC, Rivera GK, Hudson M, Mulhern RK, Hancock ML, et al. (1995) An intensive re-treatment protocol for children with an isolated CNS relapse of acute lymphoblastic leukemia. Journal of Clinical Oncology 13: 333–338.
20. Ritchey AK, Pollock BH, Lauer SJ, Andejeski Y, Barredo J, et al. (1999) Improved survival of children with isolated CNS relapse of acute lymphoblastic leukemia: a pediatric oncology group study. Journal of Clinical Oncology 17: 3745–3752.
21. Yoshihara T, Morimoto A, Kuroda H, Imamura T, Ishida H, et al. (2006) Allogeneic stem cell transplantation in children with acute lymphoblastic leukemia after isolated central nervous system relapse: our experiences and review of the literature. Bone marrow transplantation 37: 25–31.
22. Parker C, Waters R, Leighton C, Hancock J, Sutton R, et al. (2010) Effect of mitoxantrone on outcome of children with first relapse of acute lymphoblastic leukaemia (ALL R3): an open-label randomised trial. Lancet 376: 2009–2017.
23. Hagedorn N, Acquaviva C, Fronkova E, von Stackelberg A, Barth A, et al. (2007) Submicroscopic bone marrow involvement in isolated extramedullary relapses in childhood acute lymphoblastic leukemia: a more precise definition of "isolated" and its possible clinical implications, a collaborative study of the Resistant Disease Committee of the International BFM study group. Blood 110: 4022–4029.
24. Moorman AV, Ensor HM, Richards SM, Chilton L, Schwab C, et al. (2010) Prognostic effect of chromosomal abnormalities in childhood B-cell precursor acute lymphoblastic leukaemia: results from the UK Medical Research Council ALL97/99 randomised trial. The lancet oncology 11: 429–438.
25. Mitchell CD, Richards SM, Kinsey SE, Lilleyman J, Vora A, et al. (2005) Benefit of dexamethasone compared with prednisolone for childhood acute lymphoblastic leukaemia: results of the UK Medical Research Council ALL97 randomized trial. British Journal of Haematology 129: 734–745.
26. Vora A, Goulden N, Wade R, Mitchell C, Hancock J, et al. (2013) Treatment reduction for children and young adults with low-risk acute lymphoblastic leukaemia defined by minimal residual disease (UKALL 2003): a randomised controlled trial. The Lancet Oncology 14: 199–209.
27. Moorman AV, Chilton L, Wilkinson J, Ensor HM, Bown N, et al. (2010) A population-based cytogenetic study of adults with acute lymphoblastic leukemia. Blood 115: 206–214.
28. Huguet F, Leguay T, Raffoux E, Thomas X, Beldjord K, et al. (2009) Pediatric-inspired therapy in adults with Philadelphia chromosome-negative acute

lymphoblastic leukemia: the GRAALL-2003 study. Journal of Clinical Oncology 27: 911–918.

29. Pui CH, Pei D, Campana D, Bowman WP, Sandlund JT, et al. (2011) Improved prognosis for older adolescents with acute lymphoblastic leukemia. Journal of Clinical Oncology 29: 386–391.

30. Rijneveld AW, van der Holt B, Daenen SM, Biemond BJ, de Weerdt O, et al. (2011) Intensified chemotherapy inspired by a pediatric regimen combined with allogeneic transplantation in adult patients with acute lymphoblastic leukemia up to the age of 40. Leukemia 25: 1697–1703.

31. EU-project IntReALL website. Available: http://www.intreall-fp7.eu/. Accessed 2014 Sep 10.

32. Holland M, Castro FV, Alexander S, Smith D, Liu J, et al. (2011) RAC2, AEP, and ICAM1 expression are associated with CNS disease in a mouse model of pre-B childhood acute lymphoblastic leukemia. Blood 118: 638–649.

33. Akers SM, Rellick SL, Fortney JE, Gibson LF (2011) Cellular elements of the subarachnoid space promote ALL survival during chemotherapy. Leukemia research 35: 705–711.

20

Detection of the G17V RHOA Mutation in Angioimmunoblastic T-Cell Lymphoma and Related Lymphomas Using Quantitative Allele-Specific PCR

Rie Nakamoto-Matsubara[1], Mamiko Sakata-Yanagimoto[1,2,3], Terukazu Enami[1], Kenichi Yoshida[4], Shintaro Yanagimoto[5], Yusuke Shiozawa[4], Tohru Nanmoku[6], Kaishi Satomi[7], Hideharu Muto[1,2,3], Naoshi Obara[1,2,3], Takayasu Kato[1,2,3,8], Naoki Kurita[1,2,3], Yasuhisa Yokoyama[1,2,3], Koji Izutsu[9,10], Yasunori Ota[11], Masashi Sanada[4], Seiichi Shimizu[3,12], Takuya Komeno[3,13], Yuji Sato[14], Takayoshi Ito[15], Issay Kitabayashi[16], Kengo Takeuchi[17], Naoya Nakamura[18], Seishi Ogawa[4], Shigeru Chiba[1,2,3,8]*

1 Department of Hematology, Graduate School of Comprehensive Human Sciences, University of Tsukuba, Tsukuba, Ibaraki, Japan, 2 Department of Hematology, Faculty of Medicine, University of Tsukuba, Tsukuba, Ibaraki, Japan, 3 Department of Hematology, University of Tsukuba Hospital, Tsukuba, Ibaraki, Japan, 4 Department of Pathology and Tumor Biology, Graduate School of Medicine, Kyoto University, Sakyo-ku, Kyoto, Japan, 5 Division for Health Service Promotion, The University of Tokyo, Bunkyo-ku, Tokyo, Japan, 6 Department of Clinical Laboratory, University of Tsukuba Hospital, Tsukuba, Ibaraki, Japan, 7 Department of Pathology, University of Tsukuba Hospital, Tsukuba, Ibaraki, Japan, 8 Life Science Center, Tsukuba Advanced Research Center, University of Tsukuba, Tsukuba, Ibaraki, Japan, 9 Department of Hematology, Toranomon Hospital, Minato-ku, Tokyo, Japan, 10 Okinaka Memorial Institute for Medical Research, Minato-ku, Tokyo, Japan, 11 Department of Pathology, Toranomon Hospital, Minato-ku, Tokyo, Japan, 12 Department of Hematology, Tsuchiura Kyodo General Hospital, Tsuchiura, Ibaraki, Japan, 13 Department of Hematology, Mito Medical Center, National Hospital Organization, Ibaraki-machi, Ibaraki, Japan, 14 Department of Hematology, Tsukuba Memorial Hospital, Tsukuba, Ibaraki, Japan, 15 Department of Hematology, JA Toride Medical Center, Toride, Ibaraki, Japan, 16 Division of Hematological Malignancy, National Cancer Center Research Institute, Chuo-ku, Tokyo, Japan, 17 Pathology Project for Molecular Targets, The Cancer Institute, Japanese Foundation for Cancer Research, Koto-ku, Tokyo, Japan, 18 Department of Pathology, Tokai University School of Medicine, Isehara, Kanagawa, Japan

Abstract

Angioimmunoblastic T-cell lymphoma (AITL) and peripheral T-cell lymphoma, not otherwise specified (PTCL-NOS) are subtypes of T-cell lymphoma. Due to low tumor cell content and substantial reactive cell infiltration, these lymphomas are sometimes mistaken for other types of lymphomas or even non-neoplastic diseases. In addition, a significant proportion of PTCL-NOS cases reportedly exhibit features of AITL (AITL-like PTCL-NOS). Thus disagreement is common in distinguishing between AITL and PTCL-NOS. Using whole-exome and subsequent targeted sequencing, we recently identified G17V *RHOA* mutations in 60–70% of AITL and AITL-like PTCL-NOS cases but not in other hematologic cancers, including other T-cell malignancies. Here, we establish a sensitive detection method for the G17V *RHOA* mutation using a quantitative allele-specific polymerase chain reaction (qAS-PCR) assay. Mutated allele frequencies deduced from this approach were highly correlated with those determined by deep sequencing. This method could serve as a novel diagnostic tool for 60–70% of AITL and AITL-like PTCL-NOS.

Editor: Kristy L. Richards, University of North Carolina at Chapel Hill, United States of America

Funding: This work was supported by Grants-in-Aid for Scientific Research (KAKENHI) (24390241, 23659482, 23118503, and 22130002 to S.C.; 25461407 to M.S.-Y.), and the Adaptable and Seamless Technology Transfer Program through target-driven R and D (A-STEP) to M.S.-Y. from the Ministry of Education, Culture, Sports, Science and Technology of Japan. This work was also supported by the Mochida Memorial Foundation for Medical and Pharmaceutical Research, and the Uehara Memorial Foundation to M.S.-Y. The funders had no role in study design, data collection and analysis, decision to publish, or preparation of the manuscript.

Competing Interests: The authors have declared that no competing interests exist.

* Email: schiba-tky@umin.net

Introduction

Based on the classification proposed by the World Health Organization (WHO), Angioimmunoblastic T-cell lymphoma (AITL) is a distinct subtype of T-cell lymphoma that accounts for 20% of peripheral T-cell lymphoma cases [1]. AITL is characterized by generalized lymphadenopathy, hyperglobulinemia, and autoimmune-like manifestations [1,2]. Pathologic examination of AITL tumors reveals polymorphous infiltration of reactive cells, including endothelial venules and follicular dendritic cells [3,4]. Based on gene expression profiling and immunohistochemical staining, the normal counterparts of AITL tumor cells are proposed to be follicular helper T cells (TFHs) [5]. Peripheral T-cell lymphoma, not otherwise specified (PTCL-NOS) is a more heterogenous type of lymphoma, one that shows variation even in CD4 and CD8 expression. Some PTCL-NOS cases share features of AITL, such as immunohistochemical

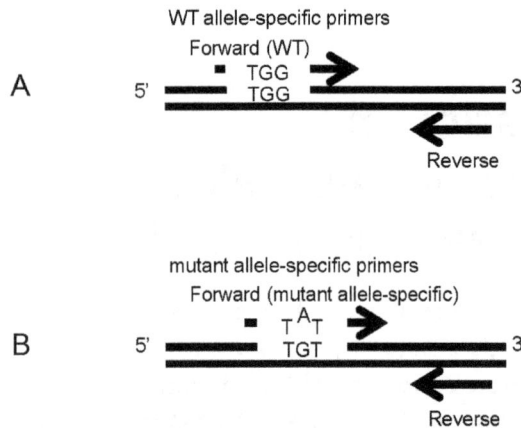

Figure 1. Design of primers used in the study. A WT allele-specific primer forward primer (Upper), a mutant allele-specific forward primer (Lower), and a common primer were designed. The 3′ end of the forward mutant primer was specific to the mutant site (G to T) and an internal mismatch at the second nucleotide from 3′ end (G to A) was introduced to improve specificity.

staining patterns resembling those seen in AITL (AITL-like PTCL-NOS) [6].

Expertise is required to diagnose AITL and PTCL-NOS because generally low tumor cell content obscures the neoplastic nature of some cases, and large reactive B-cells are often confused with tumor cells [7]. Clonal rearrangement of the T-cell receptor gene is undetectable in 10–25% of AITL cases due to low tumor cell frequency [1]. In addition, clonal growth of Epstein-Bar virus-infected B-cells is not uncommon in these kinds of cancers, causing detection of clonal immunoglobulin gene rearrangement in 20% of these case. [1].

Mutations in *TET2, IDH2,* and *DNMT3A* are frequently seen in AITL and AITL-like PTCL-NOS [8,9], although these mutations are also common to various myeloid malignancies [10,11]. We and others reported a large cohort of AITL and PTCL-NOS patients revealing that the G17V *RHOA* mutation was highly specific to AITL and AITL-like PTCL-NOS and very frequent (seen in 60–70% of cases) in these T-cell lymphomas [12,13]. This observation suggests that detection of the G17V *RHOA* mutation could serve as a new diagnostic tool to discriminate these lymphomas from other diseases. One difficulty, however, is that *RHOA* mutation allele frequencies in these lymphomas are generally as low as <0.2 or often <0.1, reflecting low tumor cell content. Therefore, diagnosis of these conditions requires development of sensitive and cost-efficient methods that are as accurate as deep sequencing, which is expensive and not commonly used in most clinical testing facilities.

To meet this need, we developed a quantitative allele-specific polymerase chain reaction (qAS-PCR) method that sensitively

detects the G17V *RHOA* mutation in a highly accurate manner. This assay should provide a realistic way to conduct laboratory testing to diagnose AITL and AITL-like PTCL-NOS.

Materials and Methods

Primer design

We designed two forward primers that discriminate wild-type (WT) from G17V *RHOA* for use with one common reverse primer. The mutant forward primer was designed using a previously described algorithm [14]. The 3′ end is specific to the mutant site and an internal mismatch at the second nucleotide from the 3′ end was introduced to improve specificity (Figure 1 and Table 1). We performed local alignment analysis using the BLAST program (http://www.ncbi.nlm.nih.gov/tools/primer-blast/) to confirm primer specificity.

Preparation of plasmids containing WT and mutant cDNA and standard curve generation

WT or G17V mutant *RHOA* cDNA was subcloned into pBluescript (pBS/wtRHOA or pBS/mutRHOA, respectively; Agilent Technologies, Santa Clara, CA). qPCR reactions were performed in a final volume of 20 μl using 10 nM primers and the SYBR-Green mix (Roche Applied Science, Mannheim, Germany), and amplicons were subjected to either the ABI7500 or 7900 Fast Sequence Detection Systems (Life Technologies, Carlsbad, CA). Use of either the WT or mutant forward primer plus the common primer generated a 73-bp PCR product. The following PCR conditions were used: 10 min at 95°C, followed by 40 cycles of 15 sec at 95°C and 60 sec at 60°C.

Standard curves of amplicon levels were created by qPCR using serially-diluted pBS/wtRHOA or pBS/mutRHOA with WT or mutant primers, respectively.

Preparation of template plasmid DNA mixtures

pBS/mutRHOA was mixed with pBS/wtRHOA in 100, 10, 1.0, 0.1, 0.01 and 0% ratios. Overall DNA concentration was adjusted to 1.0 ng/well of a plate. All mixtures were then serially-diluted 1:10 for 4 cycles. qPCR was performed with these templates plus primers using conditions described above.

Patients and samples

Tumor samples were collected from 53 patients with AITL, 55 with PTCL-NOS, 19 with B-cell malignancies, 129 with myeloid malignancies, and 5 with another T-cell lymphoma (for a total of 261), according to WHO classification. Twenty-seven non-tumor samples, including bone marrow mononuclear cells and buccal cells from lymphoma patients, were also analyzed as controls. The Ethics Committee University of Tsukuba Hospital approved the protocol and consent procedure, according to which written informed consent was provided by the participants. Genomic DNA was extracted from 13 formalin-fixed/paraffin-

Table 1. Sequence of allele-specific primers used for this study.

Primer	Sequence
Forward (WT*[1])	ATTGTTGGTGATGGAGCCTGTGG
Forward (MUT*[2])	ATTGTTGGTGATGGAGCCTGTAT
Reverse (common)	ACACCTCTGGGAACTGGTCCT

*[1] WT, wild-type; *[2] MUT, mutant.

Table 2. Analysis of genomic DNA samples.

Disease	Frozen amp*[1]	Frozen not-amp*[2]	PLP not-amp	FFPE not-amp	Total
AITL	14	10	19	10	53
PTCL-NOS	16	8	28	3	55
B-cell lymphoma	1	18			19
Myeloid malignancies	129				129
Other T-cell lymphomas		5			5
Control samples	27				27
Total	187	41	47	13	288

*[1]amp, amplified; *[2]not-amp, not-amplified.

embedded (FFPE), 47 periodate/lysine/paraformaldehyde (PLP)-fixed, and 228 fresh frozen specimens, using an FFPE tissue kit (QIAGEN, Hilden, Germany) for FFPE and PLP samples and a Puregene DNA blood kit (QIAGEN) for fresh frozen specimens, according to manufacturer's instructions.

One hundred and one DNA samples were original, while 187 were whole genome-amplified by either GenomiPhi (GE, Fairfield, CT) or a RepliG mini kit (Qiagen) (Table 2). For DNA extracted from FFPE samples, we also prepared PCR amplicon with AmpliTaq Gold 360 (Life technologies) in a final volume of 20 μl with 20 ng genomic DNA, 5 nM primers (Table 3), 5 μl of AmpliTaq gold master mix, and 0.3 μl of 360 GC Enhancer. For this amplicon preparation, the following PCR conditions were used: one cycle of 15 min at 95°C, 4 min at 60°C, and 1 min at 72°C, next 35 cycles of 1 min at 95°C, 1 min at 60°C, and 1 min at 72°C, and finally 10 min at 72°C and kept at 4°C. Amplicons were purified using PCR purification kit (QIAGEN).

Each DNA sample was quantified using the Qubit dsDNA HS Assay kit and a Qubit fluorometer (Life Technologies, Carlsbad, CA). Extracted DNA samples were stored at −20°C until use.

For 108 of the total 288 genomic DNA samples, data sets for mutant allele frequencies obtained by deep sequencing using the MiSeq System (Illumina, San Diego, CA), which were used in our previous report [12], were reanalyzed.

qPCR of patient samples

qPCR reactions using duplicate patient samples were performed in a final volume of 20 μl with 50 ng of original or whole genome-amplified genomic DNA or 1.0×10^{-2} ng PCR-amplified DNA as a template, 10 nM primers, and the SYBR-Green mix (Roche, Basel, Switzerland) in conditions similar to those used for plasmid templates described above.

Levels of amplicons generated using either the WT or mutant primer, calculated with reference to respective standard curves, were designated [wt] and [mut], respectively.

Table 3. Primer sequences for making PCR amplicons of FFPE samples.

Primer	Sequence
Forward	GCCCCATGGTTACCAAAGCA
Reverse	GCTTTCCATCCACCTCGATA

Statistical analysis

Statistical analysis was conducted using SPSS software (Japan International Business.

Machines Corporation, Tokyo). A P-value <0.05 was considered statistically significant.

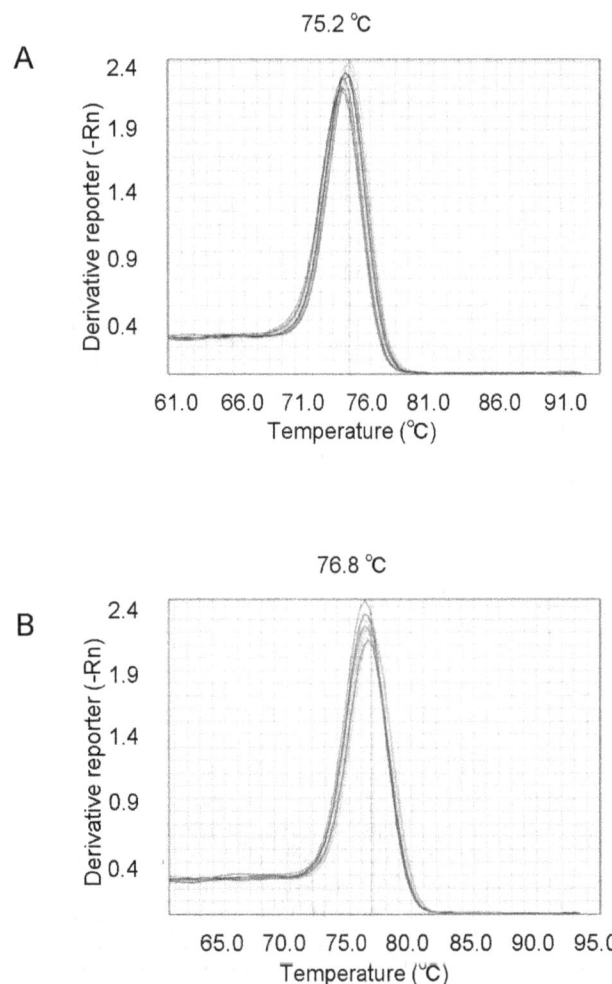

Figure 2. Melting curve analysis. A. Melting curve constructed using WT allele-specific primers. B. Melting curve constructed using mutant allele-specific primer set.

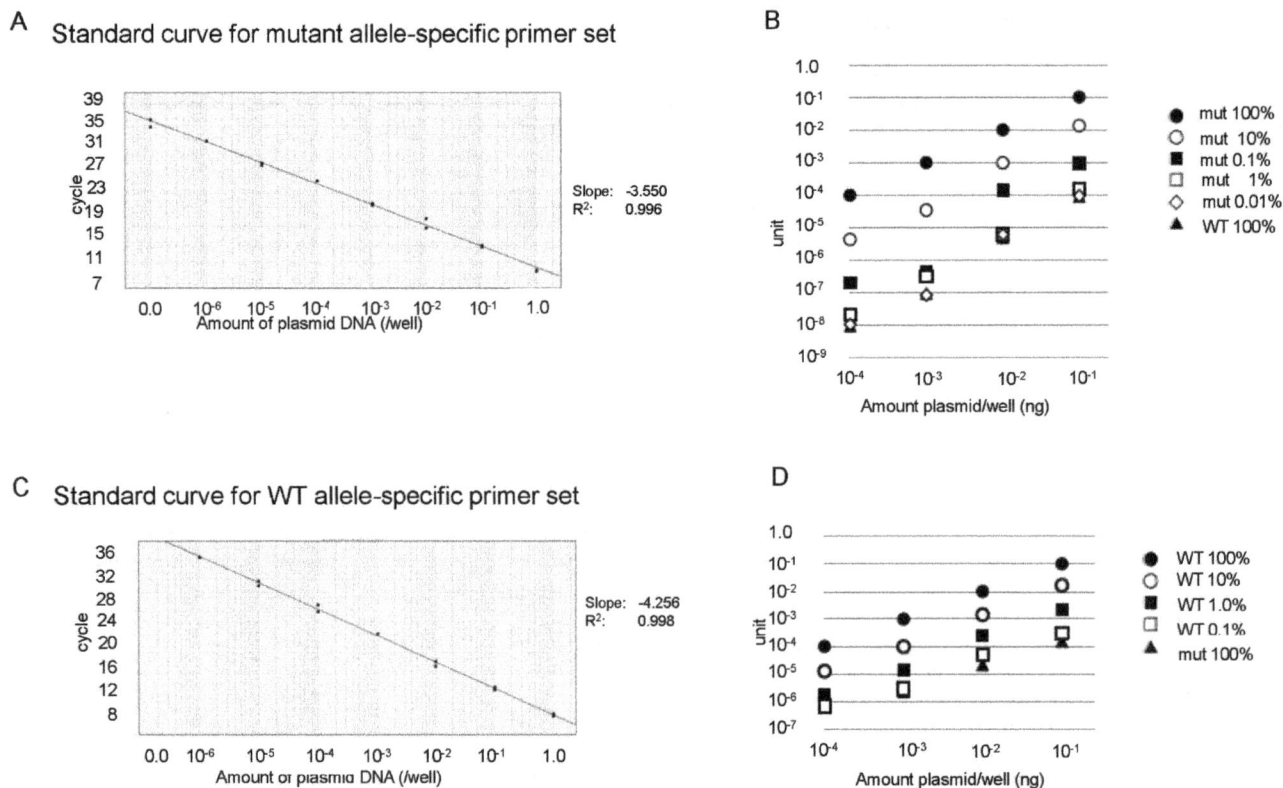

Figure 3. Standard curve showing linearity of quantitative allele-specific PCR. A standard curve was generated by serial dilution of WT or G17V cDNA that had been subcloned into pBluescript. A. Serial dilution of pBS/mutRHOA. Black dots correspond to $1.0 \times 10^{-9} \sim 1.0$ unit of mutant plasmid (duplicate samples). The titration slope is -3.550 and R^2 is 0.996. B. pBS/mutRHOA was mixed with pBS/wtRHOA at 100%, 10%, 1.0%, 0.1%, 0.01% and 0%. Mix concentrations were adjusted to 1.0 ng/well and diluted 1:10 4 times for quantitative PCR analysis with allele-specific mutant primers. Horizonal axis indicates the amount of DNA per well. Vertical axis indicates unit for each sample. Black dot, MUT 100%; open dot, MUT 10%; square, MUT 1%; open square, MUT 0.1%; diamond, MUT 0.01%; triangle, MUT 0% (WT 100%) C. Serial dilution of pBS/wtRHOA. Black dots correspond to $1.0 \times 10^{-6} \sim 1.0$ unit of WT cDNA (duplicate samples). The titration slope is -4.256, and R^2 is 0.998. D. pBS/wtRHOA was mixed with pBS/mutRHOA at 100%, 10%, 1.0%, 0.1%, 0.1% and 0%. Mix concentrations were adjusted to 1.0 ng/well and diluted 1:10 4 times for quantitative PCR analysis with WT allele-specific primers. Black dot, WT 100%; open dot, WT 10%; square, WT 1%; open square, WT 0.1%; triangle, WT 0% (MUT 100%).

Results

Primer specificity

Melting curve analysis revealed that amplicons generated using either WT or mutant primers melted at 76.8°C or 75.3°C, respectively. Non-specific amplicons were not observed in either pBS/wtRHOA/WT primer or pBS/mutRHOA/mutant primer combinations (Figures 2A and 2B).

Linearity of amplicon generation

We then varied either the ratio of pBS/mutRHOA to pBS/wtRHOA or the concentration of total input DNA, and measured the amounts of PCR product generated using the mutant primer. Because we observed a nearly linear relationship between the amounts of generated amplicon and input DNA in the range of 10^4 (1–0.0001 ng DNA/well) at each ratio of pBS/mutRHOA to pBS/wtRHOA (Figure 3A), we defined the amount of amplicon derived from 100% pBS/mutRHOA template at 0.1 ng/well as 0.1 unit, and tested whether linearity was maintained with varying ratios of pBS/mutRHOA to pBS/wtRHOA. The template samples of 0.1 ng/well containing 10, 1, 0.1, and 0.01% pBS/mutRHOA were measured as 1.0×10^{-2} unit (C.I. (confidence interval), $0.8–1.3 \times 10^{-2}$; S.F. (scaling factor), 0.95–1.06), 1.2×10^{-3} unit (C.I., $0.8–1.6 \times 10^{-3}$; S.F., 0.96–1.07), 2.2×10^{-4} unit (C.I., $1.5–3.0 \times 10^{-4}$; S.F., 1.05–1.14), and

1.0×10^{-5} unit (C.I., $0.4–1.6 \times 10^{-5}$; S.F., 0.92–1.04), indicative of linearity in the range of 10^4 (100–0.01%). Taken together, linearity was maintained in the range of 10^9 (Figures 3A and 3B).

Similarly, when we assessed the WT primer using various ratios of pBS/wtRHOA to pBS/mutRHOA and concentrations of input DNA, linearity between the amounts of amplicon and template were maintained between 100–0.1% (a range of 10^3) and 1–0.001 ng DNA/well (a range of 10^3). This analysis indicated a total dynamic range of 10^6 (Figures 3C and 3D).

qAS-PCR of T-cell lymphoma samples

qAS-PCR with 50 ng of genomic DNA was performed using 106 AITL and PTCL-NOS samples including 11 FFPE samples. The [wt] and [mut] values were distributed between 7.9×10^{-5} and 1.8×10^{-1} units, and 2.0×10^{-7} and 7.6×10^{-2} units, respectively. Nevertheless, it was not possible to use absolute values of [mut] for levels of G17V *RHOA* alleles, due to variation in DNA quality. Therefore, we undertook relative measures to assess G17V *RHOA* allele frequency. To do so, we calculated a [mut]/([wt]+[mut]) value and compared it with mutant variant allele frequencies determined by MiSeq. [mut]/([wt]+[mut]) values were distributed between 3.2×10^{-4} and 3.0×10^{-1}. Among samples judged to harbor a G17V *RHOA* mutation by deep sequencing using the MiSeq System (cut-off level, 0.02), which was defined in previous paper [12], [mut]/([wt]+[mut]) values of DNA

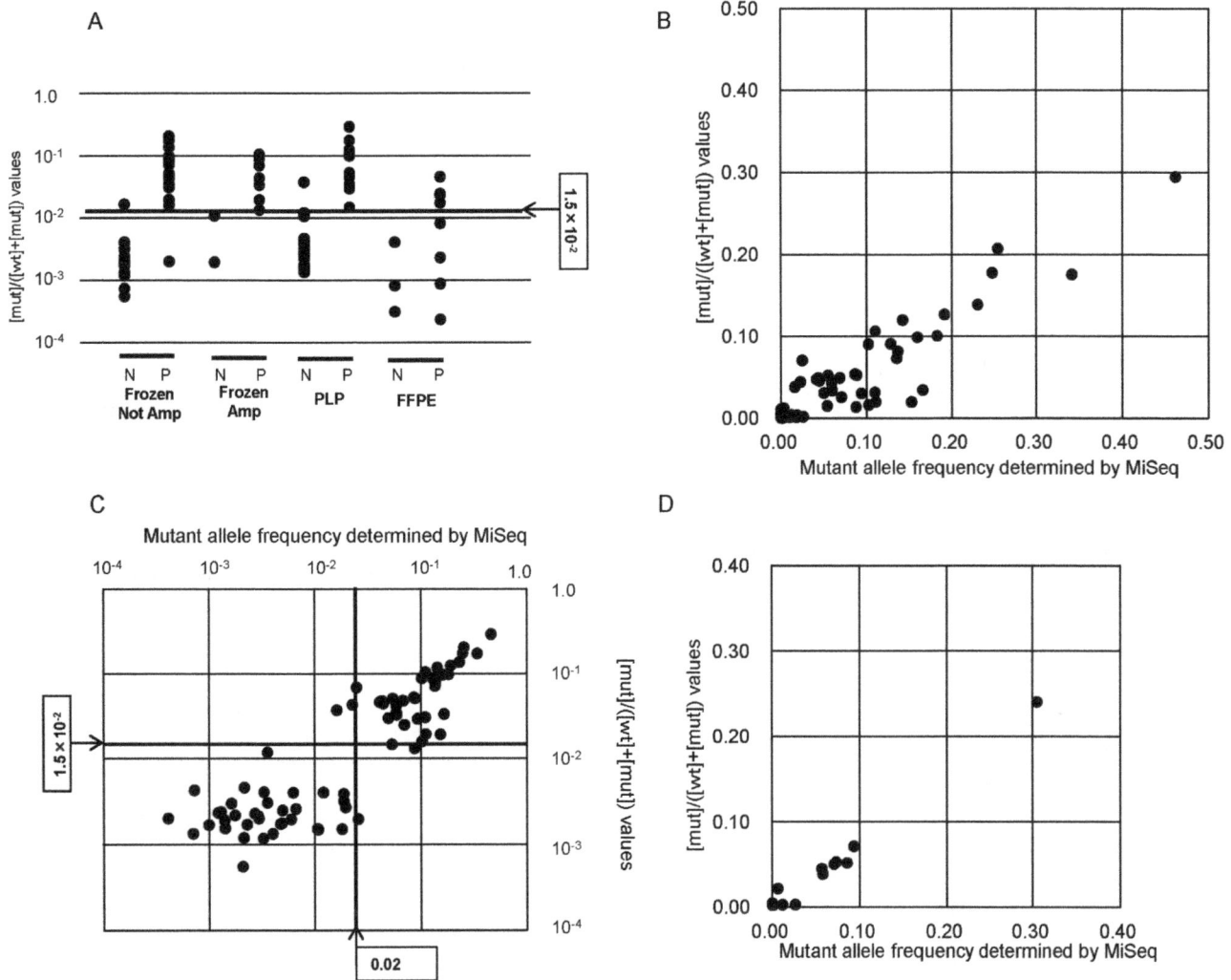

Figure 4. qAS-PCR of AITL and PTCL-NOS samples. A, Shown are [mut]/([wt]+[mut]) values for each sample. N, mutation negative determined by MiSeq; P, mutation positive determined by MiSeq; Amp, amplified; PLP, periodate/lysine/paraformaldehyde-fixed; FFPE, formalin-fixed/paraffin-embedded. B, Comparison of [mut]/([wt]+[mut]) values by qAS-PCR and mutant allele frequencies as determined by MiSeq for 95 original or whole genome-amplified DNA samples, including 43 AITL and 52 PTCL-NOS. Cut-off values were determined as 1.5×10^{-2} for [mut]/([wt]+[mut]) by qAS-PCR and as 0.02 for mutant allele frequencies as determined by MiSeq. C, Comparison of [mut]/([wt]+[mut]) values by qAS-PCR and mutant allele frequencies as determined by MiSeq for 95 DNA samples in a log scales. D, Comparison of [mut]/([wt]+[mut]) values by qAS-PCR and mutant allele frequencies as determined by MiSeq for 13 FFPE PCR-amplicon samples.

from MiSeq-positive FFPE samples were significantly lower than those from other MiSeq-positive samples (Miseq-positive FFPE vs MiSeq-positive other samples; 1.56×10^{-2} vs. 9.38×10^{-2}, p< 0.05, Student's t-test) (Figure 4A). Four out of all 8 MiSeq-positive FFPE samples were negative by qAS-PCR. Therefore, we excluded FFPE samples and analyzed data from 95 DNA samples that had been purified from PLP-fixed or frozen tissues.

When [mut]/([wt]+[mut]) values were compared with mutant variant allele frequencies determined by MiSeq, the rank correlation coefficient was 0.785 (Spearman's correlation P< 0.001) (Figure 4B and C). Among the 95 samples analyzed, 38 (29 AITL and 9 PTCL-NOS) were judged positive and 57 (14 AITL and 43 PTCL-NOS) were judged negative by MiSeq. By comparison, when the cut-off level for [mut]/([wt]+[mut]) values was set at 1.5×10^{-2}, according to ROC curve (Supplemental Figure 1), 38 cases were judged positive for the G17V *RHOA* mutation, including 29 AITL and 9 PTCL-NOS. Overall, 91 of 95 specimens showed concordant results using both methods,

while 4 cases showed discordant results (Figure 4B and C). If we assume that data generated by MiSeq is accurate, then the sensitivity and specificity of qAS-PCR were as high as 94.7% and 96.5%, respectively. Positive and negative concordance rates of the two methods were 94.7% and 96.5%, respectively (Table 4, Table S1 in File S1).

The four cases showing discordant results provided us with an insight into the comparison between MiSeq and aAS-PCR. Two samples were positive only based on MiSeq, and two were positive only by qAS-PCR. When we performed HISEQ2000 sequencing [12] for all these four samples, we observed ≥ 0.02 mutation allele frequencies in two samples. One had been deemed positive only by qAS-PCR and the other only by MiSeq. The other two samples showed <0.02 mutation allele frequencies by HISEQ2000. One of them was judged as negative only by qAS-PCR and the other only by MiSeq. Overall, accuracy with qAS-PCR and MiSeq was comparable.

Table 4. Correlation between qAS-PCR and MiSeq.

Method	Standard	Samples			N[1]	RCC[2]	Sensitivity	Specificity	PPV[3]	NPV[4]
qAS-PCR	MiSeq	AITL and PTCL-NOS	non-FFPE	all	95	0.785	94.7	96.5	94.7	96.5
				original	66	0.735	100.0	95.5	91.7	100.0
				WGA[5]	29	0.822	87.5	100.0	100	86.7
			FFPE[6]		13	0.919	87.5	80.0	87.5	80.0

[1]N, number; [2]RCC, rank correlation coefficient; [3]PPV, positive predictive value; [4]NPV, negative predictive value; [5]WGA, whole-genome amplification. [6]FFPE, formalin-fixed/paraffin-embedded.

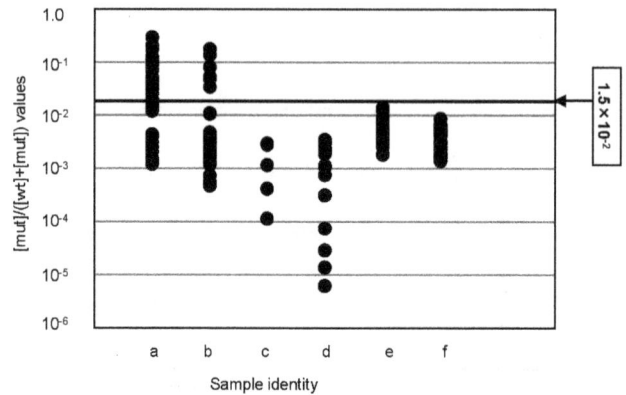

Figure 5. qAS-PCR for 275 tumor and control samples. qAS-PCR was performed for tumor samples, including 43 AITL (a), 52 PTCL-NOS (b), 5 T-cell lymphoma other than AITL and PTCL-NOS (c), 19 B-cell lymphomas (d), 129 myeloid malignancies (e) and 27 control samples (f).

The qAS-PCR method using 50 ng of whole-genome-amplified DNA did not provide a robust correlation with the Miseq data for FFPE samples. The main reason was likely to be fragmentation of genomic DNA. To overcome this limitation, DNA prepared from the 13 FFPE samples was pre-amplified by PCR prior to performing qAS-PCR. Sensitivity and specificity for FFPE samples using amplicon was 87.5% and 80.0%, respectively, based on the mutation allele frequencies determined by MiSeq. (Figure 4D, Table S2 in File S1). Therefore, even for FFPE samples, the qAS-PCR method could robustly estimate the G17V RHOA mutation allele frequencies.

Effect of whole-genome amplification for qAS-PCR

When we divided the 95 samples into original DNA and whole-genome-amplified DNA cohort, sensitivity and specificity were 100% and 95.5% for original DNA cohort, and 87.5% and 100% for whole-genome-amplified DNA cohort, respectively (Supplemental Figure 2A-D, Table S3A and B in File S1).

In order to determine whether amplification influences the evaluation of mutation allele frequency by qAS-PCR, we compared the data for 15 pairs of original and whole-genome-amplified samples. Fourteen out of 15 pairs showed concordant results with each other (Table S3C and D in File S1, Figure S2E in File S1). One sample, which was judged positive by MiSeq, showed discordant results by qAS-PCR; positive for the original DNA and negative for the whole-genome-amplified DNA. As a summary, with some limitations, whole-genome-amplified DNA could provide robust results in most cases.

qAS-PCR for myeloid, B-cell and other T-cell malignancies

We performed qAS-PCR for buccal cells and non-tumor samples including bone marrow cells without lymphoma infiltration obtained from lymphoma patients, and confirmed that the qAS-PCR values were below the cut-off level in all samples. Then, we applied qAS-PCR for 153 tumor samples other than AITL and PTCL-NOS, including 129 myeloid, 19 B-cell, and 5 T-cell malignancies. Sanger sequencing also showed no mutant signals for any of these samples. All qAS-PCR values calculated using these samples were below the cut-off level (Figure 5).

Discussion

Our recent discovery of the highly frequent G17V *RHOA* mutation in AITL and AITL-like PTCL-NOS led us to develop a novel method to detect this mutation [12]. The results of qAS-PCR analysis described here are correlated well with those derived from deep sequencing (Table 4), while qAS-PCR is superior to deep sequencing in terms of the cost and convenience. There is a pressing clinical need for a well-validated *RHOA* testing method with optimal analytical performance using the least amount of difficult-to-obtain patient specimens. We show here that even DNA samples subjected to whole-genome amplification or low quality/concentration DNA extracted from FFPE samples can serve as reliable material for our qAS-PCR method, if appropriate PCR procedure and primers are used. Allele-specific PCR for G17V *RHOA* mutation was mentioned in other report [13], although sensitivity and specificity of the methods were not described.

In a previous study, we defined the cut-off level of mutant allele frequencies determined by MiSeq as 0.02 [12]. In this study, we defined the cut-off level as 1.5×10^{-2} for qAS-PCR, but it remains to be determined whether these cut-off levels are sufficient to detect AITL. Given our finding that the mutated *RHOA* allele frequencies distributed below 0.05 in many AITL samples [12], the tumor cell content might be very low and could be detected in some cases only when the cut-off levels of qAS-PCR and deep sequencing are lowered. If we set the cut-off value lower, the sensitivity should be improved with the increase of false-positive results, raising a dilemma common to other clinical testings.

Several hotspot mutations that reveal distinct hematologic malignancies have been identified in conditions other than T-cell lymphomas. For example, detection of the V617F *JAK2* mutation is a part of the diagnostic criteria for myeloproliferative neoplasms in the latest version of WHO classification [1], although consensus is not reached about the detection methods and cut-off levels. Methods have been developed to detect this mutation including allele-specific PCR and a PCR-restriction fragment length polymorphism (RFLP) approach utilizing mutation sequence specificity for a restriction enzyme[15–18]. More recently, a V600E *BRAF* mutation in hairy cell leukemia [19], an L265P *MYD* mutation in Waldenström macrogloblinemia [20], and several mutations in *STAT3* in large granular lymphocytic

leukemia [21] have been identified as diagnostics of these tumor types. In the future, it is likely that molecular alterations, including the G17V *RHOA* mutation, will be increasingly incorporated into the diagnostic criteria for hematologic malignancies. In summary, our novel method to detect the G17V *RHOA* mutation could provide an important clinical tool to diagnose AITL and AITL-like PTCL-NOS and in the future serve as a means to classify AITL and PTCL-NOS.

Supporting Information

File S1 Figures S1–S2 and Tables S1–S4. Figure S1. ROC curve for data of qAS-PCR and MiSeq. Horizontal axis shows 1-specificity and Vertical axis shows sensitivity of qAS-PCR method compared to the data of MiSeq. Figure S2. Effect of whole-genome amplification for qAS-PCR A, Comparison of [mut]/([wt]+[mut]) values by qAS-PCR and mutant allele frequencies as determined by MiSeq for 66 original samples (linear). B, Comparison of [mut]/([wt]+[mut]) values by qAS-PCR and mutant allele frequencies as determined by MiSeq for 66 original samples (log scale). C, Comparison of [mut]/([wt]+[mut]) values by qAS-PCR and mutant allele frequencies as determined by MiSeq for 29 whole-genome amplified samples (linear). D, Comparison of [mut]/([wt]+[mut]) values by qAS-PCR and mutant allele frequencies as determined by MiSeq for 29 whole-genome amplified samples (log scale). E, Comparison of [mut]/([wt]+[mut]) values by qAS-PCR for 15 pairs of original and whole-genome amplified samples in a log scale.

Acknowledgments

We thank T Arinami for licensing the machine.

Author Contributions

Conceived and designed the experiments: RN-M MS-Y SC. Performed the experiments: RN-M. Analyzed the data: RN-M MS-Y KY SY Y. Shiozawa TN KS MS SO KT NN. Contributed reagents/materials/analysis tools: TE HM NO T. Kato NK YY KI YO SS T. Komeno Y. Sato TI IK. Contributed to the writing of the manuscript: RN-M MS-Y SC.

References

1. Swerdlow SH, Campo E, Harris NL, Jaffe ES, Pileri SA, et al. (2008) WHO classification of tumors of haematopoietic and lymphoid tissues. 4th ed. Lyon, France. IARC Press: 306–311.
2. de Leval L, Gisselbrecht C, Gaulard P (2010) Advances in the understanding and management of angioimmunoblastic T-cell lymphoma. Br J Haematol 148: 673–689.
3. Frizzera G, Moran EM, Rappaport H (1974) Angio-immunoblastic lymphadenopathy with dysproteinaemia. Lancet 1: 1070–1073.
4. Dogan A, Attygalle AD, Kyriakou C (2003) Angioimmunoblastic T-cell lymphoma. Br J Haematol 121: 681–691.
5. de Leval L, Rickman DS, Thielen C, Reynies A, Huang YL, et al. (2007) The gene expression profile of nodal peripheral T-cell lymphoma demonstrates a molecular link between angioimmunoblastic T-cell lymphoma (AITL) and follicular helper T (TFH) cells. Blood 109: 4952–4963.
6. Piccaluga PP, Fulligni F, De Leo A, Bertuzzi C, Rossi M, et al. (2013) Molecular profiling improves classification and prognostication of nodal peripheral T-cell lymphomas: results of a phase III diagnostic accuracy study. J Clin Oncol 31: 3019–3025.
7. Papadi B, Polski JM, Clarkson DR, Liu-Dumlao TO (2012) Atypical angioimmunoblastic T-cell lymphomas masquerading as systemic polyclonal B-immunoblastic proliferation. Virchows Arch 461: 323–331.
8. Couronne L, Bastard C, Bernard OA (2012) TET2 and DNMT3A mutations in human T-cell lymphoma. N Engl J Med 366: 95–96.
9. Cairns RA, Iqbal J, Lemonnier F, Kucuk C, de Leval L, et al. (2012) IDH2 mutations are frequent in angioimmunoblastic T-cell lymphoma. Blood 119: 1901–1903.

10. Delhommeau F, Dupont S, Della Valle V, James C, Trannoy S, et al. (2009) Mutation in TET2 in myeloid cancers. N Engl J Med 360: 2289–2301.
11. Langemeijer SM, Kuiper RP, Berends M, Knops R, Aslanyan MG, et al. (2009) Acquired mutations in TET2 are common in myelodysplastic syndromes. Nat Genet 41: 838–842.
12. Sakata-Yanagimoto M, Enami T, Yoshida K, Shiraishi Y, Ishii R, et al. (2014) Somatic RHOA mutation in angioimmunoblastic T cell lymphoma. Nat Genet 46: 171–175.
13. Palomero T, Couronne L, Khiabanian H, Kim MY, Ambesi-Impiombato A, et al. (2014) Recurrent mutations in epigenetic regulators, RHOA and FYN kinase in peripheral T cell lymphomas. Nat Genet 46: 166–170.
14. Wangkumhang P, Chaichoompu K, Ngamphiw C, Ruangrit U, Chanprasert J, et al. (2007) WASP: a Web-based Allele-Specific PCR assay designing tool for detecting SNPs and mutations. BMC Genomics 8: 275.
15. Zapparoli GV, Jorissen RN, Hewitt CA, McBean M, Westerman DA, et al. (2013) Quantitative threefold allele-specific PCR (QuanTAS-PCR) for highly sensitive JAK2 V617F mutant allele detection. BMC Cancer 13: 206.
16. Shammaa D, Bazarbachi A, Halas H, Greige L, Mahfouz R (2010) JAK2 V617F mutation detection: laboratory comparison of two kits using RFLP and qPCR. Genet Test Mol Biomarkers 14: 13–15.
17. Frantz C, Sekora DM, Henley DC, Huang CK, Pan Q, et al. (2007) Comparative evaluation of three JAK2V617F mutation detection methods. Am J Clin Pathol 128: 865–874.
18. Wu Z, Yuan H, Zhang X, Liu W, Xu J, et al. (2011) Development and inter-laboratory validation of unlabeled probe melting curve analysis for detection of JAK2 V617F mutation in polycythemia vera. PLoS One 6: e26534.

21

Synthesis and Characterization of Novel 2-Amino-Chromene-Nitriles that Target Bcl-2 in Acute Myeloid Leukemia Cell Lines

Hosadurga K. Keerthy[1]⑨, Manoj Garg[2]⑨, Chakrabhavi D. Mohan[3], Vikas Madan[2], Deepika Kanojia[2], Rangappa Shobith[4], Shivananju Nanjundaswamy[3], Daniel J. Mason[5], Andreas Bender[5], Basappa[1]*, Kanchugarakoppal S. Rangappa[3]*, H. Phillip Koeffler[2,6]

1 Laboratory of Chemical Biology, Department of Chemistry, Bangalore University, Bangalore, India, 2 Genomic Oncology Programme, Cancer Science Institute of Singapore, National University of Singapore, Singapore, Singapore, 3 Department of Studies in Chemistry, University of Mysore, Manasagangotri, Mysore, India, 4 Interdisciplinary Research Group of Infectious Diseases, Singapore-MIT Alliance for Research & Technology Centre (SMART), Singapore, Singapore, 5 Unilever Centre for Molecular Science Informatics, Department of Chemistry, University of Cambridge, Cambridge, United Kingdom, 6 Division of Hematology and Oncology, Cedar-Sinai Medical Centre, Los Angeles, California, United States of America

Abstract

The anti-apoptotic protein Bcl-2 is a well-known and attractive therapeutic target for cancer. In the present study the solution-phase T3P-DMSO mediated efficient synthesis of 2-amino-chromene-3-carbonitriles from alcohols, malanonitrile and phenols is reported. These novel 2-amino-chromene-3-carbonitriles showed cytotoxicity in human acute myeloid leukemia (AML) cell lines. Compound **4g** was found to be the most bioactive, decreasing growth and increasing apoptosis of AML cells. Moreover, compound **4g** (at a concentration of 5 μM) increased the G2/M and sub-G1 (apoptosis) phases of AML cells. The AML cells treated with compound **4g** exhibited decreased levels of Bcl-2 and increased levels of caspase-9. In silico molecular interaction analysis showed that compound **4g** shared a similar global binding motif with navitoclax (another small molecule that binds Bcl-2), however compound **4g** occupies a smaller volume within the P2 hot spot of Bcl-2. The intermolecular π-stacking interaction, direct electrostatic interactions, and docking energy predicted for **4g** in complex with Bcl-2 suggest a strong affinity of the complex, rendering **4g** as a promising Bcl-2 inhibitor for evaluation as a new anticancer agent.

Editor: Alessio Lodola, University of Parma, Italy

Funding: This work was supported by grants from USA National Institutes of Health (R01CA02603830); the Singapore Ministry of Health's National Medical Research Council (NMRC) under its Singapore Translational Research (STaR) Investigator Award; and the Singapore Ministry of Education (to HPK.). This research was also supported by University Grants Commission (41-257-2012-SR), Vision Group Science and Technology, Department of Science and Technology (NO. SR/FT/LS-142/2012) to B. KSR thanks Department of Science and Technology (F.NO.SR/SO/HS-006/2010 [G]) and University Grant Commission (F.No.39-106/2010 [SR Dated 24-12-2010]) for funding. HKK, CDM, and B are thankful to UGC, DST-INSPIRE, and PAVATE foundation for providing fellowships respectively. The funders had no role in study design, data collection and analysis, decision to publish, or preparation of the manuscript.

Competing Interests: The authors have declared that no competing interests exist.

* Email: salundibasappa@gmail.com (B); rangappaks@gmail.com (KSR)

⑨ These authors contributed equally to this work.

Introduction

Programmed cell death, or apoptosis, is the primary mechanism for the removal of aged and damaged cells. Cancer cells can gain a growth advantage over their normal counterpart by either dividing more quickly, not undergoing terminal differentiation and thus remaining in the proliferative pool, or not undergoing apoptosis [1]. On the functional level, interactions between pro-apoptotic proteins such as Bax, Bak, Bad, Bim, Noxa, Puma, and pro-survival proteins such as Bcl-2, Bcl-xL, Bcl-w, Mcl-1, and Bfl-1 control the regulation of programmed cell death. Cancer cells alter the balance among these opposing factions to undermine normal apoptosis, and thus gain a survival advantage [2,3]. The first identified apoptotic regulator, Bcl-2, was cloned from human follicular B cell lymphoma cells which nearly invariably have a chromosomal t(14;18) translocation, placing the Bcl-2 gene under the control of the powerful IgG heavy chain promoter [4,5] with the consequence of elevated levels of Bcl-2 promoting increased cell survival [6]. A common feature in many human tumors is overexpression of the pro-survival Bcl-2 family members Bcl-2 and Bcl-xL, which make tumor cells resistant to conventional cancer therapeutic agents.

Numerous synthetic small molecules targeting Bcl-2 protein have been studied extensively and few of them have advanced to clinical trials (**Figure 1**). Structure-based drug design approaches have previously yielded small molecules that bind to Bcl-2 such as navitoclax (ABT-263) [7]. This molecule binds to Bcl-2 and Bcl-xL; unfortunately in clinical trials it caused severe thrombocytopenia due to binding and inhibiting Bcl-xL [8]. Another structure-based synthesis has produced BM-957, a potent small-molecule inhibitor

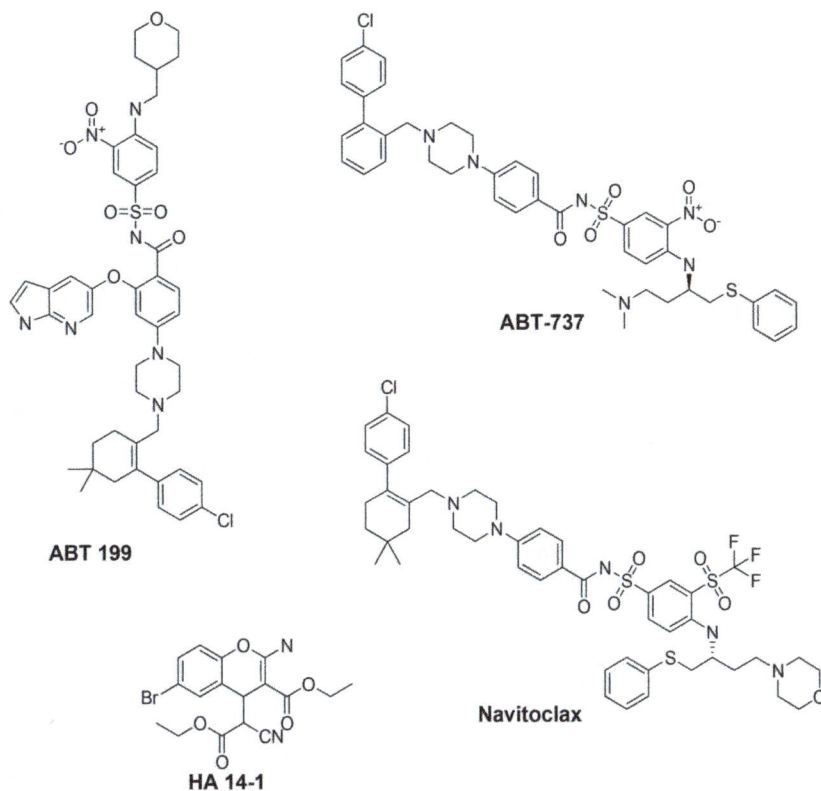

Figure 1. Known small molecules that target Bcl-2. As can be seen, different bioactive scaffolds have been established, however both efficacy and avoiding off-target effects of this class of compounds still remains a challenge.

of Bcl-2 and Bcl-xL, which was capable of achieving complete tumor regression in a small lung cancer xenograft model [9]. Similarly, the co-crystal structure of Bcl-2 resulted in identification of a small molecule called ABT-199; a Bcl-2–selective inhibitor approved by the FDA for cancer therapy [10]. The above study strongly suggested that an indole based carbinol inhibited the growth of prostate cancer cells by arresting them in the G1 phase of the cell cycle, leading to apoptosis *via* down-regulation of Bcl-2.

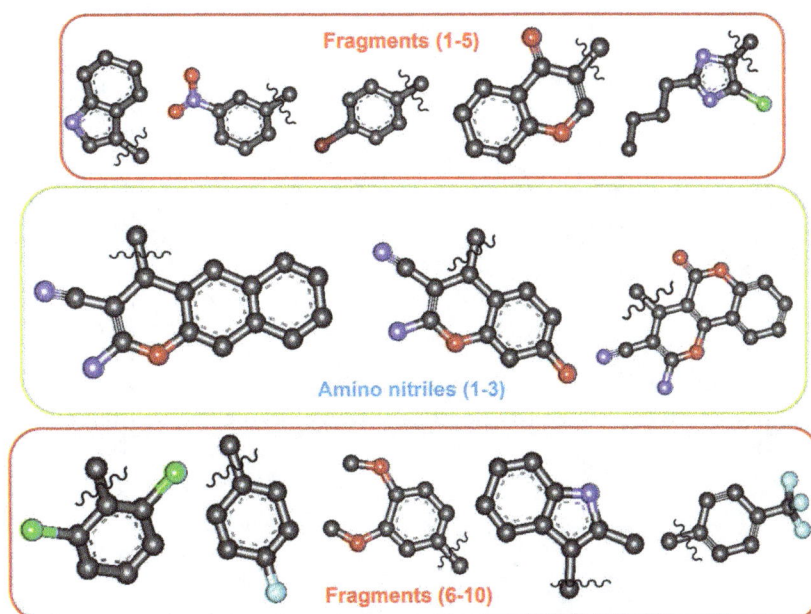

Figure 2. Molecular diversity of amino-nitrils. Structural representation (ball and stick model) of the combinatorial libraries of Bcl-2 inhibitors that depicts top and bottom row side chains, which are incorporate to three amino nitrile scaffolds.

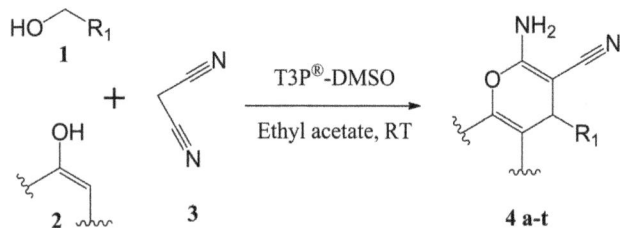

Figure 3. Synthesis of a library of 2-amino-chromene-3-carbonitriles from alcohols.

Chromene-based natural and synthetic compounds have contributed substantially to the development of therapeutics as anti-neoplastic agents against various human malignancies [11,12]. Sesilin, tephrosin, calanone and acronycine are some of the naturally occurring chromene derivatives with a very good anti-cancer activity. An important breakthrough in the development of 4H-chromenes as anti-cancer agents was given by the discovery of HA 14-1, which targets the Bcl-2 protein. It is reported to inhibit Bcl-2 by abrogating the interaction of Bax/Bcl-2, and it has also shown synergistic effect when combined with flavopiridol [13–15]. Therefore, the design of new chromene derivatives against anti-apoptotic members of the Bcl-2 family provides a plausible target in cancer therapeutics [16]. We recently reported the synthesis and explored the biological property of chromene-containing benzoxazines and other biologically important heterocyclic libraries [17,18].

In order to improve the efficacy of chromene-based small molecules as selective inhibitors of Bcl-2, we have in the current work synthesized a library of 2-amino chromene-3-carbonitriles to quantify and compare the molecular diversity between different types of libraries that would interact with Bcl-2 (**Figure 2**). We also outline the simple graphical approach for describing and comparing molecular diversity within the library of amino-nitriles.

Materials and Methods

Synthesis and characterization of various 2-amino-chromene-nitriles were provided as supplementary data (**Data S1** and **Table S1**)

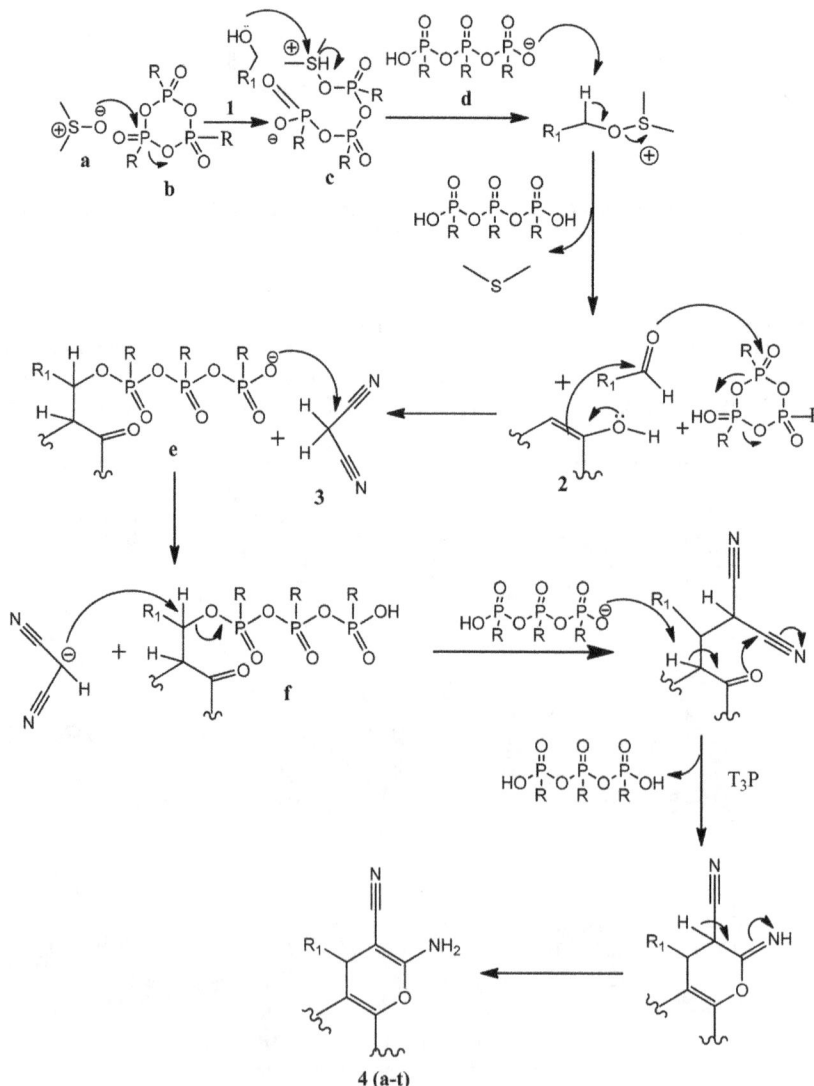

Figure 4. Plausible mechanism of the T3P-DMSO mediated synthesis of title compounds.

Table 1. Physical characteristics of the synthesized 2-amino-chromene-3-carbonitriles.

Entry	1 (Alcohol)	3 (Phenols)	Title compounds (4a-t)	Time (Hr)	Yield (%)	MP (^{O}C)
4a	(3-nitrophenyl)methanol	naphthalen-2-ol	2-amino-4-(3-nitrophenyl)-4H-benzo[g]chromene-3-carbonitrile	3–4	95[a]	179 –182
4b	(4-bromophenyl)methanol	naphthalen-2-ol	2-amino-4-(4-bromophenyl)-4H-benzo[g]chromene-3-carbonitrile	4.5	96[a]	138–140
4c	(1H-indol-3-yl)methanol	naphthalen-2-ol	2-amino-4-(1H-indol-3-yl)-4H-benzo[g]chromene-3-carbonitrile	5	92[a]	198–200
4d	3-(hydroxymethyl)-4H-chromen-4-one	naphthalen-2-ol	2-amino-4-(4-oxo-4H-chromen-3-yl)-4H-benzo[g]chromene-3-carbonitrile	9	84	-
4e	(2-butyl-4-chloro-1H-imidazol-5-yl)methanol	naphthalen-2-ol	2-amino-4-(2-butyl-4-chloro-1H-imidazol-5-yl)-4H-benzo[g]chromene-3-carbonitrile	12	79	-
4f	(2-nitrophenyl)methanol	naphthalen-2-ol	2-amino-4-(2-nitrophenyl)-4H-benzo[g]chromene-3-carbonitrile	4-5	89[a]	-
4g	(2,6-dichlorophenyl)methanol	naphthalen-2-ol	2-amino-4-(2,6-dichlorophenyl)-4H-benzo[g]chromene-3-carbonitrile	8	91	-
4h	(4-fluorophenyl)methanol	naphthalen-2-ol	2-amino-4-(4-fluorophenyl)-4H-benzo[g]chromene-3-carbonitrile	4.5	93[a]	187–189
4i	(4-fluorophenyl)methanol	resorcinol	2-amino-4-(4-fluorophenyl)-7-hydroxy-4H-chromene-3-carbonitrile	6	96[a]	218–220
4j	(1H-indol-3-yl)methanol	resorcinol	2-amino-7-hydroxy-4-(1H-indol-3-yl)-4H-chromene-3-carbonitrile	5	92[a]	-
4k	3-(hydroxymethyl)-4H-chromen-4-one	resorcinol	2'-amino-7'-hydroxy-4-oxo-4H, 4'H-[3,4'-bichromene]-3'-carbonitrile	9.5	82	-
4l	(2-butyl-4-chloro-1H-imidazol-5-yl)methanol	resorcinol	2-amino-4-(2-butyl-4-chloro-1H-imidazol-5-yl)-7-hydroxy-4H-chromene-3-carbonitrile	14	74	-
4m	(4-bromophenyl)methanol	4-hydroxy-2H-chromen-2-one	2-amino-4-(4-bromophenyl)-5-oxo-4,5-dihydropyrano[3,2-c]chromene-3-carbonitrile	3.5	97[a]	254–256
4n	(1H-indol-3-yl)methanol	4-hydroxy-2H-chromen-2-one	2-amino-4-(1H-indol-3-yl)-5-oxo-4,5-dihydropyrano[3,2-c]chromene-3-carbonitrile	5.5	86[a]	215–217
4o	3-(hydroxymethyl)-4H-chromen-4-one	4-hydroxy-2H-chromen-2-one	2-amino-5-oxo-4-(4-oxo-4H-chromen-3-yl)-4,5-dihydropyrano[3,2-c]chromene-3-carbonitrile	10	72	-
4p	(2-butyl-4-chloro-1H-imidazol-5-yl)methanol	4-hydroxy-2H-chromen-2-one	2-amino-4-(2-butyl-4-chloro-1H-imidazol-5-yl)-5-oxo-4,5-dihydropyrano[3,2-c]chromene-3-carbonitrile	9	81	-
4q	(3,4-dimethoxyphenyl)methanol	4-hydroxy-2H-chromen-2-one	2-amino-4-(3,4-dimethoxyphenyl)-5-oxo-4,5-dihydropyrano[3,2-c]chromene-3-carbonitrile	2.5	82[a]	228–230
4r	(2-methyl-1H-indol-3-yl)methanol	4-hydroxy-2H-chromen-2-one	2-amino-4-(2-methyl-1H-indol-3-yl)-5-oxo-4,5-dihydropyrano[3,2-c]chromene-3-carbonitrile	6	69	-
4s	(3,4-dimethoxyphenyl)methanol	4-hydroxy-6,7-dimethyl-2H-chromen-2-one	2-amino-4-(3,4-dimethoxyphenyl)-8,9-dimethyl-5-oxo-4,5-dihydropyrano[3,2-c]chromene-3-carbonitrile	3.5	84	-
4t	(4-(trifluoromethyl)phenyl)methanol	4-hydroxy-6,7-dimethyl-2H-chromen-2-one	2-amino-8,9-dimethyl-5-oxo-4-(4-(trifluoromethyl)phenyl)-4,5-dihydropyrano[3,2-c]chromene-3-carbonitrile	4	89	-

[a] Isolated yield.
MP- Melting point.

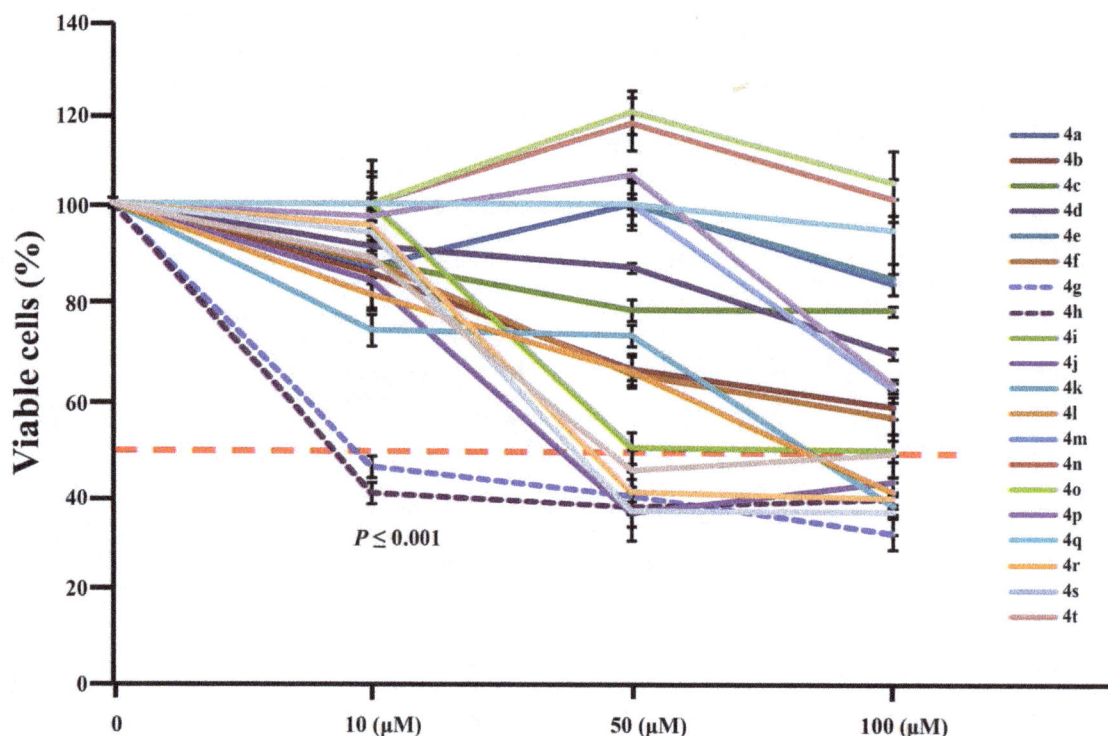

Figure 5. Screening of active compounds affecting the proliferation of HL-60 AML cells from a library of 2-amino-chromene-nitriles derivatives. MTT assays were performed after incubation of HL-60 cells with indicated concentrations of chromene derivatives 4 (a-y) for 72 hr. For each concentration, percent inhibition values were calculated and data was normalized to diluent controls. The scale X-axis is non-linear and the data represent mean ±SD from three independent experiments done in quadruplicates. ** $P \leq 0.001$ (Student's t-test).

Cell Culture

Myeloid leukemia cell lines; MOLM13 and MV4-11 were kind gifts by Dr. Martin Grundy (Department of Academic Haematology, University of Nottingham) [28]. MOLM14 cells were generously provided by Dr. Didier Bouscary (Department of Hematology-Immunology, Institut Cochin, Paris, France) [29]. The HL-60 cell line was purchased from ATCC. Cell lines were cultured and maintained in RPMI medium containing 10% fetal bovine serum (FBS), 1% penicillin-streptomycin (Invitrogen, Carlsbad, CA) at 37°C in a humidified atmosphere with 5% CO_2. All cell lines were regularly screened for absence of mycoplasma. Bone marrow cells from C57BL/6 mice were cultured in IMDM supplemented with 20% FBS and cytokines (10 ng/ml recombinant mouse IL-3, 10 ng/ml recombinant mouse IL-6 and 50 ng/ml recombinant mouse Stem Cell Factor (SCF). Antibodies against Bcl-2, Bcl-xL, Cleaved caspase-9 and GAPDH were purchased from Cell Signalling. ABT-737 was used as a reference compound for all the experiments.

Cell proliferation assay

Cellular proliferation of AML cell lines was measured by using methylthiazolyl-diphenyl-tetrazolium bromide (MTT; sigma-aldrich). 8,000 cells per well were seeded in triplicate, 96-well plates (Corning, Lowell, MA, USA) in 100 µl of medium having 2-amino-chromene-nitriles derivatives. Cells were incubated overnight at 37°C in a CO_2 incubator. At the end of the culture duration, 3-(4, 5-dimethylthiazol-2-yl)-2, 5-diphenyltetrazolium bromide (MTT) was added into each well, and the final concentration of MTT in each

well was 0.5 mg/ml. MTT plates were incubated at 37°C in a CO_2 incubator for 3 hr. After incubation, Formazan crystals were dissolved in 100 µl of stop solution (SDS-HCl). Absorbance was measured at 570 nm using a Tecan Infinite 200 PRO spectrophotometer (Mannedorf, Switzerland).

Annexin V and propidium iodide (Annexin V–PI) apoptosis assays

HL-60, MOLM13, MOLM14 and MV4-11 (1×10^5) cells were seeded into each well of a 6-well plate and treated with **4g** at the IC_{50} concentration for 48 and 72 hours. Staining was performed using FITC Annexin V Apoptosis Detection Kit II, BD Pharmingen (BD Biosciences, USA) according to the manufacturer protocol. Briefly, cells were washed with PBS at least three times, re-suspended in $1 \times$ binding buffer, and FITC-conjugated annexin V and propidium iodide (PI) was added for 15 min in the dark. Samples were analyzed by a LSR-II flow cytometer (Becton-Dickinson, San Jose, CA, USA).

Immunoblot analysis

Cell lysates were prepared using the ProteoJET Mammalian Cell lysis reagent (Fermentas) and the $1 \times$ protease inhibitor mixture (Roche Molecular Biochemicals, Pleasanton, CA). Immunoblotting was performed as described earlier [30]. Monoclonal antibodies against Bcl-2, GAPDH and cleaved caspase-9 (Cell Signalling, Boston, MA, USA) were used.

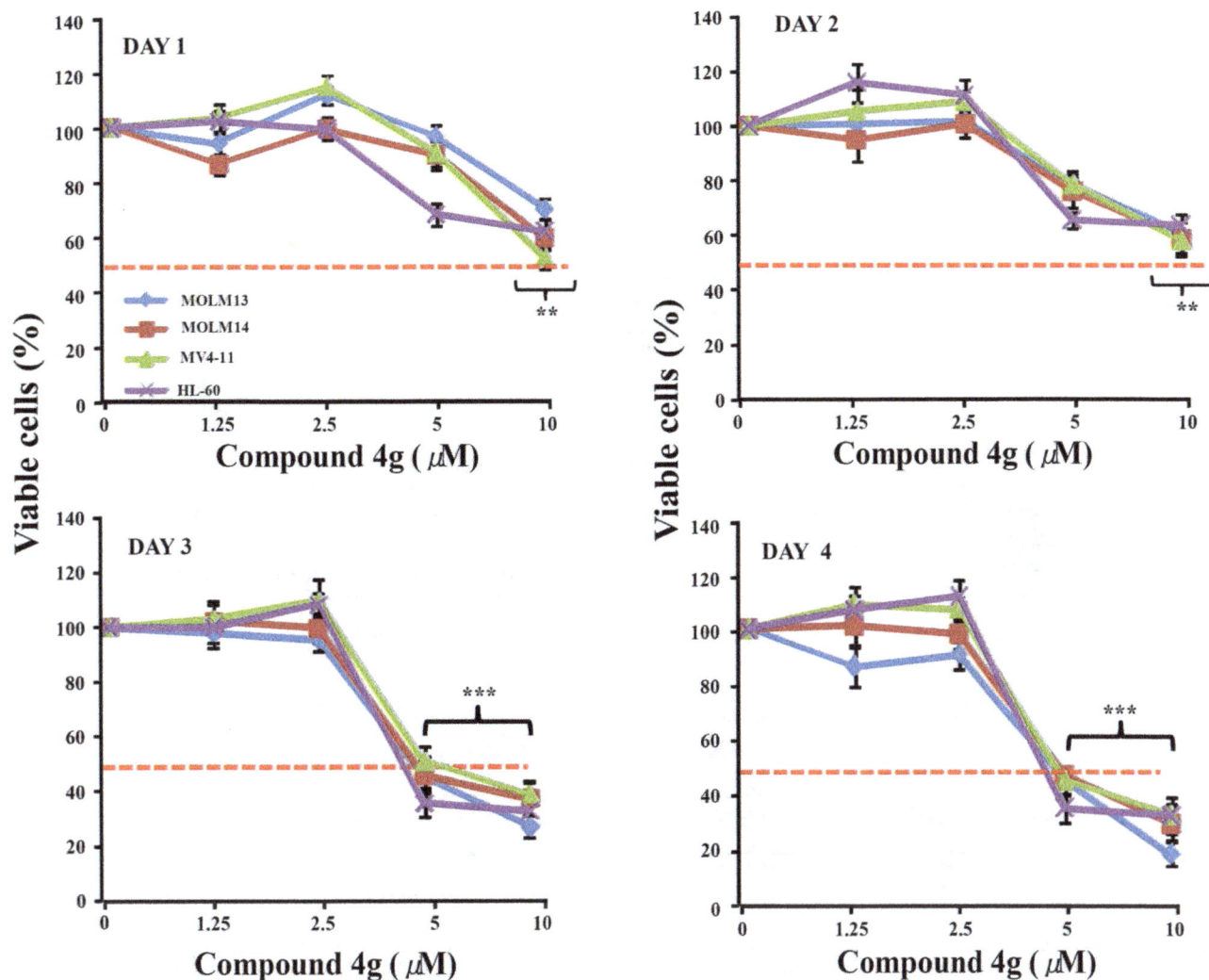

Figure 6. Anti-proliferative effect of 4g tested against AML cell lines in liquid culture. Panels (A–D): MTT assay determined cell viability of AML cells. 8,000 cells per well were seeded for MOLM13, MOLM14, MV4-11 and HL-60 cells in 96 well plates in quadruplicates. A series of dilutions (starting from 1.25 μm to 10 μm) of **4g** were added into the wells. Cell proliferation was measured after compound **4g** treatment relative to diluents controls. Results represent the mean ±SD of three independent experiments with quadruplicate wells per experiment point. ** $P \leq 0.001$; *** $P \leq 0.0001$ (Student's t-test).

In Vitro analysis of the effect of amino-nitriles against Bcl-2

Zymed Bcl-2 ELISA kit was used for the evaluation of the binding of small molecules to Bcl-2. Initially various concentrations of small molecules and the human Bcl-2 was incubated for 5 minutes and transferred the mixture to the mAb coated 96-well plate. The bound Bcl-2 was tagged with anti-Bcl-2 that conjugated with biotin. The biotin conjugate was bound with streptauvidin-HRP. The Streptavidin-HRP was reacted with TM and the absorbance is measured at 450 nm. A standard curve is prepared to determine the Bcl-2 concentration and% inhibition of the Bcl-2 binding to its antibody was presented.

Molecular docking analysis

The molecular modeling was achieved with commercially available InsightII, Discovery Studio (DS) Version 2.5 software packages. Initially, the 3D structure of Bcl-2 was cleaned and the navitoclax binding site was considered for further analysis. All of the calculations were performed using the CHARMM force field

as reported previously [31]. Each energy-minimized final docking position of the individual apigenin structural analogues was evaluated using the interaction score function in the CDOCKER module of DS version 2.5 as reported previously from our group [32]. Based on the low CDOCKER energy value, compound **4g** was selected for further studies.

Results and Discussion

Synthesis of novel 2-amino chromene-3-carbonitriles derivatives

Naturally occurring 2-amino-carbonitriles containing pyrano[3,2-c]pyridine-based structural motifs are commonly found in alkaloids and exhibit diverse biological activities, including anticancer activity [19]. A series of pyrano[3,2-c]pyridine based flavone and coumarin isosteres containing a 2-amino carbonitrile moiety have also exhibited a broad spectrum of antitumor activity against breast cancer cells [20]. In continuation of our efforts to develop efficient solution phase synthesis of novel small molecules

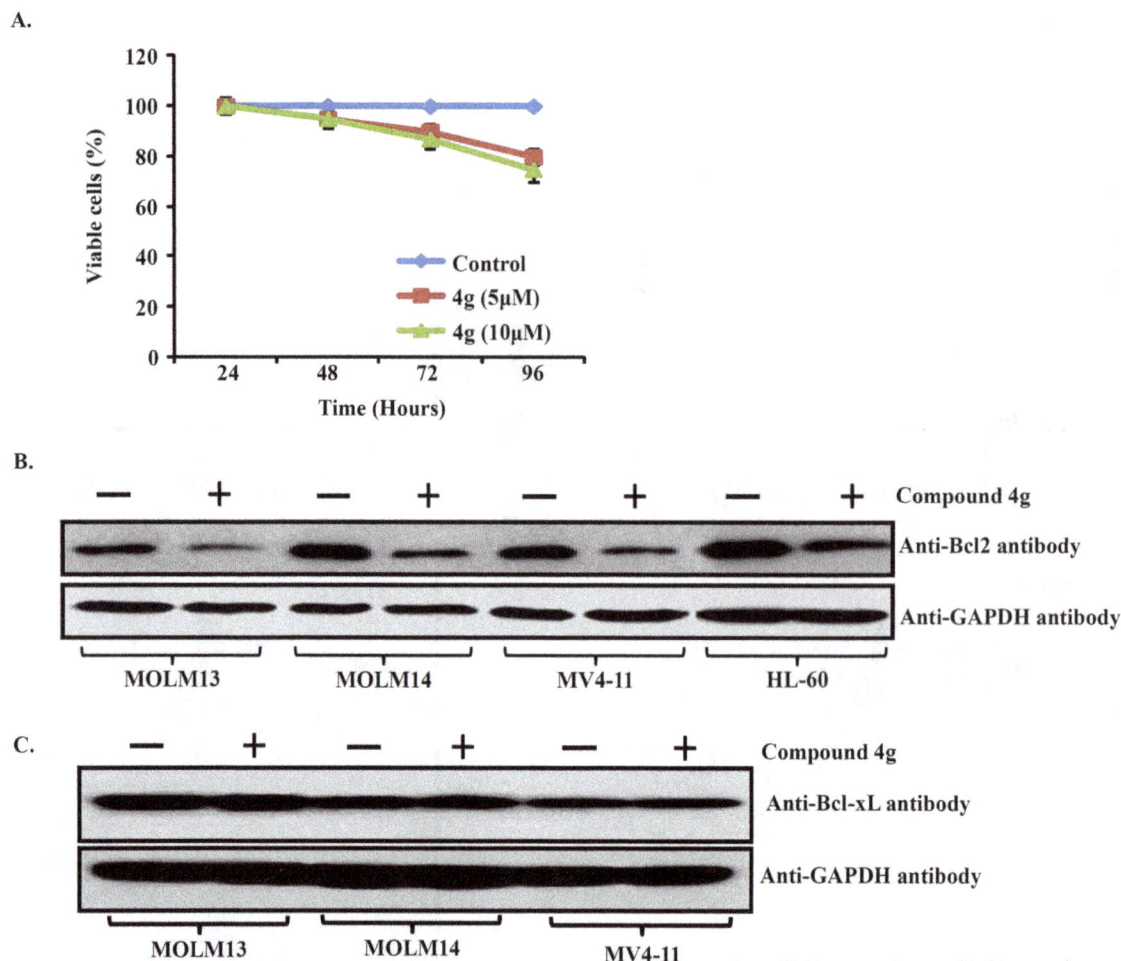

Figure 7. Expression of Bcl-2 proteins in human AML cell lines and anti-proliferative effect of compound 4g (5, 10 μm against C57BL/6 mouse bone marrow cells in liquid culture. A. MTT assay determined cell viability of C57BL/6 mouse total bone marrow cells. Results represent the mean ±SD of three independent experiments with quadruplicate wells per experiment point. **B**. MOLM13, MOLM14, MV4-11 and HL-60 AML cells were cultured either with compound **4g** (5 μM, 24 hr) or diluents control, and levels of Bcl-2 and Bcl-xL were examined by western blot. GAPDH was used as an internal loading control.

with anti-cancer agents, we reported before the synthesis of 2-amino-chromene-3-carbonitriles [21,22], where solution phase T3P-DMSO mediated the efficient synthesis using alcohols, malanonitrile and phenols (**Figure 3**). The possible mechanism involves the reaction of DMSO with T3P to give an electrophilic sulphur species (c), followed by a substitution reaction of alcohol to form an arylsulphonium salt. This is followed by a hydrogen abstraction of the arylsulphonium salt by hydrolyzed T3P (d) to create a carbonyl compound after elimination of dimethyl sulfide. Next, the phenolic hydroxyl group (2) attacks the carbonyl carbon, and the oxygen on the carbonyl group attacks one more T3P to form an intermediate (e), which in turn attacks malanonitrile (3) to give an anion. This anion attacks intermediate (f), which upon further cyclization converts to compound 4(a-t) (**Figure 4**). In addition, a variety of aromatic and heterocyclic alcohols, β-naphthol/resorcinol/4-hydroxycoumarin and malanonitrile were added to T3P (50% solution in ethylacetate), DMSO and ethyl acetate as a solvent medium, in order to obtain compounds **4a-t**. The reaction between **1**, **2** and **3** in the presence of T3P (2.5 equiv) DMSO generally resulted in a product of appreciable yield (see **Table 1**) as well as being rather versatile with regard to the choice of substrates. It was observed during the reaction that an

increase in temperature resulted in the gradual decrease in yield of the product.

2-amino chromene-3-carbonitrile derivatives elicit an anti-proliferative effect against AML cells

4*H*-chromenes are potent cytotoxic agents which have been tested against a panel of human cancer cell lines, and a chromene analog, Crolibulin (EPC2407) is currently in Phase I/II clinical trials for the treatment of advanced solid tumors [23]. We initially tested a series of 20 chromene derivatives 4(a-t) for their cytotoxic effects against a human acute myeloid leukemia (AML) cell line (HL-60), using three different concentrations (10, 50 and 100 μM) of 2-amino-chromene-carbonitriles. Among the tested compounds, **4g** significantly (*P*≤**0.001**) decreased proliferation of the AML cells, even at 10 μM concentrations. Other derivatives of these compounds showed either no or very low effect at 10 μM concentrations (**Figure 5**).

Additional studies were performed for compound **4g**, which was the most active among the structurally related compounds tested in culture. The anti-proliferative activity of compound **4g** against three additional AML cell lines (MOLM13, MOLM14 and MV4-11) was examined. Again, compound **4g** significantly decreased

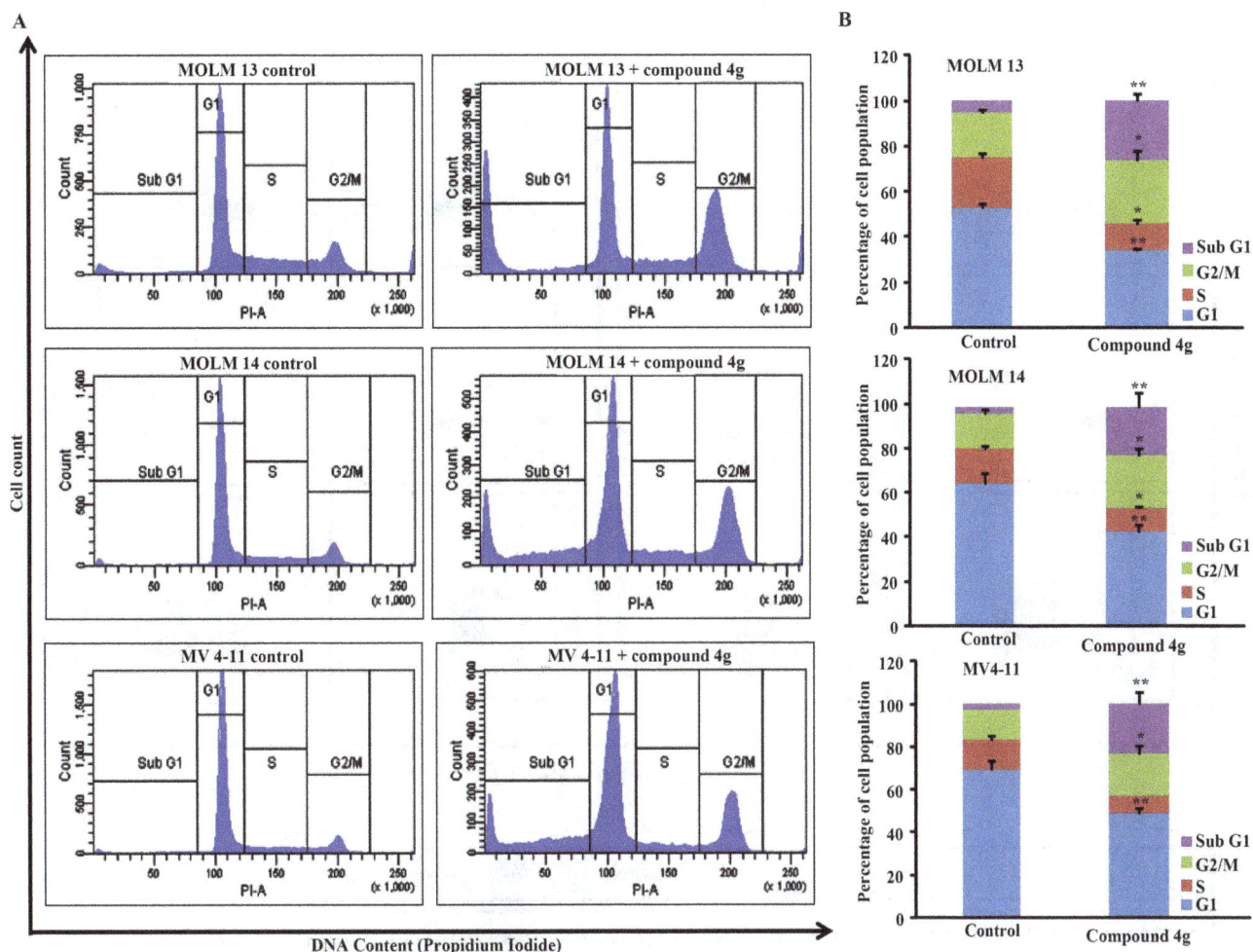

Figure 8. Cell cycle analysis of AML cell lines treated with compound 4g (5 μM, 72 hr). Panel (A), fluorescent activated cell sorter analyzed the percent cells in each phase of the cell cycle. Cell cycle analysis of three cell lines (MOLM14, MOLM14 and MV4-11) treated with diluents control and compound **4g** (5 μM) for 72 h. The figures are representative of three independent experiments. Data are presented in histograms as mean ±SD of three independent experiments. * $P \leq 0.005$; ** $P \leq 0.001$.

the proliferation of the AML cells with an ED_{50} of 5 to 10 μM after 48, 72 and 96 hours of culture (**Figures 6**). Compound **4g** inhibited proliferation of the AML cells with an IC_{50} of 5 μM. Further, C57BL/6 mouse bone marrow cells were treated with 5, 10 μM compound **4g** to assess the effect on normal hematopoietic cells. As shown in **Figure 7A**, compound **4g** (5, 10 μM) treatment displayed minimal anti-proliferative response against the normal bone cells suggesting that compound **4g** decreases proliferation of the AML cells, and has little effect on proliferation of normal bone marrow cells.

Compound 4g inhibits Bcl-2 protein and triggers cell cycle arrest at G2/M phase in AML cells

HA14-1 is a cell permeable Bcl-2 inhibitor, and acts by binding to the surface pocket of Bcl-2 [24] and disrupts the Bax/Bcl-2 interaction, resulting in induction of apoptosis of tumour cells. Interestingly, treatment of HL-60, MOLM13, MOLM14, MV4-11 cell lines with compound **4g** (5 μM, 24 hr) decreased levels of Bcl-2 (**Figure 7B**). Moreover, we checked the effect of compound 4g on the expression of the Bcl-xL. Our western blotting results showed that compound **4g** does not inhibit the expression of Bcl-xL protein (**Figure 7C**).

The effect of compound **4g** (5 μM, 72 hr) on the cell cycle analysis of MOLM13, MOLM14, and MV4-11 AML cells using flow cytometry showed significant increase in the G2/M and sub-G1 phases (apoptosis), as compared to the diluents control cells (**Figures 8A and 8B**). The cell population in the G1 phase of the cell cycle decreased.

Compound 4g induces apoptosis of AML cells

Core scaffolds such as flavones or chromenes induce apoptosis in human myeloid tumor cells [25]. Therefore, the HL-60, MOLM13, MOLM14, and MV4-11 cells were treated with compound **4g** (5 μM for 48 and 72 hr) and analysed for the induction of apoptosis using FITC-conjugated annexin V (AV) and propidium iodide (PI). Both early ($AV^{+}PI^{-}$), as well as, late ($AV^{+}PI^{+}$) apoptosis occurred in AML cells (**Figure 9A**). Detailed percentage of apoptotic cells in cell lines are summarized in supplementary data (**Table S1**). This was associated with increased levels of cleaved caspase-9 in these cell lines (**Figure 9B**), which is an enzyme known to be activated during programmed cell death.

A

B

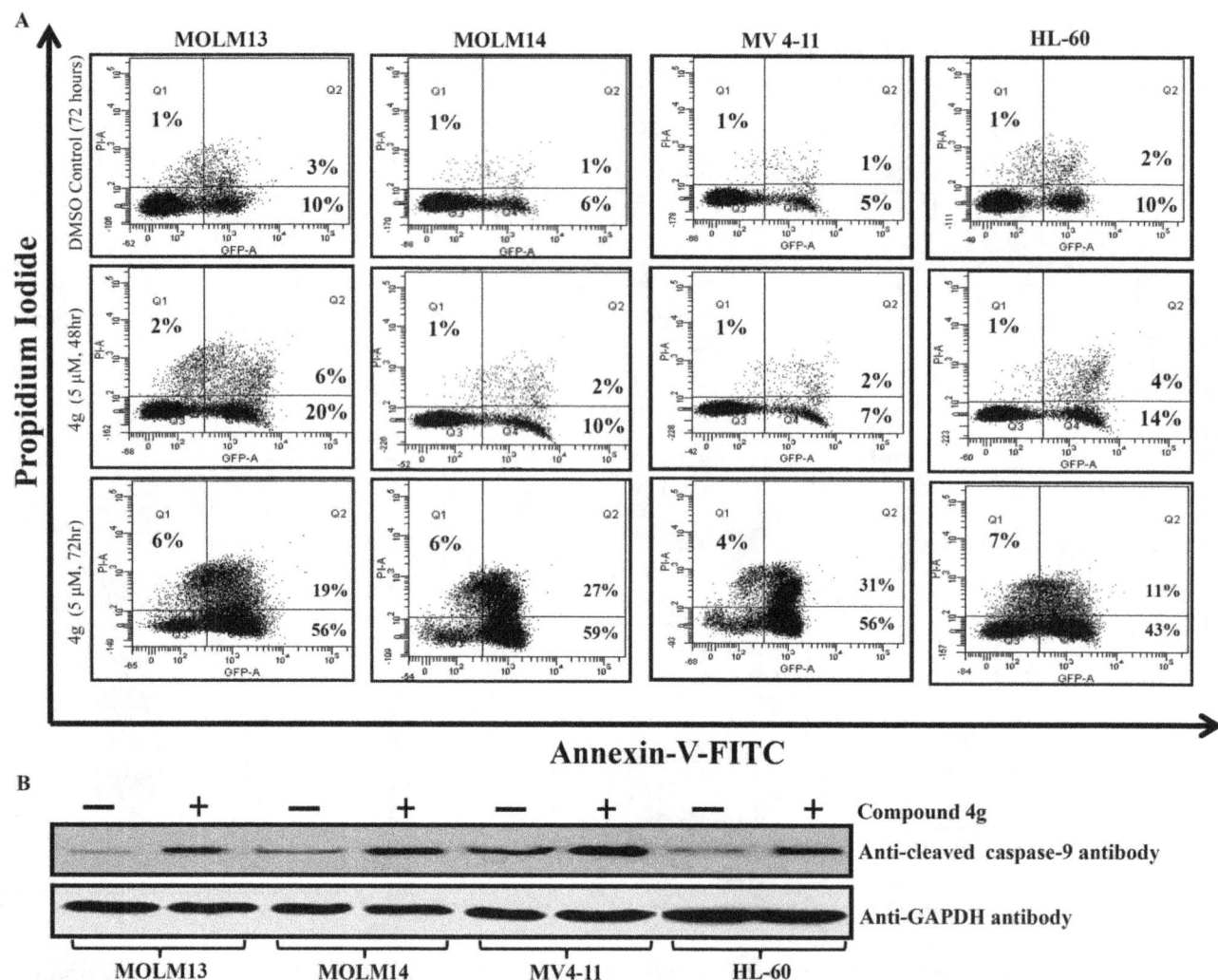

Figure 9. Compound 4g induces apoptosis of AML cells in a time-dependent manner. A. Flow cytometry profile represents Annexin V-FITC staining on the X-axis and PI staining on the Y-axis. The upper left quadrants display the necrotic cells, upper right quadrants show the late apoptotic cells, lower left quadrants display the live cells and lower right quadrants show the early apoptotic cells. **B.** Western blot showed increased expression of cleaved caspase-9 protein in compound 4g treated AML cells compared to control cells.

In Vitro analysis of the effect of amino-nitriles against Bcl-2

Bcl-2 ELISA kit from Zymed was used to determine the inhibitory activity of most active of small molecule towards Bcl-2. Among the four tested compounds, **4a**, **4h**, and **4f** at 30 μM concentration, inhibited the Bcl-2 binding to its antibody by 37.8, 53.0, 61.9% respectively (**Figure 10**). The most active compound **4g** inhibited the Bcl-2 binding to its antibody effectively with an IC_{50} value of 17.8 μM, indicate its strong affinity towards Bcl-2 compared to structurally related chromenes. Among the tested small molecules, 2,6- dichlorophenyl, 2-nitrophenyl, 4-fluorophenyl and 3-nitrophenyl side chain containing amino-nitrils displayed significant binding affinity towards Bcl-2 indicating that electron withdrawing group favors the effective binding to Bcl-2.

In silico docking analysis of chromene based small molecule (4g) that targets Bcl-2

Bcl-2 appears to be a possible target for compound **4g** as it induced the apoptosis by decreasing the level of anti-apoptotic protein Bcl-2 in AML cell lines. Hence, we performed *in silico*

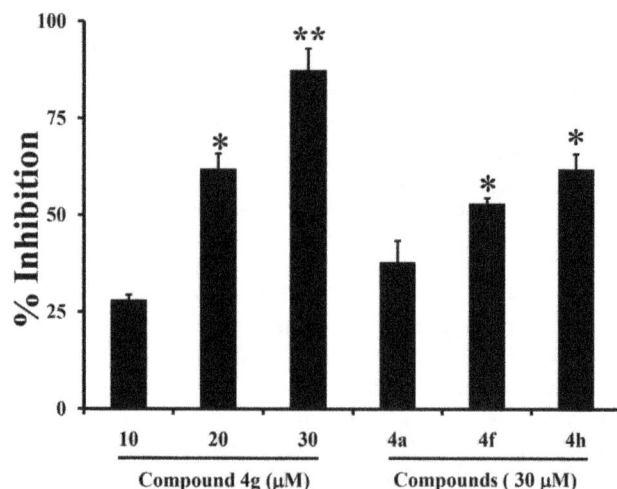

Figure 10. Amino-nitriles inhibit Bcl-2 *in vitro*. Most active small molecules 4a, 4f, 4g and 4h were analysed for their Bcl-2 inhibitory activity. **4g** displayed higher percentage of Bcl-2 inhibition in a dose dependent manner and presented as the most potent inhibitor of Bcl-2.

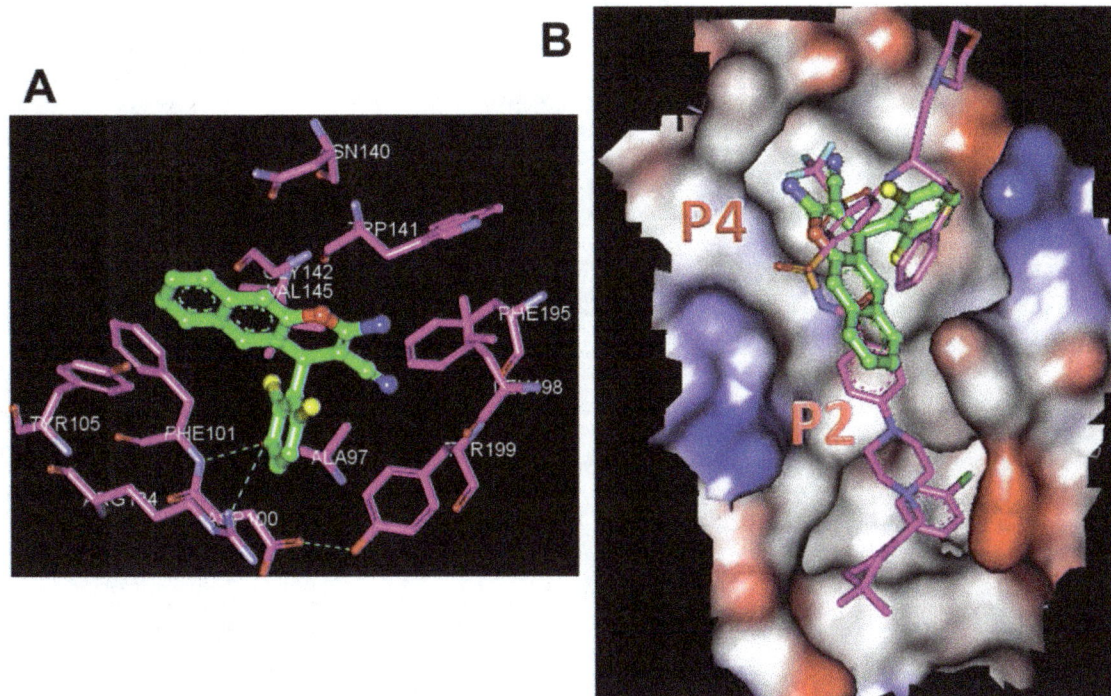

Figure 11. Molecular docking analysis of the compound 4g in the navitoclax binding site of Bcl-2. A. The 3-dimensional orientation of compound **4g** in the navitoclax binding site of Bcl-2. Amino acid side chains are shown as stick (elements are purple color except for carbon-pink), the inhibitor is shown as a ball and stick (elements are green color except for carbon-green). The hydrogen bonding is represented as a green dotted line. **B**. Navitoclax and compound 4g bound surface view of the Bcl-2, showing the interaction at the P2 and P4 hotspot of the protein. The electrostatic potential of the key amino acids is shown. The bound ball and stick version of the compound **4g** and navitoclax are represented.

molecular docking using the three-dimensional structures of Bcl-2, which consists of two central primarily hydrophobic α-helices surrounded by amphipathic helices. Our study was aided by the recent definition of the X-ray crystal structure of Bcl-2–navitoclax (PDB ID: 4LVT) [10]. Navitoclax engages the two hydrophobic 'hot spots' regions termed P2 and P4 that are known to show a high-affinity binding by proapoptotic peptides [26,27]. All docking calculations were performed using Accelrys Discovery Studio Version 2.5 and the automated docking program CDOCKER, which utilises a molecular dynamics-based simulated annealing algorithm. The active site of the enzyme was defined, and CDOCKER docked the most active compound against the navitoclax binding hotspot of Bcl-2. **Figure 10** shows the best-docked conformation of compound **4g** and navitoclox in Bcl-2 obtained from the CDOCKER program. Docking energies of the best configuration of compound **4g** and navitoclax against Bcl-2 were 4.55 and 5.45 kcal/mol, respectively. In addition, we also carried out the molecular docking analysis for the other bioactive amino nitriles with Bcl-2 and its CDOCKER energies are provided in the supplementary data (**Table S2**). The 3-dimensional illustrations of the interaction map of Bcl-2 with compound **4g**, and navitoclax, were produced using the Accelrys visualization tool (**Figure 11A**), and an intermolecular π-stacking interaction of napthyl group with Phe101 and Tyr105 of P4 host spot of Bcl-2 was observed. The 2,6-dichlorophenyl group of compound **4g** showed electrostatic interactions with the conserved arginine (Arg104) and in turn made a unique contact with the intra-molecular hydrogen bond formed by Ala97, Asp100, Phe101, and Tyr199 (**Figure 11A**). In addition to this, the amino-chromene scaffold was buried in the hydrophobic pocket of Gly142, Val145, Trp141, Asn140, Phe195, Leu198, and Tyr199.

The analysis of compound **4g** bound to the novitoclox binding site showed that it shares a similar global binding motif with navitoclax, but occupies a smaller volume within the P2 hot spot (**Figure 11B**).

Conclusions

We report for the first time the solution phase, T3P-DMSO mediated, efficient synthesis of 2-amino-chromene-3-carbonitriles from alcohols, malanonitrile and phenols. These 2-amino-chromene-3-carbonitriles were tested for their cytotoxicity using human AML cell lines. Compound **4g** was the most bioactive among the structurally related compounds. It decreased proliferation, increased caspase-9 mediated apoptosis, and caused G2/M arrest of the MOLM13, MOLM14, and MV4-11 AML cells. Our docking analysis of **4g** suggests Bcl-2 as a reasonable target, hence rendering compound **4g** as a promising Bcl-2 inhibitor for future studies as a new anticancer agent.

Supporting Information

Table S1 Quantification of early apoptotic and late apoptotic cells (%). AML cells were cultured with 4g (5 µM) for either 48 or 72 hours and propidium iodide (PI) and FITC conjugated Annexin V positive cells were enumerated. Results are a representative experiment. The experiments were done three times in triplicates.

Table S2 Computational analysis of the binding of amino nitriles against Bcl-2.

Data S1   General procedure for one pot synthesis of 2-amino chromene-3-carbonitriles.
(DOCX)

Author Contributions

Conceived and designed the experiments: MG B KSR HPK. Performed the experiments: HKK CDM MG VM DK DJM RS B. Analyzed the data: B MG SN HPK AB KSR. Contributed reagents/materials/analysis tools: B HPK KSR. Wrote the paper: MG DJM B KSR HPK.

References

1. Hanahan D, Weinberg RA (2000) The hallmarks of cancer. Cell 100: 57–70.
2. Adams JM, Cory S (2007) The Bcl-2 apoptotic switch in cancer development and therapy. Oncogene 26: 1324–1337.
3. Youle RJ, Strasser A (2008) The BCL-2 protein family: opposing activities that mediate cell death. Nat Rev Mol Cell Biol 9: 47–59.
4. Tsujimoto Y, Cossman J, Jaffe E, Croce CM (1985) Involvement of the bcl-2 gene in human follicular lymphoma. Science 228: 1440–1443.
5. Cleary ML, Smith SD, Sklar J (1986) Cloning and structural analysis of cDNAs for bcl-2 and a hybrid bcl-2/immunoglobulin transcript resulting from the t (14;18) translocation. Cell 47: 19–28.
6. Vaux DL, Cory S, Adams JM (1988) Bcl-2 gene promotes haemopoietic cell survival and cooperates with c-myc to immortalize pre-B cells. Nature 335: 440–442.
7. Park CM, Bruncko M, Adickes J, Bauch J, Ding H, et al. (2008) Discovery of an orally bioavailable small molecule inhibitor of prosurvival B-cell lymphoma 2 proteins. J Med Chem 51: 6902–6915.
8. Schoenwaelder SM, Jackson SP (2012) Bcl-xL-inhibitory BH3 mimetics (ABT-737 or ABT-263) and the modulation of cytosolic calcium flux and platelet function. Blood 119: 1320–1321; author reply 1321–1322.
9. Chen J, Zhou H, Aguilar A, Liu L, Bai L, et al. (2012) Structure-based discovery of BM-957 as a potent small-molecule inhibitor of Bcl-2 and Bcl-xL capable of achieving complete tumor regression. J Med Chem 55: 8502–8514.
10. Souers AJ, Leverson JD, Boghaert ER, Ackler SL, Catron ND, et al. (2013) ABT-199, a potent and selective BCL-2 inhibitor, achieves antitumor activity while sparing platelets. Nat Med 19: 202–208.
11. Kemnitzer W, Drewe J, Jiang S, Zhang H, Zhao J, et al. (2007) Discovery of 4-aryl-4H-chromenes as a new series of apoptosis inducers using a cell- and caspase-based high-throughput screening assay. 3. Structure-activity relationships of fused rings at the 7,8-positions. J Med Chem 50: 2858–2864.
12. Gourdeau H, Leblond L, Hamelin B, Desputeau C, Dong K, et al. (2004) Antivascular and antitumor evaluation of 2-amino-4-(3-bromo-4,5-dimethoxyphenyl)-3-cyano-4H-chromenes, a novel series of anticancer agents. Mol Cancer Ther 3: 1375–1384.
13. Pei XY, Dai Y, Grant S (2004) The small-molecule Bcl-2 inhibitor HA14-1 interacts synergistically with flavopiridol to induce mitochondrial injury and apoptosis in human myeloma cells through a free radical-dependent and Jun NH2-terminal kinase-dependent mechanism. Mol Cancer Ther 3: 1513–1524.
14. Fischer U, Schulze-Osthoff K (2005) Apoptosis-based therapies and drug targets. Cell Death Differ 12 Suppl 1: 942–961.
15. Doshi JM, Tian D, Xing C (2006) Structure-activity relationship studies of ethyl 2-amino-6-bromo-4-(1-cyano-2-ethoxy-2-oxoethyl)-4H-chromene-3-carboxylate (HA 14-1), an antagonist for antiapoptotic Bcl-2 proteins to overcome drug resistance in cancer. J Med Chem 49: 7731–7739.
16. Kirkin V, Joos S, Zornig M (2004) The role of Bcl-2 family members in tumorigenesis. Biochim Biophys Acta 1644: 229–249.
17. Bharathkumar H, Sundaram MS, Jagadish S, Paricharak S, Hemshekhar M, et al. (2014) Novel benzoxazine-based aglycones block glucose uptake in vivo by inhibiting glycosidases. PLoS One 9: e102759.
18. Rangappa KS (2005) New cholinesterase inhibitors: synthesis and structure-activity relationship studies of 1, 2-benzisoxazole series and novel imidazolyl-d2-isoxazolines. Journal of physical organic chemistry 18: 773–778.
19. Magedov IV, Manpadi M, Ogasawara MA, Dhawan AS, Rogelj S, et al. (2008) Structural simplification of bioactive natural products with multicomponent synthesis. 2. antiproliferative and antitubulin activities of pyrano[3,2-c]pyridones and pyrano[3,2-c]quinolones. J Med Chem 51: 2561–2570.
20. El-Subbagh HI, Abu-Zaid SM, Mahran MA, Badria FA, Al-Obaid AM (2000) Synthesis and biological evaluation of certain alpha, beta-unsaturated ketones and their corresponding fused pyridines as antiviral and cytotoxic agents. J Med Chem 43: 2915–2921.
21. Basappa, Sadashiva MP, Mantelingu K, Swamy SN, Rangappa KS (2003) Solution-phase synthesis of novel delta2-isoxazoline libraries via 1,3-dipolar cycloaddition and their antifungal properties. Bioorg Med Chem 11: 4539–4544.
22. Basappa, Murugan S, Kavitha CV, Purushothaman A, Nevin KG, et al. (2010) A small oxazine compound as an anti-tumor agent: a novel pyranoside mimetic that binds to VEGF, HB-EGF, and TNF-alpha. Cancer Lett 297: 231–243.
23. Patil SA, Patil R, Pfeffer LM, Miller DD (2013) Chromenes: potential new chemotherapeutic agents for cancer. Future Med Chem 5: 1647–1660.
24. Manero F, Gautier F, Gallenne T, Cauquil N, Gree D, et al. (2006) The small organic compound HA14-1 prevents Bcl-2 interaction with Bax to sensitize malignant glioma cells to induction of cell death. Cancer Res 66: 2757–2764.
25. Piedfer M, Bouchet S, Tang R, Billard C, Dauzonne D, et al. (2013) p70S6 kinase is a target of the novel proteasome inhibitor 3,3'-diamino-4'-methoxyflavone during apoptosis in human myeloid tumor cells. Biochim Biophys Acta 1833: 1316–1328.
26. Sattler M, Liang H, Nettesheim D, Meadows RP, Harlan JE, et al. (1997) Structure of Bcl-xL-Bak peptide complex: recognition between regulators of apoptosis. Science 275: 983–986.
27. Lee EF, Czabotar PE, Smith BJ, Deshayes K, Zobel K, et al. (2007) Crystal structure of ABT-737 complexed with Bcl-xL: implications for selectivity of antagonists of the Bcl-2 family. Cell Death Differ 14: 1711–1713.
28. Grundy M, Seedhouse C, Shang S, Richardson J, Russell N, et al. (2010) The FLT3 internal tandem duplication mutation is a secondary target of the aurora B kinase inhibitor AZD1152-HQPA in acute myelogenous leukemia cells. Mol Cancer Ther 9: 661–672.
29. Chapuis N, Tamburini J, Green AS, Vignon C, Bardet V, et al. (2010) Dual inhibition of PI3K and mTORC1/2 signaling by NVP-BEZ235 as a new therapeutic strategy for acute myeloid leukemia. Clin Cancer Res 16: 5424–5435.
30. Hayano T, Garg M, Yin D, Sudo M, Kawamata N, et al. (2013) SOX7 is down-regulated in lung cancer. J Exp Clin Cancer Res 32: 17.
31. Sukhorukov AY, Nirvanappa AC, Swamy J, Ioffe SL, Nanjunda Swamy S, et al. (2014) Synthesis and characterization of novel 1,2-oxazine-based small molecules that targets acetylcholinesterase. Bioorg Med Chem Lett 24: 3618–3621.
32. Sugahara K, Thimmaiah KN, Bid HK, Houghton PJ, Rangappa KS (2012) Anti-tumor activity of a novel HS-mimetic-vascular endothelial growth factor binding small molecule. PLoS One 7: e39444.

22

Global Epigenetic Regulation of MicroRNAs in Multiple Myeloma

Wenjing Zhang[1,2], **Yaoyu E. Wang**[3], **Yu Zhang**[1,4], **Xavier Leleu**[1,5], **Michaela Reagan**[1], **Yong Zhang**[1], **Yuji Mishima**[1], **Siobhan Glavey**[1], **Salomon Manier**[1], **Antonio Sacco**[1], **Bo Jiang**[2], **Aldo M. Roccaro**[1]*¶, **Irene M. Ghobrial**[1]*¶

1 Department of Medical Oncology, Dana-Farber Cancer Institute, Harvard Medical School, Boston, Massachusetts, United States of America, 2 Nanfang Hospital, Southern Medical University, Guangzhou, China, 3 Center for Cancer Computational Biology, Dana-Farber Cancer Institute, Harvard Medical School, Boston, United States of America, 4 The First People's Hospital of Yunnan Province, Kunming University of Science and Technology, Kunming, China, 5 Department of Hematology, Hopital Claude Huriez, Hospital of Lille (CHRU), Lille, France

Abstract

Epigenetic changes frequently occur during tumorigenesis and DNA hypermethylation may account for the inactivation of tumor suppressor genes in cancer cells. Studies in Multiple Myeloma (MM) have shown variable DNA methylation patterns with focal hypermethylation changes in clinically aggressive subtypes. We studied global methylation patterns in patients with relapsed/refractory MM and found that the majority of methylation peaks were located in the intronic and intragenic regions in MM samples. Therefore, we investigated the effect of methylation on miRNA regulation in MM. To date, the mechanism by which global miRNA suppression occurs in MM has not been fully described. In this study, we report hypermethylation of miRNAs in MM and perform confirmation in MM cell lines using bisulfite sequencing and methylation-specific PCR (MSP) in the presence or absence of the DNA demethylating agent 5-aza-2'-deoxycytidine. We further characterized the hypermethylation-dependent inhibition of miR-152, -10b-5p and -34c-3p which was shown to exert a putative tumor suppressive role in MM. These findings were corroborated by the demonstration that the same miRNAs were down-regulated in MM patients compared to healthy individuals, alongside enrichment of miR-152-, -10b-5p, and miR-34c-3p-predicted targets, as shown at the mRNA level in primary MM cells. Demethylation or gain of function studies of these specific miRNAs led to induction of apoptosis and inhibition of proliferation as well as down-regulation of putative oncogene targets of these miRNAs such as DNMT1, E2F3, BTRC and MYCBP. These findings provide the rationale for epigenetic therapeutic approaches in subgroups of MM.

Editor: Yan Zhang, Harbin Medical University, China

Funding: This study was supported by the Research Project Grant (National Institutes of Health/RO1CA154648), and by the Multiple Myeloma Research Foundation (MMRF; www.themmrf.org). The funders had no role in study design, data collection and analysis, decision to publish, or preparation of the manuscript.

Competing Interests: The authors have declared that no competing interests exist.

* Email: irene_ghobrial@dfci.harvard.edu (IMG); aldo_roccaro@dfci.harvard.edu (AMR)

¶ AMR and IMG are co-last authors on this work.

Introduction

Gene promoter DNA hypermethylation is one of the major epigenetic mechanisms responsible for silencing of tumor suppressor genes in a variety of malignancies [1], suggesting DNA methylation as a target for novel therapeutic agents. DNA methylation occurs at cytosine residues mainly in CpG islands, which represent specific genomic regions containing a high frequency of CpG sites [2]. Most CpG islands are located in the proximal promoter regions of genes and are usually methylated in tumor cells, mediating the inactivation of genes [3]. Recent studies have also highlighted the importance of miRNAs in supporting tumorigenesis [4–11].

MicroRNAs (miRNAs) are small non-coding RNAs of 19–25 nucleotides in length. In animals, miRNAs interact with specific target mRNAs, via complementary binding to sequences within the 3′ UTR, where they induce mRNA degradation or translational inhibition [5,9]. In the vast majority of tumors, miRNAs are down-regulated in clonal cells, thus suggesting their ability to act as tumor suppressors [6,7,10,11]. However, the mechanisms that control the expression of miRNAs are largely unknown. Prior studies have shown that miRNAs can be regulated by aberrant methylation of CpG islands encompassing miRNAs or adjacent to miRNAs [4]. For example, methylation-dependent silencing of the tumor suppressor-miR-127 and -124a has been identified in different tumor types [8,12].

Aberrant promoter methylation has been described in multiple myeloma (MM) [13–17]. Specifically, p16 methylation represents one of the epigenetic aberrations that contribute to MM disease progression [18]. In addition, methylation-dependent silencing of multiple soluble Wnt antagonists, such as WIF1, DKK3, and APC has been reported in MM, thus explaining at least in part, the constitutive activation of Wnt signaling in clonal MM cells [19]. Moreover, epigenetic inactivation of the tumor suppressive miRmiR-194-2-192 cluster and miR-203 is implicated in the pathogenesis of MM [20,21]. However, these studies highlight the methylation status of single genes or miRNAs, with highly variable prevalence of promoter hypermethylation within the same gene.

Herein, we used chromatin immunoprecipitation (ChIP) and array-based hybridization (ChIP-chip) to examine enrichment patterns of CpG islands in primary CD138+ bone marrow (BM) cells isolated from both MM patients and healthy donors (HD) and identified hypermethylation adjacent to miR-152, -10b-5p and miR-34c-3p. Moreover, by treating MM cells with a DNA demethylating agent 5-aza-2'-deoxycytidine (5-aza-CdR) we identified up-regulated miRNAs. Further validation experiments showed that miR-152, miR-10b-5p and miR-34c-3p were highly methylated, which may explain, at least in part, their low expression levels in MM. Finally, we showed that these three miRNAs act as putative tumor suppressor miRNAs by modulating several oncogenes in MM.

Methods

Cell lines and Tissue samples

The human MM cell lines MM.1S, RPMI 8226, OPM2, U266, IM9 and H929 were obtained from the American Type Culture Collection and grown in RPMI 1640 supplemented with 10% fetal bovine serum (FBS), 2 mM/ml L-glutamine, 100 U/mL penicillin, 100 µg/mL streptomycin (Invitrogen) as described previously [22]. Cells were treated with 5 µM of 5-aza-CdR (Sigma Aldrich) for 4 days, replacing the drug and medium every 24 hours [23]. Primary bone marrow stromal cells (BMSCs) were obtained from the bone marrow of patients with MM as described previously [22] and cultured in DMEM plus 20% FBS. Primary plasma cells were obtained from BM samples from patients with relapsed-refractory MM (N = 8). 5 males and 3 females were studied; median age 60 years old (range 48–75 years old). All the MM cases evaluated in these studies were patients with relapsed-refractory disease, who were off-therapy when bone marrow aspirates were collected. Previous therapies included either lenalidomide- or bortezomib-based regimens. Plasma cells were also collected from HD (N = 6). HD samples were then collected as 2 pooled control samples. Plasma cells were obtained using CD138+ microbead selection (Miltenyi Biotec, Auburn, CA) as previously described [22]. Approval for these studies was obtained from the Dana-Farber Cancer Institute Institutional Review Board. Informed consent was obtained from all patients and healthy volunteers in accordance with the Declaration of Helsinki protocol.

ChIP-chip-based DNA methylation analysis

ChIP and ChIP-chip was performed according to described protocols [24] with some modifications. CD138+ plasma cells were obtained from MM patient bone marrow. 5 males and 3 females were studied; median age 60 years old (range 48–75 years). All the MM cases evaluated in these studies were patients with relapsed-refractory disease, who were off-therapy when bone marrow aspirates were collected (i.e., at the time of progression). Previous therapies included either lenalidomide- or bortezomib-based regimens. CD138+ plasma cells were collected from 6

healthy donors and used for ChIP as 2 pooled controls. Cells were allowed to crosslink with 1% formaldehyde. After washing with ice-cold PBS, the cell suspension, in SDS lysis buffer, was disrupted by sonication on ice to gain genomic DNA fragments between 200 and 1000 bp. ChIP was performed with anti-5'-methyl-cytosine. Immunoprecipitated complexes were sequentially eluted and cross-link reversed. DNA fragments were purified using a PCR purification kit (Qiagen). The ChIPed DNA was amplified and hybridized to the Affymetrix GeneChip Human Tiling 2.0R Array Set as previously described [25]. DNA without immunoprecipitation was used as the input control. Microarray data was normalized by quantile normalization using Bioconductor [26]. The normalized data was then analyzed using the model-based analysis of tiling (MAT) array algorithm to identify genomic regions with the highest mean histone methylation scores [27]. Default parameters were used for each algorithm to find ChIP regions from all samples. The MAT library and mapping files were annotated with the nearest reference gene (1 kb distance) using the refseq annotation file based on Human Genome Assembly version 18 (hg18) which was downloaded from UCSC genome browser. Methylation peaks, with a fold change less than 10 compared to input, were filtered out for both MM and HD samples. Differential methylation was determined by the presence or absence of overlapping methylation peaks. Peaks that did not overlap with any peaks found in the contrasting condition were considered to be unique. The peaks were plotted using Circos (http://circos.ca/). MicroRNA coordinates were obtained from NanoString technologies (Seattle, WA), and the peaks overlapping microRNA regions were identified.

miRNA isolation and microRNA expression analysis

miRNAs were isolated from six MM cell lines with or without 5-aza-CdR treatment (5 µM for 4 days) by miRNase mini kit (Qiagen) [28]. Quality control was done using RNA6000 Nano assay on the Aligent 2100 Bioanalyzer (Santa Clara, CA). miRNA detection was conducted using the nCounter human miRNA expression analysis system (Nanostring technologies, Seattle, WA) and performed according to the manufacturer's instructions. Briefly, 100 ng of miRNA was used as input material, with 3 µl of the threefold-diluted sample. A specific DNA tag was ligated onto the 3' end of each mature miRNA, providing exclusive identification of each miRNA species in the sample. The tagging was performed in a multiplexed ligation reaction utilizing reverse complementary bridge oligonucleotides to dispose the ligation of each miRNA to its designated tag. All hybridization reactions were incubated at 64°C for 20 hours and then applied to the nCounter Preparation Station for automated removal of excel probes and immobilization of probe-transcript complexes on a streptavidin-coated cartridge. Data collection was carried out in the nCounter Digital Analyzer by counting individual fluorescent barcodes and quantifying target miRNA molecules present in each sample. Data normalization was performed by nSolver Analysis Software according to the manufacturer's instructions. Six internal positive spike controls were used to account for minor differences in hybridization and purification efficiencies, and six negative controls were used for the consideration of background hybridization.

Bisulfate treatment and PCR conditions

Genomic DNA (gDNA) was isolated from MM cells with DNeasy Blood & Tissue Kit (Qiagen, Valencia, CA) as previously described [23]. 500 ng of gDNA was modified by treatment with sodium bisulfate using the EZ DNA Methylation-Gold Kit (Zymo Research, Orange County, CA), which induces chemical

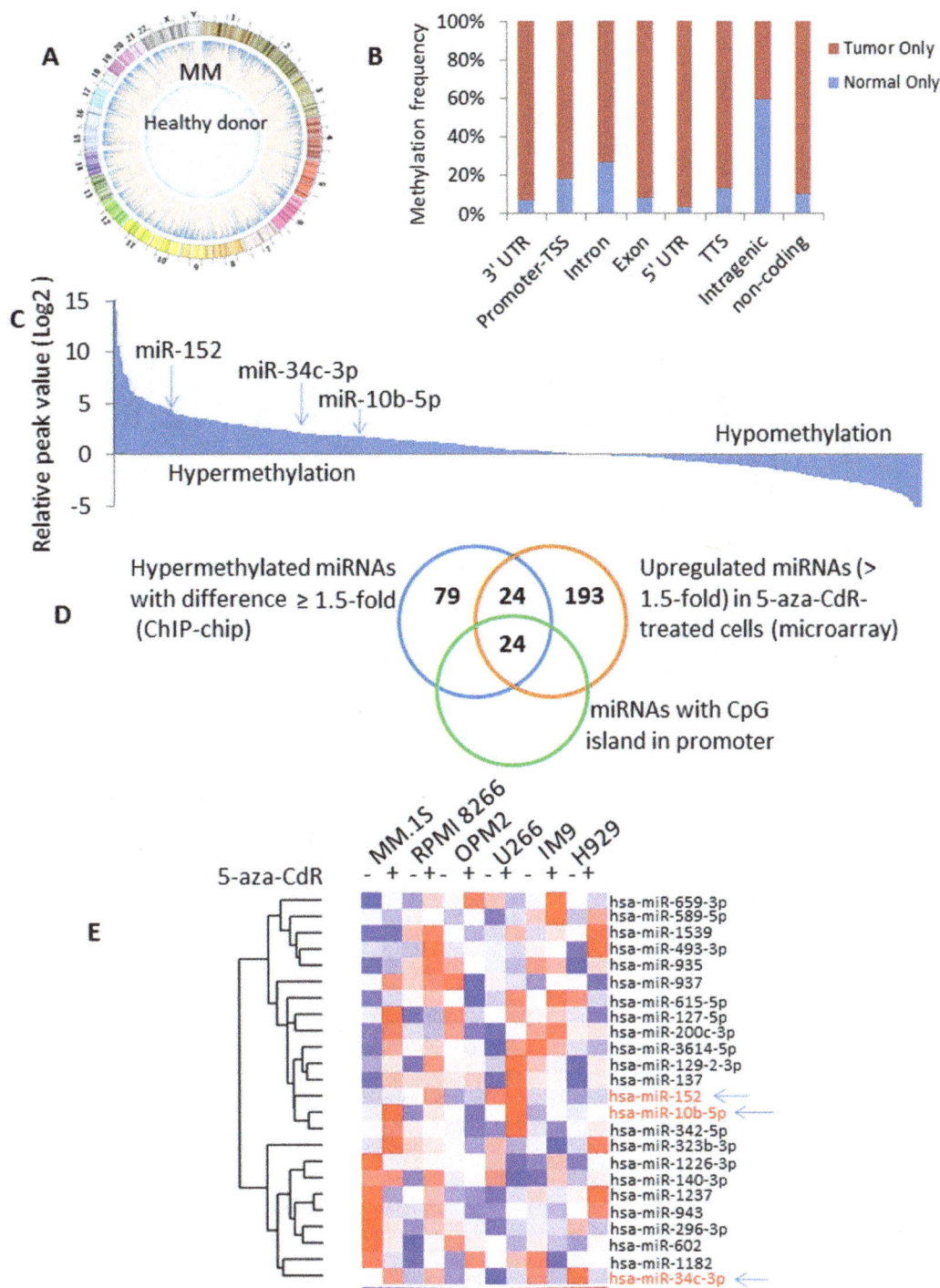

Figure 1. Methylation status of whole-genome sequencing data in MM and healthy donors. (A) Circular representation of DNA methylation levels in whole genome regions for MM and healthy donors (HD). (B) Genome-wide distribution of methylation peaks by gene regions in HD/MM only. (C) Methylation levels of regions around all known miRNAs in MM patients in decreasing order by peak intensity. Data was presented as log$_2$ values. (D) Venn diagram compared ChIP-chip and miRNA microarray data, as well as miRNAs being present with CpG island. Left, miRNAs identified as high potential methylation with the definition of a difference ≥1.5-fold between MM and HD; Right: miRNAs up-regulated by more than 1.5-fold in at least two cell lines with 5-aza-CdR treatment; Bottom: miRNAs with CpG island. (E) Heatmap of the 24 overlay miRNAs in six MM cell lines with or without 5-aza-CdR treatment. Red, high expression; blue, low expression.

conversion of unmethylated cytosines into uracils, whit methylated cytosines being protected from this conversion [29]. The sequences of miRNA and its promoter were analyzed by using miRBase and the University of California at Santa Cruz Human Genome Browser (UCSC). CpG islands and specific primers for MSP and bisulfite-sequencing PCR (BSP) were designed by MethPrimer Tools (http://www.urogene.org/methprimer/) [30]. MSP analysis was performed with primers specific for either the

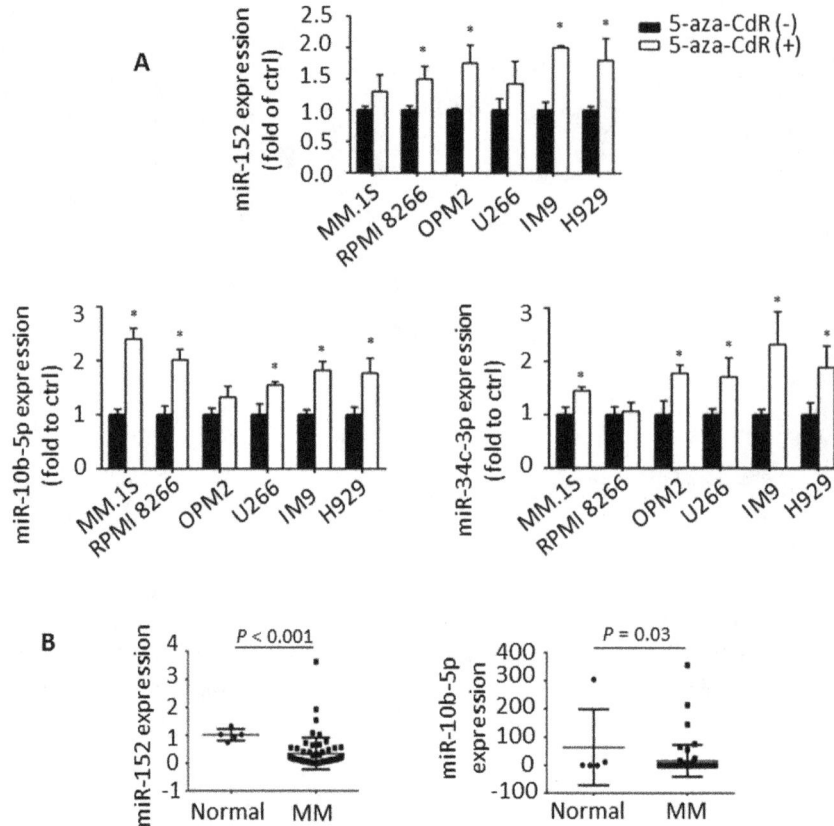

Figure 2. Identification and expression of miRNA candidates in MM. (A) Effect of 5-aza-CdR on the expression of miR-152, -10b-5p and miR-34c-3p in six MM cell lines by real-time PCR. Experiments were performed in triplicate and RNU6B was used as the internal control. Data were shown as means ± SD. *$P<0.05$ compared with cells without 5-aza-CdR. (B) Expression levels of miR-152 and miR-10b-5p in MM and healthy donor in GSE16558.

methylated or unmethylated DNA. To verify sufficient DNA quality and successful DNA modification, human genomic DNA, with methylated CpG sites, was used as the positive control; H_2O was used as the negative control. Amplified bisulfate PCR products were subcloned into the pGEM-T Easy vector (Promega, Madison, WI). Eight independent clones for each sample were selected and the T7 primers were used to sequence inserted fragments. Primers used are shown in File S1.

Quantitative Real-time PCR

Quantitative Real-time PCR was performed as described previously [28]. Briefly, total RNA or miRNA from cells was isolated with RNeasy or miRNeasy Mini kit (QIAGEN). cDNA was synthesized using the SuperScript cDNA synthesis kit (Invitrogen) or High Capacity cDNA Reverse Transcription Kit (Life Technologies, Grand Island, NY) and quantitative RT-PCR (qRT-PCR) reactions were performed using SYBR MasterMix (Qiagen) by StepOnePlus Real-Time PCR System (Applied Biosystems, Foster city, CA) in triplicate. 18S or RNU6B was used to normalize the miRNA and mRNA data, respectively. Expression was calculated using the $2^{-\Delta\Delta Ct}$ method. Primers used are described in File S1.

miRNA transfection

MM.1S, RPMI 8226, IM9 and H929 cell lines were transfected with hsa-miR-152, -10b-5p and -34c-3p mirVana miRNA or

negative control mimics (Life Technologies, Grand Island, NY) at a final concentration of 50 nM, using Lipofectamine 2000 following manufacturer's instructions. Efficiency of transfection was validated by real-time PCR.

Cell proliferation assays

Cell proliferation was measured by the incorporation of [³H] thymidine uptake assay (Perkin Elmer, Boston, MA), as described previously [22]. MM cells were incubated in 96-well plates transfected with miR-152, -10b-5p and miR-34c-3p and negative control mimics, respectively, following by being pulsed with [³H] thymidine (0.5 μCi/well) for at least 8 h of 48 h cultures. Cells were harvested onto glass filters with an automatic cell harvester (Cambridge Technology, Cambridge, MA), and counted using the LKB Betaplate scintillation counter (Wallac, Gaithersburg, MD). All experiments were performed in four-well repeat.

Immunoblotting

Sodium dodecyl sulfate-polyacrylamidegel electrophoresis (SDS-PAGE) and western blotting were performed as previously described [23]. In brief, whole-cell lysates were separated using 10–12% gels and transferred to polyvinyldenefluoride (PVDF) membranes (Bio-Rad Laboratories, Hercules, CA). The antibodies used for immunoblotting included anti-PARP, -caspase 9, caspase 3 and α-tubulin (Cell Signaling Technology, Danvers, MA).

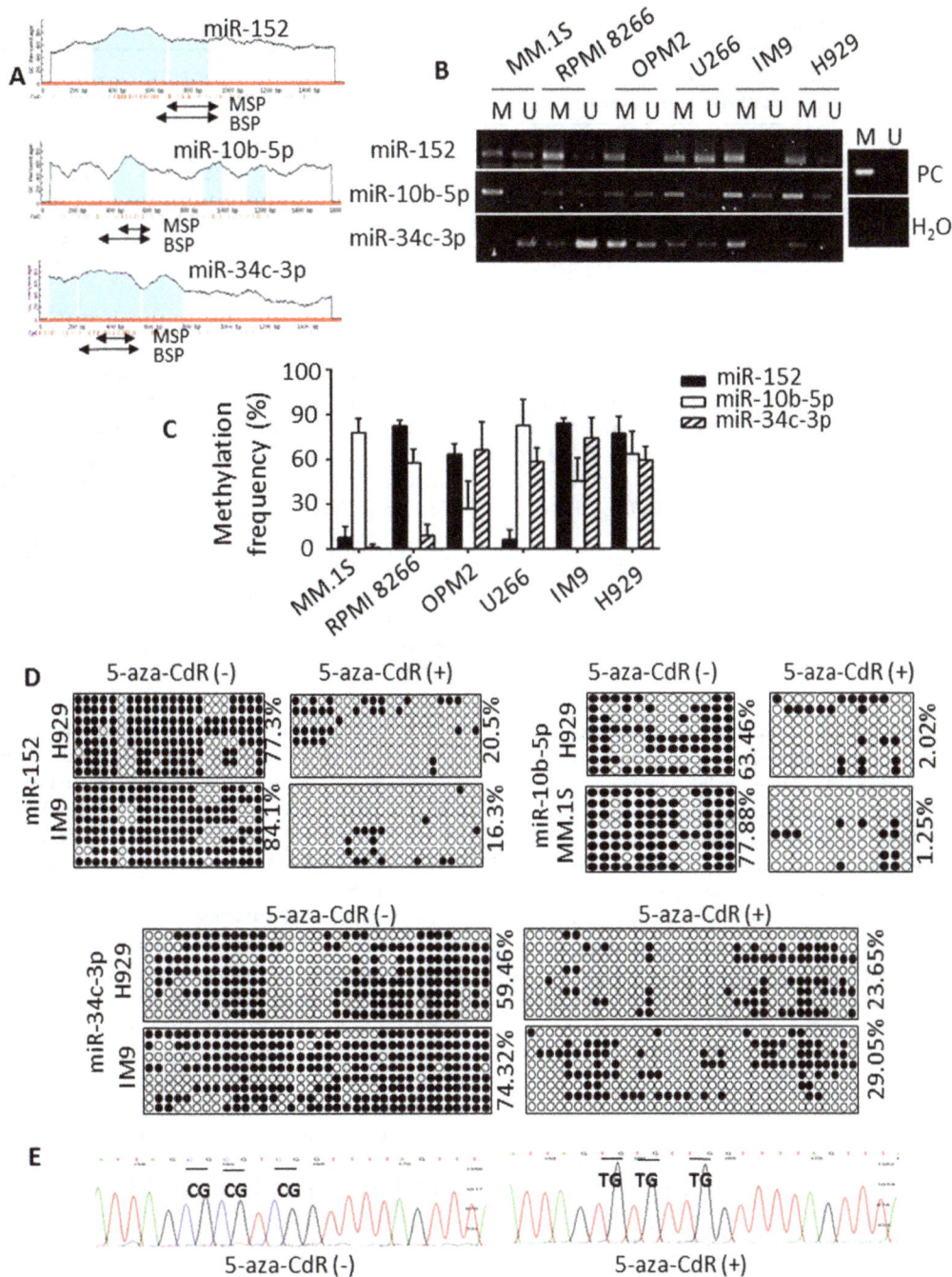

Figure 3. Methylation of miR-152, -10b-5p and miR-34c-3p in MM cells. (A) Schematic illustration of the percentage of C + G nucleotides (CG%) and the density of CpG olinucleotides were shown for a region spanning 1000 bp upstream and 500 bp downstream of miR-152, miR-10b-5p and miR-34c-3p, respectively. Specific primers for these CpG islands were designed (arrows) and used to amplify these DNA fragments in MM cell lines. The CpG island was depicted, and each vertical bar illustrated a single CpG. (B) Representative MSP results of the three miRNAs methylation inMM1S, RPMI 8266, OPM2, U266, IM9 and H929 cell lines. M: methylated primers; U: unmehtylated primers. PC: positive control. (C) Bisulfite sequencing analysis showed relative methylation frequencies of miR-152, -10b-5p and miR-34c-3p in six MM cell lines. Eight single clones for each sample were selected and T7 primers were used for sequencing. (D) Bisulfite sequencing analysis showed methylation frequencies of miR-152 and miR-34c-3p in H929 and IM9, and miR-10b-5p in H929 and MM1S, treated with or without 5'-aza-CdR (5 μM) for 4 days. Black and white circle represented methylated and unmethylated CpG, respectively. (E) Representative sequencing results showed that the cytosine (C) residues of CpG dinucleotides were converted into thymidine (T).

Expression profiling and GSEA of available datasets

miR-152 and miR-10b-5p expression was analyzed using publicly available dataset where primary bone marrow selected CD138+ cells were obtained from either MM patients or HDs (GSE16558). Similarly, the expression levels of DNMT1, E2F3, BTRC and MYCBP were analyzed using publicly available datasets where primary bone marrow selected CD138+ cells obtained from either MM patients or healthy individuals were

Table 1. Methylation frequency of miR-152, -10b-5p and miR-34c-3p in MM cell lines.

	Methylation frequency (%)					
	MM1S	**RPMI 8266**	**OPM2**	**U266**	**IM9**	**H929**
miR-152	8.0	82.4	63.6	6.3	84.1	77.3
miR-10b-5p	77.9	57.7	26.9	82.7	45.2	63.5
miR-34c-3p	1.2	9.2	66.2	58.5	74.3	59.5

studied (GSE5900; GSE 2658) [31]. Gene Sets Enrichment Analysis (GSEA) was performed by using gene sets publicly available from the Broad Institute (Cambridge, MA; http://www.broadinstitute.org/gsea/index.jsp), as previously reported [32,33]. Specifically, the following gene sets were used: TGCACTG, MIR-148A, MIR-152, MIR-148B; ACAGGGT, MIR-10A, MIR-10B and CACTGCC, MIR-34A, MIR-34C, MIR-449.

We used the easy-to-use graphical user interface of GSEA with gene set permutation to derive significance, with signal-to-noise as the distance metric and maximum expression to collapse probe sets to genes.

Statistical analysis

miRNA expression data were normalized according to manufacturer's instructions (Nanostring technologies, Seattle, WA). To further define those miRNAs differentially expressed between groups (with vs without 5-aza-CdR treatment), the expression patterns of normalized data were analyzed and hierarchical clustering was performed using dChip (http://www.hsph.harvard.edu/cli/complab/dchip/) [34]. The enrichment analysis of targeted mRNAs of miR-152, -10b-5p and miR-34c-3p in GEO datasets was performed using GSEA, and considered significant with false discovery rate (FDR) <0.25, as previously reported (31). Mann-Whitney U rank ranksum test with GraphPad software was applied to describe the distribution of miRNAs and gene levels in MM patients compared with HDs. Statistical tests were unpaired, 2-sided t-tests comparing two conditions. P values less than 0.05 were considered significant. Data were presented for the purpose of figures as means and error bars.

Results

Global changes in DNA methylation occur in MM patients

We first interrogated genome-wide methylation patterns in relapsed/refractory MM patients and HDs, and found a significant increase in global methylation in relapsed MM compared to HDs; circular representation of DNA methylation levels per each chromosome in MM and healthy donor is represented in Fig. 1A. The majority of methylation peaks were located in the intronic and intragenic regions in MM samples. Over half of the methylation peaks were identified within in intron regions (51.9% in HD and 59.6% in MM), without significant differences between HDs and MM. However, there were more significant regions differentially methylated in the 3′-UTR, promoter-TSS, exon, 5′-UTR, TTS and non-coding regions in MM compared with HDs (Fig. 1B). Of note, an 8.5-fold increase of non-coding regions was observed in MM compared to HDs. This leads us to hypothesize that methylation of miRNAs can be critical for the regulation of expression patterns of miRNAs in MM. We, therefore, mapped probe values of all known miRNAs

to determine whether miRNA-related regions were differentially methylated in MM. As shown in Fig. 1C, there was a significant increase in the number of hypermethylated miRNAs compared to the number of miRNAs with hypomethylation. Specifically, 127 miRNAs were identified as highly methylated miRNAs with ≥1.5-fold change increase in MM compared to HDs ($\log_2$) (File S2). These findings suggested that miRNAs are highly methylated in MM and may therefore explain in part the global decrease in miRNA expression in these tumor cells.

To further examine the role of methylation in miRNA regulation in tumor cells, MM cell lines (MM.1S, RPMI 8266, OPM2, U266, IM9 and H929) were treated with the DNA methyltransferase inhibitor 5-aza-CdR and the global level of miRNAs was examined. Hierarchical clustering analysis of cell lines was performed and demonstrated up-regulation of miRNAs in response to treatment with 5-aza-CdR treatment with a>1.5-fold difference. Overall, 241 miRNAs were up-regulated in at least two cell lines with 5-aza-CdR (File S3), 77 miRNAs were up-regulated in three cell lines and 7 miRNAs were up-regulated in four cell lines treated.

To further identify the most critically regulated miRNAs, we identified 48 miRNAs that were present in the methylation sites of MM patient samples and were also up-regulated in response to 5-aza-CdR treatment in MM cell lines (Fig. 1D). Among them, 4 miRNAs, miR-3605-5p, -4461, -4516 and miR-4531, were not present in UCSC and were excluded; 44 miRNAs remained. We then assessed the status of CpG islands for these 44 miRNAs and found that only 24 miRNAs were present in one or more CpG island upstream regulatory sequences (Fig. 1D&E).

Identification and expression analysis of miRNA candidates in MM

Among the 24 miRNAs, miR-152 was the most frequently up-regulated miRNA with 5-aza-CdR treatment (in all six cell lines). In addition, miR-10b-5p was up-regulated by more than 2.0-fold in at least three cell lines following treatment with 5′-aza-CdR. Therefore, we further examined the functional significance of miR-152 and miR-10b-5p in parallel with miR-34c-3p, which was also included in the 24 miRNAs and has been reported to be methylated in MM [35].

Further validation of the re-expression of these miRNAs was performed by real-time PCR and indeed confirmed that miR-152, -10b-5p and miR-34c-3p were significantly increased following exposure to 5-aza-CdR (Fig. 2A). Of note, all of the regions around these three miRNAs were highly methylated in MM patients as previously shown in Fig. 1C. We next analyzed the expression levels of these miRNAs in MM using GSE16558, and found that both miR-152 and miR-10b-5p were significantly down-regulated in MM patients compared to HD (Fig. 2B).

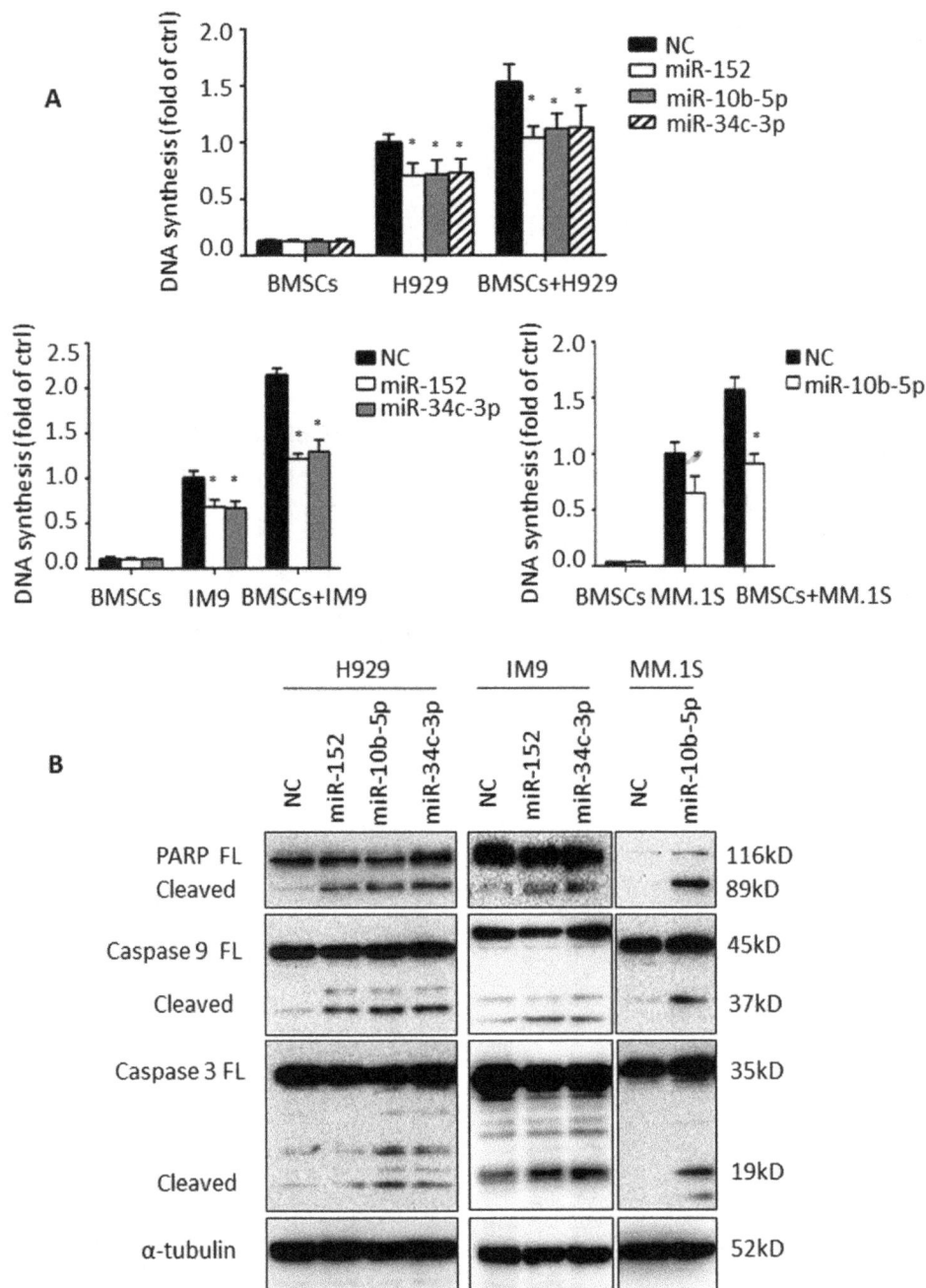

Figure 4. miR-152, -10b-5p and miR-34c-3p modulated proliferation and apoptosis of MM cells. Since the three miRNAs have different methylation frequencies and expression levels in MM cell lines, H929 cells were transfected with miR-152, -10b-5p and -34c-3p mirVana miRNA respectively; IM9 cells were transfected with miR-152 and -34c-3p mirVana miRNA respectively; MM1S cells were used to overexpress miR-10b-5p. All of the cells transfected with negative control mimics used as control cells. (A) The indicated transfected cells were cultured in presence or absence with primary BMSCs for 72 hours, following by $[H]^3$ thymidine uptake assay. NC-transfected cells in absence with BMSCs were defined as 1.0 and regarded as the control group. $^*P<0.05$. (B) MM cells (NC-, miR-152-, -10b-5p-, or miR-34c-3p-transfected) were harvested at 48 or 72 hours after transfection. Whole cell lysates were subjected to western blotting using anti-PARP, -Caspase 9, -Caspase 3 and -α-tubulin antibodies.

Methylation analyses of miR-152, -10b-5p and miR-34c-3p in MM cells

miR-152, -10b-5p and miR-34c-3p present with 2, 3 and 3 distinct CpG islands in their upstream chromosomal regions, respectively (1000 bp upstream and 500 bp upstream) as shown in Fig. 3A. We further examined the methylation status of these miRNAs using MSP analysis and showed that the miR-152

upstream promoter region was methylated in RPMI 8266, OPM2, IM9 and H929 cells; while partial/no methylation was detected in MM.1S and U266 cells. Moreover, miR-10b-5p methylation was observed in all MM cell lines tested. Complete methylation of miR-34c-3p was observed in IM9 and H929; while partial methylation was found in OPM2 and U266; in contrast with MM.1S and RPMI 8266 that were unmethylated (Fig. 3B). To demonstrate the frequency of CpG island methylation in these

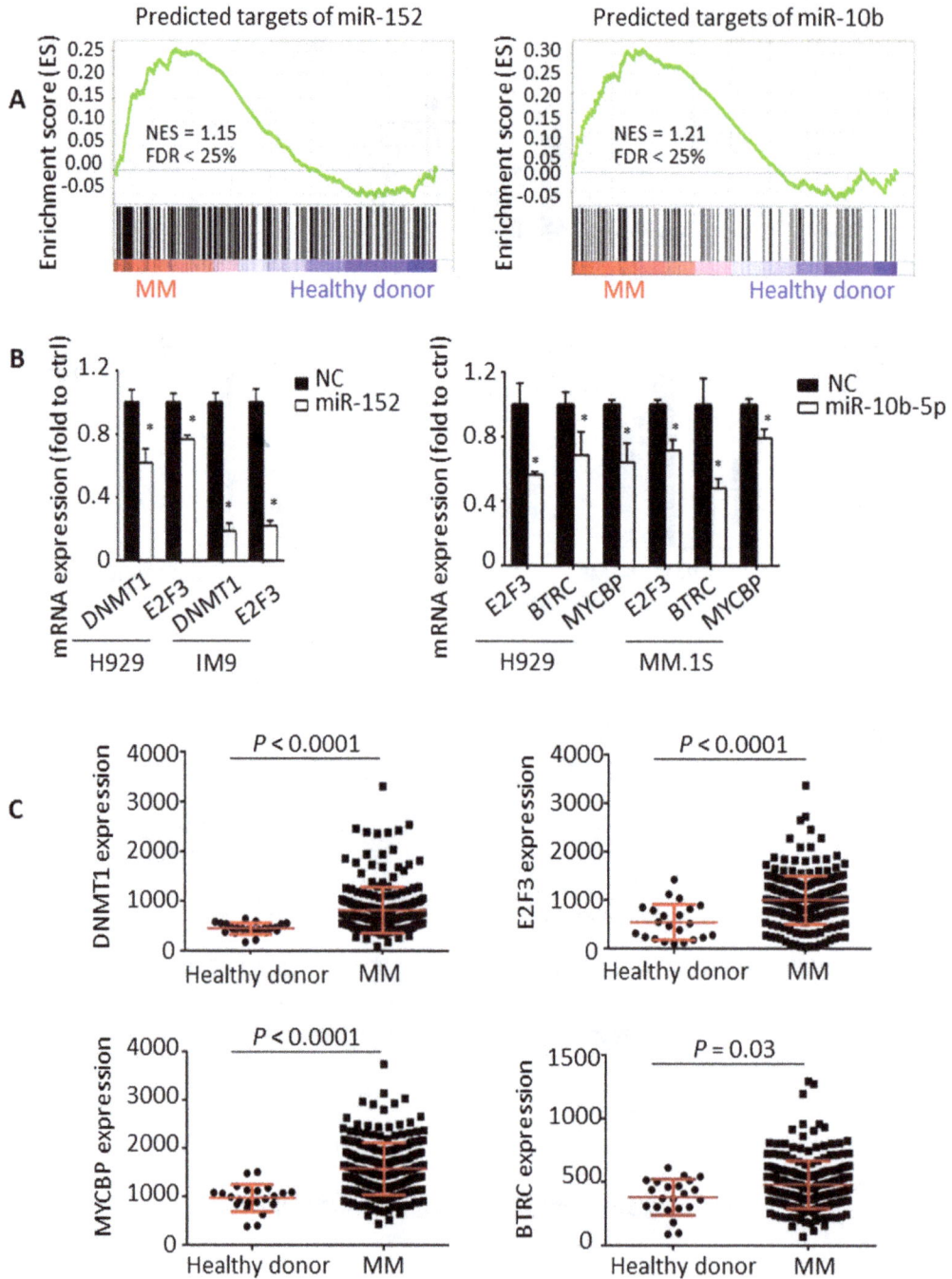

Figure 5. Effect of miR-152 and miR-10b-5p on the expression of putative targets. (A) GSEA established that predicated targets of miR-152 and miR-10b-5p was positively correlated with MM, and negatively correlated with HD. NES: normalized enrichment score; FDR: false discovery rate. (B) The expression of predicted targets of miR-152 (DNMT1 and E2F3) and miR-10b-5p (E2F3, BTRC and MYCBP) in miR-152-, -10b-5p- or NC-transfected MM cells by real-time PCR with normalization to the reference 18S expression. *P<0.05 compared with NC-transfected cells. (C) The expression of DNMT1, E2F3, BTRC and MYCBP in healthy donor and MM (GSE5900 and GSE2658).

three miRNAs, we undertook bisulfite sequencing of multiple clones (Fig. 3C). Detailed analysis has been provided in Table 1. These results support that miR-152, miR-10b-5p and miR-34c-3p hypermethylation frequently occurs in MM cells. In addition, the results of MSP and BSP suggest that the methylation of miRNAs is cell-type specific.

To determine whether 5-aza-CdR may modulate miRNA methylation status in MM cells, bisulfite sequencing was further performed in H929, IM9 and MM1S cells for specific miRNAs respectively, which was based on their different methylation frequencies in each cell line. As shown in Fig. 3D, the methylation frequencies of miR-152 decreased from 77.3% to 20.5% in H929, and 84.1% to 16.3% in IM9 cells after 5-aza-CdR treatment. Similar results were found for miR-10b-5p in H929 (63.46% to 2.02%) and MM1S (77.88% to 1.25%) cells, as well as for miR-34c-3p in H929 (59.46% to 23.65%) and IM9 (74.32% to

29.05%). The representative sites with the conversion from cytosines (C) to uracil (T) are shown in Fig. 3E. Taken together, these findings suggest that the CpG-rich promoter regions of miR-152, -10b-5p and miR-34c-3p are hypermethylated and present with low expression in MM cells.

MiR-152, -10b-5p and miR-34c-3p act as tumor suppressors in MM

We next examined the potential functional relevance of miR-152, -10b-5p and -34c-3p in MM. We therefore, examined the role of these 3 miRNAs in the growth of tumor cells alone or in the presence of bone marrow stromal cells (BMSCs) using gain of function studies. Efficiency of transfection with miR-152, -10b-5p and miR-34c-3p was first demonstrated using real-time PCR (Figure S1). There was a significant inhibition of proliferation of MM cells in response to re-expression of miR-152, -10b-5p and -34c-3p in MM cells, even in the presence of BMSCs, indicating that these miRNAs are critical for the growth and proliferation of MM cells even in the presence of the bone marrow microenvironment (Figure 4A, $P<0.05$). The effects of these miRNAs in modulating MM cell apoptosis was also investigated; re-expression of miR-152, -10b-5p and miR-34c-3p mimics induced cleavage of PARP- and caspase-9 and -3, compared to normal control-transfected cells (Fig. 4B). These findings suggest that miR-152, -10b-5p and miR-34c-3p may act as putative tumor suppressors in MM by inhibiting cell proliferation and inducing apoptosis.

MiR-152 and miR-10b-5p mediate the activation of oncogenic target genes

Given that miRNAs inhibit mRNA expression, we hypothesized that the predicted target genes of these specific miRNAs are highly expressed in CD138$^+$ bone marrow-derived MM cells. We therefore screened publically available mRNA datasets (GSE5900; GSE2658) and found that MM patients present with a significant enrichment of miR-152- and miR-10b-target genes, as shown by GSEA (FDR<0.25; Fig. 5A), whereas no significant differences were observed for miR-34c-predicted targeted genes. We next focused on the predicted genes of miR-152- and miR-10b-5p. DNA-methyltransferase 1 (DNMT1), a predicted target of miR-152; beta-transducin repeat containing E3 ubiquitin protein ligase (BTRC) and Myc binding protein (MYCBP), predicted targets of miR-10b-5p and E2F transcription factor 3 (E2F3), predicted target of both miR-152 and miR-10b-5p were examined in MM cells (Figure S2). Enhanced expression of miR-152 induced a significant reduction of DNMT1 and E2F3 expression. In addition, E2F3, BTRC and MYCBP were significantly increased after miR-10b-5p mimic transfection (Fig. 5B). Moreover, we confirmed that the expression of these genes is significantly up-regulated in MM patients compared to healthy donors using GSE5900 and GSE2658 as shown in Fig. 5C. These results suggest that methylation of miR-152 and miR-10b-5p enhances MM progression through increased expression of specific oncogenes, such as DNMT1, BTRC, MYCBP and E2F3.

Discussion

Aberrant promoter hypermethylation has been described in tumors for specific gene clusters in MM [4,35]. In addition, recent studies have shown that MM is characterized by highly variable DNA methylation patterns that exceed the methylation variability seen in several solid cancers, with focal hypermethylation changes in clinically aggressive subtypes, such as plasma cell leukemia and patients with translocation t(4;14), suggesting that methylation changes can affect disease biology [36]. Moreover, Kaiser et al

[16] identified epigenetically repressed tumor suppressor genes that were associated with prognostic relevance in myeloma. In our study, we found that the majority of methylation peaks were located in the intronic and intragenic regions in MM samples. Therefore, we investigated the effect of methylation on miRNA regulation in MM.

miRNAs act as tumor suppressors or oncogenic activators in many cancers, however, the majority of cancers present with global suppression of miRNAs including MM [6,7,10,11,36–38]. To date, the mechanism of global miRNA suppression in cancers, and specifically in MM, has not been investigated. In this study, we showed that hypermethylation occurred in regions of miRNAs in MM, compared to HDs indicating that miRNAs are highly methylated in MM, which could explain the global decrease of miRNA expression in MM cells. These studies were confirmed in MM cell lines using bisulfite sequencing and MSP in the presence or absence of the demethylating agent 5-aza-CdR.

Our studies describe the presence of hypermethylation-dependent inhibition of miR-152, -10b-5p and -34c-3p, which were shown to exert a putative tumor suppressive role in MM. We identified these miRNAs though global methylation studies in patient samples as well as providing functional validation in MM cell lines with bisulfite sequencing and MSP in the presence or absence of 5-aza-CdR. These findings were corroborated by the demonstration that the same miRNAs were present at lower level in MM patients compared to healthy individuals, together with enrichment of miR-152-, -10b-5p, and -34c-3p-predicted targets as shown at the mRNA level in primary MM cells. Demethylation or re-expression of these specific miRNAs led to induction of apoptosis and inhibition of proliferation as well as down-regulation of putative oncogene targets of these miRNAs.

MiR-10b may exert a bifunctional role, as shown by its activity as oncogene or tumor suppressor depending on the specific tumor type. For instance, it may positively regulate cell invasion and metastasis in breast cancer through Twist modulation [39,40]. In pancreatic cancer, miR-10b has been reported to enhance cell invasion by suppressing TIP30 expression and promoting EGF- and TGF-β-mediated pathways and it can be also considered as a novel diagnostic biomarker [41]. In contrast, miR-10b has been shown to play a tumor suppressive role in gastric cancer and endometrial serous adenocarcinomas [42,43]. In our studies, we found that miR-10b-5p (previous ID: miR-10b) was down-regulated via promoter methylation, resulting in inhibition of MM cell proliferation. Importantly, methylation of miR-10b-5p occurred in the MM patient samples based on a global methylation analysis [16]. These findings suggest that miR-10b-5p is regulated through different mechanisms, such as transcription regulation and promoter methylation, thereby presenting different expression profiles and functions in different types of tumors.

Aberrant methylation of miR-152 has been reported in both solid tumors and hematological malignancies. Previous studies show that miR-152 is methylated and inhibits cell growth and proliferation in breast and endometrial cancer [44,45]. In addition, methylation of miR-152 contributes to its down-regulation in hepatitis B virus-related hepatocellular carcinoma (HCC) [46]. miR-152, among others, is down-regulated in t(4;11) positive ALL, as a consequence of CpG methylation [47]. Moreover, an association between miR-152 expression and lower survival in patients with MM has been previously demonstrated [48]. Interestingly, it has been reported miR-152 is down-regulated in hyperdiploid MM compared with non-hyperdiploid disease, leading to the up-regulation of several oncogenes [49].

Since each single miRNA has a large number of predicted or established target genes, we selected several putative oncogenes to study, such as DNMT1, E2F3, BTRC and MYCBP. Among them, DNMT1 is a major enzyme responsible for maintenance of DNA methylation patternspatter. Its aberrant expression is the dominant mechanism for the genome instability, which associates with tumorigenesis and cancer development [50]. E2F3 functions as a transcription factor which is involved in the regulation of cell proliferation [51]. In fact, it has been observed that DNMT1 and E2F3 are candidate targets of miR-152 in HCC, endometrial and breast cancer [44–46]; BTRC has been shown to ubiquitinate phosphorylated NFKBIA, targeting it for degradation and thus activating NF-κB [52]. MYCBP is able to enhance c-Myc'sMyc ability to activate E box-dependent transcription [53]. The activation of both NF-κB and c-Myc partly contributes to the progression of MM. In our study, we found that down-regulation of miR-152 and miR-10b-5p is supported by over-expression of DNMT1, E2F3, BTRC and MYCBP in MM patients. More importantly, ectopic expression of miR-152 or miR-10b-5p significantly down-regulated the mRNA level of these genes. Hence, we conclude that MM cell proliferation may be mediated, at least in part, through methylation and down-regulation of miR-152- and miR-10b-5p which in turn lead to activation of DNMT1, E2F3, BTRC and MYCBP.

In conclusion, our studies indicate that global miRNA suppression in MM may be due to hypermethylation of non-coding regions in the MM genome. More specifically, miR-152, -10b-5p and miR-34c-3p are epigenetically silenced in MM through CpG island methylation; and act as potential tumor suppressor miRNAs in this disease. Re-expression of these miRNAs led to suppression of oncogenes and the inhibition of proliferation and induction of apoptosis in MM cells. These findings establish an important mechanism of miRNA deregulation in MM. Specifically, we suggest that miR-152, -10b-5p and miR-34c-3p promoter methylation may represent useful molecular biomarkers for assessing the risk of MM development. Most importantly, our study might provide a mechanistic and molecular basis for a new therapeutic use for pharmacological compounds with DNA demethylating activity in the treatment of MM patients.

Supporting Information

Figure S1   Validation of miRNA expression by real-time PCR. The indicted cells were transfected with miR-152, -10b-5p, -34c-3p or negative control (NC) respectively. miRNA levels were detected by real-time PCR, and normalized to RNU6B control. Data were shown as means ± SD. *P<0.05 compared with NC-transfected cells.

Figure S2   Binding of miR-152 or miR-10b-5p to the indicated target mRNAs at different sites. Complementary sites between miR-152 and DNMT1 and E2F3, and between miR-10b-5p and E2F3, BTRC and MYCBP according to Targetscan 6.2.

File S1   List of primer sequences and PCR products.

File S2   MM patients present with higher miRNA methylation as compared to healthy individuals.

File S3   5-aza-CdR-dependent modulation of miRNAs in MM cell lines.

Author Contributions

Conceived and designed the experiments: WZ AMR IMG. Performed the experiments: WZ Yu Zhang AS. Analyzed the data: YEW SM MR. Contributed reagents/materials/analysis tools: XL Yong Zhang YM SG BJ AS. Wrote the paper: WZ AMR IMG.

References

1. Jones PA, Baylin SB (2002) The fundamental role of epigenetic events in cancer. Nature reviews Genetics 3: 415–428.
2. Bird A (2002) DNA methylation patterns and epigenetic memory. Genes & development 16: 6–21.
3. Esteller M (2008) Epigenetics in cancer. The New England journal of medicine 358: 1148–1159.
4. Agirre X, Martinez-Climent JA, Odero MD, Prosper F (2012) Epigenetic regulation of miRNA genes in acute leukemia. Leukemia 26: 395–403.
5. Bartel DP (2004) MicroRNAs: genomics, biogenesis, mechanism, and function. Cell 116: 281–297.
6. Formosa A, Markert EK, Lena AM, Italiano D, Finazzi-Agro E, et al. (2013) MicroRNAs, miR-154, miR-299-5p, miR-376a, miR-376c, miR-377, miR-381, miR-487b, miR-485-3p, miR-495 and miR-654-3p, mapped to the 14q32.31 locus, regulate proliferation, apoptosis, migration and invasion in metastatic prostate cancer cells. Oncogene.
7. Kureel J, Dixit M, Tyagi AM, Mansoori MN, Srivastava K, et al. (2014) miR-542-3p suppresses osteoblast cell proliferation and differentiation, targets BMP-7 signaling and inhibits bone formation. Cell death & disease 5: e1050.
8. Lopez-Serra P, Esteller M (2012) DNA methylation-associated silencing of tumor-suppressor microRNAs in cancer. Oncogene 31: 1609–1622.
9. Lu J, Getz G, Miska EA, Alvarez-Saavedra E, Lamb J, et al. (2005) MicroRNA expression profiles classify human cancers. Nature 435: 834–838.
10. Song SJ, Ito K, Ala U, Kats L, Webster K, et al. (2013) The oncogenic microRNA miR-22 targets the TET2 tumor suppressor to promote hematopoietic stem cell self-renewal and transformation. Cell stem cell 13: 87–101.
11. Wei J, Wang F, Kong LY, Xu S, Doucette T, et al. (2013) miR-124 inhibits STAT3 signaling to enhance T cell-mediated immune clearance of glioma. Cancer research 73: 3913–3926.
12. Lujambio A, Esteller M (2007) CpG island hypermethylation of tumor suppressor microRNAs in human cancer. Cell cycle (Georgetown, Tex) 6: 1455–1459.
13. Agnelli L, Bicciato S, Mattioli M, Fabris S, Intini D, et al. (2005) Molecular classification of multiple myeloma: a distinct transcriptional profile characterizes patients expressing CCND1 and negative for 14q32 translocations. Journal of clinical oncology: official journal of the American Society of Clinical Oncology 23: 7296–7306.
14. Fernandez de Larrea C, Martin-Antonio B, Cibeira MT, Navarro A, Tovar N, et al. (2013) Impact of global and gene-specific DNA methylation pattern in relapsed multiple myeloma patients treated with bortezomib. Leukemia research 37: 641–646.
15. Hatzimichael E, Benetatos L, Dasoula A, Dranitsaris G, Tsiara S, et al. (2009) Absence of methylation-dependent transcriptional silencing in TP73 irrespective of the methylation status of the CDKN2A CpG island in plasma cell neoplasia. Leukemia research 33: 1272–1275.
16. Kaiser MF, Johnson DC, Wu P, Walker BA, Brioli A, et al. (2013) Global methylation analysis identifies prognostically important epigenetically inactivated tumor suppressor genes in multiple myeloma. Blood 122: 219–226.
17. Martinez-Garcia E, Popovic R, Min DJ, Sweet SM, Thomas PM, et al. (2011) The MMSET histone methyl transferase switches global histone methylation and alters gene expression in t(4;14) multiple myeloma cells. Blood 117: 211–220.
18. Scheiermann C, Kunisaki Y, Frenette PS (2013) Circadian control of the immune system. Nature reviews Immunology 13: 190–198.
19. Chim CS, Pang R, Fung TK, Choi CL, Liang R (2007) Epigenetic dysregulation of Wnt signaling pathway in multiple myeloma. Leukemia 21: 2527–2536.
20. Pichiorri F, Suh SS, Rocci A, De Luca L, Taccioli C, et al. (2010) Downregulation of p53-inducible microRNAs 192, 194, and 215 impairs the p53/MDM2 autoregulatory loop in multiple myeloma development. Cancer cell 18: 367–381.
21. Bueno MJ, Perez de Castro I, Gomez de Cedron M, Santos J, Calin GA, et al. (2008) Genetic and epigenetic silencing of microRNA-203 enhances ABL1 and BCR-ABL1 oncogene expression. Cancer cell 13: 496–506.
22. Roccaro AM, Sacco A, Thompson B, Leleu X, Azab AK, et al. (2009) MicroRNAs 15a and 16 regulate tumor proliferation in multiple myeloma. Blood 113: 6669–6680.

23. Liu Y, Quang P, Braggio E, Ngo H, Badalian-Very G, et al. (2013) Novel tumor suppressor function of glucocorticoid-induced TNF receptor GITR in multiple myeloma. PloS one 8: e66982.

24. Yang J, Chai L, Fowles TC, Alipio Z, Xu D, et al. (2008) Genome-wide analysis reveals Sall4 to be a major regulator of pluripotency in murine-embryonic stem cells. Proceedings of the National Academy of Sciences of the United States of America 105: 19756–19761.

25. Carroll JS, Liu XS, Brodsky AS, Li W, Meyer CA, et al. (2005) Chromosome-wide mapping of estrogen receptor binding reveals long-range regulation requiring the forkhead protein FoxA1. Cell 122: 33–43.

26. Toedling J, Huber W (2008) Analyzing ChIP-chip data using bioconductor. PLoS computational biology 4: e1000227.

27. Johnson WE, Li W, Meyer CA, Gottardo R, Carroll JS, et al. (2006) Model-based analysis of tiling-arrays for ChIP-chip. Proceedings of the National Academy of Sciences of the United States of America 103: 12457–12462.

28. Zhang Y, Roccaro AM, Rombaoa C, Flores L, Obad S, et al. (2012) LNA-mediated anti-miR-155 silencing in low-grade B-cell lymphomas. Blood 120: 1678–1686.

29. Wang F, Ma YL, Zhang P, Shen TY, Shi CZ, et al. (2013) SP1 mediates the link between methylation of the tumour suppressor miR-149 and outcome in colorectal cancer. The Journal of pathology 229: 12–24.

30. Li LC, Dahiya R (2002) MethPrimer: designing primers for methylation PCRs. Bioinformatics (Oxford, England) 18: 1427–1431.

31. Zhan F, Barlogie B, Arzoumanian V, Huang Y, Williams DR, et al. (2007) Gene-expression signature of benign monoclonal gammopathy evident in multiple myeloma is linked to good prognosis. Blood 109: 1692–1700.

32. Subramanian A, Tamayo P, Mootha VK, Mukherjee S, Ebert BL, et al. (2005) Gene set enrichment analysis: a knowledge-based approach for interpreting genome-wide expression profiles. Proceedings of the National Academy of Sciences of the United States of America 102: 15545–15550.

33. Mootha VK, Lindgren CM, Eriksson KF, Subramanian A, Sihag S, et al. (2003) PGC-1alpha-responsive genes involved in oxidative phosphorylation are coordinately downregulated in human diabetes. Nature genetics 34: 267–273.

34. Schadt EE, Li C, Ellis B, Wong WH (2001) Feature extraction and normalization algorithms for high-density oligonucleotide gene expression array data. Journal of cellular biochemistry Supplement Suppl 37: 120–125.

35. Wong KY, Yim RL, So CC, Jin DY, Liang R, et al. (2011) Epigenetic inactivation of the MIR34B/C in multiple myeloma. Blood 118: 5901–5904.

36. Walker BA, Wardell CP, Chiecchio L, Smith EM, Boyd KD, et al. (2011) Aberrant global methylation patterns affect the molecular pathogenesis and prognosis of multiple myeloma. Blood 117: 553–562.

37. Fonseca R, Bergsagel PL, Drach J, Shaughnessy J, Gutierrez N, et al. (2009) International Myeloma Working Group molecular classification of multiple myeloma: spotlight review. Leukemia 23: 2210–2221.

38. Morgan GJ, Walker BA, Davies FE (2012) The genetic architecture of multiple myeloma. Nature reviews Cancer 12: 335–348.

39. Ma L, Teruya-Feldstein J, Weinberg RA (2007) Tumour invasion and metastasis initiated by microRNA-10b in breast cancer. Nature 449: 682–688.

40. Yigit MV, Ghosh SK, Kumar M, Petkova V, Kavishwar A, et al. (2013) Context-dependent differences in miR-10b breast oncogenesis can be targeted for the prevention and arrest of lymph node metastasis. Oncogene 32: 1530–1538.

41. Ouyang H, Gore J, Deitz S, Korc M (2013) microRNA-10b enhances pancreatic cancer cell invasion by suppressing TIP30 expression and promoting EGF and TGF-beta actions. Oncogene.

42. Kim K, Lee HC, Park JL, Kim M, Kim SY, et al. (2011) Epigenetic regulation of microRNA-10b and targeting of oncogenic MAPRE1 in gastric cancer. Epigenetics: official journal of the DNA Methylation Society 6: 740–751.

43. Hiroki E, Akahira J, Suzuki F, Nagase S, Ito K, et al. (2010) Changes in microRNA expression levels correlate with clinicopathological features and prognoses in endometrial serous adenocarcinomas. Cancer science 101: 241–249.

44. Xu Q, Jiang Y, Yin Y, Li Q, He J, et al. (2013) A regulatory circuit of miR-148a/152 and DNMT1 in modulating cell transformation and tumor angiogenesis through IGF-IR and IRS1. Journal of molecular cell biology 5: 3–13.

45. Tsuruta T, Kozaki K, Uesugi A, Furuta M, Hirasawa A, et al. (2011) miR-152 is a tumor suppressor microRNA that is silenced by DNA hypermethylation in endometrial cancer. Cancer research 71: 6450–6462.

46. Huang J, Wang Y, Guo Y, Sun S (2010) Down-regulated microRNA-152 induces aberrant DNA methylation in hepatitis B virus-related hepatocellular carcinoma by targeting DNA methyltransferase 1. Hepatology (Baltimore, Md) 52: 60–70.

47. Stumpel DJ, Schotte D, Lange-Turenhout EA, Schneider P, Seslija L, et al. (2011) Hypermethylation of specific microRNA genes in MLL-rearranged infant acute lymphoblastic leukemia: major matters at a micro scale. Leukemia 25: 429–439.

48. Wu P, Agnelli L, Walker BA, Todoerti K, Lionetti M, et al. (2013) Improved risk stratification in myeloma using a microRNA-based classifier. British journal of haematology 162: 348–359.

49. Rio-Machin A, Ferreira BI, Henry T, Gomez-Lopez G, Agirre X, et al. (2013) Downregulation of specific miRNAs in hyperdiploid multiple myeloma mimics the oncogenic effect of IgH translocations occurring in the non-hyperdiploid subtype. Leukemia 27: 925–931.

50. Hermann A, Gowher H, Jeltsch A (2004) Biochemistry and biology of mammalian DNA methyltransferases. Cellular and molecular life sciences: CMLS 61: 2571–2587.

51. Rady B, Chen Y, Vaca P, Wang Q, Wang Y, et al. (2013) Overexpression of E2F3 promotes proliferation of functional human beta cells without induction of apoptosis. Cell cycle (Georgetown, Tex) 12: 2691–2702.

52. Spiegelman VS, Stavropoulos P, Latres E, Pagano M, Ronai Z, et al. (2001) Induction of beta-transducin repeat-containing protein by JNK signaling and its role in the activation of NF-kappaB. The Journal of biological chemistry 276: 27152–27158.

53. Xiong J, Du Q, Liang Z (2010) Tumor-suppressive microRNA-22 inhibits the transcription of E-box-containing c-Myc target genes by silencing c-Myc binding protein. Oncogene 29: 4980–4988.

23

Non-Hodgkin Lymphoma Risk and Insecticide, Fungicide and Fumigant Use in the Agricultural Health Study

Michael C. R. Alavanja[1]*, Jonathan N. Hofmann[1], Charles F. Lynch[2], Cynthia J. Hines[3], Kathryn H. Barry[1], Joseph Barker[4], Dennis W. Buckman[4], Kent Thomas[5], Dale P. Sandler[6], Jane A. Hoppin[6], Stella Koutros[1], Gabriella Andreotti[1], Jay H. Lubin[1], Aaron Blair[1], Laura E. Beane Freeman[1]

1 Division of Cancer Epidemiology and Genetics, National Cancer Institute, Rockville, Maryland, United States of America, 2 College of Public Health, University of Iowa, Iowa City, Iowa, United States of America, 3 National Institute for Occupational Safety and Health, Cincinnati, Ohio, United States of America, 4 IMS, Inc, Calverton, Maryland, United States of America, 5 National Exposure Research Laboratory, U.S. Environmental Protection Agency, Research Triangle Park, North Carolina, United States of America, 6 Epidemiology Branch, National Institute for Environmental Health Sciences, Research Triangle Park, North Carolina, United States of America

Abstract

Farming and pesticide use have previously been linked to non-Hodgkin lymphoma (NHL), chronic lymphocytic leukemia (CLL) and multiple myeloma (MM). We evaluated agricultural use of specific insecticides, fungicides, and fumigants and risk of NHL and NHL-subtypes (including CLL and MM) in a U.S.-based prospective cohort of farmers and commercial pesticide applicators. A total of 523 cases occurred among 54,306 pesticide applicators from enrollment (1993–97) through December 31, 2011 in Iowa, and December 31, 2010 in North Carolina. Information on pesticide use, other agricultural exposures and other factors was obtained from questionnaires at enrollment and at follow-up approximately five years later (1999–2005). Information from questionnaires, monitoring, and the literature were used to create lifetime-days and intensity-weighted lifetime days of pesticide use, taking into account exposure-modifying factors. Poisson and polytomous models were used to calculate relative risks (RR) and 95% confidence intervals (CI) to evaluate associations between 26 pesticides and NHL and five NHL-subtypes, while adjusting for potential confounding factors. For total NHL, statistically significant positive exposure-response trends were seen with lindane and DDT. Terbufos was associated with total NHL in ever/never comparisons only. In subtype analyses, terbufos and DDT were associated with small cell lymphoma/chronic lymphocytic leukemia/marginal cell lymphoma, lindane and diazinon with follicular lymphoma, and permethrin with MM. However, tests of homogeneity did not show significant differences in exposure-response among NHL-subtypes for any pesticide. Because 26 pesticides were evaluated for their association with NHL and its subtypes, some chance finding could have occurred. Our results showed pesticides from different chemical and functional classes were associated with an excess risk of NHL and NHL subtypes, but not all members of any single class of pesticides were associated with an elevated risk of NHL or NHL subtypes. These findings are among the first to suggest links between DDT, lindane, permethrin, diazinon and terbufos with NHL subtypes.

Editor: Suminori Akiba, Kagoshima University Graduate School of Medical and Dental Sciences, Japan

Funding: This work was supported by the Intramural Research Program of the NIH, National Cancer Institute, Division of Cancer Epidemiology and Genetics (Z01CP010119) and The National Institutes of Environmental Health Sciences (Z01ES049030). The funders had no role in study design, data collection and analysis, decision to publish, or preparation of the manuscript. IMS, Inc, provided support in the form of salaries for authors Joseph Barker and Denis W Buckman, but did not have any additional role in the study design, data collection and analysis, decision to publish, or preparation of the manuscript. The specific roles of these authors are articulated in the 'author contributions' section.

Competing Interests: The authors have the following interests. Joseph Barker and Dennis W. Buckman are employed by IMS, Inc. There are no patents, products in development or marketed products to declare.

* Email: alavanjm@mail.nih.gov

Introduction

Since the 1970s, epidemiologic studies of non-Hodgkin lymphoma (NHL) and multiple myeloma (MM) have shown increased risk among farmers and associations with the type of farming practiced [1–6]. While farmers are exposed to many agents that may be carcinogenic [7]; there has been a particular focus on pesticides. Studies from around the world have suggested increased risk of NHL or MM [8,9] and other NHL subtypes [10] in relation to the use of specific pesticides in different functional classes (i.e., insecticides, fungicides, fumigants and herbicides). A

meta-analysis of 13 case-control studies published between 1993–2005 observed an overall significant meta-odds ratio (OR) between occupational exposure to pesticides and NHL (OR = 1.35; 95% CI: 1.2–1.5) [11]. This risk was greater among individuals with more than 10 years of exposure (OR = 1.65; 95% CI: 1.08–1.95) [11], but the meta-analysis lacked details about the use of specific pesticides and other risk factors [11]. Although the International Agency for Research on Cancer (IARC) has classified "Occupational exposures in spraying and application of non-arsenical insecticides" as "probably carcinogenic to humans", the human evidence for the 17 individual pesticides evaluated in this monograph was determined to be inadequate for nine and there were no epidemiological studies for eight pesticides [12]. Since then, more studies have focused on cancer risk from specific pesticides, although the information is still relatively limited for many cancer-pesticide combinations [8,9].

To help fill the current information gap we evaluated the relationships between the use of specific insecticides, fungicides and fumigants and NHL in the Agricultural Health Study (AHS), a prospective cohort of licensed private (i.e., mostly farmer) and commercial pesticide applicators. Because the etiology of NHL and its B and T cell subtypes may differ by cell type[13], we also evaluated risk by subtype while controlling for potential confounding factors suggested from the literature [13], and the AHS data.

Novelty and Impact

These findings on occupationally exposed pesticide applicators with high quality exposure information are among the first to suggest links between DDT, lindane, permethrin, diazinon and terbufos and specific NHL subtypes in a prospective cohort study.

Materials and Methods

Study Population

The AHS is a prospective cohort study of 52,394 licensed private pesticide applicators (mostly farmers) in Iowa and North Carolina and 4,916 licensed commercial applicators in Iowa (individuals paid to apply pesticides to farms, homes, lawns, etc.), and 32,346 spouses of private applicators. Only applicators are included in this analysis. The cohort has been previously described in detail [14,15] and study questionnaires are available on the AHS website (www.aghealth.nih.gov). Briefly, individuals seeking licenses to apply restricted use pesticides were enrolled in the study from December 1993 through December 1997 (82% of the target population enrolled). At enrollment, subjects did not sign a written informed consent form. However, the cover letter of the questionnaire booklet informed subjects of the voluntary nature of participation, the ability to not answer any question, and it provided an assurance of confidentiality (including a Privacy Act Notification statement). The letter also included a written summary of the purpose of research, time involved, benefits of research, and a contact for questions about the research. The cover letter to the take-home questionnaire included all of the above and also informed the participant that they had the right to withdraw at any time. Finally, subjects were specifically informed that their contact information (including Social Security Number) would be used to search health and vital records in the future. The participants provided consent by completing and returning the questionnaire booklet. These documents and procedures were approved in 1993 by all relevant institutional review boards (i.e., National Cancer Institute Special Studies Institutional Review Board, Westat Institutional Review Board, and the University of Iowa Institutional Review Board-01).

Excluded from this analysis were study participants who had a history of any cancer at the time of enrollment (n = 1094), individuals who sought pesticide registration in Iowa or North Carolina but did not live in these states at the time of registration (n – 341) and were thus outside the catchment area of these cancer registries and individuals that were missing information on potential confounders (i.e., race or total herbicides application days [n = 1,569]). This resulted in an analysis sample of 54,306. We obtained cancer incidence information by regular linkage to the population-based cancer registry files in Iowa and North

Carolina. In addition, we linked cohort members to state mortality registries of Iowa and North Carolina and the nation-wide National Death Index to determine vital status, and to the nation-wide address records of the Internal Revenue Service, state-wide motor vehicle registration files, and pesticide license registries of state agricultural departments to determine residence in Iowa or North Carolina. The current analysis included all incident primary NHL, as well as CLL and MM (which are now classified as NHL) [13] (n = 523) diagnosed from enrollment (1993–1997) through December 31, 2010 in North Carolina and from enrollment (1993–1997) through December 31, 2011 in Iowa, the last date of complete cancer incidence reports in each state. We ended follow-up and person-year accumulation at the date of diagnosis of any cancer, death, movement out of state, or December 31, 2010 in North Carolina and December 31, 2011 in Iowa, whichever was earlier.

Tumor Characteristics

Information on tumor characteristics was obtained from state cancer registries. We followed the definition of NHL and six subtypes of NHL used by the Surveillance Epidemiology and End Results (SEER) coding scheme [16] which was based on the Pathology Working Group of the International Lymphoma Epidemiology Consortium (ICD-O-3 InterLymph modification) classification (Table S1 in File S1, [17], i.e., 1. Small B-cell lymphocytic lymphomas (SLL)/chronic B-cell lymphocytic lymphomas (CLL)/mantle-cell lymphomas (MCL); 2. Diffuse large B-cell lymphomas; 3. Follicular lymphomas; 4. 'Other B-cell lymphomas' consisting of a diverse set of B-cell lymphomas; 5. Multiple myeloma; and 6. T-cell NHL and undefined cell type). There were too few T-cell NHL cases available for analysis [n = 19] so this cell type was not included in the subtype analysis). The ICD-O-3 original definition (used in many earlier studies of pesticides and cancer) of NHL [18] was also evaluated in relation to pesticide exposure to allow a clearer comparison of our results with previous studies.

Exposure Assessment

Initial information on lifetime use of 50 specific pesticides (Table S2 in File S1), including 22 insecticides, 6 fungicides and 4 fumigants was obtained from two self-administered questionnaires [14,15] completed during cohort enrollment (Phase 1). All 57,310 applicators completed the first enrollment questionnaire, which inquired about ever/never use of 50 pesticides, as well as duration (years) and frequency (average days/year) of use for a subset of 22 pesticides including 9 insecticides, 2 fungicides and 1 fumigant. In addition, 25,291 (44%) of the applicators returned the second (take-home) questionnaire, which inquired about duration and frequency of use for the remaining 28 pesticides, including 13 insecticides, 4 fungicides and 3 fumigants.

A follow-up questionnaire, which ascertained pesticide use since enrollment, was administered approximately 5 years after enrollment (1999–2005, Phase 2) and completed by 36,342 (63%) of the original participants. The full text of the questionnaires is available at www.aghealth.nih.gov. For participants who did not complete the Phase 2 questionnaire (20,968 applicators, 37%), a data-driven multiple imputation procedure which used logistic regression and stratified sampling [19] was employed to impute use of specific pesticides in Phase 2. Information on pesticide use from Phase 1, Phase 2 and imputation for Phase 2 was used to construct three cumulative exposure metrics: (i) lifetime days of pesticide use (i.e., the product of years of use of a specific pesticide and the number of days used per year); (ii) intensity-weighted lifetime days of use (i.e., the product of lifetime days of use and a measure of exposure intensity) and (iii) ever/never use data for each pesticide. Intensity was derived from an exposure-algorithm, which was based on exposure measurements from the literature and individual information on pesticide use and practices (e.g., whether or not they mixed pesticides, application method, whether or not they repaired equipment and use of personal protective equipment) obtained from questionnaires completed by study participants [20].

Statistical Analyses

We divided follow-up time into 2-year intervals to accumulate person-time and update time-varying factors, such as attained age and pesticide use. We fit Poisson models to estimate rate ratios (RRs) and 95% confidence intervals (95% CI) to evaluate the effects of pesticide use on rates of overall NHL and the five NHL subtypes.

We evaluated pesticides with 15 or more exposed cases of total NHL, thereby excluding aluminum phosphide, carbon tetrachloride/carbon disulfide, ethylene dibromide, trichlorfon, and ziram leaving 26 insecticides, fungicides and fumigants for analysis (permethrin for animal use and crop use were combined into one category, all insecticides, fungicides and fumigants are listed in Table S2 in File S1). For each pesticide, we evaluated ever vs. never exposure, as well as tertiles of exposure which were created based on the distribution of all NHL exposed cases and compared to those unexposed. In the NHL subtype analysis and in circumstances where multiple pesticides were included in the model we categorized exposure for each pesticide into unexposed (i.e., never users) and two exposed groups (i.e., low and high) separated at the median exposure level. The number of exposed cases included in the ever/never analysis and in the trend analysis can differ because of the lack of information necessary to construct quantitative exposure metrics for some individuals.

Several lifestyle and demographic factors associated with NHL in the AHS cohort or previously suggested as possible confounders in the NHL literature[13] were evaluated as potential confounders in this analysis. These included: age at enrollment, gender, race, state, license type, education, autoimmune diseases, family history of lymphoma in first-degree relatives, body mass index, height, cigarette smoking history, alcohol consumption per week and several occupational exposures[1-13] including number of livestock, cattle, poultry, whether they raised poultry, hogs or sheep, whether they provided veterinary services to their animals, number of acres planted, welding, diesel engine use, number of years lived on the farm, total days of any pesticide use, and total days of herbicide use. However, since most of these variables did not change the risk estimates for specific pesticides, we present results adjusted for age, race, state and total days of herbicide use, which impacted risk estimates by more than 10% for some subtypes. We also performed analyses adjusting for specific insecticides, fungicides and fumigants shown to be associated with NHL or a specific NHL subtype in the current analysis. Tests for trend used the median value of each exposure category. All tests were two-sided and conducted at $\alpha = 0.05$ level. Analysis by NHL subtype was limited to insecticides, fungicides, and fumigants with 6 or more exposed cases.

We also fit polytomous logit models, where the dependent variable was a five-level variable (i.e., five NHL subtypes) and a baseline level (i.e., no NHL) to estimate exposure-response odds ratios (ORs) and 95% confidence intervals (CIs) for each subtypes of NHL. We then used polytomous logit models to estimate exposure-response trend while adjusting for age, state, race and total days of herbicide use, as in the Poisson models, and tested homogeneity among the 5 NHL subtypes.

Poisson models were fit using the GENMOD procedure and polytomous logit models were fit using the LOGISTIC procedure of the SAS 9.2 statistical software package (SAS Institute, Cary, NC). Summary estimates of NHL and NHL subtype risks for both Poisson models and polytomous logit models incorporated imputed data and were calculated along with standard error estimates, confidence intervals, and p-values, using multiple imputation methods implemented in the MIANALYZE procedure of SAS 9.2.

We also evaluated the impact of the additional pesticide exposure information imputed for Phase 2 on risk estimates. We compared risk estimates for those who completed both the phase 1 enrollment and take-home questionnaires and the phase 2 questionnaires (n = 17,545) with risk estimates obtained from the combined completed questionnaire data plus the imputed phase 2 data (n = 54,306). We also explored the effect of lagging exposure data 5 years because recent exposures may not have had time to have an impact on cancer development. For comparison to previous studies, we also assessed the exposure-response association for NHL using the original ICD-O-3 definition of NHL [18] and the new definition [16] in Table S3 in File S1. Unless otherwise specified, reported results show un-lagged exposure information from both Phase 1 and Phase 2 including Phase 2 imputed data for lifetime exposure-days and intensity-weighted lifetime days of use and NHL defined by the InterLymph modification of ICD-O-3 [17]. Data were obtained from AHS data release versions P1REL201005.00 (for Phase 1) and P2REL201007.00 (for Phase 2).

Results

The 54,306 applicators in this analysis contributed 803,140 person-years of follow-up from enrollment through December 31, 2010 in North Carolina and December 31, 2011 in Iowa (Table 1). During this period, there were 523 incident cases of NHL, including 148 SLL/CLL/MCL, 117 diffuse large B-cell lymphomas, 67 follicular lymphomas, 53 'other B-cell lymphomas' (consisting of a diverse set of B-cell lymphomas) and 97 cases of MM. Another 41 cases consisting of T-cell lymphomas (n = 19) and non-Hodgkin lymphoma of unknown lineage (n = 22) were excluded from cell type-specific analyses because of small numbers of cases with identified cell types. Between enrollment and the end of follow-up, 6,195 individuals were diagnosed with an incident cancer other than NHL, 4,619 died without a record of cancer in the registry data, and 1,248 cohort members left the state and could not be followed-up for cancer. Person-years of follow-up accumulated for all of these study participants after enrollment until they were censored for the incident cancer, death or moving out of the state (data not shown). The risk of NHL increased significantly and monotonically with age in the AHS cohort in this analysis (p = 0.001) and age-adjusted risks were significant for state and NHL overall and race for multiple myeloma (data not shown). Total days of herbicide use had a small but significant effect on the risk of some NHL subtypes, but not on NHL overall. No other demographic or occupational factors showed evidence of confounding so they were not included in the final models.

In Table 2 we present ever/never results for 26 insecticides, fungicides and fumigants by total NHL and by NHL subtype adjusted for age, race, state and herbicide use (total life-time days). Terbufos was the only pesticide associated with an increased risk of total NHL in the ever/never use analysis (RR = 1.2 [1.0–1.5]), although the trend for increasing use and risk of total NHL was not significant (p trend = 0.43) (Table 3). In contrast, there were a few chemicals that were not associated with ever/never use, but

Table 1. Baseline characteristics of AHS study participants in the NHL incidence analysis[1,2].

Variables	All NHL cases (%)	Cohort Person-years.
Age at Enrollment		
<45	84 (16.1)	426,288
45–49	51 (9.8)	101,018
50–54	75 (14.3)	84,998
55–59	90 17.2)	74,440
60–64	78 (14.9)	56,978
65–69	79 (15.1)	35,071
≥70	66 (12.6)	24,347
Race		
White	509 (97.3)	787,799
Black	14 (2.7)	15,341
State		
IA	332 (63.5)	537,252
NC	191 (36.5)	265,888
Lifetime Total Herbicide Exposure Days		
0–146 days	170 (32.5)	251,401
147–543 days	169 (32.3)	273,107
544–2453 days	184 (35.2)	278,632

[1]During the period from enrollment (1993–1997) to December 31, 2010 in NC and December 31, 2011 in Iowa.
[2]Individuals with missing ever/never exposure information or missing confounding variable information were not included in the table.

did show evidence of an exposure-response association. Lindane was the only pesticide that showed a statistically significant increasing trend in risk for NHL with both exposure metrics, for lifetime-days of lindane use the RR were = 1.0 (ref), 1.2 (0.7–1.9), 1.0 (0.6–1.7), 2.5 (1.4–4.4); p trend = 0.004 and intensity-weighted lifetime-days of use the: RR were: = 1.0 (ref), 1.3 (0.8–2.2), 1.1 (0.7–1.8), 1.8 (1.0–3.2); p trend = 0.04. DDT showed a significant trend for NHL risk with life-time days of use RR = 1.0 (ref), 1.3 (0.9–1.8), 1.1 (0.7–1.7), 1.7 (1.1–2.6); p trend = 0.02, while the intensity weighted lifetime days of use of DDT was of borderline significance: RR = 1.0 (ref), 1.2 (0.8–1.8), 1.1 (0.8–1.7), 1.6 (1.0–2.3); p trend = 0.06. The number of lifetime days of use of lindane and DDT was weakly correlated (coefficient of determination = 0.04), and the pattern of NHL risk showed little change when both were included in the model. The results for lindane adjusted for DDT were, RR = 1.0 (ref), 1.2 (0.7–2.0), 1.0 (0.5–1.8), 1.6 (0.9–3.3); p trend = 0.07 and the results for DDT adjusted for lindane were, RR = 1.0 (ref), 1.3 (0.9–2.0), 0.9 (0.6–1.6), 1.6 (0.9–2.6); p trend = 0.08).

We also evaluated pesticides by NHL sub-type. In the ever/never analyses (Table 2), permethrin was significantly associated with multiple myeloma, RR = 2.2 (1.4–3.5) and also demonstrated an exposure-response trend (RR = 1.0 (ref), 1.4 (0.8–2.7), 3.1 (1.5–6.2); p trend = 0.002) (Table 4). Similarly, there was an elevated risk of SLL/CLL/MCL with terbufos in ever/never analyses RR = 1.4 (0.97–2.0) and an exposure response trend (RR = 1.0 (ref), 1.3 (0.8–2.0), 1.6 (1.0–2.5); p trend = 0.05). For follicular lymphoma, lindane showed an elevated but non-significant association for ever use, RR = 1.7 (0.96–3.2) and a significant exposure-response association (RR = 1.0 (ref), 4.9 (1.9–12.6), 3.6 (1.4–9.5); p trend = 0.04). There were also two chemicals with evidence of exposure-response that were not associated with specific subtypes in the ever/never analyses: DDT (Dichlorodiphenyltrichloroethane) with SLL/CLL/MCL (RR = 1.0 (ref), 1.0

(0.5–1.8), 2.6 (1.3–4.8; p trend = 0.04); and diazinon with follicular lymphoma (RR = 1.0 (ref), 2.2 (0.9–5.4), 3.8 (1.2–11.4); p trend = 0.02) (Table 4).

The pattern of increased CLL/SLL/MCL risk with increased use of DDT and terbufos remained after both insecticides were placed in our model concurrently. CLL/SLL/MCL risk increased with DDT use (RR = 1.0 (ref), 0.9 (0.5–4.7); 2.4 (1.1–4.7); p trend = 0.04), and a pattern of increased CLL/SLL/MCL risk was also observed with terbufos use (RR = 1.0 (ref), 1.1 (0.6–2.1), 1.7 (0.9–3.3) p trend = 0.07), although the trend was not significant for terbufos. Similarly, the pattern of increased follicular lymphoma risk with lindane use and diazinon use remained after both insecticides were placed in our model concurrently. Follicular lymphoma risk increased with diazinon use (RR = 1.0 (ref), 4.1 (1.5–11.1); 2.5 (0.9–7.2); p trend = 0.09), and a similarly, pattern of increased follicular lymphoma risk was observed with lindane use (RR = 1.0 (ref), 1.6 (0.6–4.1), 2.6 (0.8–8.3) p trend = 0.09), although neither remained statistically significant (Table 4).

Three chemicals showed elevated risks in ever/never analyses for certain subtypes, with no apparent pattern in exposure-response analyses: metalaxyl and chlordane with SLL/CLL/MCL, RR = 1.6 (1.0–2.5) and RR = 1.4 (0.97–2.0) respectively, and methyl bromide with diffuse large B-cell lymphoma RR = 1.9 (1.1–3.3). Although there was evidence of association by subtype, and polytomous logit models indicated homogeneity across subtypes for lindane (p = 0.54), DDT (p = 0.44) and any other pesticide evaluated in this study (e.g., permethrin (p = 0.10), diazinon (p = 0.09), terbufos (p = 0.63), (last column in Table 4).

There was no evidence of confounding of the total NHL associations with either lindane or DDT. We also calculated RR for those who completed both the phase 1 enrollment and take-home questionnaires and the phase 2 questionnaire (n = 17,545) and found no meaningful difference in the RR that also included imputed exposures, although there was an increase in precision of

Table 2. Pesticides exposure (ever/never) and adjusted Relative Risk of total NHL and NHL Subtype[1].

Insecticide

Pesticide (chemical-functional class)	Total NHL Cases[2]			SLL/CLL/MCL Cases[2]			Diffuse Large B-Cell Cases[2]			Follicular B-Cell Cases[2]			Other B-cell Cases[2]			Multiple Myeloma Cases[2]		
	Ever/Never Exposed	RR[3,4]	(95% CI)	Ever/Never Exposed	RR[3,4]	(95% CI)	Ever/Never Exposed	RR[3,4]	(95% CI)	Ever/Never Exposed	RR[3,4]	(95% CI)	Ever/Never Exposed	RR[3,4]	(95% CI)	Ever/Never Exposed	RR[3,4]	(95% CI)
Aldicarb (carbamate-insecticide)	47/435	1	(0.7-1.4)	14/124	1.1	(0.6-1.8)	8/98	0.7	(0.4-1.5)	6/54	0.9	(0.3-2.2)	7/41	1.6	(0.7-3.5)	10/82	1.2	(0.6-2.2)
Carbofuran (carbamate-insecticide)	147/317	1.1	(0.9-1.3)	48/86	1.2	(0.8-1.8)	26/78	0.8	(0.5-1.3)	18/39	1	(0.5-1.7)	13/31	0.8	(0.4-1.6)	31/56	1.3	(0.8-2.1)
Carbaryl (carbamate-insecticide)	272/225	1	(0.8-1.2)	75/66	1	(0.7-1.5)	58/53	0.8	(0.5-1.3)	37/24	0.8	(0.5-1.3)	24/28	0.9	(0.5-1.6)	58/34	0.9	(0.6-1.4)
Chlorpyrifos (organophosphate-insecticide)	210/300	1	(0.8-1.2)	62/84	1	(0.7-1.4)	44/70	0.9	(0.6-1.4)	32/33	1.3	(0.8-2.2)	21/31	0.8	(0.5-1.5)	36/58	1	
Coumaphos (organophosphate-insecticide)	46/411	1.1	(0.8-1.5)	15/120	1.2	(0.7-2.1)	10/93	1	(0.5-2.1)	8/48	1.6	(0.8-3.5)	5/40	xxx		7/78	1	
DDVP (dimethyl phosphate-insecticide)	55/407	1.1	(0.8-1.5)	13/124	0.8	(0.5-1.5)	10/93	1	(0.5-1.9)	8/48	1.3	(0.6-2.7)	6/39	1		12/73	1.7	(0.9-3.2)
Diazinon (organophosphorous-insecticide)	144/342	1	(0.8-1.3)	46/93	1.3	(0.9-1.9)	30/78	0.9	(0.6-1.4)	22/38	1.3	(0.7-2.3)	12/37	0.8	(0.4-1.6)	27/64	1	
Fonofos (organophosphorous-insecticide)	115/349	1.1	(0.8-1.3)	35/100	1.1	(0.7-1.6)	25/81	1.2	(0.7-1.9)	13/45	0.9	(0.5-1.7)	15/30	1.3	(0.7-2.5)	19/66	1.3	(0.8-2.3)
Malathion (organophosphorous-insecticide)	332/163	0.9	(0.9-1.4)	99/43	1	(0.7-1.4)	72/37	0.9	(0.6-1.4)	46/14	1.3	(0.7-2.4)	30/21	0.6	(0.3-1.0)	61/32	0.9	(0.6-1.5)
Parathion (ethyl or methyl) (organophosphorous insecticide)	69/411	1.1	(0.8-1.4)	20/117	1	(0.7-1.4)	14/91	1	(0.6-1.4)	10/48	1.1	(0.8-1.5)	7/44	1.1	(0.7-1.5)	14/77	1	
Permethrin (animal and crop applications) (pyrethroid insecticide)	112/363	1.1	(0.8-1.4)	32/106	1	(0.7-1.4)	18/81	0.7	(0.4-1.2)	18/81	1.1	(0.6-2.0)	9/14	0.8	(0.4-1.6)	20/72	**2.2**	**(1.4-3.5)**
Phorate (organophosphorous-insecticide)	160/325	1	(0.8-1.2)	53/87	1.1	(0.8-1.6)	31/76	0.9	(0.5-1.3)	20/40	0.9	(0.5-1.6)	19/31	0.9	(0.5-1.6)	26/64	1	
Terbufos (organophosphorous-insecticide)	201/267	**1.2**	**(1.0-1.5)**	64/72	1.4	(0.97-2.0)	42/63	1.1	(0.7-1.7)	31/26	1.2	(0.7-2.1)	26/19	1.8	(0.94-3.2)	32/59	1.2	(0.7-1.9)
Chlorinated Insecticides																		
Aldrin (chlorinated insecticide)	116/364	0.9	(0.7-1.1)	53/99	0.9	(0.6-1.4)	15/91	0.8	(0.4-1.6)	13/45	0.8	(0.4-1.6)	12/37	0.6	(0.3-1.3)	29/62	1.5	(0.9-2.5)
Chlordane (chlorinated insecticide)	136/344	1	(0.8-1.3)	49/90	1.4	(0.99-2.1)	20/86	0.6	(0.4-1.0)	18/41	1.2	(0.7-2.1)	13/36	1	(0.7-2.0)	31/60	1.2	(0.7-1.9)
DDT	182/300	1		59/79	1.2		34/73	0.8		18/41	0.9		20/31	1.1		40/50	1.1	

Table 2. Cont.

Pesticide (chemical-functional class)	Total NHL Cases[2]			SLL/CLL/MCL Cases[2]			Diffuse Large B-Cell Cases[2]			Follicular B-Cell Cases[2]			Other B-cell Cases[2]			Multiple Myeloma Cases[2]		
	Ever/Never Exposed	RR[3,4]	(95% CI)	Ever/Never Exposed	RR[3,4]	(95% CI)	Ever/Never Exposed	RR[3,4]	(95% CI)	Ever/Never Exposed	RR[3,4]	(95% CI)	Ever/Never Exposed	RR[3,4]	(95% CI)	Ever/Never Exposed	RR[3,4]	(95% CI)
Insecticide																		
Dieldrin (chlorinated insecticide)	35/442	0.9	(0.6–1.2)	5/130	xxx		4/101	xxx		4/54	xxx		7/42	1	(0.7–2.0)	10/81	0.9	(0.5–1.4)
Heptachlor (chlorinated insecticide)	90/384	1	(0.7–1.2)	33/104	1.1	(0.7–3.0)	10/95	1.1	(0.3–3.1)	9/48	1.1	(0.5–3.2)	13/36	0.9	(0.5–2.7)	17/72	1.1	(0.6–2.0)
Lindane (chlorinated insecticide)	85/396	1	(0.8–1.2)	27/113	1.2	(0.6–1.5)	12/95	0.6	(0.3–1.1)	16/41	1.7	(0.96–3.2)	9/40	0.7	(0.4–1.2)	13/73	1.1	(0.5–2.0)
Toxaphene (chlorinated insecticide)	79/397	1	(0.7–1.2)	21/116	0.9	(0.5–1.5)	14/90	0.8	(0.4–1.4)	9/47	1	(0.6–2.0)	10/40	1.1	(0.6–2.0)	19/73	1.1	(0.6–1.9)
Fungicides																		
Benomyl (carbamate fungicide)	54/428	1.1	(0.8–1.5)	18/123	1.2	(0.7–2.0)	12/95	1.1	(0.6–1.9)	4/51	xxx		4/51	xxx		11/80	1.1	(0.6–2.0)
Captan (phthalimide fungicide)	60/406	1.1	(0.8–1.4)	18/118	1.1	(0.6–1.8)	12/91	0.9	(0.5–1.8)	5/51	xxx		6/39	1.1	(0.5–2.7)	12/76	1.2	(0.6–2.2)
Chloro-thalonil (poly-chlorinated aromatic thalonitrile fungicide)	35/474	0.8	(0.5–1.2)	9/135	0.9	(0.4–1.9)	6/107	0.5	(0.2–1.3)	5/60	xxx		2/50	xxx		11/84	1.2	(0.6–2.3)
Maneb/ Mancozeb (dithiocarbamate fungicide)	44/437	0.9	(0.7–1.3)	13/127	1.1	(0.6–2.1)	12/95	1.1	(0.6–2.1)	4/60	xxx		5/49	xxx		10/79	0.8	(0.4–1.7)
Metalaxyl (acylalanine fungicide)	108/381	1	(0.8–1.3)	34/106	**1.6**	**(1.0–2.5)**	27/82	1.1	(0.6–1.8)	10/48	0.7	(0.4–1.4)	10/40	0.9	(0.4–1.7)	21/71	0.8	(0.4–1.3)
Fumigant																		
Methyl bromide (methyl halide fumigant)	85/425	1.1	(0.9–1.5)	18/126	0.9	(0.5–1.7)	28/86	**1.9**	**(1.1–3.3)**	7/58	0.6	(0.2–1.4)	8/44	2.2	(0.9–5.7)	19/76	1	(0.6–1.8)

[1] During the period from enrollment (1993–1997) to December 31, 2010 in NC and December 31, 2011 in Iowa.
[2] Numbers of cases by NHL subtype do not sum to total number of NHL cases (n=523) due to missing data.
[3] Adjusted RR: age (<45, 45–49, 50–54, 55–59, 60–64, 65–69, ≥70), State (NC vs. IA), Race (White vs. Black), AHS herbicides (tertiles of total herbicide use-days). Statistically significant RR and 95% confidence limits are bolded.
[4] RR was not calculated if the number of exposed cases in a pesticide-NHL subtype cell was <6 and the missing RR was marked with an XXX. Statistically significant RRs and 95% confidence limits are bolded.

Table 3. Pesticide exposure (lifetime-days & intensity weighted life-time days) and adjusted risks of total NHL incidence[1].

Insecticides

Pesticide (chemical-functional class) [days of lifetime exposure for each category]	NHL Cases[2]	Non-Cases[2]	RR[3,4] (95% CI) by Total Days of Exposure	NHL Cases[2,]	Non-Cases	RR[3,4] (95% CI) Intensity-weighted days of exposure
Aldicarb (carbamate-insecticide)						
None	238	21557	1.0 (ref)	238	21557	1.0 (ref)
Low [≤8.75]	7	633	1.1 (0.5–2.3)	6	383	1.3 (0.6–3.3))
Medium [>8.75–25.5]	5	522	0.9 (0.3–2.5)	6	853	0.9 (0.4–1.9)
High [>25.5–224.75]	5	1266	0.5 (0.2–1.3)	5	1183	0.5 (0.2–1.3)
			P trend = 0.23			P trend = 0.22
Carbofuran (carbamate-insecticide)						
None	317	36296	1.0 (ref)	317	36296	1.0 (ref)
Low [≤8.75]	63	4775	1.2 (0.9–1.6)	46	3695	1.2 (0.9–1.6)
Medium [>8.75–38.75]	32	3648	0.8 (0.6–1.2)	46	4590	1.0 (0.7–1.3)
High [>38.75–767.25]	44	4370	0.97 (0.7–1.4)	45	4477	1.0 (0.7–1.4)
			P trend = 0.69			P trend = 0.74
Carbaryl (carbamate-insecticide)						
None	128	12864	1.0 (ref)	128	12864	1.0 (ref)
Low [≤8.75]	54	4128	1.1 (0.7–1.6)	46	3962	1.0 (0.7–1.5)
Medium [8.75–56]	43	5096	0.9 (0.6–1.2)	45	4433	0.9 (0.7–1.5)
High [>56–737.5]	39	3281	1.0 (0.7–1.6)	44	4029	1.0 (0.6–1.5)
			P trend = 0.87			P trend = 0.94
Chlorpyrifos (organophosphate-insecticide)						
None	300	30393	1.0 (ref)	300	30393	1.0 (ref)
Low [≤8.75]	71	6493	1.1 (0.9–1.5)	61	6383	1.1 (0.8–1.4)
Medium [>8.75–44]	65	6892	1.1 (0.8–1.4)	60	7549	0.9 (0.7–1.2)
High [>44–767.25]	67	9380	0.8 (0.6–1.1)	60	7044	1.0 (0.7–1.3)
			P trend = 0.11			P trend = 0.85
Coumaphos (organophosphate-insecticide)						
None	411	44846	1.0 (ref)	411	44846	1.0 (ref)
Low [<8.75]	16	1510	1.0 (0.6–1.7)	15	1132	1.3 (0.8–2.1)
Medium [>8.75–38.75]	14	1076	1.2 (0.7–2.1)	14	1452	1.0 (0.6–1.6)
High [>38.75–1627.5]	13	1175	1.2 (0.7–2.0)	14	1170	1.2 (0.7–2.1)
			P for trend = 0.50			P trend = 0.48
DDVP (dimethyl phosphate-insecticide)						
None	407	44551	1.0 (ref)	407	44551	1.0 (ref)
Low [≤8.75]	19	1342	1.4 (0.9–2.1)	18	1281	1.4 (0.9–2.3)
Medium [>8.75–87.5]	17	1519	1.2 (0.7–1.9)	18	1633	1.1 (0.7–1.8)
High [>87.5–2677.5]	17	1893	0.9 (0.6–1.5)	17	1824	1.0 (0.6–1.6)
			P trend = 0.78			P trend = 0.83
Diazinon (organophosphorous-insecticide)						
None	187	17943	1.0 (ref)	187	17943	1.0 (ref)
Low [≤8.75]	28	2506	1.1 (0.7–1.6)	23	2047	1.1 (0.7–1.8)
Medium [>8.75–25]	19	1515	1.0 (0.6–1.8)	24	2246	0.9 (0.5–1.5)
High [>25–457.25]	23	1990	1.2 (0.7–1.9)	22	1708	1.3 (0.8–2.1)
			P trend = 0.52			P trend = 0.33

Table 3. Cont.

Insecticides

Pesticide (chemical-functional class) [days of lifetime exposure for each category]	NHL Cases[2]	Non-Cases[2]	RR[3,4] (95% CI) by Total Days of Exposure	NHL Cases[2,]	Non-Cases	RR[3,4] (95% CI) Intensity-weighted days of exposure
Fonofos (organophosphorous-insecticide)						
None	349	39570	1.0 (ref)	349	39570	1.0 (ref)
Low [≤20]	47	3812	1.3 (0.96–1.8)	37	2906	1.4 (0.97–1.9)
Medium [>20–50.75]	28	2819	1.1 (0.7–1.6)	38	3487	1.1 (0.8–1.6)
High [>50.75–369.75]	37	3385	1.1 (0.7–1.5)	36	3606	1.0 (0.7–1.4)
			P trend = 0.83			P trend = 0.87
Malathion (organophosphorous-insecticide)						
None	90	8368	1.0 (ref)	90	8368	1.0 (ref)
Low [≤8.75]	75	7284	0.97 (0.7–1.3)	60	5535	1.0 (0.7–1.4)
Medium [>8.75–38.75]	47	5779	0.7 (0.5–1.1)	59	6899	0.8 (0.6–1.1)
High [>38.75–737.5]	57	5037	0.9 (0.6–1.3)	59	5588	0.9 (0.6–1.2)
			P trend = 0.63			P trend = 0.46
Parathion (ethyl or methyl) (organophosphorous insecticide)						
None	228	21457	1.0 (ref)	228	21457	1.0 (ref)
Low [≤8.75]	9	693	1.0 (0.5–2.0)	7	612	0.9 (0.4–2.0)
Medium [>8.75–24.5]	6	351	1.4 (0.6–3.2)	8	462	1.4 (0.7–2.9)
High [>.24.5–1237.5]	6	652	0.8 (0.3–1.8)	6	621	0.8 (0.4–1.9)
			P trend = 0.64			P trend = 0.74
Permethrin (animal and crop applications) (pyrethroid insecticide)						
None	371	37496	1.0 (ref)	371	37496	1.0 (ref)
Low [≤8.75]	38	4315	1.1 (0.8–1.5)	33	4263	0.9 (0.6–1.3)
Medium [>8.75–50.75]	31	4611	0.8 (0.5–1.2)	33	4200	1.0 (0.7–1.4)
High [>50.75–1262.25]	33	4121	1.2 (0.8–1.7)	32	4553	1.0 (0.7–1.5)
			P trend = 0.54			P trend = 0.99
Phorate (organophosphorous-insecticide)						
None	171	16834	1.0 (ref)	171	16834	1.0 (ref)
Low [≤8.75]	27	2621	0.8 (0.5–1.2)	26	2320	0.9 (0.6–1.4)
Medium [8.75–24.5]	33	1819	1.4 (0.96–2.1)	27	1951	1.1 (0.7–1.7)
High [>24.5–224.75]	18	2246	0.6 (0.4–1.1)	25	2409	0.8 (0.5–1.3)
			P trend = 0.25			P trend = 0.44
Terbufos (organophosphorous-insecticide)						
None	267	31076	1.0 (ref)	267	31076	1.0 (ref)
Low [≤24.5]	82	8410	1.2 (0.9–1.5)	64	6895	1.1 (0.9–1.5)
Medium [>24.5–56]	54	3925	1.6 (1.2–2.1)	64	4642	1.6 (1.2–2.2)
High [>56–1627.5]	57	6080	1.1 (0.8–1.5)	63	6842	1.1 (0.8–1.5)
			P trend = 0.43			P trend = 0.44
Chlorinated Insecticides						
Aldrin (chlorinated insecticide)						
None	193	19743	1.0 (ref)	193	19743	1.0 (ref)
Low [≤8.75]	27	1613	0.9 (0.6–1.4)	20	1212	0.9 (0.6–1.4)
Medium [>8.75–24.5]	16	1002	0.8 (0.5–1.3)	20	1279	0.8 (0.5–1.3)

Table 3. Cont.

Insecticides

Pesticide (chemical-functional class) [days of lifetime exposure for each category]	NHL Cases[2]	Non-Cases[2]	RR[3,4] (95% CI) by Total Days of Exposure	NHL Cases[2,]	Non-Cases	RR[3,4] (95% CI) Intensity-weighted days of exposure
High [>24.5–457.25]	17	903	0.9 (0.5–1.5)	19	1026	0.9 (0.6–1.5)
			P trend = 0.58			P trend = 0.74
Chlordane (chlorinated insecticide)						
None	179	19115	1.0 (ref)	179	19115	1.0 (ref)
Low [≤8.75]	47	2687	1.3 (0.97–1.9)	23	1303	1.4 (0.9–2.2)
Medium[5]	0	0	xxx	24	1747	1.0 (0.6–1.5)
High [>8.75–1600]	23	1450	1.1 (0.7–1.7)	22	1085	1.4 (0.9–2.2)
			P trend = 0.43			P trend = 0.16
DDT (chlorinated insecticide)						
None	152	18543	1.0 (ref)	152	18543	1.0 (ref)
Low [≤8.75]	43	2121	1.3 (0.9–1.8)	33	1601	1.2 (0.8–1.8)
Medium [>8.75–56]	28	1598	1.1 (0.7–1.7)	32	1760	1.1 (0.8–1.7)
High [>56–1627.5]	27	953	1.7 (1.1–2.6)	32	1305	1.6 (1.0–2.3)
			P trend = 0.02			P trend = 0.06
Dieldrin (chlorinated insecticide)						
None	235	22510	1.0 (ref)	235	22510	1.0 (ref)
Low [≤8.75]	7	472	0.7 (0.3–1.5)	6	363	0.8 (0.4–1.8)
Medium [>8.75–24.5]	8	154	2.3 (1.1–4.7)	5	106	2.2 (0.9–5.3)
High [>24.5–224.75]	2	140	0.7 (0.2–2.9)	5	298	0.8 (0.3–2.0)
			P trend = 0.47			P trend = 0.84
Heptachlor (chlorinated insecticide)						
None	205	20844	1.0 (ref)	205	20844	1.0 (ref)
Low [≤8.75]	21	1261	1.0 (0.6–1.6)	15	1110	0.8 (0.5–1.4)
Medium [>8.75–24.5]	18	679	1.5 (0.9–2.4)	16	425	2.0 (1.2–3.4)
High [>24.5–457.25]	7	600	0.7 (0.3–1.4)	14	1001	0.8 (0.5–1.4)
			P trend = 0.82			P trend = 0.88
Lindane (chlorinated insecticide)						
None	205	20375	1.0 (ref)	205	20375	1.0 (ref)
Low [≤8.75]	18	1285	1.2 (0.7–1.9)	15	976	1.3 (0.8–2.2)
Medium [>8.75–56]	13	1103	1.0 (0.6–1.7)	16	1205	1.1 (0.7–1.8)
High [>56–457.25]	14	467	2.5 (1.4–4.4)	14	673	1.8 (1.0–3.2)
			P trend = 0.004			**P trend = 0.04**
Toxaphene (chlorinated insecticide)						
None	214	20911	1.0 (ref)	214	20911	1.0 (ref)
Low [≤8.75]	14	1198	0.8 (0.5–1.4)	11	630	1.3 (0.7–2.3)
Medium [>8.75–24.5]	13	564	1.5 (0.9–2.7)	12	931	0.9 (0.5–1.6)
High [>24.5–457.25]	6	686	0.6 (0.3–1.4)	10	886	0.8 (0.4–1.5)
			P trend = 0.50			P trend = 0.38
Fungicides						
Benomyl (carbamate fungicide)						
None	219	21425	1.0 (ref)	219	21425	1.0 (ref)
Low [≤12.25]	14	896	1.7 (0.9–2.9)	9	432	2.2 (1.1–4.3)
Medium [>12.25–24.5]	4	214	2.4 (0.9–6.6)	10	732	1.7 (0.9–3.2)

Table 3. Cont.

Insecticides						
Pesticide (chemical-functional class) [days of lifetime exposure for each category]	NHL Cases[2]	Non-Cases[2]	RR[3,4] (95% CI) by Total Days of Exposure	NHL Cases[2,]	Non-Cases	RR[3,4] (95% CI) Intensity-weighted days of exposure
High [>24.5–457.25]	8	834	1.0 (0.5–2.1)	7	779	0.9 (0.4–2.0)
			P trend = 0.93			P trend = 0.75
Captan (phthalimide fungicide)						
None	407	43433	1.0 (ref)	407	43433	1.0 (ref)
Low [≤0.25]	15	2334	0.8 (0.5–1.4)	15	2108	0.9 (0.6–1.5)
Medium [>0.25–12.25]	16	1004	1.5 (0.8–2.6)	15	1171	1.2 (0.7–2.2)
High [>12.25–875]	14	1823	0.8 (0.5–1.5)	14	1805	0.8 (0.5–1.5)
			P trend = 0.69			P trend = 0.52
Chlorothalonil (polychlorinated aromatic thalonitrile fungicide)						
None	474	48442	1.0 (ref)	474	48442	1.0 (ref)
Low [≤12.25]	13	1509	0.9 (0.5–1.6)	10	1800	0.6 (0.3–1.2)
Medium [>12.25–64]	9	1492	0.8 (0.4–1.6)	11	1501	0.9 (0.5–1.7)
High [>64–395.25]	9	1678	0.6 (0.3–1.3)	9	1362	0.8 (0.4–1.6)
			P trend = 0.16			PP trend = 0.52
Maneb/Mancozeb (dithiocarbamate fungicide)						
None	228	21512	1.0 (ref)	228	21512	1.0 (ref)
Low [≤7]	8	400	1.9 (0.9–3.9)	8	486	1.6 (0.8–3.3)
Medium [>7–103.25]	9	990	0.9 (0.4–1.7)	9	680	1.3 (0.6–2.6)
High [>103.25–737.5]	7	454	1.4 (0.6–2.9)	7	677	0.9 (0.4–1.9)
			P trend = 0.49			P trend = 0.78
Metalaxyl (acylalanine fungicide)						
None	209	18833	1.0 (ref)	209	18833	1.0 (ref)
Low [≤6]	16	1439	1.0 (0.6–1.8)	15	1079	1.3 (0.8–2.2)
Medium [>6–28]	15	2182	0.7 (0.4–1.3)	15	2203	0.8 (0.4–1.3)
High [>28–224.75]	13	1566	1.1 (0.6–2.1)	14	1893	0.9 (0.5–1.6)
			P trend = 0.76			P trend = 0.63
Fumigant						
Methyl bromide (methyl halide fumigant)						
None	425	45265	1.0 (ref)	425	45265	1.0 (ref)
Low [≤8]	37	2060	2.0 (1.4–2.9)	26	1680	1.8 (1.2–2.7)
Medium [>8–28]	24	3011	0.9 (0.6–1.4)	25	2501	1.1 (0.7–1.8)
High [>28–387.5]	17	2768	0.6 (0.4–1.0)	25	3571	0.8 (0.5–1.2)
			P trend = 0.04			P trend = 0.10

[1]During the period from enrollment (1993–1997) to December 31, 2010 in NC and December 31, 2011 in Iowa.
[2]Numbers of cases in columns do not sum to total number of NHL cases (n = 523) due to missing data. In the enrollment questionnaire, lifetime-days & intensity weighted life-time days of pesticide use was obtained for the insecticides: carbofuran, chlorpyrifos, coumaphos, DDVP, fonofos, permethrin and terbufos; the fungicides: captan, chlothalonil and the fumigant: methyl bromide. In the take home questionnaire lifetime-days & intensity weighted life-time days of pesticide use were obtained for the insecticides: aldicarb, carbaryl, diazinon, malathion, parathion, and phorate, the chlorinated insecticides: aldrin, chlordane, DDT, dieldrin, heptachlor, lindane, and toxaphene, the fungicides: benomyl, maneb/mancozeb and metalaxyl, therefore, numbers of NHL cases can vary among pesticides listed in the table.
[3]Adjusted RR: age (<45, 45–49, 50–54, 55–59, 60–64, 65–69, ≥70), State (NC vs. IA), Race (White vs. Black), AHS herbicides (tertiles of total herbicide use-days). Statistically significant P trends are bolded.
[4]Permethrin for animal use and crop use were combined into one category.
[5]The distribution of life-time days of chlordane exposure was clumped into two exposed groups those who with, ≤8.75 life-time days of exposure and those with >0.75 life-time days of exposure.

Table 4. Pesticide exposure (Lifetime-Days of Exposure) and adjusted risks for NHL Subtypes.

Insecticides

	SLL, CLL, MCL		Diffuse Large B-cell		Follicular B-cell		Other B-cell types		Multiple Myeloma		NHL subtype Homogeneity Test (p-value)
	RR[3,4] (95% CI)	N²	RR[3,4] (95% CI)	N²	RR[3,4] (95% CI)	N²	RR[3,4] (95% CI)	N²	RR[3,4] (95% CI)	N²	
Carbaryl											
None	1.0 (ref)	42	1.0 (ref)	29	1.0 (ref)	11	1.0 (ref)	14	1.0 (ref)	22	
Low	1.1 (0.6–2.2)	19	0.8 (0.4–1.6)	17	1.6 (0.6–3.9)	10	1.8 (0.7–4.3)	10	0.7 (0.3–1.4)	14	
High	0.6 (0.3–1.3)	15	1.3 (0.6–2.8)	15	2.8 (1.0–7.4)	10	0.4 (0.1–1.5)	3	1.1 (0.7–1.8)	13	
	p trend = 0.16		p trend = 0.33		p trend = 0.06		p trend = 0.63		p trend = 0.98		0.19
Carbofuran											
None	1.0 (ref)	87	1.0 (ref)	78	1.0 (ref)	39	1.0 (ref)	33	1.0 (ref)	56	
Low	1.1 (0.7–1.8)	28	0.9 (0.5–1.7)	13	1.3 (0.7–2.4)	15	0.8 (0.4–1.8)	8	1.9 ((1.1–3.3)	16	
High	1.5 (0.9–2.5)	19	0.8 (0.5–1.3)	13	0.4 (0.1–1.4)	3	0.7 (0.2–2.0)	4	0.9 (0.4–1.6)	12	
	p trend = 0.16		p trend = 0.37		p trend = 0.31		p trend = 0.46		p trend = 0.57		0.52
Chlorpyrifos											
None	1.0 (ref)	84	1.0 (ref)	70	1.0 (ref)	33	1.0 (ref)	31	1 (ref)	58	
Low	1.2 (0.8–1.8)	31	0.9 (0.6–1.5)	22	1.6 (0.9–2.9)	20	1.2 (0.6–2.2)	14	1.0 (0.6–1.8)	17	
High	0.9 (0.6–1.3)	30	1.1 (0.6–1.7)	22	1.0 (0.5–2.1)	11	0.5 (0.2–1.3)	7	0.7 (0.4–1.3)	14	
	p trend = 0.45		p trend = 0.80		p trend = 0.94		p trend = 0.13		p trend = 0.27		0.90
Coumaphos											
None	1.0 (ref)	120	1.0 (ref)	92	1.0 (ref)	48	1.0 (ref)	40	1.0 (ref)	78	
Low	1.1 (0.5–2.2)	8	0.7 (0.3–1.9)	4	2.1 (0.7–5.8)	4	xxx-	4	0.7 (0.2–2.2)	3	
High	1.5 (0.6–3.4)	6	1.6 (0.6–4.5)	4	1.4 (0.5–4.0)	4	xxx-	1	1.2 (0.4–4.0)	3	
	p trend = 0.35		p trend = 0.42		p trend = 0.47		p trend = xxx		p trend = 0.84		0.63
Diazinon											
None	1.0 (ref)	53	1.0 (ref)	40	1.0 (ref)	15	1.0 (ref)	20	1.0 (ref)	41	
Low	1.4 (0.7–2.7)	14	1.5 (0.7–3.2)	9	2.2 (0.9–5.4)	8	xxx	3	0.4 (0.1–1.2)	4	
High	1.9 (0.98–3.6)	12	1.1 (0.5–2.4)	8	3.8 (1.2–11.4)	7	xxx	2	0.5 (0.2–1.7)	3	
	p trend = 0.06		p trend = 0.72		**p trend = 0.02**		p trend = xxx		p trend = 0.35		0.09
DDVP											
None	1.0 (ref)	124	1.0 (ref)	93	1.0 (ref)	48	1.0 (ref)	39	1.0 (ref)	73	
Low	0.8 (0.4–1.9)	6	1.1 (0.4–2.7)	5	1.5 (0.6–3.9)	5	1.1 (0.4–3.7)	3	2.7 (1.2–5.8)	7	
High	0.7 (0.3–1.7)	6	0.9 (0.4–2.3)	5	1.0 (0.3–3.4)	3	0.9 (0.3–3.1)	3	1.0 (0.3–2.7)	4	
	p trend = 0.49		p trend = 0.87		p trend = 0.90		p trend = 0.91		p trend = 0.81		0.96
Fonofos											
None	1.0 (ref)	100	1.0 (ref)	81	1.0 (ref)	45	1.0 (ref)	30	1.0 (ref)	66	
Low	1.2 (0.7–2.0)	20	1.2 (0.7–2.2)	13	1.5 (0.8–3.0)	11	1.4 (0.6–3.1)	8	1.2 (0.6–2.5)	9	
High	1.0 (0.6–1.8)	15	1.2 (0.6–2.3)	11	0.3 (0.1–1.2)	2	1.1 (0.4–2.7)	6	1.4 (0.7–3.0)	9	
	p trend = 0.96		p trend = 0.65		p trend = 0.19		p trend = 0.84		p trend = 0.33		0.35
Malathion											
None	1.0 (ref)	27	1.0 (ref)	20	1.0 (ref)	6	1.0 (ref)	11	1.0 (ref)	17	
Low	0.7 (0.4–1.3)	29	0.96 (0.5–1.8)	23	1.0 (0.4–2.9)	12	1.0 (0.5–2.4)	11	1.0 (0.5–2.1)	18	
High	1.0 (0.6–1.8)	22	1.0 (0.5–2.0)	20	1.6 (0.6–4.4)	11	0.3 (0.1–0.8)	6	1.0 (0.5–2.0)	17	
Ever/Never	1.0 (0.7–1.4)		0.9 (0.6–1.4)		1.3 (0.7–2.4)		0.6 (0.3–1.0)		0.9 (0.6–1.5)		
	p trend = 0.65		p trend = 0.88		p trend = 0.25		p trend = 0.17		p trend = 0.86		0.33
Permethrin											

Table 4. Cont.

Insecticides	SLL, CLL, MCL		Diffuse Large B-cell		Follicular B-cell		Other B-cell types		Multiple Myeloma		
	RR[3,4] (95% CI)	N[2]	RR[3,4] (95% CI)	N[2]	RR[3,4] (95% CI)	N[2]	RR[3,4] (95% CI)	N[2]	RR[3,4] (95% CI)	N[2]	NHL subtype Homogeneity Test (p-value)
None	1.0 (ref)	108	1.0 (ref)	89	1.0 (ref)	41	1.0 (ref)	38	1.0 (ref)	64	
Low	1.1 (0.6–2.0)	15	0.6 (0.3–1.2)	8	1.3 (0.6–2.7)	8	0.9 (0.3–2.7)	5	1.4 (0.8–2.7)	13	
High	0.8 (0.5–1.5)	15	1.0 (0.5–2.1)	8	1.0 (0.5–2.4)	8	0.5 (0.2–1.7)	4	3.1 (1.5–6.2)	12	
	p trend = 0.53		p trend = 0.99		p trend = 0.88		p trend = 0.28		**p trend = 0.002**		0.10
Phorate											
None	1.0 (ref)	48	1.0 (ref)	37	1.0 (ref)	20	1.0 (ref)	16	1.0 (ref)	36	
Low	1.0 (0.6–1.9)	14	1.4 (0.7–2.7)	15	1.1 (0.4–3.0)	5	0.9 (0.3–2.2)	6	0.7 (0.3–1.8)	6	
High	0.8 (0.4–1.6)	11	0.7 (0.3–2.1)	4	0.8 (0.3–2.2)	5	1.1 (0.4–3.5)	4	0.8 (0.3–2.4)	4	
	p trend = 0.51		p trend = 0.80		p trend = 0.67		p trend = 0.91		p trend = 0.73		0.77
Terbufos											
None	1.0 (ref)	72	1.0 (ref)	63	1.0 (ref)	31	1.0 (ref)	19	1.0 (ref)	59	
Low	1.3 (0.8–2.0)	32	1.2 (0.8–1.9)	29	1.6 (0.9–3.1)	15	1.8 (0.9–3.6)	17	1.1 (0.6–1.9)	12	
High	1.6 (1.0–2.5)	31	1.0 (0.5–2.0)	12	0.8 (0.4–1.7)	10	1.6 (0.7–3.9)	8	1.3 (0.7–2.7)	5	
	p trend = 0.05		p trend = 0.90		p trend = 0.48		p trend = 0.29		p trend = 0.42		0.63
Chlorinated Insecticides											
Aldrin											
None	1.0 (ref)	53	1.0 (ref)	46	1.0 (ref)	22	1.0 (ref)	20	1.0 (ref)	34	
Low	1.0 (0.5–2.0)	11	xxx	2	1.2 (0.4–3.8)	4	0.4 (0.1–1.5)	3	2.1 (0.9–4.7)	8	
High	1.0 (0.5–2.0)	10	xxx	3	0.8 (0.3–2.5)	4	1.1 (0.3–3.9)	3	1.2 (0.5–3.2)	6	
	p trend = 0.70		p trend = xxx		p trend = 0.21		p trend = 0.67		p trend = 0.40		0.98
Chlordane											
None	1.0 (ref)	48	1.0 (ref)	42	1.0 (ref)	20	1.0 (ref)	21	1.0 (ref)	32	
Low	1.8 (1.0–3.1)	16	1.0 (0.5–2.2)	8	1.7 (0.7–4.3)	6	xxx	2	1.7 (0.9–3.3)	13	
High	1.5 (0.7–3.3)	8	1.4 (0.6–3.3)	7	1.3 (0.4–4.6)	3	xxx	2	0.7 (0.2–2.2)	3	
	p trend = 0.34		p trend = 0.69		p trend = 0.70		p trend = xxx		p trend = 0.57		0.85
DDT											
None	1.0 (ref)	42	1.0 (ref)	34	1.0 (ref)	17	1.0 (ref)	16	1.0 (ref)	28	
Low	1.0 (0.5–1.8)	16	1.6 (0.4–3.1)	2	3.3 (1.4–8.1)	9	0.4 (0.3–2.5))	5	1.2 (0.6–2.6)	10	
High	2.6 (1.3–4.8)	15	1.4 (0.6–3.5)	3	1.1 (0.3–3.6)	4	2.1 (0.7–6.5)	5	0.8 (0.4–1.8)	9	
	p trend = 0.04		P trend = 0.17		p trend = 0.80		p trend = 0.64		p trend = 0.37		0.44
Heptachlor											
None	1.0 (ref)	58	1.0 (ref)	47	1.0 (ref)	24	1.0 (ref)	21	1.0 (ref)	40	
Low	1.1 (0.5–2.3)	9	xxx	3	xxx	2	xxx	3	1.3 (0.4–3.8)	4	
High	1.4 (0.7–3.0)	9	xxx	1	xxx	1	xxx	2	1.2 (0.4–3.6)	4	
	p trend = 0.16		p trend = xxx		p trend = xxx		p trend = xxx		p trend = 0.91		0.68
Lindane											
None	1.0 (ref)	57	1.0 (ref)	49	1.0 (ref)	16	1.0 (ref)	21	1.0 (ref)	43	
Low	1.2 (0.6–2.5)	10	0.6 (0.2–1.7)	4	4.9 (1.9–12.6)	6	xxx	2	xxx	3	
High	2.6 (1.2–5.6)	9	2.0 (0.6–6.5)	3	3.6 (1.4–9.5)	6	xxx	1	xxx	2	
	p trend = 0.13		p trend = 0.96		**p trend = 0.04**		p trend = xxx		p trend = xxx		0.54
Toxaphene											
None	1.0 (ref)	68	1.0 (ref)	47	1 (ref)	23	1.0 (ref)	22	1.0 (ref)	40	

Table 4. Cont.

Insecticides	SLL, CLL, MCL		Diffuse Large B-cell		Follicular B-cell		Other B-cell types		Multiple Myeloma		NHL subtype
	RR[3,4] (95% CI)	N²	RR[3,4] (95% CI)	N²	RR[3,4] (95% CI)	N²	RR[3,4] (95% CI)	N²	RR[3,4] (95% CI)	N²	Homo-geneity Test (p-value)
Low	0.9 (0.4–2.3)	5	1.3 (0.5–3.3)	5	xxx	2	xxx	3	0.7 (0.2–2.0)	4	
High	0.4 (0.1–1.6)	2	0.9 (0.3–3.0)	3	xxx	2	xxx	2	0.7 (0.2–2.9)	2	
	p trend = 0.08		p trend = 0.77		p trend = xxx		p trend = xxx		p trend = 0.64		0.34
Fungicides											
Captan											
None	1.0 (ref)	118	1.0 (ref)	91	1.0 (ref)	52	1.0 (ref)	39	1.0 (ref)	76	
Low	0.9 (0.4–1.9)	7	1.1 (0.5–2.4)	7	xxx	2	xxx	3	1.4 (0.5–3.4)	5	
High	1.1 (0.5–2.6)	7	0.7 (0.1–3.1)	4	xxx	1	xxx	2	1.2 (0.5–2.9)	5	
	p trend = 0.78		p trend = 0.58		p trend = xxx		p trend = xxx		p trend = 0.75		0.92
Chlorothalonil											
None	1.0 (ref)	135	1.0 (ref)	107	1.0 (ref)	60	1.0 (ref)	50	1.0 (ref)	84	
Low	0.9 (0.4–2.3)	5	1.1 (0.4–3.1)	4	xxx	3	−xxx	1	1.1 (0.4–2.8)	5	
High	1.1 (0.4–3.3)	4	0.3 (0.1–1.2)	2	xxx	2	−xxx	1	0.7 (0.6–2.3)	3	
	p trend = 0.83		p trend = 0.09		p trend = xxx		p trend = xxx		p trend = 0.56		0.76
Metalaxyl											
None	1.0 (ref)	60	1.0 (ref)	45	1.0 (ref)	25	1.0 (ref)	23	1.0 (ref)	39	
Low	2.8 (1.4–5.8)	9	1.1 (0.4–2.6)	7	xxx	3	−xxx	2	0.4 (0.1–1.1)	4	
High	1.1 (0.4–2.8)	6	1.0 (0.4–2.7)	5	xxx	2	−xxx	1	1.1 (0.4–3.2)	4	
	p trend = 0.99		p trend = 0.97		p trend = xxx		p trend = xxx		p trend = 0.87		0.92
Maneb/ Mancozeb											
None	1.0 (ref)	69	1.0 (ref)	49	1.0 (ref)	25	1.0 (ref)	26	1.0 (ref)	41	
Low	2.1 (0.7–6.0)	4	4.0 (1.4–11.6)	4	xxx	2	−xxx	0	1.0 (0.4–2.5)	5	
High	1.2 (0.3–4.0)	3	0.9 (0.3–3.1)	3	−xxx	1	−xxx	0	2.2 (0.5–9.5)	2	
	p trend = 0.84		p trend = 0.74		p trend = xxx		p trend = xxx		p trend = 0.28		0.82
Fumigant											
Methyl Bromide											
None	1.0 (ref)	126	1.0 (ref)	86	1.0 (ref)	58	1.0 (ref)	44	1.0 (ref)	76	
Low	1.1 (0.5–2.2)	9	4.0 (2.2–7.4)	15	1.4 (0.5–4.2)	4	3.6 (1.3–9.8)	5	1.0 (0.5–2.1)	8	
High	0.8 (0.4–1.8)	8	1.0 (0.5–2.1)	11	0.3 (0.1–1.1)	3	1.3 (0.3–5.0)	3	0.8 (0.4–1.8)	8	
	p trend = 0.58		p trend = 0.67		p trend = 0.08		p trend = 0.56		p trend = 0.63		0.59

[1]During the period from enrollment (1993–1997) to December 31, 2010 in NC and December 31, 2011 in Iowa.
[2]Numbers of cases in columns do not sum to total number of NHL cases (n = 523) due to missing data. Ever/never use of all 26 pesticides (table 3) do not always match with exposure-response data in table 4 because of missing data to calculate lifetime-days of use.
[3]Adjusted for age (<45, 45–49, 50–54, 55–59, 60–64, 65–69, ≥70), State (NC vs. IA), Race (White vs. Black), AHS herbicides (in tertiles of total herbicide use-days). Significant RR and 95% confidence limits are bolded.
[4]RR was not calculated if the number of exposed cases for any NHL subtype was <6 and these cells are marked XXX. Four pesticides included in Table 2 (i.e., aldicarb, benomyl, dieldrin and parathion) were not included in Table 4 because no NHL subtype included ≥6 cases of a specific cell types with lifetime-days of exposure.

risk estimates (i.e., narrower confidence intervals) when we included phase 2 imputed data (n = 54,306) (data not shown). Lagging exposures by five years did not meaningfully change the association between lindane or DDT and total NHL (data not shown). The significant exposure-response trends linking use of a particular pesticide to NHL and certain NHL subtypes did not always correspond to a significant excess risk among those who ever used the same pesticide. For chemicals for which the detailed information was only asked about in the take-home questionnaire, we evaluated potential differences between the ever/never analyses based on the enrolment questionnaire and data from the same sub-set of participants who completed the exposure-response in the take-home questionnaire and found no meaningful differences in the results. We also evaluated the impact of using an updated definition of NHL; when using the original ICD-O-3 definition of NHL[19], lifetime-days of lindane use remained significantly associated with NHL risk (RR = 1.0 (ref), 1.3 (0.7–2.6), 1.2 (0.6–2.8), 2.7 (1.3–5.4), p trend = 0.006). The trend between total NHL and lifetime-days of DDT, however, was less clear and not statistically significant (RR = 1.0 (ref) 1.3 (0.9–1.8), 1.1 (0.5–2.1), 1.4 (0.8–2.6), p trend = 0.32) [Table S3 in File S1]. Carbaryl and diazinon showed non-significant trends with the older definition of NHL, but not with the newer definition used here.

Discussion

A significant exposure–response trend for total NHL was observed with increasing lifetime-days of use for two organochlorine insecticides, lindane and DDT, although RRs from ever/never comparisons were not elevated. On the other hand, terbufos use showed a significant excess risk with total NHL in ever vs. never exposed analysis, but displayed no clear exposure-response trend. Several pesticides showed significant exposure-response trends with specific NHL subtypes however, when polytomous models were used to test the difference in parametric estimates of trend among the five NHL subtypes, there was no evidence of heterogeneity in the sub-types for specific chemicals. The subtype relationships that looked particularly interesting were DDT and terbufos with the SLL/CLL/MCL subtype, lindane and diazinon with the follicular subtype, and permethrin with MM. These pesticide-NHL links should be evaluated in future studies.

Lindane (gamma-hexachlorocyclohexane) is a chlorinated hydrocarbon insecticide. Production of lindane was terminated in the United States in 1976, but imported lindane was used to treat scabies and lice infestation and for agricultural seed treatment [21] until its registration was cancelled in 2009 [22], the same year production was banned worldwide [23]. In our study, 3,410 people reporting ever using lindane (6%) prior to enrollment, 433 reported use at the phase 2 questionnaire (1%), indicating that use had dropped substantially. Oral administration of lindane has increased the incidence of liver tumors in mice and less clearly, thyroid tumors in rats [24]. Lindane produces free radicals and oxidative stress (reactive oxygen species [ROS]) [25] and has been linked with chromosomal aberrations in human peripheral lymphocytes in vitro [26].

Lindane has been linked with NHL in previous epidemiologic studies. A significant association between lindane use and NHL was observed in a pooled analysis of three population-based case-control studies conducted in the Midwestern US, with stronger relative risks observed for greater duration and intensity of use [27]. NHL was also associated with lindane use in a Canadian case-control study [28]. Lindane was significantly associated with NHL risk in an earlier report from the AHS [29]. We are not aware of any previous study that assessed the association between a NHL subtype and lindane use. The exposure-response pattern with total NHL and the follicular lymphoma subtype indicates a need for further evaluation of lindane and NHL.

DDT is an organochlorine insecticide that was used with great success to control malaria and typhus during and after World War II [29] and was widely used for crop and livestock pest control in the United States from the mid-1940s to the 1960s [30]. Its registration for crop use was cancelled in the US in 1972 [30] and banned worldwide for agricultural use in 2009, but continues to be used for disease vector control in some parts of the world [23]. In our study, 12,471 participants (23%) reported ever using DDT

prior to enrollment; 12%, 8.7% and 2.3% responding to the take-home questionnaire reported their first use occurred prior to the 1960s, during the 1960s, and during the 1970s, respectively. The National Toxicology Program classifies DDT as "reasonably anticipated to be a human carcinogen" [31] and IARC classifies DDT as a "possible human carcinogen (2B)" [12], both classifications were based on experimental studies in which excess liver tumors were observed in two rodent species. Epidemiology data on the carcinogenic risk of DDT is inconsistent. NHL was not associated with use of DDT in a pooled analysis of three case-control studies in the U.S. where information on exposure was obtained from farmers by questionnaire [32]. There also was no association between the use of DDT and NHL in our study when we used an earlier definition of NHL [18], suggesting some of the inconsistency may be due to disease definition. In the large Epilymph study, no meaningful links between DDT and the risk of NHL, or diffuse large B cell lymphoma were observed, and only limited support was found for a link to CLL [33], although a case-control study of farmers in Italy suggested increased risk of NHL and CLL with DDT exposure [34]. NHL was not associated with serum levels of DDT in a prospective cohort study from the U.S. [35], but NHL was associated with the DDT-metabolite p, p'-DDE, as well as chlordane and heptachlor-related compounds (oxychlordane, heptachlor epoxide) and dieldrin, in a study with exposure measured in human adipose tissue samples [36]. In a Danish cohort, a higher risk of NHL was associated with higher prediagnostic adipose levels of DDT, cis-nonachlor, and oxychlordane [37]. In a Canadian study, analytes from six insecticides/insecticide metabolites (beta-hexachlorocyclohexane, p, p'-dichloro-DDE, hexachlorobenzene (HCB), mirex, oxychlordane and transnonachlor) were linked with a significant increased risk with NHL [38]. However, in an analysis of plasma samples from a case-control study in France, Germany and Spain, the risk of NHL did not increase with plasma levels of hexachlorobenzene, beta-hexachlorobenzene or DDE [39]. In this analysis, NHL was significantly associated with reported use of DDT, but not with the other organochlorine insecticides studied (i.e., aldrin, chlordane, dieldrin, heptachlor, toxaphene). Our findings add further support for an association between DDT and total NHL and our results on SLL/CLL/MCL are novel and should be further explored.

Permethrin is a broad-spectrum synthetic pyrethroid pesticide widely used in agriculture and in home and garden use as an insecticide and acaricide, as an insect repellant, and as a treatment to eradicate parasites such as head lice or mites responsible for scabies [40]. This synthetic pyrethroid was first registered for use in the United States in 1979 [40]. The U.S. Environmental Protection Agency classified permethrin as "likely to be carcinogenic to humans" largely based on the observed increase incidence of benign lung tumors in female mice, liver tumors in rats and liver tumors in male and female mice [41]. Permethrin was not associated with NHL overall in our study, nor in pooled case-control studies of NHL from the U.S (the NHL definition in use at the time of the study did not include MM) [42]. In our analysis, however, the risk of MM increased significantly with lifetime-days of exposure to permethrin, as had been noted in an earlier analysis of AHS data [43]. We are unaware of other studies that have found this association.

Terbufos is an organophosphate insecticide and nematicide first registered in 1974 [44]. The EPA classifies terbufos as Group E, i.e., "Evidence of Non-Carcinogenicity for Humans" [44]. We found some evidence for an association between terbufos use and NHL, particularly for the SLL/CLL/MCL subtype. NHL was not associated with terbufos in the pooled case-control studies from the

U.S. [42] but there was a non-significant association between terbufos and small cell lymphocytic lymphoma [10].

Diazinon is an organophosphate insecticide registered for a variety of uses on plants and animals in agriculture [45]. It was commonly used in household insecticide products until the EPA phased out all residential product registrations for diazinon in December 2004 [45.46]. In an earlier evaluation of diazinon in the AHS, a significant exposure-response association was observed for leukemia risk with lifetime exposure-days [47]. While there was no link between diazinon and NHL overall in this analysis, there was a statistically significant exposure-response association between diazinon and the follicular lymphoma subtype and an association with the SLL/CLL/MCL subtype that was not statistically significant. Diazinon was previously associated with NHL in pooled case-control studies from the U.S. and particularly with SLL [10].

Several other insecticides, fungicides and fumigants cited in recent reviews of the pesticide-cancer literature suggested etiological associations with total NHL [8,9], these include: oxychlordane, trans-nonachlor, and cis-nonachlor which are metabolites of chlordane; and dieldrin and toxaphene among NHL cases with t(14,18) translocations. We did not find a significant association between chlordane and total NHL nor with any NHL subtype, but we did not have information about chlordane metabolites to make a more direct comparison. Similarly we did not observe a significant association between dieldrin nor toxaphene and total NHL nor with any NHL subtypes. Mirex (1,3-cyclopentadiene), an insecticide, and hexachlorobenzene, a fungicide, were also associated with NHL risk [8,9] but we did not examine these compounds in the AHS.

This study has a number of strengths. It is a large population of farmers and commercial pesticide applicators who can provide reliable information regarding their pesticide use history [48]. Information on pesticide use and application practices was obtained prior to onset of cancer. An algorithm that incorporated several exposure determinants which predicted urinary pesticide levels was used to develop an intensity-weighted exposure metric in our study [20]. Exposure was ascertained prior to diagnosis of disease, which should eliminate the possibility of case-response bias [14]. Because of the detailed information available on pesticide use, we were able to assess the impact for the use of multiple pesticides. For example, we evaluated total pesticide use-days, and specific pesticides found to be associated with NHL or its subtypes in the AHS. We found no meaningful change in the associations with DDT, lindane, permethrin, diazinon and terbufos from such adjustments. Information on many potential NHL risk factors was available and could be controlled in the analysis.

Most epidemiological investigations of NHL prior to 2007 [17] did not include CLL and MM as part of the definition. These two subtypes made up 37% (193/523) of the NHL cases in this analysis. This is a strength of our study in that the definition of NHL used here is based on the most recent classification system [16,17] and will be relevant for comparisons with future studies. On the other hand, the inclusion of MM and CLL in the recent definition of NHL makes comparisons of our findings with earlier literature challenging, because the NHL subtypes may have different etiologies. For example, DDT was not significantly associated with NHL using the older definition, but was significantly associated with the NHL using the most recent definition of NHL because of its association with the SLL/CLL/MCL subtype (Table S1 in File S1). On the other hand, carbaryl and diazinon were associated with the old definition of NHL (although non-significantly) but not with the new definition. Lindane, however, was associated with both definitions of NHL.

Lindane was significantly associated with the follicular lymphoma subtype and this subtype was included in the older and newer definition of NHL. No other pesticides were significantly associated with NHL under the old definition (Table S3 in File S1).

Although this is a large prospective study, limitations should be acknowledged. A small number of cases exposed to some specific pesticides could lead to false positive or negative findings. We also had reduced statistical power to evaluate some pesticides for total days of use and intensity-weighted days of use because some participants did not complete the phase one take-home questionnaire and the tests of homogeneity between specific pesticides and specific NHL subtypes were underpowered. Some chance associations could occur because of multiple testing, i.e., a number of pesticides, several NHL subtypes, and more than one exposure metric. Despite the generally high quality of the information on pesticide use provided by AHS participants [48,50], misclassification of pesticide exposures can occur and can have a sizeable impact on estimates of relative risk, which in a prospective cohort design would tend to produce false negative results [49].

Conclusion

Our results showed pesticides from different chemical and functional classes were associated with an excess risk of NHL and NHL subtypes, but not all members of any single class of pesticides were associated with an elevated risk of NHL or NHL subtypes, nor were all chemicals of a class included on our questionnaire. Significant pesticide associations were between total NHL and reported use of lindane and DDT. Links between DDT and terbufos and SLL/CLL/MCL, lindane and diazinon and follicular lymphoma, and permethrin and MM, although based on relatively small numbers of exposed cases, deserve further evaluation. The epidemiologic literature on NHL and these pesticides is inconsistent and although the findings from this large, prospective cohort add important information, additional studies that focus on NHL and its subtypes and specific pesticides are needed. The findings from this large, prospective cohort add important new information regarding the involvement of pesticides in the development of NHL. It provides additional information regarding specific pesticides and NHL overall and some new leads regarding possible links with NHL subtypes that deserve evaluation in future studies.

Supporting Information

File S1   This file contains Table S1, Table S2, and Table S3. Table S1, Frequency of NHL in Agricultural Health Study applicators using New (Interlymph hierarchical classification of lymphoid neoplasms) and Older Definitions (ICD-O-3). Table S2, Pesticides included in the Agricultural Health Study questionnaires by Chemical/Functional Class. Table S3, Pesticide exposure (lifetime-days) and adjusted risks of total NHL incidence (Older definition [ICD-O-3]).

Acknowledgments

Disclaimer: The findings and conclusions in this report are those of the author(s) and do not necessarily represent the views of the National Institute for Occupational Safety and Health. The United States Environmental Protection Agency through its Office of Research and Development partially funded and collaborated in the research described here under Contracts 68-D99–011 and 68-D99–012, and through Interagency Agreement DW-75–93912801-0. It has been subjected to Agency review and approved for publication.

This work was supported by the Intramural Research Program of the NIH, National Cancer Institute, Division of Cancer Epidemiology and

Genetics (Z01CP010119) and the National Institutes of Environmental Health Science (Z01ES049030). The authors have no conflicts of interest in connection with this manuscript.

Ms. Marsha Dunn and Ms. Kate Torres, (employed by Westat, Inc. Rockville, Maryland) are gratefully acknowledged for study coordination. The ongoing participation of the Agricultural Health Study participants is indispensable and sincerely appreciated.

Author Contributions

Conceived and designed the experiments: MCA DPS AB. Performed the experiments: MCA CFL KT CJH. Analyzed the data: MCA JNH CFL CJH KHB JB DWB KT DPS JAH SK GA JHL AB LEB. Contributed reagents/materials/analysis tools: MCA JB DWB CFL. Wrote the paper: MCA LEBF JNH CFL CJH KT AB DWB JHL. Designed the software: JB DWB.

References

1. Milham S (1971) Leukemia and multiple myeloma in farmers. Am J Epidemiol 94: 507–510.
2. Cantor KP (1982) Farming and mortality from non-Hodgkin's lymphoma: a case-control study. Int J Cancer 29: 239–247.
3. Blair A, Malker H, Cantor KP, Burmeister L, Wiklund K (1985) Cancer among farmers: A review. Scand J Work Environ Health 11: 397–407.
4. Pearce NE, Smith AH, Fischer DO (1985) Malignant lymphoma and multiple myeloma linked with agricultural occupation in a New Zealand cancer registration-base-study. Am J Epidemiol 121: 235–237.
5. Baris D, Silverman DT, Brown LM, Swanson GM, Hayes RB, et al. (2004) Occupation, pesticide exposure and risk of multiple myeloma. Scand J Work Environ Health 30(3): 215–222.
6. Beane Freeman LE, DeRoos AJ, Koutros S, Blair A, Ward MH, et al. (2012) Poultry and livestock exposure and cancer risk among farmers in the agricultural health study. Cancer Causes Control 23: 663–670.
7. Cordes DH, Rea DF (1991) Farming: A Hazardous Occupation. In: Health Hazards of Farming. Occupational Medicine: State of the Art Reviews. Vol6(3). Hanley & Belfus, Inc., Philadelphia, PA.
8. Alavanja M, Bonner M (2012) Occupational pesticide exposure and cancer risk. A Review. J. Toxicol Environ Health B Critic Review. 1594: 238–263.
9. Alavanja MCR, Ross MK, Bonner MR (2013) Increased cancer burden among pesticide applicators and others due to pesticide exposure. CA, Cancer J Clin; 63(2): 120–142.
10. Waddell BL, Zahm SH, Baris D, Weisenburger DD, Holmes F, et al. (2001). Agricultural use of organophosphate pesticides and the risk of non-Hodgkin's lymphoma among male farmers (United States). Cancer Causes and Control 12: 509–517.
11. Merhi M, Raynal H, Cahuzac E, Vinson F, Cravedi JP, et al. (2007) Occupational exposure to pesticides and risk of hematopoietic cancers: meta-analysis of case-control studies. Cancer Causes Control. 18: 1209–1226.
12. IARC (1991) International Agency for Research on Cancer (IARC). Occupational Exposures in Insecticide applications and some pesticides. Lyon, France: IARC, 1991. Monographs on the Evaluation of Carcinogenic Risk to Humans, volume 53.
13. Morton LM, Slager SL, Cerhan JR, Wang SS, Vajdic CM, et al. (2014) Etiologic Heterogeneity Among NHL Subtypes: The InterLymph NHL Subtypes Project. J Natl Cancer Institute 48: 130–144.
14. Alavanja MCR, Sandler DP, McMaster SB, Zahm SH, McDonnell CJ, et al. (1996) The Agricultural Health Study. Environ Health Perspect 104: 362–369.
15. Alavanja MC, Samanic C, Dosemeci M, Lubin J, Tarone R, et al. (2003) Use of agricultural pesticides and prostate cancer risk in the Agricultural Health Study Cohort. Am J Epidemiol 157(9): 800–814.
16. SEER Program, National Cancer Institute. Available: http://seer.cancer.gov/lymphomarecode Accessed September 15, 2013.
17. Morton LM, Turner JJ, Cerhan JR, Linet MS, Treseler PA, et al. (2007) Proposed classifciation of lymphoid neoplasms for epidemiologic research from the Pathology Working Group of the International Lymphoma Epidemiology Consortium (InterLymph). Blood 110(2): 695–708.
18. Percy C, Fritz A, Ries L (2001) Conversion of neoplasms by topography and morphology from the International Classification of Disease for Oncology, second edition, to International Classification of Diseases for Oncology, 3rd ed. Cancer Statistics Branch, DCCPS, SEER Program, National Cancer Institute; 2001.
19. Heltshe SL, Lubin JH, Koutros S, Coble JB, Ji B-T, et al. (2012) Using multiple imputation to assign pesticide use for non-respondents in the follow-up questionnaire in the Agricultural Health Study J. Exp Sci Environ Epidemiol 22(4): 409–416.
20. Coble J, Thomas KW, Hines CJ, Hoppin JA, Dosemeci M, et al. (2011) An updated algorithm for estimation of pesticide exposure intensity in the Agricultural Health Study. Int J Environ Res Public Health. 8(12): 4608–4622.
21. ATSDR (2005) Agency for Toxic Substances and Disease Registry. Toxicological profile for Alpha-, Beta-, Gamma- and Delta- Hexahlorcyclohexane, August, 2005. Available: http://www.atsdr.cdc.gov/Toxprofiles/tp43.pdf. Accessed 2013 Sep 15.
22. EPA (2006a) US Environmental Protection Agency (2006). Lindane; Cancellation Order December 13, 2006. Federal Register/Vol 71, number 239, page 74905.
23. Stockholm Convention Report (2009) Report of the conference of the Parties of the Stockholm Convention on Persistent Organic Pollutants on the work of its fourth meeting. Convention on Persistent Organic Pollutants. Fourth Meeting, Geneva, 4–8 May 2009. Available: http://chm.pops.int/Portals/0/Repository/COP4/UNEP-POPS-COP.4–38.English.pdf.

24. IARC (1987) International Agency for Research on Cancer (IARC). Overall evaluation of carcinogenicity: an updating of IARC monographs volume 1 to 42. Lyon, France: IARC, 1987. Monographs on the Evaluation of Carcinogenic Risk to Humans, Supplement 7.
25. Piskac-Collier AL, Smith MA (2009) Lindane-induced generation of reactive oxygen species and depletion of glutathione do not result in necrosis in renal distal tube cells. J Toxicol and Environ Health, Part A. 72: 1160–1167.
26. Rupa DS, Reddy PP, Reddi OS (1989). Genotoxic effect of benzene hexachloride in cultured human lymphocytes. Hum Genet 83: 271–273.
27. Blair A, Cantor KP, Zahm SH (1998) Non-Hodgkin's lymphoma and agricultural use of the insecticide lindane. Am J Ind Med 33: 82–87.
28. McDuffie HH, Pahwa P, Mclaughlin JR, Spinelli JJ, Fincham S, et al. (2001) Non-Hodgkin's lymphoma and specific pesticide exposures in Men: Cross-Canada Study of Pesticides and Health. Cancer, Epidemiology, Biomarkers & Prevention 10: 1155–1163.
29. Purdue MP, Hoppin JA, Blair A, Dosemeci M, Alavanja MCR (2007) Occupational exposure to organochlorine insecticides and cancer incidence in the Agricultural Health Study. Int J Cancer. 120(3): 642–649.
30. EPA (2012) US Environmental Protection Agency 2012. DDT-A Brief History and Status. Available: http://www.epa.gov/pesticides/factsheets/chemicals/ddt-brief-history-status.htm. Accessed 2013 Sep 15.
31. NTP (2011) National Toxicology Program, Report on Carcinogen- Twelfth Edition. Available: http://ntp.niehs.nih.gov/go/roc12. Accessed 2013 Sep 15.
32. Baris D, Zahm SH, Cantor KP, Blair A (1998). Agricultural use of DDT and the risk of non-Hodgkin's lymphoma: pooled analysis of three case-control studies in the United States, Occup Environ Med 55: 522–527.
33. Cocco P, Satta G, Dubois S, Pilli C, Pillieri M, et al. (2013) Lymphoma risk and occupational exposure to pesticides: results of the Epilymph study. Occupational Environ Med 70(2): 91–98.
34. Nanni O, Amadori D, Lugaresi C, Falcini F, Scarpi E, et al. (1996) Chronic lymphocytic leukaemia and non-Hodgkin's lymphomas by histological type in farming-animal breeding workers: a population case-control study based on a priori exposure matrics Occup Environ Med 53(10): 652–657.
35. Rothman N, Cantor KP, Blair A, Bush D, Brock JW, et al. (1997) A nested case-control study of non-Hodgkin lymphoma and serum organochlorine residues. The Lancet 350: 240–244.
36. Quintana PJE, Delfino RJ, Korrick S, Ziogas A, Kutz FW, et al. (2004) Adipose tissue levels of organochlorine pesticides and chlorinated biphenyls and the risk of non-Hodgkin's lymphoma. Environ Health Perspect 112: 854–861.
37. Brauner EV, Sorensen MA, Gaudreau E, LeBlanc A, Erikson KT, et al. (2012) A prospective study of organochlorines in adipose tissue and risk of non-Hodgkin lymphoma. Environ Health Perspect. 120(1): 105–111.
38. Spinelli JJ, Ng CH, Weber JP, Connors JM, Gascoyne RD, et al. (2007) Organochlorines and risk of non-Hodgkin lymphoma. Int J Cancer. 121(12): 2767–2775.
39. Cocco P, Brennan P, Ibba A, de Sanjose Llongueras S (2008) Plasma polychlorobiphenyl and organochlorine pesticide level and risk of major lymphoma subtypes. Occup Environ Med 65: 132–140.
40. EPA 2006(b). U.S. Environmental Protection Agency. 2006. Re-registration Eligibility Decision for Permethrin: Available: http://www.epa.gov/oppsrrd1/REDs/permethrin_red.pdf. Accessed 2013 Sep 15.
41. NPIC (2012). National Pesticide Information Center. Chemicals Evaluated for Carcinogenic Potential. Office of Pesticide Programs. U.S. Environmental Protection Agency. November 2012. Available: http://npic.orst.edu/chemicals_evaluated.pdf. Accessed 2013 Sep 15.
42. De Roos AJ, Zahm SH, Cantor KP, Weisenburger DD, Holmes FF, t al. (2003) Integrative assessment of multiple pesticides as risk factors for non-Hodgkin's lymphoma among men Occup Environ Med 60: E11.
43. Rusiecki JA, Patel R, Koutros S, Beane Freeman LE, Landgren O, et al. (2009) Cancer incidence among pesticide applicators exposed to permethrin in the Agricultural Health Study. Environ Health Perspect 117: 582–586.
44. EPA 2006(b). U.S. Environmental Protection Agency. 2006. Re-registration Eligibility Decision for Terbufos: Available: http://www.epa.gov/pesticides/reregistration/REDs/terbufos_red.pdf Accessed 2013 Nov 18.
45. Environmental Protection Agency, 2004. Interim registration eligibility decision: diazinon. Available: http://www.epa.gov/pesticides/reregistration/REDs/diazinon_red.pdf. Accessed 2013 Nov 18.
46. Donalson D, Kieley T, Grube A (2002) Pesticide industry sales and usage: 1998 and 1999 market estimates. Washington, DC.: US Environmental Protection Agency, 2002 (EPA-733-R-02–001).

47. Beane Freeman LE, Bonner MR, Blair A, Hoppin JA, Sandler DP, et al. (2005). Cancer incidence among male pesticide applicators in the Agricultural Health Study cohort exposed to diazinon. Am J Epidemiol. 162: 1070–1079.

48. Blair A. Tarone R, Sandler D, Lynch CF, Rowland A, et al. (2002) Reliability of reporting on life-style and agricultural factors by a sample of participants in the Agricultural Health Study from Iowa. Epidemiology 13(1): 94–99.

49. Blair A, Thomas HT, Coble J, Sandler DP, Hines CJ, et al. (2011). Impact of pesticide exposure on misclassification on estimates of relative risks in the Agricultural Health Study. Occup Environ Med 68: 537–541.

50. Thomas KW, Dosemeci M, Coble JB, Hoppin JA, Sheldon LS, et al. (2010) Assessment of a pesticide exposure intensity algorithm in the Agricultural Health Study. J Expo Sci Environ Epidemiol 20(6): 559–569.

24

Simple and Reliable Determination of Intravoxel Incoherent Motion Parameters for the Differential Diagnosis of Head and Neck Tumors

Miho Sasaki, Misa Sumi, Sato Eida, Ikuo Katayama, Yuka Hotokezaka, Takashi Nakamura*

Department of Radiology and Cancer Biology, Nagasaki University School of Dentistry, Nagasaki, Japan

Abstract

Intravoxel incoherent motion (IVIM) imaging can characterize diffusion and perfusion of normal and diseased tissues, and IVIM parameters are authentically determined by using cumbersome least-squares method. We evaluated a simple technique for the determination of IVIM parameters using geometric analysis of the multiexponential signal decay curve as an alternative to the least-squares method for the diagnosis of head and neck tumors. Pure diffusion coefficients (D), microvascular volume fraction (f), perfusion-related incoherent microcirculation (D*), and perfusion parameter that is heavily weighted towards extravascular space (P) were determined geometrically (Geo D, Geo f, and Geo P) or by least-squares method (Fit D, Fit f, and Fit D*) in normal structures and 105 head and neck tumors. The IVIM parameters were compared for their levels and diagnostic abilities between the 2 techniques. The IVIM parameters were not able to determine in 14 tumors with the least-squares method alone and in 4 tumors with the geometric and least-squares methods. The geometric IVIM values were significantly different (p<0.001) from Fit values (+2±4% and −7±24% for D and f values, respectively). Geo D and Fit D differentiated between lymphomas and SCCs with similar efficacy (78% and 80% accuracy, respectively). Stepwise approaches using combinations of Geo D and Geo P, Geo D and Geo f, or Fit D and Fit D* differentiated between pleomorphic adenomas, Warthin tumors, and malignant salivary gland tumors with the same efficacy (91% accuracy = 21/23). However, a stepwise differentiation using Fit D and Fit f was less effective (83% accuracy = 19/23). Considering cumbersome procedures with the least squares method compared with the geometric method, we concluded that the geometric determination of IVIM parameters can be an alternative to least-squares method in the diagnosis of head and neck tumors.

Editor: Sune N. Jespersen, Aarhus University, Denmark

Funding: The authors received the funds of this study from the internal source of Nagasaki University. The funders had no role in study design, data collection and analysis, decision to publish, or preparation of the manuscript.

Competing Interests: The authors have declared that no competing interests exist.

* Email: taku@nagasaki-u.ac.jp

Introduction

Diffusion occurs because of the non-ending movement of every single molecule [1]. Brown first observed this phenomenon (although Ingenhousz found the phenomenon earlier than Brown did), and Einstein later gave this phenomenon a sound mathematical description considering a free diffusion process, where the molecules only collide with other molecules in a homogeneous container without boundaries. Diffusion-weighted imaging (DWI) is based on MR signal attenuations caused by the displacement of intracellular and extracellular water molecules for a given time. In biological tissues, however, the environment of water molecules can hardly be called homogeneous: membranes, macromolecules, and fibers hamper the diffusion process [2]. Furthermore, there is other incoherent motion within a voxel that can lead to signal attenuation; in particular, the water molecules in blood capillaries exhibit a pseudorandom motion in the tortuous capillaries.

Le Bihan proposed that intravoxel incoherent motion (IVIM) imaging can distinguish between the pure molecular diffusion and motion of water molecules in the capillary network with a single

DWI acquisition technique, provided that high b-values (≥200 s/mm^2) and low b-values (<200 s/mm^2) are used [3]. The IVIM imaging can be characterized by 3 parameters: pure diffusion coefficient (D); microvascular volume fraction (f); and perfusion-related incoherent microcirculation (D*) [4]. To determine the IVIM parameters from a multiexponential signal decay curve, the least-squares method is usually used [4,5]. However, the method is cumbersome, and thus may not be suitable for routine clinical use.

Recently, some researchers have applied simplified methods for determining IVIM parameters to characterize tumors in the liver, prostate, and head and neck region [6–9]. For example, Lewin et al shoed that the perfusion fraction parameter f determined by using a geometric analysis of DW MR images can be a marker of sorafenib treatment of patients with advanced hepatocellular carcinoma [7]. However, they did not indicate how precise the geometric determination of the perfusion parameter compared with the conventional technique. In addition, Mazaheri et al noted that the linear fit of the logarithmic signal using limited numbers of b-value is statistically less appropriate than fitting the signals to exponential functions using a least-squares method [8]. The

Table 1. 105 head and neck tumors.

Tumor	n
Benign	35
Salivary gland tumor	
Pleomorphic adenoma	15
Warthin tumor	8
Odontogenic tumor	
Ameloblastoma	2
Keratcystic odontogenic tumor	2
Odontogenic fibroma	2
Odontogenic myxoma	1
Hemangioma	1
Angiomyoma	1
Myofibroma	1
Papiloma	1
Adenomatous goiter	1
Malignant	70
SCC	25
SCC node	12
Lymphoma	14
Salivary gland tumor	
Carcinoma ex. pleomorphic adenoma	2
Adenoid cystic carcinoma	1
Acinic cell carcinoma	1
Adenocarcinoma	1
Dedifferentiated carcinoma	1
Salivary duct carcinoma	1
Lymph node metastasis from malignant salivary gland tumor	4
Malignant melanoma	1
Nasopharyngeal carcinoma	1
Neuroendocrine carcinoma	1
Papillary thyroid carcinoma	1
Lymph node metastasis from papillary thyroid carcinoma	3
Ameloblastic carcinoma	1
Total	105

SCC, squamous cell carcinoma.
Of 105 tumors, 18 were excluded from the study owing to measurement errors, including 6 pleomorphic adenomas, 2 lymphomas, 2 SCCs (oropharynx and hypopharynx), 1 SCC node, 1 adenocarcinoma, 1 metastatic node from papillary thyroid carcinoma, 1 neuroendocrine carcinoma, 1 ameloblastic carcinoma, 1 hemangioma, 1 keratocystic odontogenic tumor, 1 myxoma.

authors also suggested the importance of b-value selection used for the simplified IVIM analysis. In simplified methods, the IVIM parameters are estimated by using a limited number [3–4] of b-values compared with the authentic IVIM imaging, which uses 9–13 b-values [4,5,10,11]. However, the reliability in measurements and effectiveness in diagnosing tumors with simplified IVIM techniques using limited numbers of b-value has not been fully investigated. Sasaki et al. reported the reproducibility of IVIM parameter measurements in evaluating the technique for functional assessment of the masticator muscles [12]. However, there was no published report that presented the reproducibility of IVIM parameters in diagnosing tumors. In the present study, we directly compared the IVIM parameter values that were determined by a simplified geometric method with those determined by the conventional least-squares method. We have also compared the diagnostic accuracy for diagnosing head and neck squamous cell carcinomas (SCCs) and lymphomas as well as benign and malignant salivary gland tumors between the 2 methods.

Materials and Methods

Ethics statement

The Ethics Committee of Nagasaki University approved this study. Informed consent was waived due to the retrospective

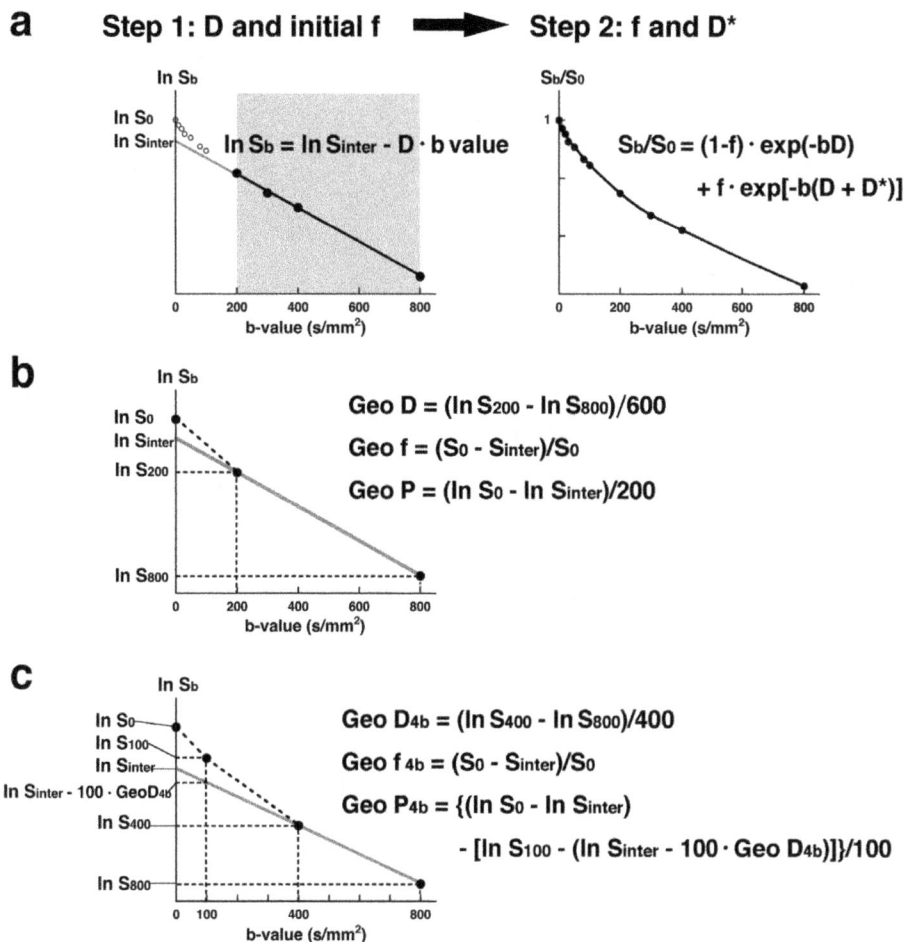

Figure 1. IVIM parameter determination by least-squares or geometric method. a, Least-squares method. Upper panel shows a representative signal decay curve obtained by using 11 b-values (0, 10, 20, 30, 50, 80, 100, 200, 300, 400, 800 s/mm^2). At first step, D (Fit D) can be obtained by least-squares method using ln S_{200}, ln S_{300}, ln S_{400}, and ln S_{800}, and initial f value is calculated as $(S_0 - S_{inter})/S_0$, where S_{inter} is the interception of the logarithmic regression line obtained by using b-values of 200, 300, 400, and 800 s/mm^2 with the y-axis. Right panel shows relationship between S_b/S_0 and varying b-values. Given D and initial f and D* values, f (Fit f) and D* (Fit D*) values can be obtained by least-squares method based on the equation: $S_b/S_0 = (1-f) \cdot \exp(-bD) + f \cdot [-b(D+D^*)]$. **b,** Geometric method. Graph shows geometric determination of IVIM parameters using 3 (0, 200, and 800 s/mm^2) of the 11 b-values. D is calculated by the equation $GeoD = (\ln S_{200} - \ln S_{800})/600$. f is estimated by the equation $Geof = (S_0 - S_{inter})/S_0$, and P is estimated by the equation $GeoP = (lnS_0 - \ln S_{inter})/200$Geo P = (ln S_0–ln S_{inter})/200. **c,** Geometric method based on 4-b-value data. Graph shows geometric determination of IVIM parameters using 4 (0, 100, 400, and 800 s/mm^2) of the 11 b-values. D is calculated by the equation $GeoD_{4b} = (\ln S_{400} - \ln S_{800})/400$, f is estimated by the equation $Geof4b = (S_0 - S_{inter})/S_0$, and P is estimated by the equation $GeoP_{4b} = \{(\ln S_0 - \ln S_{inter}) - [lnS_{100} - (\ln S_{inter} - 100 \cdot GeoD_{4b})]\}/100$.

Table 2. Inter- and intraobserver errors in measuring Geo and Fit IVIM parameters.

	IVIM parameters	%CV	
		Geo	Fit
Interobserver errors	D	0.5±0.2	0.5±0.3
	f	5.2±0.8	9.7±7.8
	P/D*	5.1±0.8	16.2±11.0
Intraobserver errors	D	0.9±0.9	1.0±0.9
	f	5.4±5.4	11.4±7.9
	P/D*	5.5±5.5[a]	19.7±8.6[a]

%CV, percent coefficient of variation; Geo, geometric measurement; Fit, least-squares method. P/D*, Geo P/Fit D*.
a, significant difference between Geo and Fit values (p = 0.0195, Wilcoxon signed-rank test).

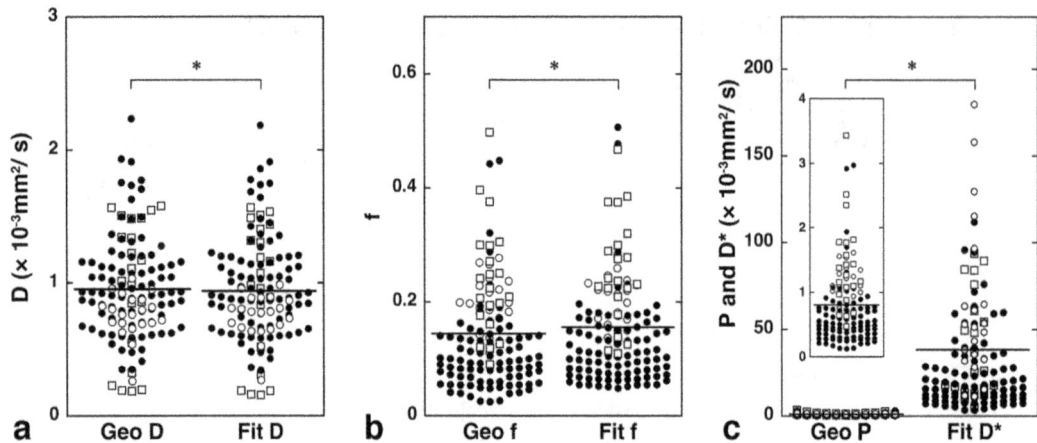

Figure 2. IVIM parameters of normal structures and tumors in the head and neck region. Plot graphs show D (Geo D), f (Geo f), and P (Geo P) values that were determined by geometric method; and D (Fit D), f (Fit f), and D* (Fit D*) values that were determined by least-squares method of normal structures (parotid glands, open circles; and masseter muscles, open squares) and head and neck tumors (closed circles). Broken white contours indicate tumor areas. Parotid gland: Geo D, Geo f and Geo P=0.76±0.17×10^{-3} mm²/s, 0.20±0.04, and 1.12±0.27×10^{-3} mm²/s, respectively; and Fit D, Fit f, and Fit D*=0.75±0.16×10^{-3} mm²/s, 0.20±0.05, and 62.96±46.78×10^{-3} mm²/s, respectively. Masseter muscle: Geo D, Geo f, and Geo P=0.99±0.51×10^{-3} mm²/s, 0.24±0.10, and 1.41±0.71×10^{-3} mm²/s, respectively; and Fit D, Fit f, and Fit D*=0.96±0.51×10^{-3} mm²/s, 0.25±0.10, and 40.50±30.13×10^{-3} mm²/s, respectively. Tumors: Geo D, Geo f, and Geo P=1.00±0.38×10^{-3} mm²/s, 0.11±0.08, and 0.61±0.48×10^{-3} mm²/s, respectively; Fit D, Fit f, and Fit D*=0.99±0.37×10^{-3} mm²/s, 0.12±0.08, and 24.14±21.15×10^{-3} mm²/s, respectively. Insert, Geo P distribution on a small scale. The values are the results of integrated signal intensities within the ROIs. *, p<0.001 (Wilcoxon signed-rank test).

nature of the study. Patient records/information was anonymized and de-identified prior to analysis.

Patients

We retrospectively studied DW MR images of patients with head and neck tumors who underwent preoperative MR examinations between March 2003 to April 2012. We selected head and neck tumors from patients (1) who underwent diffusion-weighted MR imaging as well as conventional contrast-enhanced and non-enhanced T1-weighted and fat-suppressed T2-weighted MR imaging; (2) whose tumors were excised and histologically proven; and (3) whose DW images were good in quality without any severe susceptibility artifacts that would interfere with IVIM analysis. Consequently, the study cohort included 105 head and neck tumors (35 benign and 70 malignant tumors) that arose in 94 patients (56 men and 38 women; average age, 62±15 years; age range, 3–91 years). Detailed tumor pathology is listed in Table 1.

DW MR images of the healthy parotid glands (n=21) and the masseter muscles (n=21) of the contralateral sides in patients with parotid tumor were also analyzed for comparing the IVIM parameters determined by using geometric or least-squares methods.

MR imaging

MR imaging was performed using a 1.5-T MR unit (Gyroscan Intera 1.5T Master; Philips Healthcare, Best, The Netherlands). 73 patients were scanned by using a 2-channel 17-cm×14-cm (Synergy-Flex M), 7 patients by using a 2-channel 20-cm (Synergy-Flex L) surface coil, and 14 patients by using a 3-channel head and neck coil (Synergy Head Neck).

T1- and T2-weighted MR imaging

We obtained axial T1- and fat-suppressed (spectral attenuated with inversion recovery, [SPAIR]) T2-weighted MR images (TR/TE/number of signal acquisitions=500 ms/15 ms/2 and 6385 ms/80 ms/2, respectively) by using a turbo spin-echo

(TSE) sequence (TSE factor=3 and 15, respectively). We used a 200-mm FOV, 256×204 scan and 512×512 reconstruction matrix sizes, a 4-mm slice thickness and a 0.4-mm slice gap. For contrast-enhanced T1-weighted MR imaging, a gadolinium-based agent (gadopentatate dimeglutimine, Magnevist; Bayer Healthcare, Berlin, Germany) was intravenously injected at a dose of 0.2 mL per kg of body weight and a rate of 1.5 mL/s.

DW MR imaging

Axial DW images (TR/TE=1625 ms/81 ms) were obtained using single-shot, spin-echo echo planar imaging (SE-EPI). The EPI factor was 47, and Sensitivity Encoding (SENSE) factor was 2. We used a 200-mm FOV, 4-mm slice thickness, 0.4-mm slice gap, and 112×90 matrix size. The measured pixel size was 1.79/2.28/4 mm. We used 11 b-values (0, 10, 20, 30, 50, 80, 100, 200, 300, 400, and 800 s/mm²). The total acquisition time was 1 min 53 s per 5 slices.

Regions of interest

A region of interest (ROI) was manually placed onto each tumor area such that it encompassed as much of the tumor area as possible. The mean ROI area was 3.4±2.8 cm² (0.8–18.1 cm²). Visually large cystic or necrotic areas were excluded from the present analysis. We used the contrast-enhanced T1-weighted and fat-suppressed T2-weighted MR images as references to determine tumor areas on the corresponding DW images. We compared the IVIM values between geometric and least-squares methods based on the IVIM values calculated from ROI-averaged signal intensities. We used DW image slices including the 1–3 maximal tumor areas, and the IVIM values obtained from each ROIs were averaged. For the healthy parotid glands and masseter muscles, irregular ROIs were placed so that they included as much of the gland or muscle area as possible, but did not include large vessels, such as the retromandibular vein, or intraglandular main ducts. A radiologist with 20-year experience in head and neck radiology placed ROIs and analyzed IVIM images.

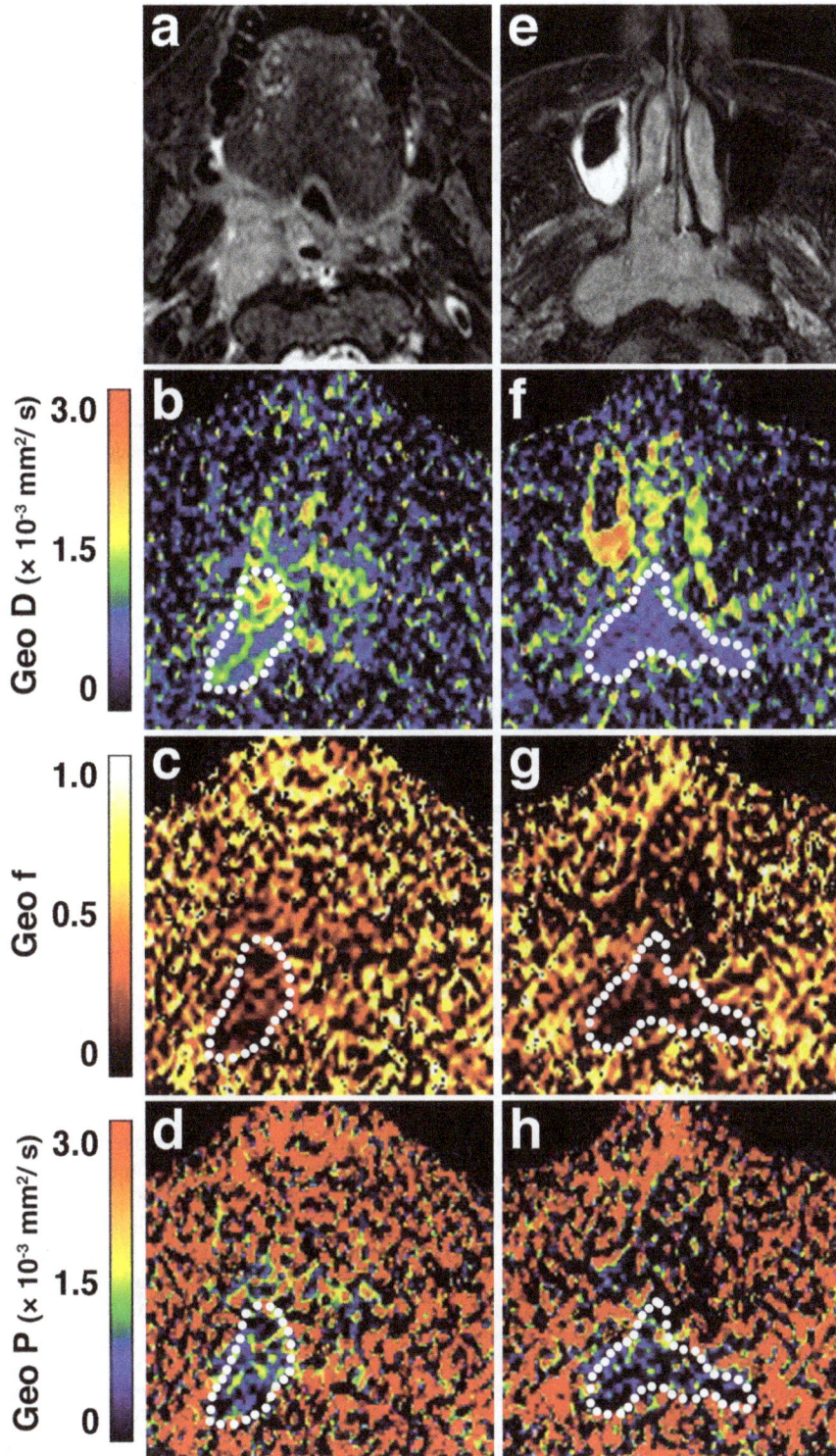

Figure 3. IVIM maps of SCC and lymphoma. a–d, Axial fat-suppressed T2-weighted MR image (**a**), and Geo D (**b**), Geo f (**c**), and Geo P (**d**) maps of 72-year-old man with SCC in oropharynx show tumor with homogeneous T2-signals and IVIM parameter values of Geo D, Geo f, and Geo P $= 1.16 \times 10^{-3}$ mm^2/s, 0.14, and 0.76×10^{-3} mm^2/s, respectively; and Fit D, Fit f, and Fit D* $= 1.14 \times 10^{-3}$ mm^2/s, 0.18, and 8.50×10^{-3} mm^2/s, respectively. **e–h**, Axial fat-suppressed T2-weighted MR image (e), and Geo D (f), Geo f (g), and Geo P (h) maps of 79-year-old man with lymphoma in nasopharynx show tumor with homogeneous T2 signals and IVIM parameter values of Geo D, Geo f, and Geo P $= 0.59 \times 10^{-3}$ mm^2/s, 0.08, and 0.41×10^{-3} mm^2/s, respectively; and Fit D, Fit f, and Fit D* $= 0.60 \times 10^{-3}$ mm^2/s, 0.07, and 17.01×10^{-3} mm^2/s, respectively. The values are the results of integrated signal intensities within the ROIs.

Table 3. IVIM parameters of SCCs and lymphomas.

IVIM parameter	SCC (n = 34)	Lymphoma (n = 12)
D (×10^{-3} mm^2/s)		
Geo	0.93±0.23[a]	0.63±0.16[a]
Fit	0.93±0.23[b]	0.62±0.15[b]
f		
Geo	0.13±0.10	0.09±0.04
Fit	0.14±0.10	0.10±0.03
P/D* (×10^{-3} mm^2/s)		
Geo	0.74±0.65	0.49±0.23
Fit	27.11±22.06	28.52±15.01

IVIM, intravoxel incoherent motion; SCC, squamous cell carcinoma; Geo, IVIM parameters determined by geometric method; Fit, IVIM parameters determined by least squares method. P/D*, Geo P/Fit D*.
[a, b] significant differences (p = 0.0002, Mann-Whitney U test).

IVIM analysis based on least squares method

The relationship between signal intensities and b-values based on the IVIM theory can be expressed using the following equation:

$$S_b/S_o = (1-f) \cdot \exp(-bD) + f \cdot \exp[-b(D+D^*)] \quad (1)$$

where f is microvascular volume fraction, D is pure diffusion coefficient, and D* represents perfusion-related incoherent microcirculation [4]; S_0 and S_b are signal intensities at b = 0 and b = 10, 20, 30, 50, 80, 100, 200, 300, 400, or 800 s/mm^2, respectively. Using logarithmic plots (Fig. 1a), D (Fit D) can be obtained with a linear regression algorithm (the least-squares methods using b-values of 200, 300, 400, and 800 s/mm^2). Given a D value, the initial f value was estimated as y-axis intersection of the linear regression (Fig. 1a). Then, the corresponding f (Fit f) and D* (Fit D*) values can be calculated using a nonlinear regression algorithm based on equation (1) (Fig. 1a). Fit f and Fit D* values were obtained after substituting initial f and D* values into the Levenberg-Marquardt algorithm [13], using SPSS software (Version 18.0, IBM incorporation). The initial values used for the least-squares method were as follows: f = −0.06–0.49 (average, 0.11±0.08); D* = 0.01 [5,7]. The convergence criterion was 0.00000001.

IVIM analysis based on geometric method

Separately, we analyzed signal decay curves by using the geometric method as described previously [6,7,9]. By using logarithmic plots, D can be estimated as a decline between b = 200–800 s/mm^2, (ln S$_{200}$–ln S$_{800}$)/600 (Fig. 1b). Given an estimated D value, we estimated the tissue perfusion by geometrically estimating the f as 1–S$_{inter}$/S$_0$ (S$_{inter}$ is the interception of the logarithmic regression line obtained using b-values of 200 and 800 s/mm^2 with the y-axis) (Fig. 1). On the other hand, perfusion property can be geometrically estimated by the formula as (ln S$_0$–ln S$_{inter}$)/200. Fit D* reflects the vascular space only. However, the geometrically defined perfusion parameter is heavily weighted towards the perfusion in the extravascular space. Therefore, the geometrically perfusion parameter is fundamentally different from Fit D*. We introduced a perfusion parameter Geo P, which reflects and averages the vascular and extravascular spaces.

Separately, we determined IVIM parameters based on 4 b-value (b = 0, 100, 400, and 800 s/mm^2) data according to the followings (Fig. 1c):

$$GeoD_{4b} = (lnS_{400} - \ln S_{800})/400$$
$$Geof_{4b} = (S_0 - S_{inter})/S_0$$
$$GeoP_{4b} =$$
$$\{(\ln S_0 - \ln S_{inter}) - [\ln S_{100} - (\ln S_{inter} - 100 \cdot GeoD_{4b})]\}/100$$
$$= (\ln S_0 - \ln S_{100} - 100 \cdot GeoD_{4b})/100$$

DW images in a DICOM format were converted to 2D color maps of geometrically determined f, D, and D* values by using the ImageJ software (NIH, http://rsweb.nih.gov/ij/index.html). We used an existing fit plug-in for ImageJ software. The color maps were generated purely for qualitative illustration and were not employed in the quantitative performance comparison of the least squares and geometrical methods for calculating IVIM parameters.

Interobserver and intraobserver errors

Separate sets of DW MR images, including conventional T1- and T2-weighted, contrast-enhanced T1-weighted, and DW MR images, from 5 patients with head and neck tumors were analyzed independently by 3 separate radiologists with 17–20-year experience. The radiologists were asked to place an ROI onto each of DW MR images at b-values of 0, 200, and 800 s/mm^2. One day after, the same radiologists were asked to repeat the same procedure with the same sets of DW MR images. Interobserver and intraobserver errors were assessed by calculating percent coefficient of variation (%CV) of IVIM parameters obtained from different ROIs placed on the same DW MR images.

Statistics

Wilcoxon signed-rank test was used for the comparison of the IVIM parameters between the 2 techniques. Steel-Dwass test was used for the comparison of the IVIM parameters between the 3 different types of salivary gland tumors. Mann-Whitney U-test was used for the comparison of the IVIM parameters between lymphomas and SCCs. Cluster analysis was used to determine the best threshold for the IVIM criteria for discriminating between different tumor groups, where the best cutoff IVIM values were determined so that the values differentiated with the highest

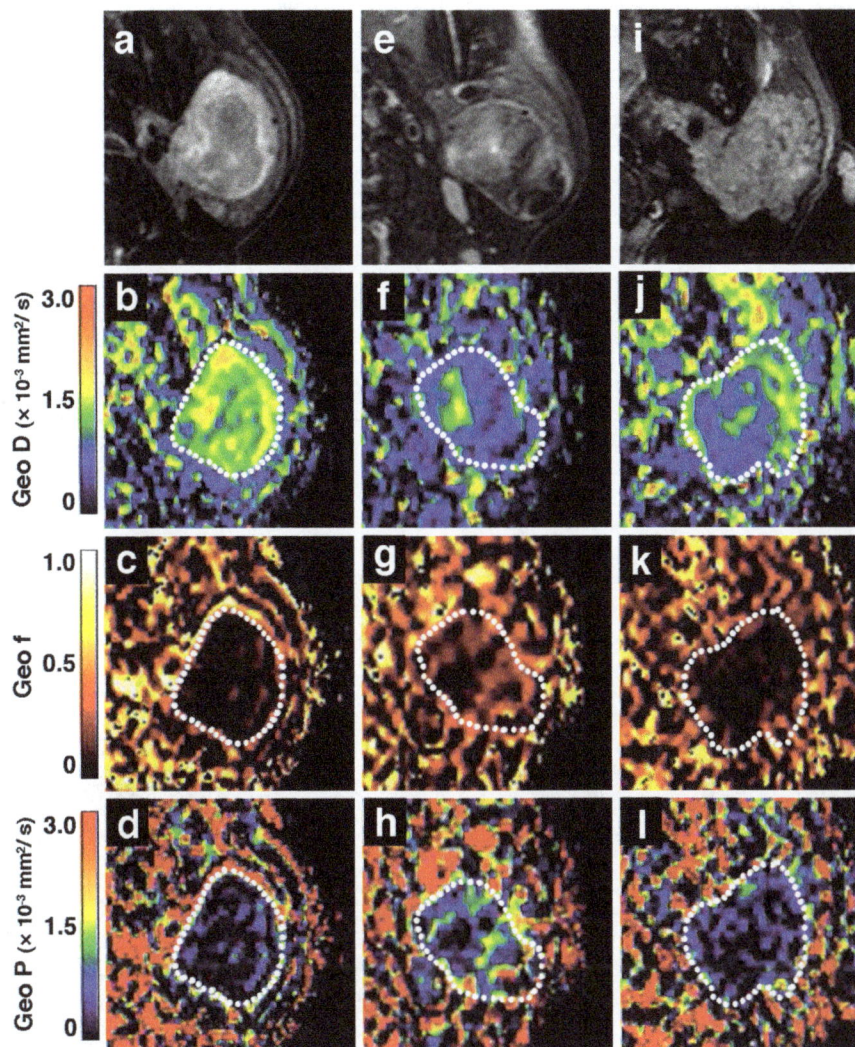

Figure 4. IVIM maps of benign and malignant salivary gland tumors. a–d, Axial fat-suppressed T2-weighted MR image (**a**), and Geo D (**b**), Geo f (**c**), and Geo P (**d**) maps of 67-year-old man with pleomorphic adenoma in left parotid gland show tumor with heterogeneous T2-signals and IVIM parameter values of Geo D, Geo f, and Geo P = 1.37×10^{-3} mm^2/s, 0.02, and 0.12×10^{-3} mm^2/s, respectively; and Fit D, Fit f, and Fit D* = 1.37×10^{-3} mm^2/s, 0.05, and 4.23×10^{-3} mm^2/s, respectively. Broken white contours indicate tumor areas. **e–h**, Axial fat-suppressed MR image (**e**), and Geo D (**f**), Geo f (**g**), and Geo P (**h**) maps of 65-year-old woman with Warthin tumor in left parotid gland show tumor with heterogeneous T2-signals and IVIM parameter values of Geo D, Geo f, and Geo P = 0.87×10^{-3} mm^2/s, 0.14, and 0.75×10^{-3} mm^2/s, respectively; and Fit D, Fit f, and Fit D* = 0.84×10^{-3} mm^2/s, 0.16, and 23.32×10^{-3} mm^2/s, respectively. Broken white contours indicate tumor areas. **i–l**, Axial fat-suppressed T2-weighted MR image (**i**), and Geo D (**j**), Geo f (**k**), and Geo P (**l**) maps of 59-year-old woman with carcinoma ex. Pleomorphic adenoma in left parotid gland show tumor with heterogeneous T2-signals and IVIM parameter values of Geo D, Geo f, and Geo P = 0.89×10^{-3} mm^2/s, 0.04, and 0.20×10^{-3} mm^2/s, respectively; and Fit D, Fit f, and Fit D* = 0.88×10^{-3} mm^2/s, 0.05, and 10.00×10^{-3} mm^2/s, respectively. Broken white contours indicate tumor areas. The values are the results of integrated signal intensities within the ROIs.

accuracy between different tumor groups that were categorized by Ward's method using dendrogram. The statistical analyses were performed using SPSS (Version 18.0, IBM Corporation) and Excel Statistics 2012 (Version 1.00; SSRI).

Results

Errors in ROI placement

Interobserver and intraobserver errors of IVIM parameters were similar between Geo and Fit methods, except for intraobserver errors of D* values (Tables 2, S1, and S3).

Computation-induced invalidity

IVIM imaging of 18 out of the 105 head and neck tumors resulted in invalid IVIM values from the whole ROI, including 4 tumors, in which f values were negative with geometric method; 3 tumors, in which initial f values were negative with least-squares method; and 17 tumors, in which obtained f or D* values were the same as the initial values with least-squares method. Consequently, IVIM parameters were not able to be determined in 14 tumors owing to computation-induced invalidity with the least-squares method alone, and 4 tumors owing to measurement errors with both methods.

Table 4. IVIM parameters of pleomorphic adenomas, Warthin tumors, and malignant SG tumors.

IVIM parameter	Pleomophic adenoma (n = 9)	Warthin tumor (n = 8)	Malignant SG tumor (n = 6)
D ($\times10^{-3}$ mm^2/s)			
Geo	1.41$\pm$0.28^{a,b}	0.80$\pm$0.27^a	0.93$\pm$0.20^b
Fit	1.40$\pm$0.28^{a,b}	0.79$\pm$0.27^a	0.94$\pm$0.22^b
f			
Geo	0.07$\pm$0.04^c	0.13$\pm$0.04^c	0.09$\pm$0.04
Fit	0.09$\pm$0.04	0.13$\pm$0.03^d	0.08$\pm$0.03^d
P/D* ($\times10^{-3}$ mm^2/s)			
Geo	0.35$\pm$0.19^e	0.70$\pm$0.20^e	0.47$\pm$0.22
Fit	15.16$\pm$17.15^f	36.23$\pm$28.61^f	18.38$\pm$17.84

IVIM, intravoxel incoherent motion; SG, salivary gland; Geo, IVIM parameters determined by geometrical method; Fit, IVIM parameters determined by least squares method. P/D*, Geo P/Fit D*.
$^{a-f}$significant differences (p<0.05, Steel-Dwass test).

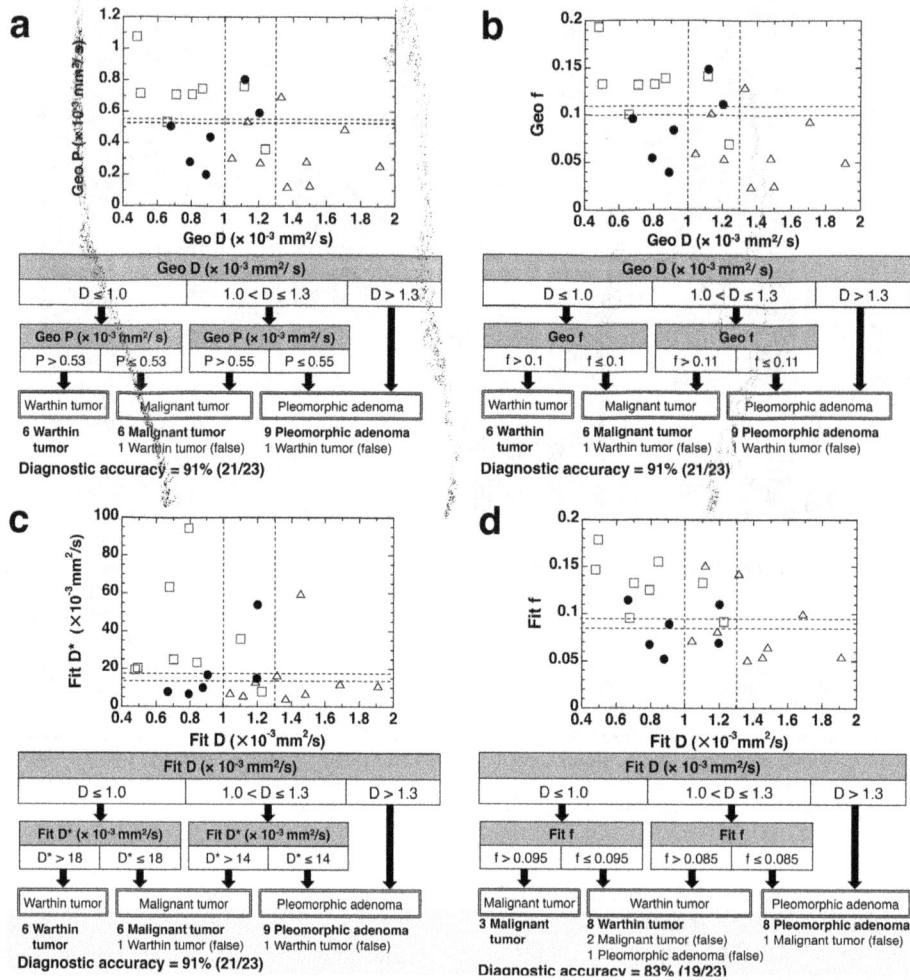

Figure 5. Stepwise differentiation between pleomorphic adenomas, Warthin tumors, and malignant salivary gland tumors using D, f, and D* or P values that were determined by geometric (Geo) or least-squares (Fit) method. Plot graphs show 2D distributions of Geo P and GeoD (**a**), Geo f and Geo D (**b**), Fit D* and Fit D (**C**), or Fit f and Fit D (**d**). Open triangles, open squares, and closed circles indicate pleomorphic adenomas, Warthin tumors, and malignant salivary gland tumors, respectively. In combinations of Geo D and Geo P (a), Geo D and Geo f, or Fit D and Fit D*, stepwise approach diagnosed 21 of 23 salivary gland tumors correctly; in these approaches, the same Warthin tumor was incorrectly diagnosed as a malignant salivary gland tumor owing to having a large Geo D (=1.11×10^{-3} mm^2/s) or Fit D values (=1.11×10^{-3} mm^2/s); or incorrectly diagnosed as a pleomorphic adenoma owing to having a large Geo D (=1.24×10^{-3} mm^2/s) or Fit D (=1.23×10^{-3} mm^2/s) and small Geo P (=0.36×10^{-3} mm^2/s) or Fit D* (=7.90×10^{-3} mm^2/s) values. The diagnostic accuracy with stepwise approach using Fit D and Fit f was lower than that using the corresponding geometric parameters (**b, d**). Diagnostic accuracy was provided for the respective classifications at the bottom of each diagram.

Table 5. IVIM parameters of 23 salivary gland tumors that were determined by least squares, 3b-geometrical, or 4b-geometrical methods.

IVIM parameters	Fit	3b-Geo	4b-Geo
D ($\times 10^{-3}$ mm²/s)	1.07±0.37	1.07±0.37	1.03±0.38
f	0.10±0.04	0.09±0.04	0.08±0.04
P/D* ($\times 10^{-3}$ mm²/s)	23.3±23.1[a,b]	0.50±0.25[a]	0.80±0.47[b]

IVIM, intravoxel incoherent motion; Fit, least squares method; 3b-Geo, geometric method using 3 b-values; 4b-Geo, geometric method using 4 b-values. P/D*, Geo P/Fit D*.
[a,b]significant differences (p<0.05) (Steel-Dwass test).

Differences in values of IVIM parameters between geometric and least-squares methods

D values determined by the geometric method (Geo D, $0.96\pm0.39\times10^{-3}$ mm²/s) were significantly (p<0.001) greater than those determined by the least squares method (Fit D, $0.94\pm0.38\times10^{-3}$ mm²/s) (Fig. 2, Tables S1 and S2). Geo f values (0.15±0.09) were significantly (p<0.001) smaller than Fit f valued (0.16±0.09). The differences were very small (2±4% for D values and −7±24% for f values) between 2 techniques.

Differences in diagnostic abilities of IVIM parameters between geometric and least-squares methods

Given the significant differences in values of IVIM parameters between geometric and least squares methods, we next tested whether these differences would affect the diagnostic abilities of IVIM parameters in differentiating SCCs and lymphomas (Fig. 3, Tables 3, S1, and S4). We found that f and P/D* values were ineffective for differentiating the 2 types of malignant tumors, resulting in 59% accuracy with Geo f and Fit f values; and 59% and 50% accuracy with Geo P and Fit D*, respectively. However, D values differentiated between SCCs and lymphomas with diagnostic abilities of 71% sensitivity, 100% specificity, and 78% accuracy with Geo D; and 74% sensitivity, 100% specificity, and 80% accuracy with Fit D.

Although significant differences in the IVIM values were found between the different types of salivary gland tumors (pleomorphic adenomas, Warthin tumors, and malignant salivary gland tumors), any single use of the parameters was ineffective in discriminating between the different tumor types (Fig. 4, Tables 4, S1, and S5). Therefore, we attempted to discriminate between the 3 different tumor types by using a stepwise approach with combined uses of the 3 IVIM parameters that were determined by the geometric or the least-squares methods (Fig. 5. Tables S1 and S5). The stepwise differentiation using Geo D and Geo P (Fig. 5a), Geo D and Geo f (Fig. 5b), or Fit D and Fit D* (Fig. 5c) differentiated 21 (91%) of the 23 salivary gland tumors correctly; consequently, the same 2 Warthin tumors were incorrectly diagnosed as malignant tumor or pleomorphic adenoma. However, a stepwise approach using Fit D and Fit f differentiated the salivary gland tumors less effectively; 3 malignant tumors were incorrectly diagnosed as Warthin tumors or pleomorphic adenoma; and 1 pleomorphic adenoma as Warthin tumor (Fig. 5d).

Lastly, we tested whether the use of 4 b-values (0, 100, 400, and 800 s/mm²) could significantly influence the IVIM parameter levels and their diagnostic abilities compared with the use of 3 b-values (0, 200, and 800 s/mm²). We found that Geo D and Geo f values of salivary gland tumors determined by the 3 b- or 4 b-values were not significantly different (Tables 5, S1, and S5). Furthermore, the use of 4 b-values resulted in less effective differentiation of salivary gland tumors compared with the IVIM

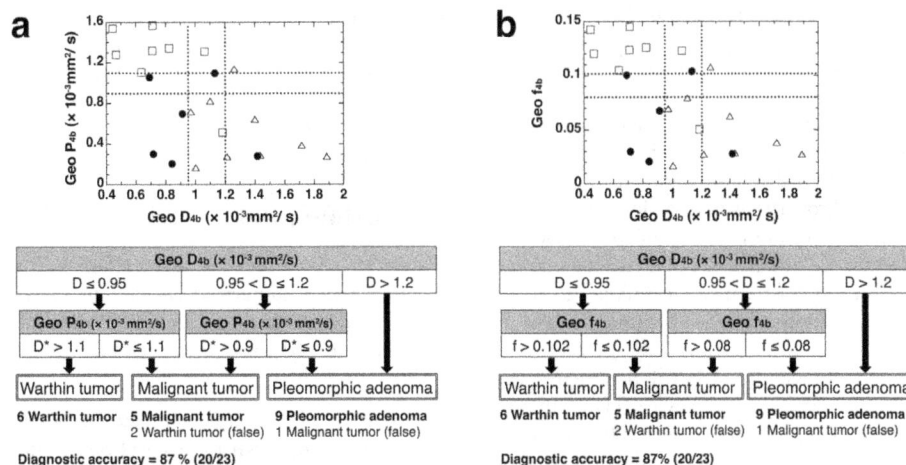

Figure 6. Stepwise differentiation between pleomorphic adenomas, Warthin tumors, and malignant salivary gland tumors using D, f, and D* or P values that were determined by geometric (Geo) method using 4 b-values (0, 100, 400, and 800 s/mm²). Plot graphs show 2D distributions of Geo P and GeoD (**a**), or Geo f and Geo D (**b**). Open triangles, open squares, and closed circles indicate pleomorphic adenomas, Warthin tumors, and malignant salivary gland tumors, respectively. Diagnostic accuracy was provided for the respective classifications at the bottom of each diagram.

parameters that were determined using 3 b-values, and 3 tumors were incorrectly diagnosed (Fig. 6, Tables S1 and S5).

Discussion

The present results showed that levels of IVIM parameters that were determined by geometric method were significantly different from those determined by least-squares method. However, differences in levels of D and f values were very small between the 2 methods, and diagnostic abilities of geometrically determined IVIM parameters were equivalent to those of IVIM parameters determined by least-squares method in differentiating between lymphomas and SCCs, and between different types of salivary gland tumors (pleomorphic adenomas, Warthin tumors, and malignant salivary gland tumors). Considering cumbersome procedures with least-squares method, the simple geometric IVIM assessment could be an alternative to least-squares method in the clinics.

By using a limited number of b-values, IVIM imaging has the advantage of achieving DW MR images that have better quality and of examining broader areas of head and neck region in a single scan compared with IVIM imaging using more b-values; for example, IVIM imaging using 11 b-values requires 1 min 53 s for obtaining 10 DW image slices per patient; on the other hand, IVIM imaging using 3 b-values requires 26 s for obtaining the same number of DW images per patient. The 3 b-value IVIM technique abandoned the idea of using low b-value (<100 s/mm^2) DWI for a fine analysis of the different vascular compartments with different sizes of vessels [14–16]. Perfusion contributes to signal decays in DWI in a biexponential mode for b-values in very low range (0–200 s/mm^2) [3,14,15]. Indeed, the significant differences in D, f, and D* values between the geometric and least-squares methods may be owing to the use of the upper limit of this b-value range (200 s/mm^2) for assessing the perfusion-related and pure molecular diffusion parameters separately in the present study. However, the use of 4 b-values did not improve the diagnostic abilities in differentiating the different tumor types. These results suggest that the use of 3 b-values (0, 200, and 800 s/mm^2) is clinically feasible for assessing perfusion and diffusion of head and neck tumors in routine examinations.

The present study showed that computation-induced invalidity occurred less frequently with the geometric method compared with the least-squares one. However, these results do not necessarily ensure the better performance of the implied IVIM technique. Basically, the least-squares method has better performance than the geometric method in terms of predicting lesional perfusion and diffusion characteristics with less artifacts and higher signal-to-noise ratios compared with the simplified technique. For example, some perfusion property may be lost during the simplified IVIM parameter calculation with limited numbers of small (<200 s/mm^2) b-values. Furthermore, many of the computation-induced errors with the least-squares technique could be avoided through the use of appropriate scan setting and/or b-values.

The 3 b-value geometric assessment of IVIM parameters was slightly less effective in the diagnosis of salivary gland tumors compared with a previous study, which achieved 100% accuracy [5]. The difference in study cohort may be a possible reason for the difference in diagnostic accuracy. In the present study, stepwise approaches using Fit D and Fit D* or Geo D and Geo P diagnosed 21 of the 23 salivary gland tumors correctly (91% accuracy). In both the combinations of Fit and Geo IVIM parameters, the 2 same Warthin tumors were incorrectly diagnosed as malignant or pleomorphic adenoma (Fig. 5). However, diagnostic accuracy with

stepwise approaches using Fit D and Fit f values was lower than that using Geo D and Geo f values (19/23 = 83% vs 21/23 = 91%), implying advantages of geometric method for the clinical use in diagnosing salivary gland tumors.

A major limitation of this study was the small patient cohort. Different or additional cutoff points might be required for effective discrimination in a larger patient cohort that is comprised of increased numbers of tumors within each tumor type and broader types of head and neck tumors. For example, the present study cohort of salivary gland tumor did not include oncocytoma, which histologically mimics Warthin tumor or malignant salivary gland tumors such as acinic cell carcinoma and clear cell carcinoma [17]. The retrospective nature, including the exclusion of patients with severe susceptibility artifacts from the study cohort, also limit the value of this study. In addition, the benefit of using the simplified IVIM technique may largely depends on disease types. Furthermore, the perfusion-related parameter Geo P defined by the simplified IVIM technique is fundamentally different from the conventional one (Fit D*). For example, in some cases where the diffusion property is important for diagnosing tumors/diseases, the simplified IVIM technique may be beneficial; however, in other cases where the perfusion assessment is essential for diagnosing tumors/disease, the simplified technique will provide perfusion parameters that are greatly different from those obtained with the least squares technique using multiple b-values and may thus mislead the diagnosis.

Another limitation of the present study may reside in ROI placement errors. We found that the interobserver and intraobserver errors were relatively small. However, there were substantial overlaps in IVIM parameters between different tumor types, and thus a small change in the value due to ROI placement may lead to a different result in tumor categorization based on IVIM imaging. In addition, distortion of tumor area due to susceptibility and motion artifacts may be critical factors against precise IVIM parameter measurements.

Conclusion

In this study, we showed that the IVIM parameters determined by geometric method were significantly different from those determined by conventional least-squares method. Nonetheless, both yielded very similar results in terms of differential diagnosis of major types of head and neck tumors, including SCCs, lymphomas, and salivary gland tumors. Therefore, we concluded that geometric determination of IVIM parameters could be an alternative to least-squares methods in the diagnosis of head and neck tumors.

Supporting Information

Table S1 All numerical data for Figs. 2, 5 and 6, and Tables 2, 3, 4 and 5 are summarized. Signal intensities relative to varying b-values (0–800 s/mm^2) are shown for each of benign (n = 26) and malignant (n = 61) head and neck tumors.

Table S2 IVIM parameters (Geo D, Geo f, Geo P, Fit D, Fit f, and Fit D*) are shown for each of benign (n = 26) and malignant (n = 61) head and neck tumors.

Table S3 IVIM parameters (Geo D, Geo f, Geo P, Fit D, Fit f, and Fit D*) determined 5 times (#1–#5) by 3 observers (1–3) are shown for 5 head and neck tumors (Cases 1–5).

Table S4   IVIM parameters (Geo D, Geo f, Geo P, Fit D, Fit f, and Fit D*) for lymphomas (n = 12), primary SCCs (n = 23), and SCC nodes (n = 11) are shown.

Table S5   IVIM parameters determined by least squares method (Fit D, Fit f, and Fit D*), geometrical method using 3 b-values (Geo D3b, Geo f3b, and Geo P3b), or geometrical method using 4 b-values (Geo D4b, Geo f4b, Geo P4b) for benign (n = 17) and malignant (n = 6) salivary gland tumors are shown.

Author Contributions

Conceived and designed the experiments: TN MS MS. Analyzed the data: MS MS SE IK YH. Wrote the paper: TN MS MS.

References

1. Nakamura T, Sumi M, Van Cauteren M (2009) Salivary gland tumors: Preoperative tissue characterization with apparent diffusion coefficient mapping. *In* Methods of Cancer Diagnosis, Therapy, and Prognosis. Hyat MA ed. Vol 7: NY, Springer: 255–269.
2. Le Bihan D (2003) Looking into the functional architecture of the brain with diffusion MRI. Nat Rev Neurosci 4: 469–480.
3. Le Bihan D, Breton E, Lallemand D, Aubin ML, Vignaud J, et al. (1988) Separation of diffusion and perfusion in intravoxel incoherent motion imaging. Radiology 168: 497–505.
4. Luciani A, Vignaud A, Cavet M, Tran Van Nhieu J, Mallat A, et al. (2008) Liver cirrhosis: Intravoxel incoherent motion MR imaging – Pilot study. Radiology 249: 891–899.
5. Sumi M, Van Cauteren M, Sumi T, Obara M, Ichikawa Y, Nakamura T (2012) Salivary gland tumors: use of intravoxel incoherent motion MR imaging for assessment of diffusion and perfusion for the differentiation of benign and malignant tumors. Radiology 263: 770–777.
6. Moteki T, Horikoshi H (2006) Evaluation of hepatic lesions and hepatic parenchyma using diffusion-weighted echo-planar MR with three values of gradient b-factor. J Magn Reson Imaging 24: 637–645.
7. Lewin M, Fartoux L, Vignaud A, Arrivé L, Menu Y, et al. (2011) The diffusion-weighted maging perfusion fraction f is a potential marker of sorafenib treatment in advanced hepatocellular carcinoma: a pilot study. Eur Radiol 21: 281–290.
8. Mazaheri Y, Vargas HA, Akin O, Goldman DA, Hricak H (2012) Reducing the influence of b-value selection on diffusion-weighted imaging of the prostate: Evaluation of a revised monoexponential model within a clinical setting. J Magn Reson Imaging 35: 660–668.
9. Sumi M, Nakamura T (2013) Head and neck tumors: Assessment of perfusion-related parameters and diffusion coefficients based on the intravoxel incoherent motion model. AJNR Am J Neuroradiol 34: 410–416.
10. Patel J, Sigmund EE, Rusinek H, Oei M, Babb JS, Taouli B (2010) Diagnosis of cirrhosis with intravoxel incoherent motion diffusion MRI and dynamic contrast-enhanced MRI alone and in combination: Preliminary experience. J Magn Reson Imaging 31: 589–600.
11. Lai V, Li X, Lee VHF, Lam KO, Chan Q, et al. (2013) Intravoxel incoherent motion MR imaging: Comparison of diffusion and perfusion characteristics between nasopharyngeal carcinoma and post-chemoradiation fibrosis. Eur Radiol 23: 2793–2801.
12. Sasaki M, Sumi M, Van Cauteren M, Obara M, Nakamura T (2013) Intravoxel incoherent motion imaging of masticatory muscles: A pilot study for the assessment of perfusion and diffusion during clenching. AJR AM J Roentgenol 201: 1101–1107.
13. Gao Q, Srinvasan G, Magin RL, Zhou XJ (2011) Anomalous diffusion measured by a twice-refocused spin echo pulse sequence: Analysis using fractional order calculus. J Magn Reson Imaging 33: 1177–1183.
14. Le Bihan D (2008) Intravoxel incoherent motion perfusion MR imaging: A wake-up call. Radiology 249: 748–752.
15. Koh DM, Collins DJ (2007) Diffusion-weighted MRI in the body: Applications and challenges in oncology. AJR Am J Roentgenol 188: 1622–1635.
16. Penner AH, Sprinkart AM, Kukuk GM, Gütgemann I, Gieseke J, et al. (2013) Intravoxel incoherent motion model-based liver lesion characterisation from three b-value diffusion-weighted MRI. Eur Radiol 23: 2773–2783.
17. Barnes L, Everson JW, Reichart P, Sidransky D (2005) Pathology and genetics of head and neck tumours. World Health Organization classification of tumors. IARC Press, Lyon, France.

25

Leukemic Stem Cell Frequency: A Strong Biomarker for Clinical Outcome in Acute Myeloid Leukemia

Monique Terwijn[1], Wendelien Zeijlemaker[1], Angèle Kelder[1], Arjo P. Rutten[1], Alexander N. Snel[1], Willemijn J. Scholten[1], Thomas Pabst[2], Gregor Verhoef[3], Bob Löwenberg[4], Sonja Zweegman[1], Gert J. Ossenkoppele[1], Gerrit J. Schuurhuis[1]*

1 Department of Hematology, VU University Medical Center, Amsterdam, The Netherlands, 2 Department of Medical Oncology, Inselspital, Bern University Hospital, University of Bern, Bern, Switzerland, 3 Department of Hematology, University Hospital Leuven, Leuven, Belgium, 4 Department of Hematology, Erasmus University Medical Center, Rotterdam, The Netherlands

Abstract

Introduction: Treatment failure in acute myeloid leukemia is probably caused by the presence of leukemia initiating cells, also referred to as leukemic stem cells, at diagnosis and their persistence after therapy. Specific identification of leukemia stem cells and their discrimination from normal hematopoietic stem cells would greatly contribute to risk stratification and could predict possible relapses.

Results: For identification of leukemic stem cells, we developed flow cytometric methods using leukemic stem cell associated markers and newly-defined (light scatter) aberrancies. The nature of the putative leukemic stem cells and normal hematopoietic stem cells, present in the same patient's bone marrow, was demonstrated in eight patients by the presence or absence of molecular aberrancies and/or leukemic engraftment in NOD-SCID IL-2Rγ-/- mice. At diagnosis (n = 88), the frequency of the thus defined neoplastic part of CD34+CD38- putative stem cell compartment had a strong prognostic impact, while the neoplastic parts of the CD34+CD38+ and CD34- putative stem cell compartments had no prognostic impact at all. After different courses of therapy, higher percentages of neoplastic CD34+CD38- cells in complete remission strongly correlated with shorter patient survival (n = 91). Moreover, combining neoplastic CD34+CD38- frequencies with frequencies of minimal residual disease cells (n = 91), which reflect the total neoplastic burden, revealed four patient groups with different survival.

Conclusion and Perspective: Discrimination between putative leukemia stem cells and normal hematopoietic stem cells in this large-scale study allowed to demonstrate the clinical importance of putative CD34+CD38- leukemia stem cells in AML. Moreover, it offers new opportunities for the development of therapies directed against leukemia stem cells, that would spare normal hematopoietic stem cells, and, moreover, enables *in vivo* and *ex vivo* screening for potential efficacy and toxicity of new therapies.

Editor: Kevin D Bunting, Emory University, United States of America

Funding: This work was supported by Netherlands Cancer Foundation KWF grant 2006-3695. The funders had no role in study design, data collection and analysis, decision to publish, or preparation of the manuscript.

Competing Interests: The authors have declared that no competing interests exist.

* Email: gj.schuurhuis@vumc.nl

Introduction

There is increasing evidence that the development of solid and hematological tumors depends on the presence of small populations of cells known as tumor-initiating cells or tumor stem cells [1]. The first proof of the stem cell concept came from studies by John Dick and colleagues in acute myeloid leukemia (AML) [2,3]. In AML, these cells are referred to as leukemia-initiating cells or leukemic stem cells (LSCs) [4]. Since the first studies on LSCs, cell compartments defined by immunophenotype (CD34/CD38 expression) and function (side population, SP, and aldehyde dehydrogenase [ALDH] activity) have been reported to contain LSCs [5–9]. The first LSC compartment that was described had

the CD34+CD38- immunophenotype [2,3]. Although immune reactivity of the CD38 antibody used in earlier studies likely caused the lack of engraftment of CD38+ cells [10], the CD34+CD38- compartment still seemed to be the most robust compartment in CD34-positive (CD34+) patients, since it was found to be the predominant compartment containing leukemia-initiating cells in less immunocompromised mouse models [3]. On the other hand, in more severely immune-compromised mouse models, CD34+CD38+ and CD34-negative compartments were also found to contain leukemia initiating cells [5,7–9,11].

In bone marrow (BM) of AML patients, leukemic and normal cells are present within one compartment. The CD34+CD38- compartment in particular, was shown to contain both CD34+

CD38- LSCs and normal hematopoietic stem cells (HSCs) [10,12]. Previous papers reported only on the role of the size of the total CD34+CD38-stem cell compartment and only at diagnosis [13–17]. However, for proper identification of LSCs, with the aim to establish the prognostic impact of their frequencies at diagnosis and to follow their fate during and after therapy, it is important to identify distinguishing features between LSCs and HSCs. We previously have found that in a substantial number of AML cases, CD34+CD38- LSCs are characterized by the expression of C-type lectin-like molecule-1 (CLL-1) and aberrant expression of several lineage markers [18,19]. Since these markers are absent on HSCs in regenerating BM after chemotherapy [18,19], for the current study we chose to use these markers to distinguish between LSCs and HSCs in both diagnosis and post-diagnosis samples. Other LSC markers have also been described for AML diagnosis (reviewed in ref [20]), but since little is known about their behavior during and after therapy, their suitability for LSC tracking remains to be established. However, despite the usefulness of CLL-1 and lineage markers, in at least 25% of the AML patients, aberrant marker expression on CD34+/CD38- cells is absent or too weak, and therefore there is a need to identify other discriminative parameters [6,19]. In the first part of this paper, we will describe such additional parameters for CD34+CD38- compartment. Now being able to discriminate neoplastic from normal CD34+CD38- cells, in the second part we will focus on the prognostic role of the CD34+CD38- stem cell compartment. This will be compared with the other CD34/CD38 defined compartments.

Moreover, another important aspect of cancer stem cells is their putative therapy resistance [21], with a subsequent ability to cause re-growth. The present study is the first to address the resistance to therapy by showing the prognostic impact of AML stem cells post-therapy in a large patient group. The results demonstrate that defining residual LSCs post-therapy has important prognostic impact. Moreover, we show that it adds important prognostic impact to a well-established immunophenotypical MRD approach, known to identify and quantify the bulk of neoplastic cells.

Patients, Material and Methods

More detailed information can be found in the supporting text (Text S1).

Patient treatment and sampling

Patients between 18 and 60 years of age with AML, except those with FAB M3 and previously untreated RAEB and RAEB-t patients (with IPSS ≥ 1.5), were included in this study. Detailed information regarding treatment can be found at http://www.hovon.nl. The HOVON/SAKK 42a and 92 studies were reviewed and approved by an institutional review board (METc) of the Erasmus MC Rotterdam for the total study (number 2000-220 for Hovon 42a) and 2008/216 for Hovon 92). In addition, the VU Amsterdam review board approved both studies with METc number 2001/50 (LUV) and 2008/292 (LUV), respectively. Patients provided their written informed consent to participate in this study. In 250 CD34-positive patients, we used a specific gating strategy to identify normal and neoplastic cells in the CD34+CD38-, CD34+CD38+ and the CD34- compartment at diagnosis. Patient details are in Table S1 (patient groups 1 and 2). Additionally, in the last part of the results, an extra patient group (n = 23) was included (details are in Table S1, patient group 3) to study combination of LSC and minimal residual disease (MRD) data after second cycle of therapy.

Flow cytometry

Methods. LSC characterisation at diagnosis and LSC monitoring during follow up was performed on fresh patient samples. Purified white blood cells were obtained from BM or PB using lysing solution (Pharm lyse, Becton Dickinson, BD, San Jose, CA, U.S.A.) to eradicate red blood cells. After washing with PBS containing 0.1% human serum albumin (HSA), cells were re-suspended in PBS containing 0.1% HSA, incubated with monoclonal antibody combinations (mAbs) for 15 minutes at room temperature and washed with PBS containing 0.1% HSA. Details on antibodies (sources, clones, fluorochromes) are written in the supporting text (Text S1). Samples were analysed using a 4-color approach on a FACSCalibur from Becton Dickinson (BD, San Jose, CA, USA) using CellQuest and Infinicyte software. Cell sorting was performed using FACSAria (BD) with FACSDiva analysis software. More details are in the supporting text (Text S1).

Marker selection for the CD34+CD38- LSC. In a previous paper [19], we have shown that particular lineage markers, i.e. CD2, CD7, CD11b, CD19, CD22, CD56, can be positive on CD34+CD38- LSC, while always negative on CD34+CD38- HSC. This is true for CLL-1 too [18]. All markers have been shown to be negative on HSCs in normal bone marrow, but also on normal stem cells present at diagnosis and at follow up [18,19]. In addition, the absence of CD13, CD33 and HLA-DR was considered aberrant, since these markers are always expressed on normal HSCs [19,22]. For each new AML case one or more of these markers may be aberrantly expressed; in a next case this may be completely different. Therefore, for each new AML case, the choice for a marker was based on screening for presence (>10% positivity) of all markers. Even more heterogeneity was seen, since part of the CD34+CD38- population might be negative for these markers, and all or not covered by another marker.

Marker selection for the more mature CD34+CD38+ and CD34- populations. For CD34+CD38+ and CD34- leukemic cells, identification had to be done using lineage markers: it is only lineage markers that are absent (or present at very low frequencies) on these more mature populations [23,24]. This property offers the basis for detection of residual leukemic cells (all leukemic cells) in MRD approaches. CLL-1, however, cannot be used as a neoplastic marker on CD34+CD38+ and CD34- cells since it is present on part of these populations in normal bone marrow [25]. For LSC identification/quantification at diagnosis and follow up, only AML samples were used that, at diagnosis, showed >1% CD34 expression relative to the total WBC count. This was done because we have previously shown that the CD34+ population in AML with <1% CD34 is of normal origin [26]. CD34 negative AML samples, together with normal bone marrow, were used as a control for FSC/SSC values in HSC (see results section I.A). For details on the gating strategy to define the CD34+CD38- compartment, see Figure 1, part I. The details how to define scatter characteristics of marker positive and marker negative populations are outlined under Results. Stem cell numbers (LSC and HSC) were defined as a percentage of total white blood cells (WBC).

Engrafting studies

Animal experiments were performed after approval of the animal ethical committee of the VU University, Amsterdam, The Netherlands under DEC number: KNO06-02. NOD/SCID IL-2Rγ -/- mice were obtained from the Jackson laboratory (Bar Harbor, ME, USA). At the age of 8-10 weeks, the mice were irradiated sub-lethally with a dose of 350 cGy, 24 hours prior to transplantation of the human AML cells. Details of irradiation, anesthesia, intravenous and intra-femoral injection are outlined in

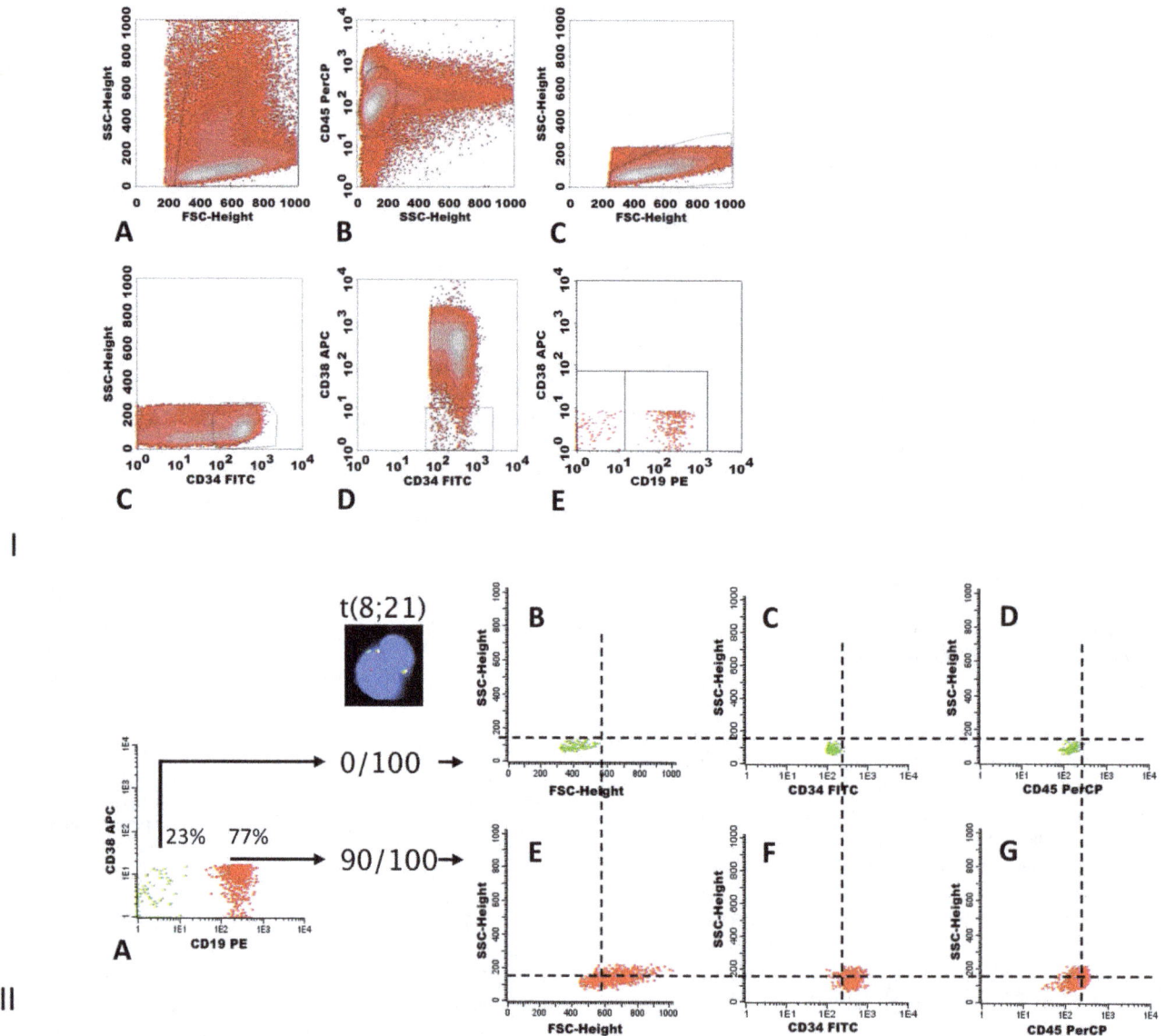

Figure 1. Gating strategy for the CD34+CD38- compartment and identification of pLSCs and HSCs in this compartment. I. Gating of CD34+CD38- AML cells. Cells were labeled with antibody-fluorochrome combinations as described in Patients, Materials and Methods. Remaining erythrocytes, debris and dead cells are largely excluded in an FSC/SSC plot (A). CD45^{dim}/SSC^{dim} blast cells (B) were gated to homogeneity in FSC/SSC plot (C). CD34 positive cells are gated (D) and the CD38- stem cells are gated within this fraction (E). The CD38-negative fraction in D may contain two stem cell populations differing in CD34 expression (details in text). F. Within the CD34+CD38- gate, CD38 is plotted against an aberrant marker (in this case CD19) to indicate presence of putative LSCs (pLSCs) and HSCs. **II. Identification of pLSCs and HSCs.** This patient (nr 317) was diagnosed with t(8;21). Primary gating was as in I. Sorted CD34+CD38-/CD19+ cells (A, in red) were t(8;21) positive; sorted CD34+CD38-/CD19- cells (A, in green) were t(8;21) negative. These two populations were backgated in FSC/SSC (B,E), CD34/SSC (C,F) and CD45/SSC (D,G) plots. The CD19- cells are shown in the upper panels and the CD19+ cells in the lower panels. Dotted vertical lines (B–D) show that normal CD19- cells are FSC^{low} (B), CD34^{low} (C) and slightly lower in CD45 (D), compared to CD19+ cells (E–G). The dotted horizontal line shows that SSC of the normal stem cells (in green) was slightly lower than that of neoplastic stem cells (in red). FISH data are from an example published previously [19]. Similar results were found in an additional series of 7 patients (Tables 1 and 2). FSC and SSC of CD19+ pLSC were factor 1.71 and 1.77 higher than lymphocyte present in the same samples. FSC and SSC of the CD19 negative cells were only 1.08 and 1.20 times lower than lymphocytes.

the supporting text (Text S1) under "Patients". Human leukemic and multi-lineage engraftment was determined based on positivity for CD45-PercP, the presence/absence of CD19-positive B-cells, CD13 and/or CD33-positive cells and, in three cases, by the presence/absence of aberrant marker expression.

Engraftment was defined as a clear clustered population in CD45 expression in a minimum of 200,000 acquired mice marrow cells. The minimum percentage of human engraftment that was detected was 0.1%, which shows up as a cluster of 200 cells on the scatterplot. Human leukemic engraftment was determined based on positivity for CD45-PercP, the absence of CD19-positive B cells and the presence of CD13 and/or CD33 positive cells: when CD13 was aberrantly absent on the AML that was injected, CD33 was used and when CD33 was absent, CD13 was used. Human multi-lineage engraftment was identified when CD45 positive cells consisted of both CD19 positive B-cells and myeloid cells with both CD13 and CD33 present (identified as monocytes and/or

Table 1. Molecular status of diagnosis total AML and sorted stem cell fractions from the same BM.

Patient nr	Molecular status of AML blasts[§]	Aberrant marker expressed onCD34+CD38- cells[*]	CD34+CD38- aberrant marker negative		CD34+CD38- aberrant marker positive	
			CD34+CD38- aberrant marker-	% aberrant marker- of CD34+CD38-[§]	CD34+CD38- aberrant marker+	% aberrant marker+ of CD34+CD38-
317[¥]	t(8;21) pos	CD19	t(8;21) neg	23	t(8;21) pos	77
808	50% FLT3-ITD[#]	CD33-	wt	67	45% ITD[#]	33
	NPM1 mut	CD33-	wt	67	NPM1 mut	33
945	NPM1 mut	CLL-1	wt	47	NPM1 mut	53
951	42% FLT3-ITD	CLL-1	wt	46	60% ITD	54
966	43% FLT3-ITD	CD7	wt	41	41% ITD	59
1263	60% FLT3-ITD	CD33-	wt	2.5	80% ITD	97.5
575	50% FLT3-ITD	CD33-	wt	58	50% ITD	42
	NPM1 mut	CD33-	wt	58	NPM1 mut	42
670	NPM1 mut	CLL-1	wt	74	NPM1 mut	26

[§]signal originating from the bulk of the leukemic blasts has been used for reference. Sorted lymphocytes from the same BM showed no molecular aberrancies.
[*]Aberrant markers with the highest coverage of the CD34+CD38- compartment were used for sorting HSC (aberrant marker negative) and pLSC (aberrant marker positive).
[¥]Shown in Figure 1.
[#]For FLT3-ITD+ cases, the percentage of ITD of the total signal is indicated.
[§]Median frequency of HSCs (46.5% of CD34+CD38- compartment) was higher than the median in a larger group of cases (median 18%), since cases in this table had to be selected on clear availability of both HSCs and pLSCs.
Abbreviations: wt, wild type: no FLT3-ITD or NPM1 peak present; mut: mutation of NPM1 (not quantitative), neg: negative, pos: positive, BM: bone marrow.

granulocytes in a FSC/SSC plot), and with absence of aberrant markers.

FISH, FLT3-ITD and NPM1 analysis

For the FISH analysis, cytospins were prepared with FACS-sorted cells. LSI AML1/ETO dual color for t(8;21) probe (Vysis, Abbott molecular, Illinois, U.S.A.) was applied to the denatured cells and incubated as previously described [17]. Genomic DNA from sorted cell populations was analyzed for the presence of an FLT3-ITD as described before [27]. Mutations in NPM1 exon 12 were analyzed by PCR using genomic DNA that had been isolated from sorted cell fractions (see Text S1).

Survival analysis

Statistical analysis of the stem cell data at follow-up was carried out using the SPSS 20.0 software program. The supplement provides details regarding the definition of overall survival (OS), event-free survival (EFS), relapse-free survival (RFS), Kaplan-Meier analyses, and Cox regression analyses for both univariate and multivariate analyses. P-values below 0.05 were considered significant.

Results

In the absence of formal proof of leukemia initiating ability in the stem cell compartments of most of the samples studied, the different stem cell compartments are referred to as *putative* LSCs (abbreviated as pLSC).

Since the aim of the study was to define the prognostic impact of the neoplastic CD34+CD38- compartment, and to compare with the neoplastic CD34+CD38+ and CD34 negative compartments, first, properties will be described that allow to discriminate between the neoplastic and the normal compartment within the CD34+CD38- compartment (Section I.A–D) and the CD34+CD38+ and the CD34- compartments (Section I.E). Proof of the

resulting concept was obtained using either molecular biological and/or murine engraftment experiments.

In Section II. the findings were used to assess the prognostic impact of the number of pLSCs at diagnosis and post-therapy for the CD34+CD38- compartment (II.A,B) and the CD34+CD38+ and CD34- compartment (II.C,D). Finally, the prognostic impact of the combination of follow up CD34+CD38- pLSC frequency, with MRD data will be described (II.E).

I. Discrimination between leukemic and normal stem cell compartments

A. CD34+CD38-: discrimination of pLSCs and HSCs can be made based on aberrant marker expression and scatter properties. We have previously shown that the expression of aberrant markers on CD34+CD38- cells indicates the leukemic nature of stem cells [18,19]. Figure 1.II illustrates the difference between CD34+CD38- pLSCs and HSCs based on aberrant marker expression and molecular aberrancies [in this example, t(8;21)]. In addition to Figure 1, Table 1 shows 7 other patients with aberrant marker positive cells, all with molecular aberrancies indicating that these are in fact neoplastic cells. The figure also shows that marker-positive pLSCs, compared to HSCs, are further characterized by a tight clustered cell population with higher forward scatter (FSC, reflecting cell size) and higher sideward scatter (SSC, reflecting granularity). This phenomenon was found in the other patients of Table 1 too (shown in Table 2). In Table 2, FSC and SSC of lymphocytes were used as internal controls to define the FSC/SSC position of pLSC and HSC. pLSC and HSC may also differ in CD34 and CD45 expression (in the case of Figure 1, CD34 expression of pLSC was higher than HSC). Such differences were not consistent but helped to define clusters of cells especially in cases with very low numbers of cells and/or small differences in aberrant marker expression and/or FSC/SSC.

Table 2. FSC/SSC position relative to lymphocytes.

Patient nr	Aberrant marker negative CD34+CD38-	Aberrant marker positive CD34+CD38-
	FSC/SSC position*	FSC/SSC position*
317[¥]	1.08/1.20	1.71/1.77
808	1.27/1.17	1.57/1.80
945	1.38/1.52	1.97/3.25
951	0.93/0.77	1.46/1.39
966	1.15/1.0	1.53/1.99
1263	1.04/1.22	1.39/2.08
575	1.06/1.02	1.34/1.77
670	1.21/1.07	1.52/1.73

[¥]Shown in Figure 1.
* FSC/SSC values are based on the position of cells in FSC/SSC relative to the
FSC/SSC position of normal lymphocytes in the same BM sample.
The molecular status of the sorted cell fractions is summarized in Table 1.

Table S2 shows the FSC/SSC position relative to lymphocytes of CD34+CD38- HSCs present in normal BM, as well as CD34+CD38- present in CD34 negative AML, which have previously been shown to be normal [26]. FSC/SSC of HSCs present in these controls are all lower than pLSC present in CD34+ AML (Table S2). Moreover, HSC present in CD34+ AML also have low FSC/SSC and altogether there is not even overlap in FSC/SSC between pLSC in CD34+ AML and the HSCs present in these three bone marrow sources. This allows accurate definition of the nature of a population especially in those cases with only a single population present.

B. CD34+CD38-: is there a role of FSC/SSC to define pLSC and HSC in aberrant marker-negative part of CD34+CD38- compartment?. Aberrant markers may cover only part of neoplastic CD34+CD38- cells [19]. We therefore investigated whether scatter differences may help to discriminate pLSCs from HSCs in aberrant marker-negative cells. This was indeed seen as illustrated for patient sample 456 in Figure 2.I. The investigation of expression of only aberrant markers would have led to an over-estimation of HSC numbers and an under-estimation of pLSC numbers. Figure 2.II provides more examples.

In approximately 25% of AML cases, there is no clear aberrant marker expression in the CD34+CD38- compartment, and in even more cases, marker expression is weak and overlaps with the marker negative cells [19]. In order to nevertheless discriminate between pLSCs and HSCs, we investigated whether scatter might replace marker expression in this respect. Figure 3 (A–D) shows that, even without clear aberrant marker expression (CD19 covers only a very low frequency CD34+CD38- population), differences in scatter can be used. Since, in this particular AML case, aberrant expression of CD7 was found (Figure 3 E–F), the validity of the scatter approach could be demonstrated (compare Figure 3 E–F with D). This shows that the scatter approach allows to discriminate pLSC and HSC in the absence of aberrant markers.

C. CD34+CD38-: discrimination between HSCs and pLSCs in a large patient group using marker and scatter differences. In cases with differences seen in FSC and SSC between pLSC and HSC, pLSC always had higher FSC/SSC than HSC. However, at this point it should be emphasized that differences in scatter were found in part of the patients. In 250 diagnosis AML cases studied, the combination of marker expression and FSC/SSC differences allowed accurate identification of both pLSCs and HSCs in 117/250 cases (47%), (outlined in

detail in Table S3 and summarized in Table S4. For reasons mentioned earlier, differences in expression of CD34 and CD45 were only used for fine-tuning. As might be expected, the pLSC compartment made up the majority of the total CD34+CD38- compartment (median of 82%, ranging from 0%–100%). Apart from these 117 cases, there was an extra group of 102 patients (41%) with only marker expression available, while 31 patients (12%) had no marker and scatter properties usable for pLSC detection (summarized in Table S4).

D. CD34+CD38-: multilineage and leukemic engraftment of CD34+CD38- HSCs and CD34+CD38- pLSCs in NOD/SCID IL-2R $\gamma^{-/-}$ mice. To provide further proof of principle for the strategy based on marker expression, secondary gating and molecular profiles, murine engraftment experiments were performed. HSCs were sorted by marker negativity, and clustering as FSC/SSC^{low}, and/or distinct CD34/CD45 clustering, injected intrafemorally and evaluated for engraftment. In 5/6 cases, multilineage engraftment was found with no signs of leukemia (Figure 4, Table S5). In accordance with our *in vitro* gating strategy, AML engraftment with low cell numbers was observed in 2/6 cases for CD34+CD38- marker-positive samples and in 1/6 cases for the CD34+CD38- marker-negative cells, the latter being identified as neoplastic based on high FSC and aberrant CD34 expression (see legends of Table S5).

E. CD34+CD38+ and CD34-: discrimination between normal and leukemic CD34+CD38+ and CD34- cells and their leukemic engraftment in NOD/SCID IL-2R $\gamma^{-/-}$ mice. Although emphasis in this paper is on the CD34+CD38- compartment, results described later for prognosis of CD34+CD38- pLSC will be compared with the other CD34/CD38 defined compartments. To enable such, neoplastic CD34+CD38+ and CD34- cells were identified by aberrant expression of markers used to define so-called Leukemia Associated (Immuno) Phenotypes established at diagnosis and used by others and us [23,24] for detection of minimal residual disease. Cells were sorted as described in Text S1. In agreement with recent reports, these cell compartments also had leukemia initiating potency since AML engraftment was found in 4/6 cases for the CD34+CD38+ compartment and in 2/6 cases using CD34- compartments (referred to in the legends of Table S5). In all but one case, this was accomplished with high cell numbers (100,000-1,000,000).

I

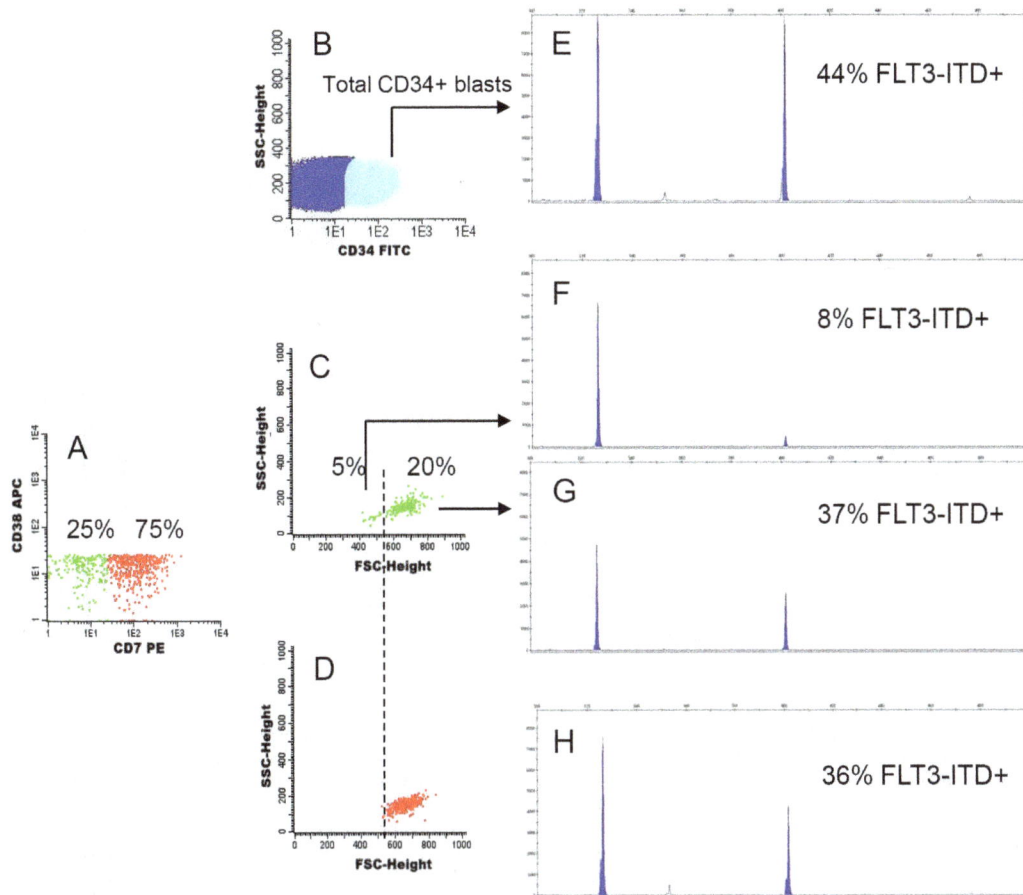

II

Patient nr	Aberrantly expressed marker	FLT-3 ITD (% of total) in cell fraction [#]					
		CD34+	Lymphocytes	CD34+CD38-/ aberrant marker+	CD34+CD38-/ aberrant marker-		
						FSC/SSC[low] [§]	FSC/SSC[high] [§]
598	CLL-1	54	0	50		0	38
1034	CLL-1	20	0	37		0	17
423	CLL-1	45	0	21		6	45
456*	CD7	44	0	36		8	37

Figure 2. Marker-negative cells may contain leukemic cells defined by aberrant scatter. I. Gating/sorting strategy and molecular analysis for patient 456. CD34+ CD38- cells (patient 456, figure 2) were gated as in figure 1. CD34+CD38- cells were either CD7-negative (green in A and C, 25% of CD34+CD38-) or CD7 positive (red in A and D, 75% of CD34+CD38-). CD7+ cells were FSC/SSC[high] (D) and of neoplastic origin (H). CD7-negative cells were further subdivided into FSC/SSC[low] (left of the broken line in C), and FSC/SSC[high] (right of the broken line in C). The CD7-negative, but FSC/SSC[high], cells were neoplastic (G), while the CD7-negative FSC/SSC[low] cells were essentially normal (F). CD34+ cells was the positive control (E). **II. Molecular analysis of stem cell subpopulations in four patients.** Sorting and analysis was done as in figure 2.I A for 3 additional patients. [#] FLT3-ITD (% of total signal: FLT3-ITD + wt) determined in cell populations sorted from CD34+ AML patients. * shown in figure 2.I A. [§] FSC/SSC[low] and FSC/SSC[high] defined as outlined in Table 2.

II. Prognostic role of putative stem cell compartments

To assess the clinical impact of our findings, we assessed the prognostic value of the size the three individual LSC compartments both at diagnosis and, where applicable, especially at clinical follow-up.

A. CD34+CD38- at diagnosis. To assess prognostic impact, different cut-off values were established to define patients with high pLSC count (above the cut-off level: referred to as pLSC+) and patients with low pLSC count (below the cut-off level: pLSC-). Patients who later turned out not to have achieved complete remission (non-CR patients) had median 6-fold higher pLSC count than patients who had achieved CR (see legends of Figure 5). Moreover, the CR patient group could be divided into two groups with significantly different prognoses at multiple cut-off points ranging from 0.002% to 1% (Figure 5A and Table S6A). Figure 5B shows that further splitting up the CR group resulted in the definition of three groups with large differences in relapse-free survival (RFS). The latter result was also found upon inclusion of non-CR patients (not shown) and replacement of RFS by EFS (Figure 5C). Multivariate analysis showed pLSC frequency to be an independent prognostic factor (Figure 5, legends).

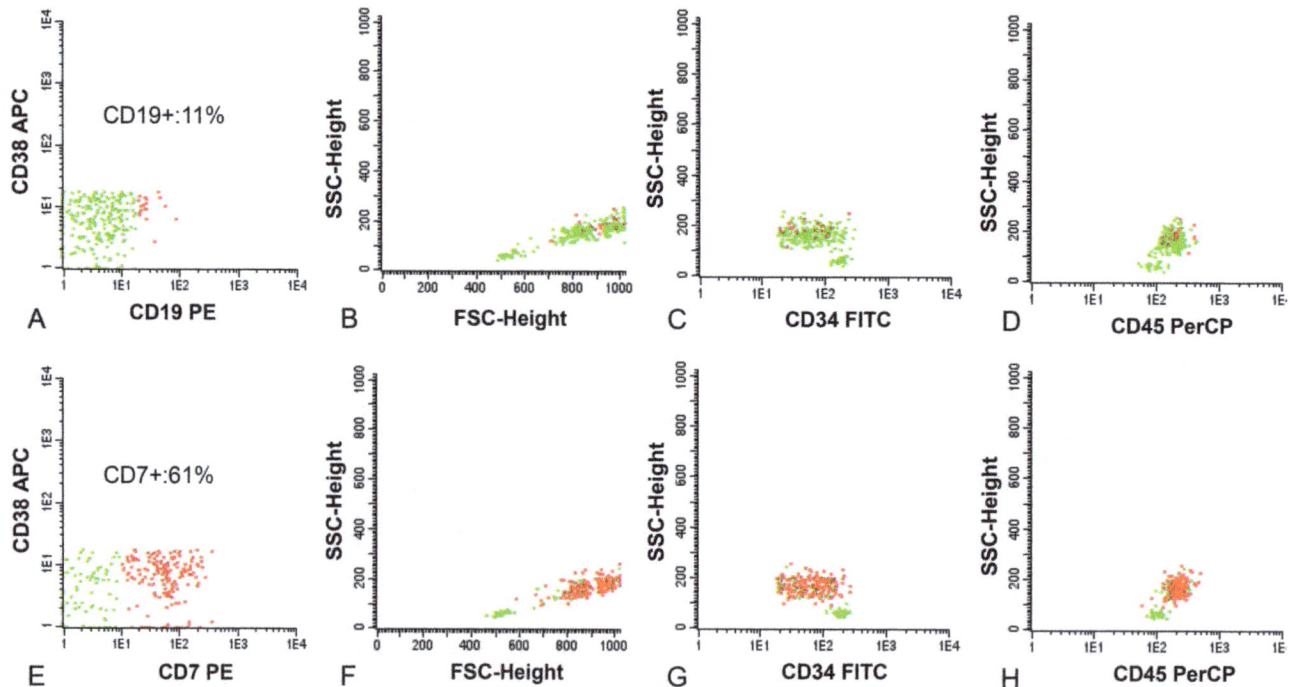

Figure 3. Marker negative pLSCs co-exist with marker positive pLSCs and are identified by scatter and CD34/CD45 expression patterns. CD34+ CD38- cells (patient 372) were identified as described in figure 1.I and gated for sub-compartments as described for figure 2.I. In the stem cell compartment of this AML case, only 11% could be identified as CD19+ (A). When back-gated in FSC/SSC (similar as performed in Figures 1 and 2), two different populations were identified based on the position in FSC/SSC: the small CD19+ fraction (events in red in A–D) is characterized by FSC/SSC^{high} (B), low CD34 expression (C) and high CD45 expression (D). CD19 negative cells (events in green in A–D), apart from a small FSC/SSC^{low}/CD34^{high}/CD45^{low} population of putative HSCs (A–D), contained a large population of cells that, similar to the CD19+ population in A–D, were FSC/SSC^{high} (B), CD34^{low} (C), and CD45^{high} (D). Apart from CD19, CD7 was an aberrant marker: 61% of the cells was CD7+ (E). Upon backgating, CD7+ cells (events in red in E–H), similar to CD19+ cells, were all FSC/SSC^{high} (F) CD34^{low} (G) and CD45^{high} (H). In contrast to CD19, CD7 negative cells (events in green in E–H) now completely consisted of a small FSC/SSC^{low} (F), CD34^{high}(G), CD45^{low} (H) fraction. CD7 thus covered the whole neoplastic CD34+CD38- population and shows perfect discrimination between HSC and pLSC. CD19 expression in the absence of both CD7 expression and other scatter and CD34/CD45 expression parameters would have under-estimated the pLSC in the CD34+CD38- compartment by a factor 5.5 (61%/11%), while the HSCs would have been over-estimated by a factor 2.3 (89%/39%). In this case CD7 was a good marker to compare with the poor CD19 marker; it can be seen, however, that in the absence of CD7 expression, but with the scatter and CD34/CD45 aberrancies present, these would have enabled a complete discrimination between putative HSC and LSC compartments. This patient was identified as NPM1-positieve and FLT3-ITD positive. Other molecular aberrancies were not detected.

B. CD34+CD38- during follow-up in CR. The gating approach shown in Figure 1 was used to follow the fate of pLSCs over time using sequential sampling (examples in Figure S1). Cox regression analysis showed a strong significant inverse correlation between the pLSC percentage after all therapy cycles and RFS and OS (for details, see legends to Table S7). Kaplan-Meier analyses showed markedly improved RFS and OS in pLSC- patients compared with pLSC+ patients (example in Figure 6, A–C), which applies for a large range of cut-off values (Table S7). Multivariate analyses with cut-off values showed that pLSC frequency after the first and second treatment cycles was an independent prognostic factor for RFS and OS (example with 0.0003% and 0.0001% shown in Table S8).

C. CD34+CD38+ and CD34- at diagnosis and at follow up. The CD34+CD38+ and CD34- compartments have been shown to contain leukemia initiating cells [5,11] (also in this paper). In order to assess whether these were clinically important, when present together with the leukemia initiating CD34+CD38- compartment, we assessed their prognostic impact.

At diagnosis, neoplastic CD34+CD38+ and CD34- blast cells were identified as described under I.B. For CD34+CD38+, there was no single cut-off value (tested in the range 2%–60%) that resulted in discrimination of two patient groups with different RFS

(Figure 5D; Table S6B), even when non-CR patients were included in the latter (data not shown). Although only borderline significant, in contrast to CD34+CD38-, the neoplastic CD34+ CD38+ compartment was even smaller in non-CR patients than in CR patients (10.8% of WBC versus 23.7% of WBC; p = 0.06). Similar results were obtained for the CD34- compartment with cut-off points ranging from 0.1%–30% (Figure 5E; Table S6C), with the neoplastic compartment size, similar to CD34+CD38+, being even smaller (albeit non-significantly) in non-CR patients than in CR patients (0.87% of WBC versus 2.41% of WBC, p = 0.48).

At follow up, the neoplastic component of the CD34+CD38+ and CD34- compartment represented a considerable portion of the total neoplastic blast compartment. This reflects the total leukemic burden, or MRD, which, in turn, has previously been shown by many authors, including ourselves, to have prognostic impact (see also next paragraph) [23,24].

D. Post-diagnosis prognostic impact of CD34+CD38- LSC combined with MRD. The burden of leukemic stem cells after chemotherapy does not always reflect the total leukemic burden (known as MRD). It can thus be argued that the combination of pLSC frequency and MRD frequency may improve prognostic information at follow up. Because this combination would divide

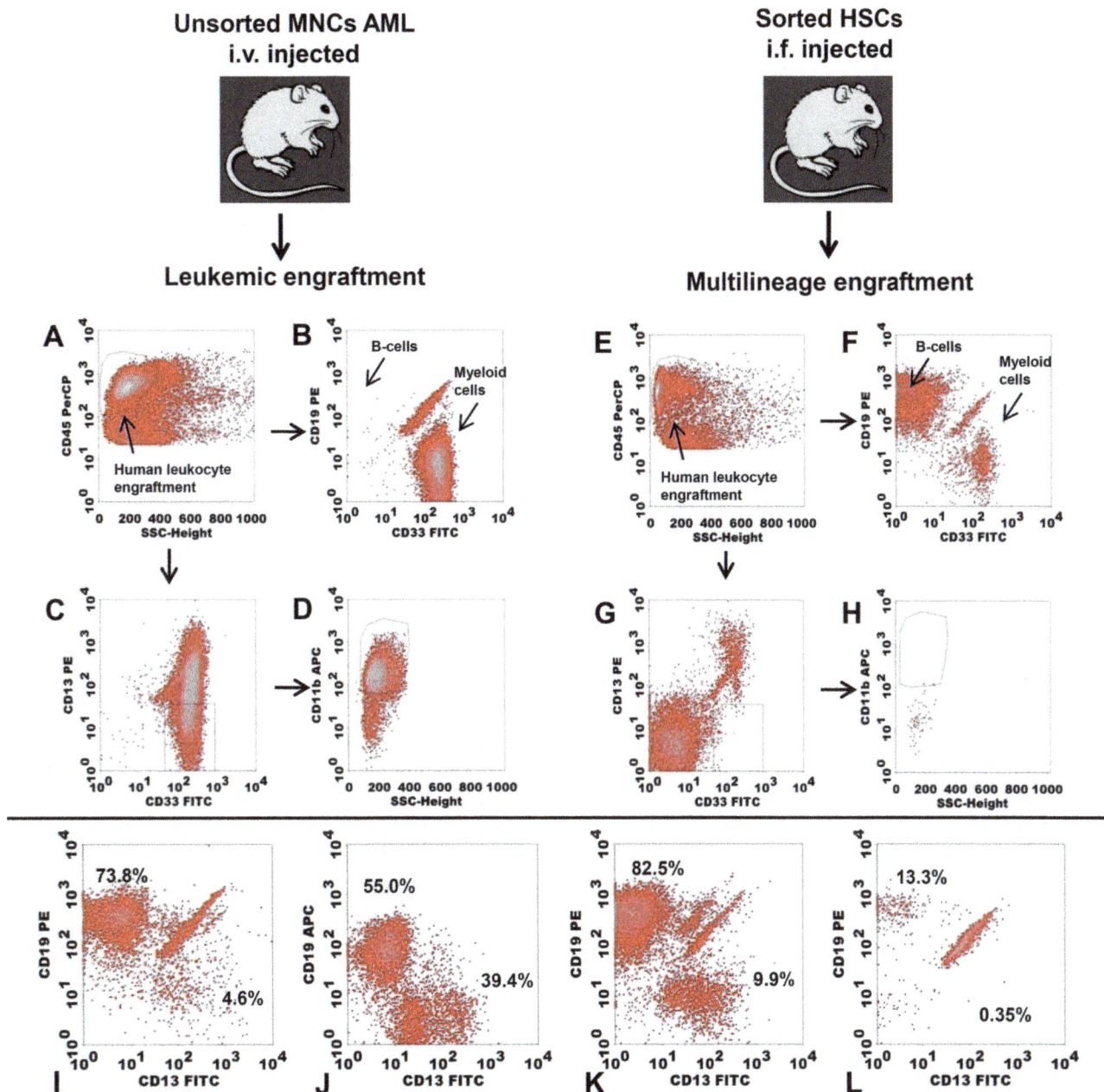

Figure 4. Multilineage engraftment of CD34/CD38 and scatter-defined putative HSCs. Unsorted mononuclear cells (MNCs) were injected intravenously and resulted in leukemic engraftment: cells were CD45+ (A) and of myeloid origin (B). In this case, the myeloid cells were positive for the diagnosis of leukemia-associated phenotype (LAP): partly CD33+CD13- (C) and CD11b+ (D). Sorted putative HSCs were injected intrafemorally (details, see Table S5). Engrafted CD45+ cells (E), contained both B-cells and myeloid cells (F), and lacked LAP (G,H). Multilineage engraftment of the sorted subpopulations was seen for patient 598 (I), 661 (J), 423 (K), and 928 (L). B-cells and myeloid cells (percentage of CD45+ cells) are in the upper left and lower right corners of the plots, respectively. The AML cells of patients 598 (I) and 661 (J) had an aberrant phenotype at diagnosis that was present in the neoplastic engrafted cells, but absent in the normal cells (not shown).

the total patient group in four relatively small sub-groups defined by both a pLSC cut-off (Figure 6, Table 3) and a fixed MRD cut-off of 0.1 [24]), we increased the size of the present patient remission group by including 23 similarly treated young adults in remission (<65 years) (details in Table S1 "Patients 3"). In the total group (n = 91) pLSC frequency again had strong prognostic impact over a range of cut-off points (from 0 in 10^6 WBC up to 10 in 10^6 WBC. As an example, the cut-off point of 0.0001% is shown in Figure 7A. For MRD, the cut-off point of 0.1% had the

expected prognostic impact (Figure 7B) [24]. When combining MRD and pLSC in Figure 7C, four groups were identified. The main conclusions from this figure are: 1) within the total MRD-group (n = 64), pLSC+ patients (n = 31) have significantly poorer prognosis than pLSC- patients (n = 33; p = 0.01); 2) within the pLSC+ group, MRD- patients, although having a relatively poor prognosis, may do better than MRD+ patients (p = 0.04); the pLSC-/MRD- group had relatively good prognosis, while the pLSC+/MRD+ group had very poor prognosis.

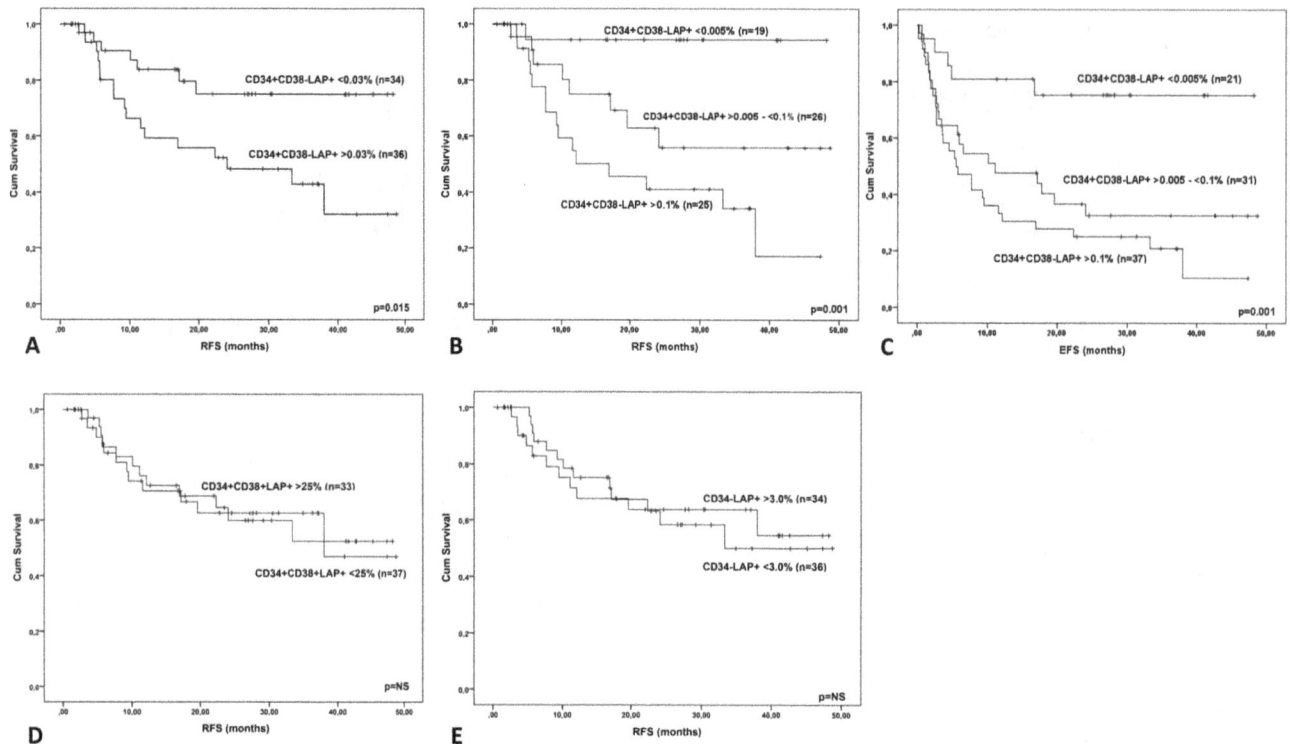

Figure 5. Prognostic value of frequencies of pLSC compartments at diagnosis. This figure shows the Kaplan-Meier analyses at diagnosis for the three compartments putatively containing pLSCs: CD34+CD38- (A,B,C), CD34+CD38+ (D) and CD34- (E). Of the 117 patients shown in Table S3, for Figures 5 and 6, 88 patients were chosen who had at least one follow-up time point. Of these, 70 entered Complete Remission, of whom 53 after the first course, 13 after the second course and 4 at later stages. Eighteen never reached CR. The size (median values) of the CD34+CD38- compartment at diagnosis was significantly (six-fold) higher in patients who did not enter CR (n = 18) compared with patients who did (n = 70): 0.225% of WBC versus 0.036% of WBC (p = 0.041). For CD34+CD38+ and CD34-, there were no significant differences (see text). Cut-off levels were defined to divide the total population into high stem cell frequencies (above cut-off) and low stem cell frequencies (below cut-off). A particular cut-off value was chosen (A, D, E) to ensure approximately equally numbers of patients in the resulting high and low stem cell frequency compartments. Results for other cut-offs for the three pLSC compartments are in Table S6. A–C: CD34+CD38-; D: CD34+CD38+; E: CD34-. A. RFS in remission patients (n = 70) with diagnosis CD34+CD38- cut-off of 0.03%; B. RFS in the same patient group (n = 70), but now with 2 cut-offs (0.005% and 0.1%); C. Event-free survival for all CR and non-CR patients (n = 88); D. RFS in remission patients (n = 70) with CD34+CD38+ cut-off of 25%; E. RFS in remission patients (n = 70) with CD34- cut-off of 3%. All relevant prognostic variables with statistical significance were investigated in a multivariate model. In this multivariate analysis it was found that risk group (according to the HOVON 102 trial) was an independent prognostic factor for OS at diagnosis (p = 0.001). For RFS, both risk group and CD34+CD38- leukemic stem cell load (using a 0.03% cut-off point) were independent prognostic factors at diagnosis (p = 0.017 and p = 0.011, respectively).

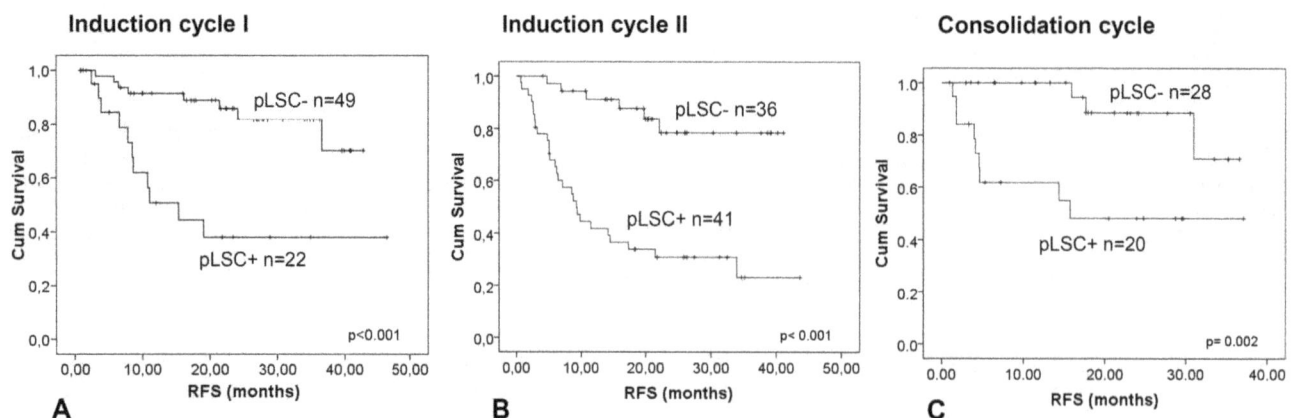

Figure 6. Prognostic value of frequencies of CD34+CD38- pLSC compartment at follow-up. This figure shows the Kaplan-Meier analyses for RFS for the CD34+CD38- pLSC compartment at follow up for three consecutive therapy cycles. The optimal cut-off levels were chosen to define pLSC + and pLSC- after 1st induction cycle (0.0003%,which is 3 pLSCs in 1,000,000 WBC) and after 2nd induction cycle and consolidation therapy 0.0001% (1 pLSC in 1,000,000 WBC). Results for other cut-offs are in Table S7. After the first induction cycle (B, 71 patients), second induction cycle (C, 77 patients), and after consolidation therapy (D, 48 patients), patients with high pLSC frequency (pLSC+) showed significantly more adverse performance compared with patients with low pLSC frequency (LSC-).

Table 3. Role of cytogenetically/molecularly defined risk groups in pLSC/MRD defined sub-groups.

Group sub-group (cytogen/mol)	N (nr per pLSC/MRD sub-group)	% per pLSC/MRD sub-group	40 months survival* (%)
pLSC-/MRD- (total)	33	100	74
good	8	24	69
intermediate	11	33	80
poor	10	30	80
very poor	4	12	50
pLSC-/MRD+ (total)	9	100	56
good	5	56	60
intermediate	3	33	67
poor	0	0	-
very poor	1	11	0
pLSC+/MRD- (total)	31	100	45
good	8	26	47
intermediate	7	23	57
poor	12	39	47
very poor	4	13	0
pLSC+/MRD+ (total)	18	100	16
good	4	22	25
Intermediate	2	11	0
Poor	7	39	15
Very poor	5	28	0

* 40 months was chosen as most survival curves had reached a plateau.
MRD cut-off: 0.1% of WBC, pLSC cut-off: 0.0001% of WBC.

When including the distribution of cytogenetically/molecularly good, intermediate, poor and very poor patients, these were all represented in the four LSC/MRD defined subgroups (Table 3). This shows that, the pLSC/MRD prognostic impact is across cytogenetic risk groups, although in the LSC+/MRD+ group poor and very poor cytogenetic/molecular risk groups are prevalent.

When including the post-diagnosis prognostic parameter "cycle after which CR is reached" in Figure 7, it turned out that there was no significant difference between the first three pLSC/MRD defined patient groups in number of cycles needed to reach CR: in the first group (pLSC-/MRD-) 29 after first cycle versus 4 after second cycle; in the third group (pLSC+/MRD-) this was 25 versus 6. The second group (pLSC-/MRD+) was too small (all patients in CR after one cycle). However, in the fourth group (pLSC+/MRD+) for 9 patients two cycles were needed, with one for the other 9 patients.

These data show that combining cytogenetic/molecular defined risk groups together and clinical parameters like cycles to CR, together with pLSC/MRD defined risk assessment may offer a very important new algorithm in risk assessment.

Discussion

One of the major challenges in the design of new therapies to eradicate leukemia stem cells is to achieve high therapeutic specificity. To this end, it is important to distinguish LSCs from the concomitantly present HSCs, and to assess whether this distinction is of prognostic value, since it would underline the clinical importance of LSCs. Consequently, it was necessary to identify parameters that allowed discrimination between these

pLSCs and HSCs, preferably in all AML cases. Recent studies have shown that pLSCs may reside not only in CD34+CD38-, but also in CD34+CD38+ and CD34- compartments [5,11]. In the present paper, we first present methods to discriminate between the neoplastic and normal portions of these compartments, and we subsequently assessed the prognostic value of these putative stem cell compartments.

With regard to the prognostic impact, using a uniquely-designed multi-parameter flow cytometry protocol, we show for the first time that the CD34+CD38- pLSC load after different cycles of therapy was highly predictive of patient survival, independent of other prognostic parameters. In addition, following our own preliminary studies [13], we identified three patient groups at diagnosis defined by CD34+CD38- pLSC with very large differences in prognosis, again independent of other prognostic parameters. By comparison with literature [13–15], it can be appreciated that the prognostic impact using our new approach, in which the pLSC compartment within the total CD34+CD38- compartment was specifically used, is much higher than using the total CD34+CD38- compartment as done in the previous studies. This is likely due to the "contamination" of the leukemic CD34+ CD38- compartment with HSCs in the earlier studies (ranges of 0%–100% of pLSC, as seen in our study, also means that HSC range from 0%–100%), as seen in Table S3. In contrast, the CD34+CD38+ and CD34- compartments at diagnosis completely lacked prognostic impact, which strongly suggests that CD34+ CD38+ and CD34- pLSCs are of minor clinical importance, at least in AML cases where these compartments are accompanied by CD34+CD38- pLSCs (as by definition is the case in our current CD34 positive patient group). However, at follow-up, leukemic

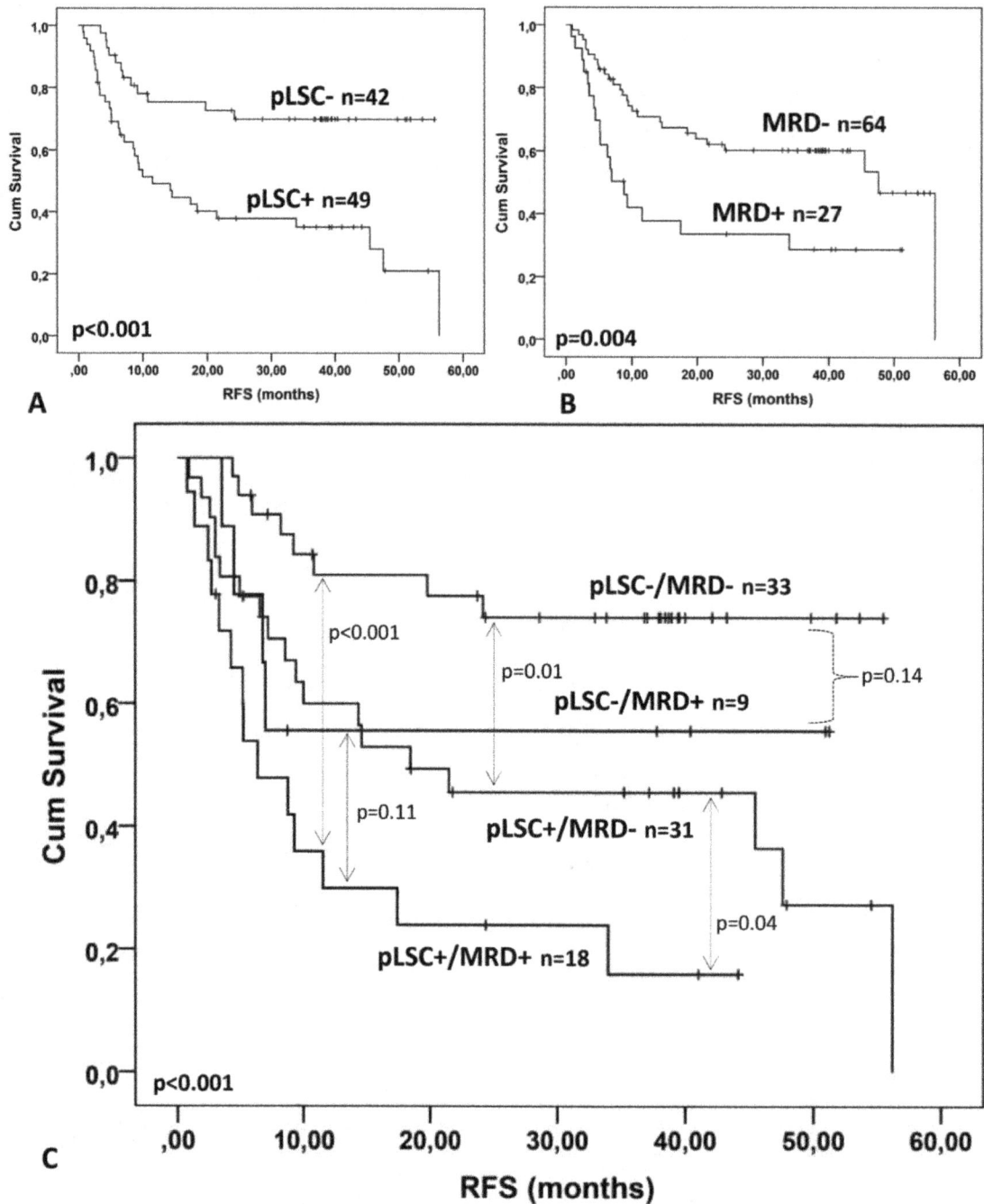

Figure 7. Prognostic value of combined p-LSC and MRD. (A) Kaplan-Meier analyses after cycle II for RFS for the pLSC data as shown in Figure 6, with an additional 23 patients (Table S1). The pLSC cut-off used is 0.0001%. (B) Kaplan Meier analysis of MRD data (cut-off 0.1%) obtained for the same patient group as in A (n = 91). (C) Combined pLSC and MRD (n = 91) data resulted in 4 patient groups: pLSC-/MRD-, pLSC-/MRD+, pLSC+/MRD- and pLSC+/MRD+.

CD34+CD38+ and CD34- compartments represent considerable portions of the total leukemic burden and thus reflect MRD cell frequency rather than pLSC frequency. Here, CD34+CD38+ and CD34- cells probably originate from (limited) differentiation of the CD34+CD38- pLSCs, a process that has been shown to occur *in vivo* by Goardon and colleagues [28].

The results are compatible with the following model: what the paper shows is that in CD34 positive AML cases, it is the percentage of the CD34+CD38- population at diagnosis that

strongly correlates with clinical outcome and not the percentage of CD34+CD38+ or CD34- cells. This does not mean that CD34+ CD38+ and CD34- cells do not contain leukemia initiating ability; it simply strongly suggests that, in the presence of CD34+CD38- cells, these CD34+CD38+ and CD34- leukemia initiating cells are either less therapy resistant and/or less malignant compared to CD34+CD38- cells. Likely, leukemia initiating ability in mouse models of CD34/CD38 defined sub-populations do not reflect clinical importance (see also next paragraph), since this ability is always assessed using purified populations, whereby the "competition" between these populations in outgrow and/or the relative therapy resistance cannot be taken into account. This model also implies that in CD34 negative AML (with only neoplastic CD34- populations present), it is the CD34- pLSC that takes over the leukemia initiating ability. Also in CD34 positive AML in the absence of CD34+CD38- cells, but with neoplastic CD34+CD38+ and CD34- populations present, the latter two populations may take over the leukemia initiating ability. As a logical consequence of the model these putatively less aggressive and/or less therapy resistant populations should define a better clinical outcome, which is indeed the case: in a separate cohort of 438 patients, survival of CD34 negative patients was significantly better than survival of CD34 positive patients (unpublished results).

The lack of correlation between prognosis and the size of the different CD34+CD38+ and CD34- compartments, while all compartments in purified form do engraft in a mouse model, may be explained as follows: the overall immune status of a patient group like that in our study, may best be represented by a less immune-restricted mouse model, where CD34+CD38- pLSCs are the predominant engrafting cells [29,30]. In line with that, in our earlier engrafting experiments using CD34+ cells (i.e., containing CD34+CD38-, CD34+CD38+ and CD34- cells) in the less immune-restricted NOD/SCID mice, it was only the size of the CD34+CD38- compartment at diagnosis that correlated with levels of engraftment [13]. More immune-restricted mouse models are useful to study LSC engraftment of probably less aggressive pLSC sub-populations [5,28]. In this respect, an important initial observation was made by Costello and co-workers, who found that, in vitro, CD34+CD38- cells were more therapy-resistant and less immunogenic than other compartments [21]. Moreover, further compelling evidence that the CD34+CD38- compartment is most important in the clinical setting comes from our clinical observations: in most cases which had low frequency mutations at diagnosis, which became predominant at relapse, these mutations were present and/or enriched in the neoplastic CD34+CD38- diagnosis compartment [31].

Survival and outgrowth of leukemia cells after therapy may depend on many factors and include the LSC load and likely specific LIC properties, but also the frequency of AML blast cells referred to as MRD. Many authors, including us, have shown that MRD is a strong independent prognostic factor [24,32,33]. In this paper we have shown that both CD34+CD38- pLSC frequency and MRD cell frequency are complementary, thereby defining a new post-diagnosis combination factor that offers strong prognostic information, even across cytogenetics/molecular defined risk groups. This will prospectively be validated in a new patient cohort of the HOVON/SAKK cooperative study group for which patient enrollment has already started.

With regard to our approach to distinguish between pLSCs and HSCs within the CD34+CD38- compartment, we have shown that aberrant expression of antigens (including CLL-1) and lineage markers, as well as additional aberrancies (including differences in CD34 and CD45 expression and differences in light scatter) allow unequivocal discrimination between pLSCs and HSCs. Moreover, this approach even allowed CD34+CD38- pLSC detection in patients lacking aberrant antigen expression. By applying the additional parameters, underestimation of pLSC numbers or overestimation of HSC numbers (often seen when using marker expression alone) is avoided. The present study thereby confirms the findings of others [29] that different CD34+CD38- pLSC markers expressed in individual AML cases may miss substantial portions of LSCs present (Figure 3). Although secondary parameters are thus very useful, it requires experience.

The number of accurately-identified pLSCs would increase with the use of additional AML markers. Such markers may include: CD123, CD96, CD44, CD47, CD25, CD32, CD33, TIM-3 [12,18,29,34–38]. In the present study, both lineage markers and CLL-1 were used to identify CD34+CD38- pLSCs and HSCs during follow-up, since these markers remained highly specific for these LSCs during and after therapy [18,19]. To date, other markers have not yet been tested and considerable efforts will be necessary to demonstrate their applicability both for pLSC quantification at diagnosis and especially at follow up, and as putative targets in antibody therapies. In particular, undesirable post-chemotherapy up-regulation on HSCs may occur for some of these markers [18,19]. Thus, our study implies that, for adequate pLSC (and HSC) tracking, a spectrum of markers and probably additional parameters should be screened for each individual AML case. Therefore, broad application of a single target antigen for diagnostic purposes, as well as for future LSC-directed antibody therapies, still seems unlikely.

Although FSC/SSC characteristics are often effective in discriminating between CD34+CD38- pLSCs and HSCs, the underlying cause of this difference is not yet known. An attractive option is that, similar to normal stem cells, CD34+CD38- AML sub-populations may exist with slightly different levels of differentiation [28]. In fact, we now have more formal proof for that: AML cases with high FSC and SSC of the CD34+CD38- cells all have expression of the differentiation marker CD45RA. It is known that this marker identifies GMP CD34+CD38+ progenitors in contrast to MEP and CMP CD34+CD38+ progenitors. We have found that CD45RA is completely absent on the real CD34+CD38- HSCs, but marked corresponding CD34+CD38- pLSC populations in roughly half of the AML cases. In the other half, the pLSC had FSC and SSC close to those of corresponding HSCs; these pLSCs were CD45RA negative. The CD45RA positive cases may indeed reflect more progenitor-like pLSCs compared to the CD45RA negative pLSCs that resemble HSCs [28].

In AML cases with no malignant CD34+CD38- compartments, the pLSCs will be located in the CD34+CD38+ and/or CD34- compartments. It is likely, however, that within these relatively large compartments, further compartmentalization will be necessary to identify the true LSC sub-compartment which likely occurs at low frequencies. One candidate fraction is the side population (SP), which does occur in low numbers (usually <1% of the WBC population) and contains both normal and AML cells at diagnosis [8,9]. Moreover, the SP has also been found to contain different CD34/CD38-defined sub-fractions [6], which may represent CD34/CD38/SP pLSCs. In the future, it would be interesting to examine the relationships between the functional phenotypes (based on SP or aldehyde dehydrogenase activity) [6–9,39,40] and the CD34/CD38 immunophenotype.

In conclusion, the present study offers tools for detecting concomitantly present pLSCs and HSCs, both at diagnosis and at disease follow-up, and provides the first proof that CD34+CD38- pLSCs are not only clinically important at diagnosis, but also at follow-up. No evidence was found to suggest that the CD34+ CD38+ and CD34- leukemic fractions contain clinically important LSCs, at least not in CD34 positive AML with leukemic CD34+ CD38- present. The combination with well-established MRD assessment likely opens a new field in prognostication in patients with AML. Ultimately, our findings may contribute to the development of new diagnostic tools and to novel, more selective therapies, including antibody-based therapies that would be highly effective against AML stem cells, while leaving the normal HSCs intact. Finally, these results may stimulate further research into the role of cancer stem cells in other cancers, such as solid tumors.

Supporting Information

Figure S1 pLSCs monitoring during sequential BM sampling. A patient (243) with AML positive for a t(8;21) showed CLL-1 expression in the CD34+CD38- compartment (A), while normal BM misses CLL-1+ CD34+CD38- cells [1]. In CR, CLL-1+ CD34+CD38- cells (B) were sorted and assessed for t(8;21): mainly neoplastic cells were present (E). Normal CD34+ CD38-CLL-1 negative cells were almost completely absent here. Shown in F-H are examples of sequential monitoring in three cases with increasing periods of complete remission until relapse (F, pt 253; G, pt 372) and in continuous remission (H, pt 572). Note the increase of pLSC frequency preceding relapse (F, G).

Table S1 Patient characteristics. *"Patients 1" are all CD34+ patients. "Patients 2" are all patients were accurate discrimination between HSC and pLSC was enabled using our extensive gating strategy. "Patients 3" are CR patients with MRD and pLSC data to enlarge the total patient group as shown in Figure 7.

Table S2 FSC and SSC position relative to lymphocytes. FSC, forward scatter; SSC, side scatter; HSC hematopoietic stem cells; pLSC, putative leukemia stem cell; NA, not applicable. * FSC and SSC values relative to those of lymphocytes present in the same sample.

Table S3 Gating details of 117 patients with a secondary gating strategy to define pLSC and HSC at diagnosis AML.

Table S4 Number of patients for different strategies in 250 CD34+ AML cases. *>20% aberrant marker expression was considered substantial to identify directly at least a substantial part of the pLSC population (179/250 patients; rows 3 and 4). In 102/179 patients (41% of all 250 CD34+ patients, row 3), pLSC frequencies may be under-estimated since additional gating strategy (with FSC/SSC etc, referred to in columns 3–7) was not possible, probably leaving part of marker negative pLSCs unidentified. In 77 of these 179 patients, an additional gating step could be performed (FSC/SSC etc, see row 4), allowing a more accurate assessment of both pLSC and HSC frequencies. #: <20% aberrant marker expression (71/250 cases) is shown in rows 5 and 6. In 31 cases (12%) only inadequate LSC assessment was possible (row 5). However, in 40 of these 71 cases HSCs could still be distinguished from pLSCs with the use of secondary parameters (row 6). Highly adequate LSC assessment, using both aberrant marker expression and secondary parameters was thus possible in 77+40 cases (47%). Columns show parameters/plots used to distinguish HSCs from pLSCs.
(DOCX)

Table S5 Multi-lineage engraftment of marker negative FSC/SSC^{low} (CD34^{high}) CD34+CD38- cells present in AML. * in the missing mouse, engraftment could not be assessed since this mouse died before examination was possible. # In the missing mouse, no human engraftment was detected. In terms of leukemic engraftment our results also confirmed the observation of Bonnet's group that purified CD34+CD38+ and CD34- were able

to engraft be it in our case after injection of high cell numbers. CD34+CD38-/CLL-1+ in pts 1 and 2 (40,000 and 130,000 cells, respectively) CD34+CD38-/CLL-1-/FSC ^{high} CD34^{low} in pt 1 (6,000 cells) CD34+CD38+ in pts 2, 4, 5, 6 (high cell numbers, 100,000-10^6 injected in pts 2, 4, 6 and 1,000 in pt 5) CD34- in pts 2 and 5 (high cell numbers injected:100,000-10^6).

Table S6 Cut-off values in the CD34+CD38-, CD34+CD38+ and CD34- cell compartment at diagnosis to identify patient groups with different survival. *p-values refer to significance of differences in RFS between patients above and patients below the indicated cut-offs.

Table S7 Relative risk of relapse determined for pLSC- and pLSC+ patients at follow up defined by different cut-off points. Not shown in the Table: for RFS and OS, without use of cut-offs, Cox regression analysis showed a strong significant inverse correlation between pLSC percentage and **RFS** after 1st cycle (n = 71, RR = 2.4, 95%CI:1.3–4.6, p = 0.008), 2nd cycle (n = 77, RR = 2.5, 95%CI:1.7–3.7, p<0.001) and consolidation cycle (n = 48, RR = 3.0, 95%CI:1.4–6.2, p = 0.004). For **OS**, these figures were RR = 1.8 (p = 0.04), RR = 2.7 (p<0.001) and RR = 2.0 (p = 0.07). Hereafter different cut offs were applied for risk on relapse. RR, relative risk of relapse using these different cut offs. Cut-offs of 0.0003% (3 in a million, 1st cycle) and 0.0001% (2nd and consolidation cycle) were used for relapse-free survival (**RFS**) in Kaplan-Meier analyses shown in Figure 6. With these cut-offs median overall survival (**OS**, not shown in Figure 6) was not reached (>42 months) for pLSC+ patients after 1st cycle, but more patients survived in the pLSC- group (p = 0.002). After 2nd cycle median **OS** in pLSC- group was>45 months versus 35 months in pLSC+ group (p<0.001). After consolidation cycle these figures were both>37 months (p = 0.05).

Table S8 Multivariate analysis$^{#}$ for impact of pLSC frequency on RFS. # in univariate analyses performed on 162 CD34+ patients, cytogenetic/molecular risk (p = 0.001, n = 162), number of chemotherapy cycles needed to achieve CR (p<0.001, n = 162), and WBC count at diagnosis (p = 0.002, n = 162) were significant. Other factors showed a trend: NPM1 mutation (p = 0.093, n = 140) and EVI-1 (p = 0.18, n = 140). n.r. not relevant since all evaluated patients achieved CR after first cycle RR, relative risk of relapse. * only the most optimal cut-offs (0.0003% after 1st cycle and 0.0001% after 2nd and consolidation cycle) are shown.

Text S1 Supporting text.

Acknowledgments

The authors would like to thank Hans Meel and Rolf Wouters for their help with the sorting and PCR experiments.

Author Contributions

Conceived and designed the experiments: MT AK ANS WZ APR SZ GJO GJS. Performed the experiments: MT AK ANS WZ APR WJS. Analyzed the data: MT AK ANS WZ APR WJS SZ GJO GJS. Contributed reagents/materials/analysis tools: SZ GJO TP GV BL GJS. Wrote the paper: MT AK ANS WZ APR WJS TP GV BL SZ GJO GJS.

References

1. Valent P, Bonnet D, De MR, Lapidot T, Copland M, et al. (2012) Cancer stem cell definitions and terminology: the devil is in the details. Nat Rev Cancer 12: 767–775.

2. Lapidot T, Sirard C, Vormoor J, Murdoch B, Hoang T, et al. (1994) A cell initiating human acute myeloid leukaemia after transplantation into SCID mice. Nature 367: 645–648.

3. Bonnet D, Dick JE (1997) Human acute myeloid leukemia is organized as a hierarchy that originates from a primitive hematopoietic cell. Nature medicine 3: 730–737.

4. Dick JE (2008) Stem cell concepts renew cancer research. Blood 112: 4793–4807.

5. Taussig DC, Vargaftig J, Miraki-Moud F, Griessinger E, Sharrock K, et al. (2010) Leukemia-initiating cells from some acute myeloid leukemia patients with mutated nucleophosmin reside in the CD34(-) fraction. Blood 115: 1976–1984.

6. Moshaver B, Van Rhenen A, Kelder A, Van der Pol M, Terwijn M, et al. (2008) Identification of a small subpopulation of candidate leukemia-initiating cells in the side population of patients with acute myeloid leukemia. Stem cells 26: 3059–3067.

7. Pearce DJ, Taussig D, Simpson C, Allen K, Rohatiner AZ, et al. (2012) Characterization of cells with a high aldehyde dehydrogenase activity from cord blood and acute myeloid leukemia samples. Stem cells 23: 752–760.

8. Wulf GG, Wang RY, Kuehnle I, Weidner D, Marini F, et al. (2001) A leukemic stem cell with intrinsic drug efflux capacity in acute myeloid leukemia. Blood 98: 1166–1173.

9. Feuring-Buske M, Hogge DE (2001) Hoechst 33342 efflux identifies a subpopulation of cytogenetically normal CD34(+)CD38(-) progenitor cells from patients with acute myeloid leukemia. Blood 9: 3882–3889.

10. Taussig DC, Miraki-Moud F, Anjos-Afonso F, Pearce DJ, Allen K, et al. (2008) Anti-CD38 antibody-mediated clearance of human repopulating cells masks the heterogeneity of leukemia-initiating cells. Blood 112: 568–575.

11. Sarry JE, Murphy K, Perry R, Sanchez P V, Secreto A, et al. (2011) Human acute myelogenous leukemia stem cells are rare and heterogeneous when assayed in NOD/SCID/IL2Rgammac-deficient mice. J Clin Invest 121: 384–395.

12. Majeti R, Chao MP, Alizadeh AA, Pang WW, Jaiswal S, et al. (2009) CD47 is an adverse prognostic factor and therapeutic antibody target on human acute myeloid leukemia stem cells. Cell 138: 286–299.

13. Van Rhenen A, Feller N, Kelder A, Westra AH, Rombouts E, et al. (2005) High stem cell frequency in acute myeloid leukemia at diagnosis predicts high minimal residual disease and poor survival. Clinical cancer research 11: 6520–6527.

14. Ran D, Schubert M, Taubert I, Eckstein V, Bellos F, et al. (2012) Heterogeneity of leukemia stem cell candidates at diagnosis of acute myeloid leukemia and their clinical significance. Experimental hematology 40: 155–165.

15. Witte KE, Ahlers J, Schafer I, Andre M, Kerst G, et al. (2011) High proportion of leukemic stem cells at diagnosis is correlated with unfavorable prognosis in childhood acute myeloid leukemia. Pediatr Hematol Oncol 28: 91–99.

16. Roshal M, Chien S, Othus M, Wood BL, Fang M, et al. (2013) The proportion of CD34(+)CD38(low or neg) myeloblasts, but not side population frequency, predicts initial response to induction therapy in patients with newly diagnosed acute myeloid leukemia. Leukemia 27: 728–731.

17. Vergez F, Green AS, Tamburini J, Sarry JE, Gaillard B, et al. (2011) High levels of CD34+CD38low/-CD123+ blasts are predictive of an adverse outcome in acute myeloid leukemia: a Groupe Ouest-Est des Leucemies Aigues et Maladies du Sang (GOELAMS) study. Haematologica 96: 1792–1798.

18. Van Rhenen A, Van Dongen GA, Kelder A, Rombouts EJ, Feller N, et al. (2007) The novel AML stem cell associated antigen CLL-1 aids in discrimination between normal and leukemic stem cells. Blood 110: 2659–2666.

19. Van Rhenen A, Moshaver B, Kelder A, Feller N, Nieuwint AW, et al. (2007) Aberrant marker expression patterns on the CD34+ CD38- stem cell compartment in acute myeloid leukemia allows to distinguish the malignant from the normal stem cell compartment both at diagnosis and in remission. Leukemia 21: 1700–1707.

20. Becker MW, Jordan CT (2011) Leukemia stem cells in 2010: current understanding and future directions. Blood Rev 25: 75–81.

21. Costello RT, Mallet F, Gaugler B, Sainty D, Arnoulet C, et al. (2000) Human acute myeloid leukemia CD34+/CD38- progenitor cells have decreased sensitivity to chemotherapy and Fas-induced apoptosis, reduced immunogenicity, and impaired dendritic cell transformation capacities. Cancer Res 60: 4403–4411.

22. Taussig DC, Pearce DJ, Simpson C, Rohatiner AZ, Lister TA, et al. (2005) Hematopoietic stem cells express multiple myeloid markers: implications for the origin and targeted therapy of acute myeloid leukemia. Blood 106: 4086–4092.

23. Feller N, Van der Pol MA, van Stijn A, Weijers GW, Westra AH, et al. (2004) MRD parameters using immunophenotypic detection methods are highly reliable in predicting survival in acute myeloid leukaemia. Leukemia 18: 1380–1390.

24. Terwijn M, Van Putten WLJ, Kelder A, Van der Velden VHJ, Brooimans RA, et al. (2013) High Prognostic Impact of Flow Cytometric Minimal Residual Disease Detection in Acute Myeloid Leukemia: Data From the HOVON/SAKK AML 42A Study. Journal of clinical oncology 31: 3889–3897.

25. Bakker AB, Van den Oudenrijn S, Bakker AQ, Feller N, van Meijer M, et al. (2004) C-type lectin-like molecule-1: a novel myeloid cell surface marker associated with acute myeloid leukemia. Cancer Res 64: 8443–8450.

26. Van der Pol MA, Feller N, Roseboom M, Moshaver B, Westra G, et al. (2006) Assessment of the normal or leukemic nature of CD34+ cells in acute myeloid leukemia with low percentages of CD34 cells. Haematologica 88: 983–993.

27. Cloos J, Goemans BF, Hess CJ, Van Oostveen JW, Waisfisz Q, et al. (2006) Stability and prognostic influence of FLT3 mutations in paired initial and relapsed AML samples. Leukemia 20: 1217–1220.

28. Goardon N, Marchi E, Atzberger A, Quek L, Schuh A, et al. (2011) Coexistence of LMPP-like and GMP-like leukemia stem cells in acute myeloid leukemia. Cancer cell 19: 138–152.

29. Jan M, Chao MP, Cha AC, Alizadeh AA, Gentles AJ, et al. (2011) Prospective separation of normal and leukemic stem cells based on differential expression of TIM3, a human acute myeloid leukemia stem cell marker. Proc Natl Acad Sci USA 108: 5009–5014.

30. Ishikawa F, Yoshida S, Saito Y, Hijikata A, Kitamura H, et al. (2007) Chemotherapy-resistant human AML stem cells home to and engraft within the bone-marrow endosteal region. Nature biotechnology 25: 1315–1321.

31. Bachas C, Schuurhuis GJ, Assaraf YG, Kwidama ZJ, Kelder A, et al. (2012) The role of minor subpopulations within the leukemic blast compartment of AML patients at initial diagnosis in the development of relapse. Leukemia 26: 1313–1320.

32. Buccisano F, Maurillo L, Del Principe MI, Del PG, Sconocchia G, et al. (2012) Prognostic and therapeutic implications of minimal residual disease detection in acute myeloid leukemia. Blood 119: 332–341.

33. Freeman SD, Virgo P, Couzens S, Grimwade D, Russell N, et al. (2013) Prognostic relevance of treatment response measured by flow cytometric residual disease detection in older patients with acute myeloid leukemia. J Clin Oncol 31: 4123–4131.

34. Hosen N, Park CY, Tatsumi N, Oji Y, Sugiyama H, et al. (2007) CD96 is a leukemic stem cell-specific marker in human acute myeloid leukemia. Proc Natl Acad Sci USA 104: 11008–11013.

35. Jordan CT (2002) Unique molecular and cellular features of acute myelogenous leukemia stem cells. Leukemia 16: 559–562.

36. Jordan CT, Upchurch D, Szilvassy SJ, Guzman ML, Howard DS, et al. (2000) The interleukin-3 receptor alpha chain is a unique marker for human acute myelogenous leukemia stem cells. Leukemia 14: 1777–1784.

37. Jin L, Hope KJ, Zhai Q, Smadja-Joffe F, Dick JE (2006) Targeting of CD44 eradicates human acute myeloid leukemic stem cells. Nat med 12: 1167–1174.

38. Saito Y, Kitamura H, Hijikata A, Tomizawa-Murasawa M, Tanaka S, et al. (2010) Identification of therapeutic targets for quiescent, chemotherapy-resistant human leukemia stem cells. Sci Transl Med 2: 17ra9.

39. Ran D, Schubert M, Pietsch L, Taubert I, Wuchter P, et al. (2009) Aldehyde dehydrogenase activity among primary leukemia cells is associated with stem cell features and correlates with adverse clinical outcomes. Exp Hematol 37: 1423–1434.

40. Cheung AMS, Wan TSK, Leung JCK, Chan LYY, Huang H, et al. (2007) Aldehyde dehydrogenase activity in leukemic blasts defines a subgroup of acute myeloid leukemia with adverse prognosis and superior NOD/SCID engrafting potential. Leukemia 2: 1423–1430.

26

Deazaneplanocin A Is a Promising Drug to Kill Multiple Myeloma Cells in Their Niche

Jérémie Gaudichon[1], Francesco Milano[1], Julie Cahu[1], Lætitia DaCosta[2¤], Anton C. Martens[3], Jack-Michel Renoir[2], Brigitte Sola[1]*

1 Equipe Associée 4652, Université de Caen, Normandie Univ, Caen, France, 2 Institut National de la Santé et de la Recherche Médicale U749, Institut Gustave Roussy, Villejuif, France, 3 Department of Immunology, University Medical Center Utrecht, Utrecht, The Netherlands

Abstract

Tumoral plasma cells has retained stemness features and in particular, a polycomb-silenced gene expression signature. Therefore, epigenetic therapy could be a mean to fight for multiple myeloma (MM), still an incurable pathology. Deazaneplanocin A (DZNep), a S-adenosyl-L-homocysteine hydrolase inhibitor, targets enhancer of zest homolog 2 (EZH2), a component of polycomb repressive complex 2 (PRC2) and is capable to induce the death of cancer cells. We show here that, in some MM cell lines, DZNep induced both caspase-dependent and -independent apoptosis. However, the induction of cell death was not mediated through its effect on EZH2 and the trimethylation on lysine 27 of histone H3 (H3K27me3). DZNep likely acted through non-epigenetic mechanisms in myeloma cells. In vivo, in xenograft models, and in vitro DZNep showed potent antimyeloma activity alone or in combination with bortezomib. These preclinical data let us to envisage new therapeutic strategies for myeloma.

Editor: Richard L. Eckert, University of Maryland School of Medicine, United States of America

Funding: This work was funded by grants from the Cancéropôle Nord-Ouest (canceropole-nordouest.org), the Ligue contre le Cancer - Comité de la Manche (ligue-cancer.net) (to BS). JC was financially supported by the Conseil Régional de Basse-Normandie. The funders had no role in the study design, data collection and analysis, decision to publish, or preparation of the manuscript.

Competing Interests: The authors have declared that no competing interests exist.

* Email: brigitte.sola@unicaen.fr

¤ Current address: Institut du cerveau et de la moelle épinière, UMRS 1127, Paris, France

Introduction

Multiple myeloma (MM) is a hematological malignancy characterized by the accumulation of abnormal plasma cells in the bone marrow. MM is the second most-common hemopathy and represents 1% of all cancers. Despite the emergence of new drugs including immunomodulators (lenalinomide) and proteasome inhibitors (bortezomib) that have significantly extended patients' survival, this disease remains incurable, with severe complications, and always leads to death [1]. This explains the need of new drugs and/or therapeutic strategies. The involvement of epigenetic alterations in oncogenesis starts to be well understood. In turn, epigenetic therapies have emerged and seemed efficient in the treatment of some hemopathies including MM [2].

The polycomb repressive complexes (PRC) are key mediators of transcriptional repression. PRC2 controls the pivotal methylation of lysine 27 of histone H3 (H3K27) catalyzed by the SET-domain containing enhancer of zest homolog 2 (EZH2) protein and its cofactors. Components of PRC2 are required for embryonic development and notably loss of *EZH2* gene is associated with a block in B- and T-cell differentiation [3]. Moreover, *EZH2* acts as an oncogene, is overexpressed in many solid cancers and lymphomas, in both advanced and metastatic diseases [4].

In a subtype of diffuse large B-cell lymphomas and follicular lymphomas, heterozygous missense mutations at Y641, within the

SET domain of *EZH2* have been described [5,6]. This mutation results in gain-of-function as the expression of the mutated allele adds up to the wild type one and increases level of H3K27me3 [7,8]. Although such mutations have not been reported so far in MM, *EZH2* is clearly overexpressed in MM cells and contributes to cell survival [9]. This is consistent with data reporting the enrichment for H3K27me3 marked genes [10] as well as the finding of prevalent mutations of the H3K27-demethylase UTX [11] in MM cells. Although the functional role of EZH2 in maintaining the survival of MM cells is unknown, it has been shown that depletion of EZH2 could trigger apoptosis. This was achieved using the 3-deazaneplanocin A (DZNep) *in vitro* on MM cell lines [10,12]. DZNep is an inhibitor of S-adenosyl-L-homocysteine (AdoHcy) hydrolase, the enzyme responsible for the reversible hydrolysis of AdoHcy to adenosine and homocysteine within the methionine cycle. Its inhibition by DZNep leads to the accumulation of AdoHcy and, in turn, *EZH2* downregulation [4]. The depletion of EZH2 and H3K27me3 triggers the apoptosis of cancer cells [13,14]. We analyzed here the effects of DZNep on MM cell lines and investigated its mode of action. We then determined the efficacy of DZNep *in vivo* by using xenograft models. Collectively, our data showed that DZNep could be effective to treat some severe forms of MM.

Materials and Methods

Chemicals, siRNAs and antibodies

Quinoyl-valyl-O-methylaspartyl-(2,6-difluoro-phenoxy)-methyl ketone or Q-VD-OPh, everolimus, propidium iodide (PI), cycloheximide (CHX) were purchased from Sigma-Aldrich (Saint-Quentin Fallavier, France), LY294002 from Biomol (Hamburg, Germany), bortezomib from Selleckchem (Houston, TX), MG-132 from Calbiochem (Gibbstown, NJ), DZNep from Cayman Chemical, (Ann Arbor, MI). Drugs were dissolved in ethanol (EtOH) or DMSO to obtain stock solutions (10–50 mM) and were diluted in serum-free culture medium before use. For control experiments using drugs, ethanol (EtOH) or dimethylsulfoxide (DMSO) were added as vehicles at the same concentration. For *in vivo* experiments, DZNep was dissolved in 10% D-mannitol (Sigma-Aldrich), then diluted at the appropriate concentration in PBS to reach 0.1% D-mannitol for i.p mice injections.

The following antibodies (Abs) were used in the study: anti-β-actin (sc-47778), anti-caspase 3 (sc-7148), and anti-caspase 8 (sc-7890) from Santa Cruz Biotechnologies (Santa Cruz, CA); anti-caspase 9 (#9508), anti-poly (ADP-ribose) polymerase or PARP (#9542) and anti-EZH2 (#3147) from Cell Signaling Technology (Danvers, MA); anti-B-cell lymphoma 2 or BCL2 (110887) from Dako (Courtaboeuf, France), anti-glyceraldehyde-3-phosphodeshydrogenase (GAPDH, #4300) from Applied Biosystems/Ambion (Austin, TX) and anti-H3K27me3 (mAb6002) from Abcam (Paris, France).

Cell cultures and cell viability determination

EJM (ACC-560), JJN3 (ACC-541), L363 (ACC-49) and RPMI 8226 (here 8226, ACC-402) cells were purchased from DSMZ (Leibniz Institute, German Collection of Microorganisms and Cell cultures, Braunschweig, Germany); LP1 [15], NCI-H929 (here H-929) [16], U266 [17] cells were provided by R Bataille (CRCNA research facility, Nantes, France) and OPM2 [18] cells from D Bouscary (Institut Cochin, Paris, France). The identity of non-commercially obtained cells was checked as described before [19]. Multiple myeloma cell lines (MMCLs) were maintained in RPMI 1640 medium supplemented with 100 U/mL penicillin, 100 U/mL streptomycin, 2 mM L-glutamine (all from Lonza, Basel, Switzerland) and 10% fetal calf serum (FCS, PAA Lab., Villacoublay, France). For cell viability studies, exponentially growing cells were seeded at a density of 2×10^5 cells/mL into six-well plates in 0.1% DMSO-containing medium or various concentrations of DZNep. The human stromal cell line HS-5 obtained from ATTCC (CRL-11882, Manassas, VA) was maintained in Dulbecco's modified eagle's medium containing antibiotics, L-glutamine and 10% FCS. Viable cells, excluding Trypan blue, were counted in a hemocytometer at various time intervals after various drug concentration treatments. The 8226 tumoral population contains both CD138^{low} and CD138^{high} cells; they were separated using anti-CD138 Ab coupled to magnetic microbeads (ref. 130-051-301, Miltenyi Biotec, Bergisch Gladbach, Germany) according to [20].

Cell proliferation determination

Cell proliferation was assayed using a ((2,3-bis(2-methoxy-4-nitro-5-sulfophenyl)-2H-tetrazolium-5-carboxanilide) inner salt) MTS assay, here the CellTiter 96 AQueous One Solution Cell Proliferation assay (Promega, Charbonnières, France). According to the supplier, 10^4 cells were seeded into 96-well plates, incubated with vehicle or various concentrations of drug for 24–144 h. Each culture condition was realized at least in triplicate. The absorbance values at 492 nm were corrected by subtracting the average absorbance from the control wells containing "no cells".

Cell cycle analysis, apoptosis determination and reactive oxygen species detection by flow cytometry sorting

For each culture condition, cultured cells were washed and suspended in ice-cold EtOH (80% in phosphate buffered saline, PBS). EtOH-fixed cells were then suspended in PBS containing 100 μg/mL RNase A (Roche Molecular Biochemicals, Meylan, France) and 20 μg/mL PI then incubated for 30 min before fluorescence-activated cell sorting (FACS) analysis. For apoptosis determination, cells were suspended in 100 μL of PBS containing 10 μL of anti-APO2.7 Ab (IOTest, Beckman Coulter) and incubated for 30 min at room temperature before FACS analysis. For the detection of reactive oxygen species (ROS), 5-(and-6)-chloromethyl-2',7'-dichlorodihydrofluoresceindiacetate acetyl ester or CM-H$_2$DCFDA (C6827, Invitrogen) staining was performed according to the manufacturer's instructions. On average, 2×10^4 cells were analyzed with a Gallios cytometer (Beckman Coulter) and data were analyzed with the Kaluza software (Beckman Coulter).

Morphological analyses of MMCLs

Cells were treated with either DZNep or vehicle, cytospun and stained with May-Grünwald-Giemsa before observation and image acquisition. A systematic uniform sampling was used in order to cover the whole slide (space between two acquisitions: 1 mm). Each image was acquired thanks to a microscope (AX70, Olympus, objective 40x) coupled to a camera (SpOt RT/KE, Diagnostics Instruments). The true-color images (24 bits RGB color) were saved in uncompressed tagged image file format (.tif) with a resolution of 1600×1200 pixels. A script was written in Python language with the specific module Mahotas to segment each cell. This script was based on color deconvolution [21] and mathematical morphology [22]. Only integral cells were kept. An interactive step was included after image processing for eliminating potential errors (bad segmentation, artifacts elements, etc.). For each cell, the perimeter, area and circularity (defined as (perimeter)^2/4×π×area) were computed. The circularity parameter allows objectivizing the shape of an object (C = 1 when the object is a circle, C = 0 when the object is a line). For transmission electronic microscopy, cells were prepared and examined with a JEOL 2011 as previously described [19].

Western blots

Whole cell lysates were obtained by incubating cells for 30 min on ice in the following buffer: 1% NP-40, 100 mM Tris-HCl (pH 7.4), 5 mM EDTA, 150 mM NaCl and a cocktail of protease inhibitors (cOmplete EDTA-free, Roche Diagnostics, Meylan, France). Proteins (50 μg) were separated by SDS/PAGE and blotted onto nitrocellulose membranes (Bio-Rad). Membranes were incubated with various Abs then exposed to a chemiluminescence detection reagent (Western Lightning Plus, PerkinElmer, Waltham, MA).

Real-time qRT-PCR

According to supplier's instruction, RNA samples were extracted with TRIzol reagent (Ambion, Austin, TX) from cultured MM cells. Total RNA was reverse-transcribed by using M-MuLV reverse transcriptase with random primers (all from Invitrogen, Life Technologies, Saint-Aubin, France). Real-time qRT-PCR was performed with a thermocycler (StepOne Plus, Applied Biosystems) using the GoTaq Master Mix (Promega). The relative expression of each gene was quantified by the comparative threshold (C_t) method ($\Delta\Delta C_t$) by using *RPLP0* gene as internal control with the StepOne v2.2.2 (Applied Biosystems) software. Specific primers produced by Eurogentec (Liege, Belgium) were the following: *EZH2*, F 5'-ATG ATG GAG ACG ATC CTG AA-3', R 5'-TCT TCT GCT GTG CCC TTA-3'; *SUZ12*, F 5'-AAA CGA AAT CGT GAG GAT GG-3', R 5'-CCA TTT CCT GCA TGG CTA CT-3'; *EED*, F 5'-ATC CGG TTG TTG CAA TCT TA-3', R 5'-TTT GGA TCT CTT GGA TGG AA-3'; *BMI1*, F5'-CTG GTT GCC CAT TGA CAG C-3', R 5'-CAG AAA ATG AAT GCG AGC CA-3'; *RPLP0*, F 5'-CCA GGC GTC CTC GTG GAA GTG-3', R 5'-TTC CCG CGA AGG GAC ATG CG-3'.

Xenograft models

Experiments were conducted in accordance with the recommendations of EEC (86/609/CEE). Experiments were approved by the Animal Experimental Ethics Committee of our Institution (Institut Gustave Roussy, France, permit n°26-2012-13). We used the RPMI 8226-Luc-GFP cell model described previously [23]. Six-week old non-obese diabetic/severe combined immunodeficiency/interleukin 2 receptor γ chain $-/-$ or NSG mice were injected in the caudal vein with 5×10^6 MM cells. Three days later, mice received either vehicle (n = 5) or were injected i.p. with 3 mg/kg DZNep twice a week (n = 5) until the end of the experiment. In a second series, using the same protocol of cells injection and engraftment, treatments started ten days later. NSG mice received vehicle (n = 5), bortezomib 0.4 mg/kg twice a week (n = 5), DZNep 1.5 mg/kg every two days (n = 5) or bortezomib in combination with DZNep 1.5 mg/kg every two days (n = 5). For bioluminescence imaging (BLI), mice were injected with 75 mg/kg of D-luciferine (Promega) and then analyzed with a Xenogen Optical In Vivo System (IVIS) coupled to Living Image Acquisition and Analysis software (Perkin Elmer, Waltham, MA). Ventral plus dorsal luminescence were determined by quantifying photon flux through the whole mouse and quantified. Mice were imaged at successive time points and were euthanized at the end of the treatment.

Tumor phenotyping by immunohistochemistry

At the end of experiments, bones were excised and immediately fixed in 4% paraformaldehyde (Electron Microscopy Sciences) prior to dehydration and paraffin inclusion for hematoxylin/eosin staining (HES) and immunohistochemistry (IHC). Acquired digital images of whole histological tumor sections were recorded using a Nikon SuperCoolscan 8000 ED slide scanner equipped with a FH-8G1 medical slide holder (Nikon, Champigny-sur-Marne, France). IHC analyzes were realized using a rabbit polyclonal Ab against phospho-H3 (p-H3, 1/50, #9701, Cell Signaling Tech.), a marker of M phase or against cleaved caspase 3 (cl. caspase 3, 1/100, #9661S, Cell signaling Tech.), a marker of apoptosis according to [24]. N-Histofine Simple Stain anti-rat and N-Histofine anti-mouse stain kits (both from Nichirei, Japan) were used for CD34 and CD138 detection, respectively. For each antibody, isotype control was included in each experiment. Micrograph images were obtained either at x100 or x630 magnification with immersion objective using a Zeiss Axiophot microscope (Carl Zeiss, Oberkochen, Deutschland).

Statistical analysis

Student's *t*-test was used to determine the significance of differences between two experimental groups. Data were analyzed with a two-sided test and $p<0.05$ (*) was considered significant.

Results

DZNep induces myeloma cells death

To study the effects of DZNep on cell growth and survival, we tested various DNZep concentrations (0.1, 0.5 and 1 μM) on eight MMCLs: 8226, U266, OPM2, H929, LP1, JJN3, EJM and L363 for several time intervals (24 to 144 h). DZNep-treated cells were analyzed for Trypan blue exclusion and compared to vehicle-treated cells. Four cell lines (U266, OPM2, H929 and LP1) were resistant to the treatment whereas the other four (8226, L363, JJN3 and EJM) were sensitive. As exemplified Figure 1a, a 1 μM- and 72 h-treatment was cytotoxic on 8226 and L363 (loss of viability of 19% and 31%, respectively). JJN3 cells were also sensitive to DZNep (loss of viability of 37% at 72 h, Figure 1a). However, because of a slower proliferation rate compared to other MMCLs, a loss of viability of 31% was reached 144 h post-treatment for EJM cells (Figure 1a). We next analyzed the proliferation capacity of cells treated with the same concentrations of DZNep and the same time intervals using a MTS assay. Again, we observed a time- and dose-dependent decrease of cell proliferation for 8226, L363 and JJN3 cells (data not shown). This assay allowed us to calculate the half maximal inhibitory concentration (IC_{50}) at 72 h: 1 μM for 8226, 0.7 μM for L363, and 1.1 μM for JJN3. Our results showed that, in good agreement with previous reports [10,12], DZNep was efficient to induce the death of MM cells.

DZNep-induced cell death is not autophagy or necroptosis

Since autophagy was recognized as a regulator of both cell viability and death in MM [25], we looked for markers of autophagy in DZNep-treated 8226 and LP1 (as control) cells. As shown Figure 1b, in treated cells, we detected neither autophagosomes nor multilamellar bodies. The absence of autophagic cell death was further confirmed by the inhibition of the phosphoinositide 3-kinase (PI3K)/AKT/mammalian target of rapamycine (mTOR) pathway that controls autophagy in MM cells [26]. The pretreatment of 8226 cells with LY294002 (an inhibitor of PI3K/AKT, 1 μM for 2 h) or everolimus (an inhibitor of mTOR, 10 nM for 2 h) did not modify the response towards DZNep (Figure 1c).

However, we observed that DZNep induced morphological changes in the responding 8226 cells. On images of transmission electronic microscopy, DZNep-treated 8226 cells adopted an "epithelioid" morphology (Figure 2a). Moreover, compared to LP1, 8226 cells tended to increase in size, at the perimeter, area and circularity levels (Figure 2b). These morphological modifications being compatible with prenecrosis swelling, we hypothesized that another type of cell death could be implicated, possibly necroptosis. ROS production is an essential event of necrosis-oriented cell death [27]. MMCLs were then treated with DZNep and the production of ROS was measured by FACS using the CM-H_2DCFDA dye. DZNep did not induce ROS production in L363 cells (Figure 2c) or LP1 cells (not shown). *TXNIP* is a key regulator of ROS generation and has been previously described to be upregulated by DZNep treatment in acute myeloid leukemia [28]. We found that DZNep did not lead to significant changes in *TXNIP* expression in responsive or resistant MM cells (Figure 3d). Taken together, our results show that the cell death triggered by DZNep in MM is neither autophagy nor necroptosis.

DZNep induces caspase-dependent and -independent apoptotic cell death

MMCLs were treated (vehicle or 1 μM DZNep for 72 h) and stained with PI or anti-APO2.7-phycoerythrin (PE) Ab before flow

a

b

c

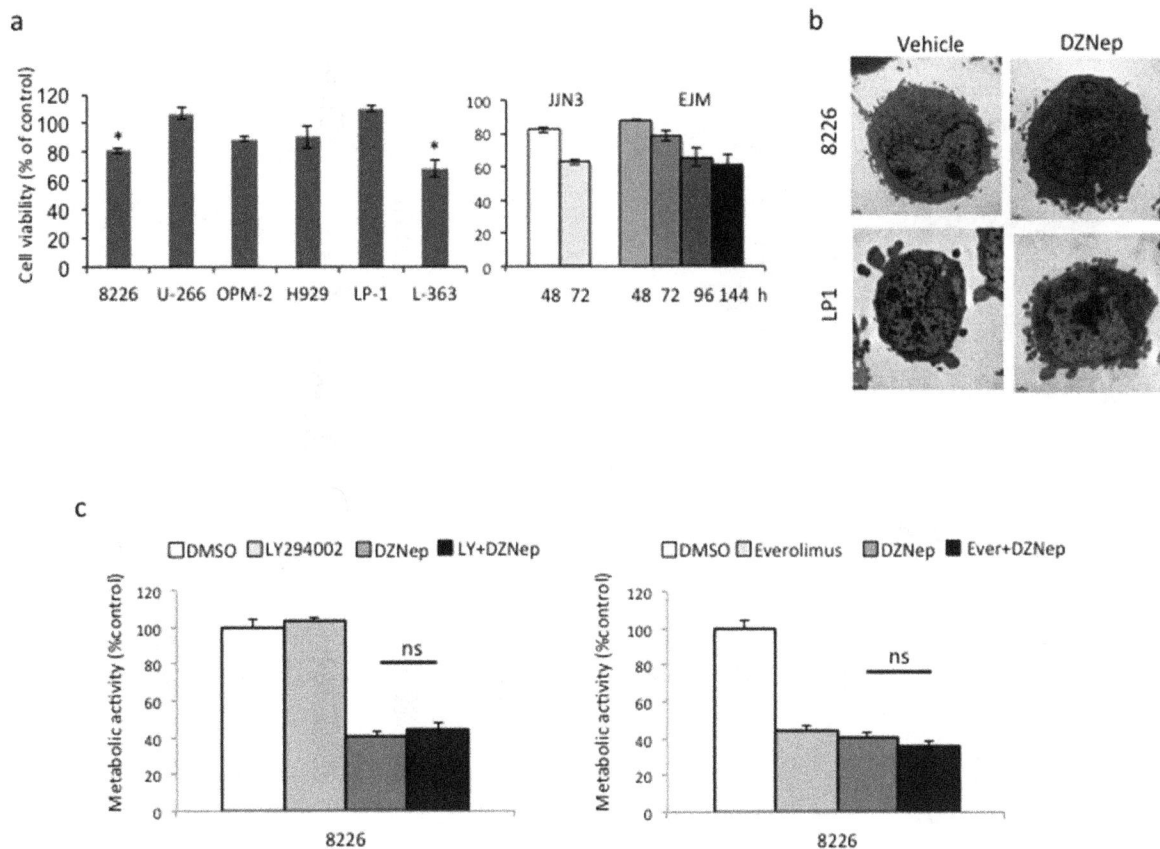

Figure 1. DZNep induces myeloma cells death. Exponentially growing MM cells were either treated with vehicle (DMSO 0.1%) or DZNep 1 μM for 72 h (**a left part**) or 48–144 h (**a right part**). (**a**) Cell viability was assessed by Trypan blue exclusion. The percentage of viable cells referred to control experiments assigned to 100%. The experiment has been repeated three times, histograms show means $\pm$ SD, *$p<0.05$. (**b**) Responsive 8226 and resistant LP1 cells were either treated with vehicle or DZNep (1 μM for 24 h) then examined by transmission electronic microscopy. (**c**) RPMI 8226 cells were treated with vehicle, the PI3K inhibitor LY94002 (1 μM for 24 h, **left part of the figure**), the mTOR inhibitor everolimus (10 nM for 24 h, **right part of the figure**), DZNep (1 μM for 24 h) or both and cell proliferation assayed by a MTS assay. For each culture condition, cells were seeded in three to five wells. The experiments have been repeated two or three times. A representative experiment is shown with the mean and SD values. ns, not significant.

cytometry sorting. As shown Figure 3a, analysis of APO2.7-positive cells demonstrated that sensitive MMCLs (8226, L363 and JJN3) underwent apoptosis after drug treatment. The triggering of apoptosis by DZNep was confirmed by the appearance of a sub-G1 phase (*i.e.* containing apoptotic cells) for PI-stained cells (data not shown). DZNep-resistant cells (U266, OPM2 and H929) were not blocked at any phase of the cell cycle excluding an entry in quiescence/senescence. In agreement, in DZNep-treated cells, we did not observe the upregulation of quiescence/senescence-associated proteins p16 and p21 (data not shown). The use of a pan-caspase inhibitor (Q-VD-OPh) restored, albeit not completely, the proliferation of JJN3 and 8226 cells after treatment (1 μM DZNep or vehicle for 24 h) as assayed by the MTS assay (Figure 3b). After APO2.7 staining of DZNep-treated sensitive 8226 and JJN3 cells and resistant LP1 cells as control, we observed that Q-VD-OPh did not abrogate completely DZNep effects (Figure 3c). We concluded that the apoptosis triggered by DZNep proceeded by both caspase-dependent and -independent mechanisms. We, finally, performed Western blotting to observe the effects of DZNep on the caspase cascade. As exemplified Figure 3d, after DZNep treatment (72 h, 1 μM), caspase-3 and -9 were activated leading to PARP cleavage. Moreover, associated with the recruitment of the intrinsic apoptotic pathway, we

observed the decrease of the anti-apoptotic protein BCL2 necessary for MM cells to enter apoptosis.

EZH2 expression level is reduced by DZNep treatment in MMCLs but not its targets

Some previous reports have shown that DZNep-induced cell death results from the reduction of EZH2 expression level due to its degradation by the proteasome, and in turn, from the reduction of the H3K27me3 expression level [13,14,29,30]. The levels of EZH2 and H3K27me3 were analyzed by Western blots in treated cells (DZNep 1 μM or vehicle for 72 h). The level of EZH2 protein decreased in a dose-dependent manner but to the same extent in resistant (U266, LP1, H929) and sensitive (L363, JJN3, 8226) cells (Figure 4a and not shown). Moreover, we did not detect any alteration of H3K27me3 levels in those cell lines (Figure 4a). This suggests that the triggering of apoptosis by DZNep is independent of EZH2 level and the global methylation status of H3K27 in MM cells. To further investigate the mechanisms of DZNep-induced EZH2 depletion, we analyzed the expression of *EZH2* gene as well as genes coding for PRC2 (*SUZ12, EED*) or PRC1 (*BMI1*) components by real-time reverse-transcription polymerase chain reaction (RT-PCR) after DZNep treatment (1 μM, 48 h). As shown Figure 4b, DZNep treatment did not lead

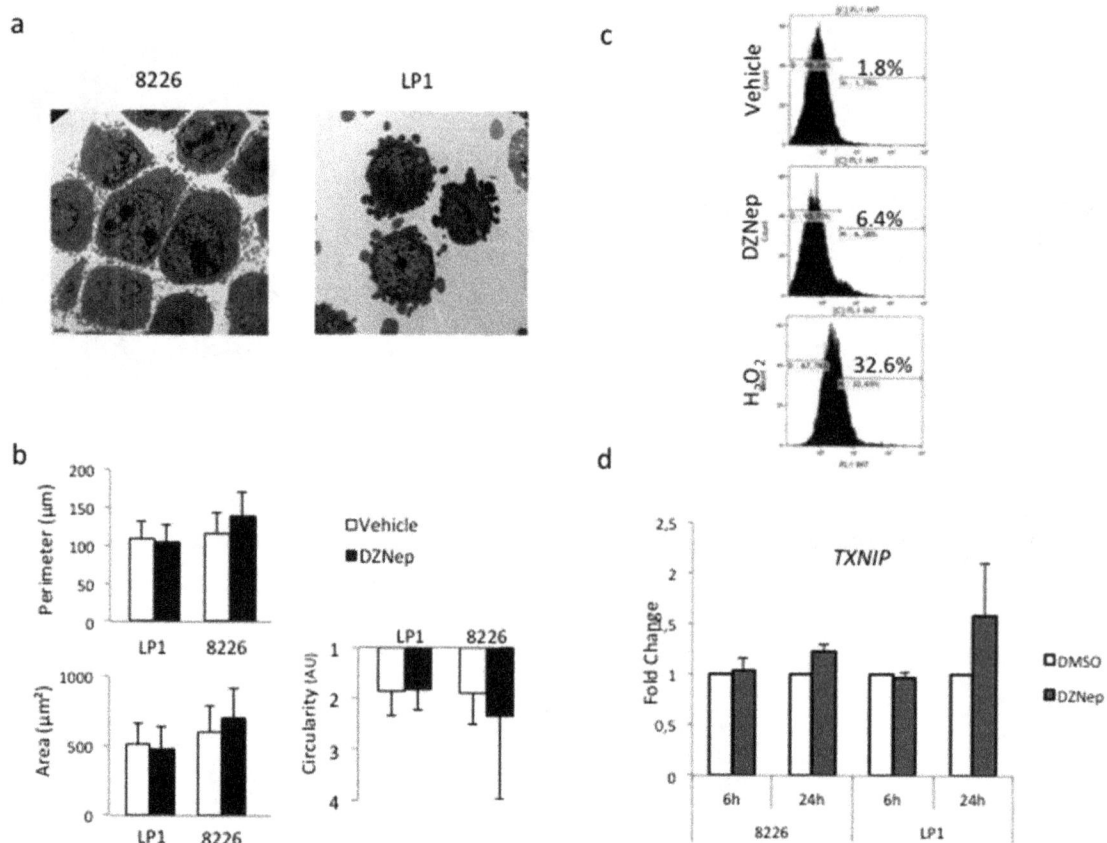

Figure 2. DZNep-induced cell death is not necroptosis. (**a**) Responsive 8226 and resistant LP1 cells were either treated with vehicle or DZNep (1 μM for 24 h) then examined by transmission electronic microscopy. (**b**) Responsive 8226 and resistant LP1 cells were either treated with vehicle or DZNep (1 μM for 24 h). The perimeter (in μm), the area (in μm^2) and the circularity (in arbitrary unit) of vehicle-(in white) or DZNep-treated (in black) LP1 and 8226 cells were determined by image analysis as described in the method section. (**c**) L363 cells were treated with vehicle, DZNep 1 μM for 24 h, or hydrogen peroxide (H$_2$O$_2$), incubated with CM-H$_2$DCFDA before FACS analysis. At least, 2×10^4 events were gated. The percentage of stained cells (*i.e.* cells producing ROS) is indicated on the graph. (**d**) Responsive 8226 and resistant LP1 cell lines were treated for 6 or 24 h with DZNep 1 μM. The transcriptional expression of *TXNIP* was determined by qRT-PCR using the $\Delta\Delta C_t$ method with *RPLP0* as internal standard. The fold change was calculated as $2^{-\Delta\Delta Ct}$. Indicated values corresponded to the mean ± SD from at least three independent experiments done with two distinct RNA preparations.

to any significant variation of the transcription of those genes in good agreement with a previous report [14]. This implies that DZNep acted on EZH2 expression at a post-transcriptional level. MMCLs were next pretreated with the proteasome inhibitor MG-132 (100 nM for 24 h or vehicle) then treated with either DZNep 1 μM or vehicle for 48 h and the level of EZH2 analyzed by Western blot. As shown Figure 4c, the inhibition of the ubiquitin/proteasome degradation pathway did not stabilize EZH2 in DZNep-treated cells. We next analyzed the turnover of EZH2 protein in cells in which protein synthesis was inhibited by CHX. As shown Figure 4d, the level of EZH2 decreased faster in DZNep-treated cells than in vehicle-treated cells. We concluded that DZNep affects EZH2 synthesis rather than degradation. In conclusion, following DZNep-treatment, EZH2 level is regulated at a post-transcriptional level but not by the proteasome degradation pathway. We suggest from those data that the anti-survival properties of DZNep in MMCLs could be due to an off-target effect.

DZNep impairs tumor cells engraftment and growth in their niche in NSG mice

To assess the activity of DZNep *in vivo*, we used the RPMI 8226-GFP-Luc cell line capable to graft into immunodeficient mice and to progress as myeloma tumor. Tumor localization and growth could be monitored by non-invasive BLI. Moreover, this model has been found pertinent for the evaluation of therapies in multiple myeloma [23]. We first confirmed that RPMI 8226-GFP-Luc cell line responded as well as the parental cell line to DZNep (data not shown). We injected RPMI 8226-GFP-Luc cells in the caudal vein of NSG mice. Two mouse groups were designed: the control one was injected with vehicle (n = 5), the other received DZNep (n = 5) as scheduled in Figure 5a. Two days post-injection, areas of luciferase activity were detected mainly in the lungs and at the basis of the tail in all mice (data not shown). As soon as three days post-injection, mice were then treated (DZNep or vehicle) twice a week and sequentially imaged as depicted in Figure 5a. In agreement with published results [23], in vehicle-treated mice, RPMI 8226-GFP-Luc cell line progressed as a myeloma tumor predominantly in the bone marrow. Foci of luciferase activity were present in the limbs (both anterior and posterior), pelvic region, skull, sternum, ribs and spinal vertebrae (Figure 5b and Table 1).

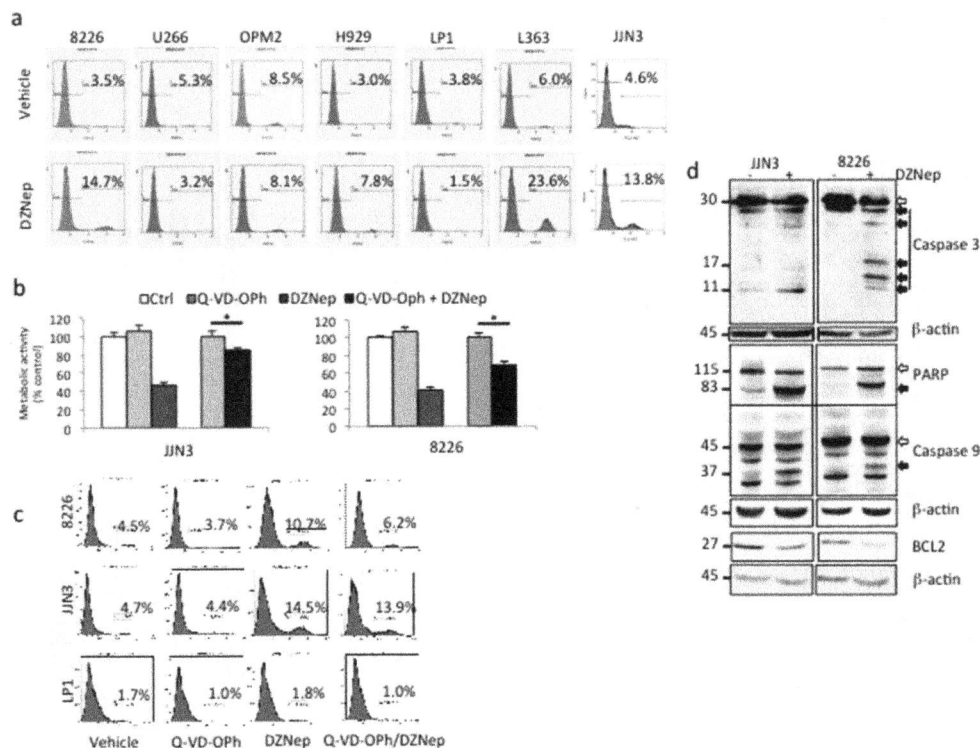

Figure 3. DZNep-induced cell death is apoptosis. (a) Exponentially growing MM cells were either treated with vehicle (DMSO 0.1%) or DZNep 1 μM for 72 h. Apoptosis was analyzed by FACS after APO2.7 staining. At least, 2×10^4 events were gated. The percentage of apoptotic cells (stained for APO2.7) is indicated on the graph. **(b)** Exponentially growing JJN3 and 8226 cells were either pretreated with vehicle or Q-VD-OPh 10 μM for 1 h then with vehicle or DZNep 1 μM for 48 h. Cell proliferation was estimated by a MTS assay. Control samples referred to 100%. Here is shown a representative example from three independent experiments; each culture condition being in triplicate. Histograms show mean $\pm$ SD, $*p<0.05$. **(c)** 8226, JJN3 and LP1 cells were treated with vehicle or Q-VD-OPh (10 μM for 1 h) and/or treated with DZNep (1 μM for 72 h). Cells were then stained with anti-APO2.7 Ab and analyzed by FACS. At least, 2×10^4 events were gated. The percentage of apoptotic cells (stained for APO2.7) is indicated on the graph. **(d)** Western blots were performed with the indicated antibodies to study the caspase cascade; β-actin Ab was used as control of charge and transfer. White arrows show proforms of PARP and caspase 3/9 and black arrows the cleaved (cl.) and activated forms of proteins.

The pattern of luciferase foci varies from one mouse to the other but was specific for each one (Figure 5b). MM growth in the bones resulted in hind legs paralysis in two out five mice in the group of vehicle-treated animals (mice #494 and 495); they were sacrificed at day 36. HES and CD138 detection by IHC further confirmed the presence of myeloma cells in the bone marrow (Figure 6a). Low levels of activated caspase 3 were present in control mice (Figure 6a). Considering the DZNep-treated group, the growth of MM tumors was delayed in two out of five mice (mice #548 and 549). At day 27, tumor localizations were the same than in the vehicle-treated group confirming that soft tissues were not the primary sites for MM engraftment (Table 1). Indeed, only two out of five mice in each series showed luciferase activity in the abdomen and/or pelvic regions. We further characterized these cells to be CD138$^+$ myeloma cells having invaded lymphatic nodes (not shown). Again the pattern of luciferase foci was specific for each mouse (Figure 5b). Importantly, in the DZNep-treated group, the ventral and dorsal luciferase activities were lower than in the vehicle-treated group. Moreover, at day 27, tumors stopped growing (Figure 5c). HES and CD138 staining confirmed the presence of myeloma cells in the bones of limbs, rachis and skull of animals (Figure 6b and c). As exemplified Figure 6b, tumor cells concentrated in well-defined foci within the femur (F) and the tibia (T) of mouse 517. Bones were invaded by CD138$^+$ tumoral cells (tc) with large and dense nuclei among a mixture of mouse hematopoietic cells (m). Although the intensity of cl. caspase 3

staining varied from one sample to the other (compare the insets (c), (f) and (i), Figure 6c), caspase 3 activity was associated with CD138 staining within disorganized bone marrow. Due to the destruction of bone and bone marrow structures caused by IHC protocols, we were unable to quantify the level of activated caspase 3. However, the analysis of several sections from various bones and various animals confirmed higher caspase 3 activities in DZNep-treated series (compare Figure 6a and c). Our data demonstrated that, *in vivo*, DZNep delayed the engraftment and impaired the growth of MM cells in their physiological niche.

DZNep shows specificity towards CD138^{high} MM cells

IHC analysis of bone sections in DZNep-treated mice showed a dramatic disorganization of bone structures (Figure 6c). This could be due to the death of stromal cells after DZNep-treatment or by the disappearance of apoptotic tumor cells that invaded bone matrix. In aiming to verify this point, we assessed the cytotoxicity of DZNep on HS-5 human stromal cells. As shown Figure 7a, DZNep, tested as before on MMCLs, had no effect on cell viability and proliferation. We concluded that DZNep acts specifically on MM cells and not on their bone marrow microenvironment.

We, and others, have characterized a sub-population of CD138^{low} cells within several MM cell lines, including 8226 cells, having the properties of cancer stem cells [20,31]. Recently, it has been reported that those clonogenic cells show an enriched pattern of stemness genes including PRC genes and could be more

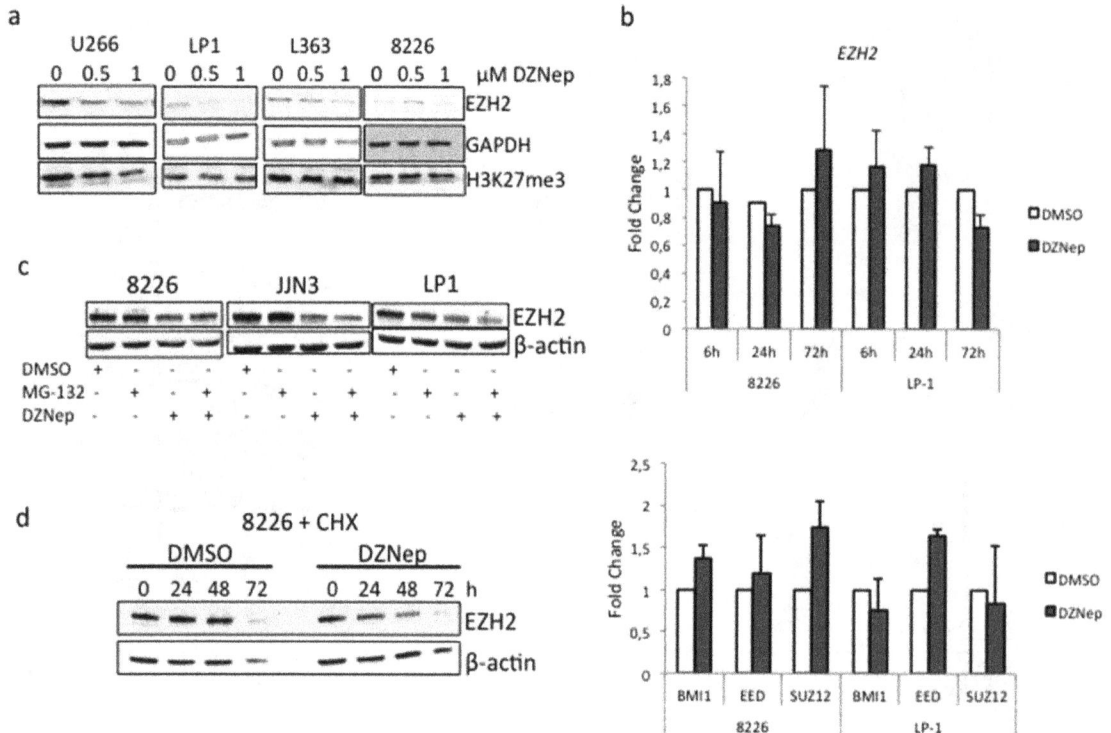

Figure 4. EZH2 expression is reduced at post-transcriptional level but is not involved in MM cells response to DZNep treatment. (a) MMCLs were treated with either vehicle (0) or indicated concentrations of DZNep for 72 h. Western blots were performed with indicated antibodies. Anti-GAPDH Ab was used for loading and transfer control. The experiment has been repeated three times. **(b)** Responsive 8226 and resistant LP1 cell lines were treated for different time intervals (**upper part**) or 72 h (**lower part**). The transcriptional expression of *EZH2* (**upper part**) or *BMI1, EED* and *SUZ12* (**lower part**) was studied by qRT-PCR using the $\Delta\Delta C_t$ method with *RPLP0* as internal standard. The fold change was calculated as $2^{-\Delta\Delta Ct}$. Indicated values corresponded to the mean $\pm$ SD from at least three independent experiments. **(c)** The responsive 8226 and JJN3 and the resistant LP1 cells were treated with vehicle, MG-132 (100 nM for 24 h), DZNep (1 µM for 24 h) or both. Cell were harvested; total proteins were purified, separated by SDS-PAGE and analyzed by Western blot with the indicated Abs. **(d)** 8226 cells were treated with CHX (100 µM for 1 h) then with vehicle or DZNep (1 µM for 24 h). Total proteins were purified, separated by SDS-PAGE and analyzed by Western blot with the indicated Abs.

sensitive than CD138^{high} cells to DZNep [32]. We analyzed the response of CD138^{high} cells purified from 8226 cells towards DZNep treatment (1 µM). As shown Figure 7b, the sensitivity of CD138^{high} cells towards DZNep was the same than the global population 72 h post-treatment leading us to conclude that CD138^{high} MM cells are able to undergo apoptosis when treated with DZNep.

DZNep co-operates with bortezomib to kill MM cells *in vivo* and *in vitro*

Combined therapies show superior efficacy in myeloma patients [33]. We analyzed the response of JJN3 and LP1 cells exposed *in vitro* to bortezomib, largely used in clinical practice, alone or in combination with DZNep. As expected, JJN3 and LP1 cells responded to bortezomib treatment (10 and 25 nM for 24 h) and were sensitive or resistant to DZNep treatment (1 µM for 24 h), respectively (Figure 7c). Importantly, we observed additive effects when cells were cotreated with drugs even in the resistant LP1

Table 1. Localization of tumoral foci in NSG mice.

Treatment	DMSO	DZNep	Global
Sternum	1/5	1/5	2/10
Rachis	3/5	2/5	5/10
Posterior limbs	5/5	4/5	9/10
Skull	0/5	2/5	2/10
Pelvic region	1/5	1/5	2/10
Abdomen	1/5	1/5	2/10

The distribution of tumoral cells was assessed by BLI in ten mice (five per group), 45 days after the inoculation of 5×10^6 RPMI 8226-GFP-Luc cells in the caudal vein of immunodeficient NSG mice.

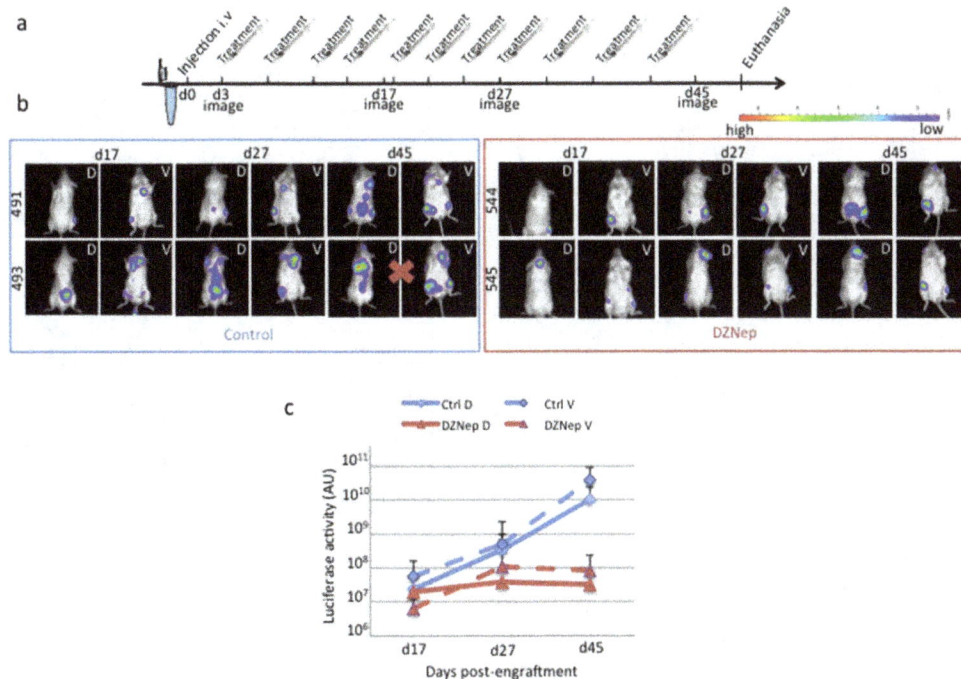

Figure 5. DZNep delays the engrafment and impairs the growth of MM cells in NSG mice. (**a**) RPMI 8226-GFP-Luc cells were injected into the caudal vein of NSG mice (n = 10) at day 1 (5×10^6 cells were injected per animal). Three days later, mice were separated into two groups (n = 5 in each group), one received vehicle for control; the other was treated with 100 µg DZNep twice a week as indicated in the scheme. At day 48, mice (except two, see below) were euthanized and tumors in soft tissues and bones removed for HES and IHC analyses. (**b**) BLI of the dorsal (D) and the ventral (V) sides of mice were taken at four sequential time points from day 3 to day 45. Both ventral and dorsal images of two mice in each group (mice #491/493 and #544/545) are shown. Mice 492 and 493 (red cross) showing hind leg paralysis were killed at day 36. (**c**) The luciferase activity of RPMI 8226-GFP-Luc cells in vehicle- (blue curves) and DZNep-treated (red curves) mice were determined into the two groups by BLI at the dorsal (plain line) and ventral (dotted line) levels.

cells, indicating that bortezomib overcomes DZNep resistance. The additivity of combined treatment on apoptosis was further confirmed on DZNep- and/or bortezomib-treated cells stained with the anti-APO2.7 Ab and analyzed by cytometry (Table 2). We finally assessed the combined bortezomib/DZNep treatment *in vivo* in the same settings than before. As previously reported [34,35], bortezomib was very efficient and inhibited tumor growth as soon as 20 days post-treatment (Figure 8a). In agreement with *in vitro* results, combined bortezomib plus DZNep treatment exerted higher growth inhibition towards 8226 xenografts but only at the end of the experiment (day 39, Figure 8a). We stopped the experiment at that time because of bortezomib toxicity in mice. IHC confirmed the co-operation between DZNep and bortezomib to kill MM cells (Figure 8b).

Discussion

The DZNep was first studied to enlarge the antiviral drugs arsenal and was further shown to induce cancer cell death [13]. DZNep became a promising anti-tumoral drug with a significant efficacy on various cell types and no evident toxicity *in vivo* [14,36,37]. Although DZNep is an inhibitor of AdoHcy, in most of cancers it acts through the reduction of EZH2 level and in turn, the re-expression of genes silenced by PRC2 *via* the demethylation of K27II3 [13,14,37]. Since MM patients exhibit a gene signature enriched for H3K27me3 marks and in particular in PRC2-silenced genes [10], the targeting of PRC2 components could be relevant for treatment. We show here that DZNep induces caspase-dependent and -independent apoptosis in a subset of MM cells *in vitro* and *in vivo*, alone or in combined therapy, but the

induction of cell death is not mediated by the downregulation of EZH2 and the subsequent re-expression of PRC2-silenced genes. One mechanism of EZH2 depletion is its degradation by the ubiquitin/proteasome degradation pathway [13,14,29,30]. However, we reported here that DZNep affects EZH2 synthesis rather than degradation suggesting that it may act through a global effect on cell metabolism as previously suggested [12].

The effects of DZNep on MM cell lines, primary cells and *in vivo* models have been reported previously in two contrasting reports. In the first one, the reactivation of silenced genes by the pharmacological depletion of EZH2 by DZNep allows the induction of apoptosis in two MMCLs and in the 5T33MM *in vivo* model [10]. By contrast, in another study, in agreement with our data, the induction of apoptosis in responsive MM cells was accompanied by the downregulation of EZH2 but not H3K27me3 [12]. Since, DZNep is a global inhibitor of histone methylation and displays no selectivity, others epigenetic marks such as trimethylation of lysine 20 on histone H4 (H4K20me3), dimethylation of lysine 9 on histone H3 (H3K9me2), trimethylation of lysine 79 on histone H3 (H3K79me3) etc., could be modified as reported in breast cancer cells [13]. DZNep treatment could induce modifications of the methylation of histones without affecting the trimethylation of H3K27 and, in turn, modifications of the global transcription, maybe by involving other epigenetic marks we did not explore.

Our results suggest that the decrease of EZH2 is probably not decisive for the apoptotic response of MM cells towards DZNep. We used siRNA to specifically induce the downregulation of *EZH2* and in turn, study the effect of decreased EZH2 on cell death. For an unknown reason, we did not obtained more than

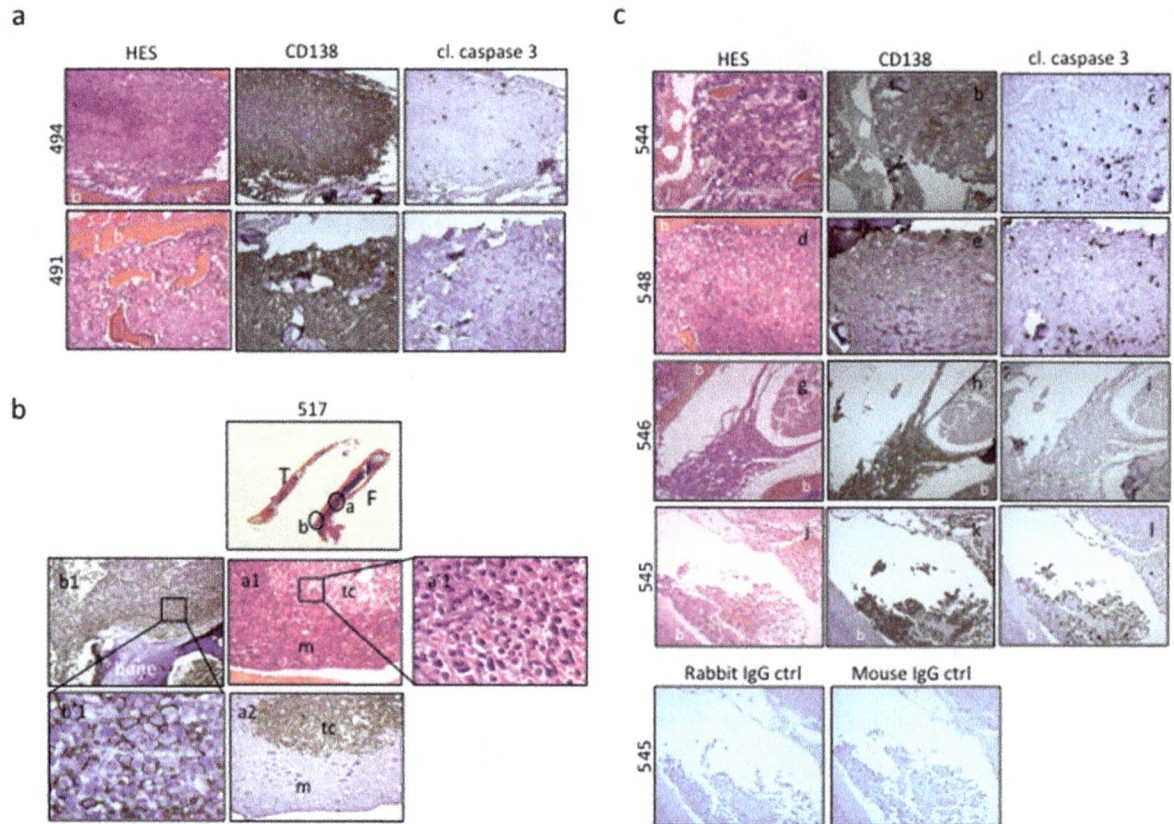

Figure 6. DZNep impairs the growth of MM cells in their niche. (a) Bones from control mice were processed and analyzed by HES and by IHC for CD138 and cleaved (cl.) caspase 3 staining. Images (x100 magnification) obtained for the femur of mouse #494 and the rachis of mouse #491, both vehicle-treated. CD138-positive cells that invaded bone marrow, caused bone (b) disorganization within the femur (#494) and the intervertebral discs (#491). Concomitantly, few cl. caspase 3 staining was noticed. **(b)** The femur (F) and tibia (T) from vehicle-treated mouse #517 were processed, scanned (x30 magnification), HE stained and analyzed for CD138 labeling by IHC (x100 magnification, a1, a2, b1; x630 magnification, a'1, b'1). Foci (a, b, c, circled regions) of typical CD138-membrane stained (b'1) MM cells tumors cells (tc) are visible within disorganized mouse bone marrow (m). MM cells mainly concentrated in trabecular areas (b, b1, b'1) but also in delineated medullae foci (a, a1, a'1, a2). **(c)** Examples of histological analyses (HES, CD138 and cl. caspase 3 staining) from rachis (mice #544 and 546), femur (mouse #548) and skull (mouse #545) samples removed from DZNep-treated series. CD138-positive *bona fide* MM cells invaded bone (b) tissues causing destruction and disorganization (puddles or ghosts associated with elevated caspase 3 activity). This high caspase 3 activity underlined DZNep therapeutic efficacy. Images of negative isotype rabbit or mouse IgG controls done on skull sections from mouse 454 are shown.

50% gene extinction with reasonable cell viability. In those experimental conditions, cell survival was not affected (data not shown). Those data underlie a probable off-target effect for DZNep. This cellular mechanism of action should be investigated further but we know from previous results that DZNep could modify deeply cell metabolism and in particular, lipid biosynthesis [12].

Xie *et al.*, reported previously no association between the sensitivity towards DZNep and the presence of the chromosomal translocation t(4;14) in MM cells [12]. In the subgroup of MM cells with t(4;14), the *MMSET* histone methyltransferase is overexpressed and in turn, the global pattern of histone methylations is modified [38]. Interestingly, in our study, all responsive cells (8226, JJN3, L363 and EJM) carry a translocation that affects a gene coding for a transcription factor of the MAF family (*c-MAF* for t(14;16) or *MAFB* for t(14;20)). This is of particular interest, since these translocations are associated with adverse prognosis in clinical practice [38]. We hypothesized that *MAF* could be directly impacted by DZNep treatment. However, it has become unlikely since the level of cyclin D2, a direct target of MAF, was not modulated after DZNep treatment as observed by RT-PCR and Western blot experiments (data not shown).

Moreover, the overexpression of *MAF* transcripts is a frequent event even in MM cells which do not carry the t(14;16) translocation [39]. And c-MAF/MAFB proteins are present in the non-responsive LP1 and OPM2 cells [40]. Nevertheless, if a direct role of MAF can be excluded, the genetic background that accompanies t(14;16) or t(14;20) translocations could be important for sensitivity towards DZNep. The *TP53* gene status regulates the sensitivity of gastric cancer cells to DZNep [41]. DZNep depleted EZH2 in almost all tested cell lines but only those with a wild-type *TP53* are sensitive and growth-inhibited. In our series, *TP53* is abnormal in three responsive cells (8226, JJN3 and L363) ruling out a common mechanism of action for gastric cancer and myeloma cells.

In prostate cancer cells, DZNep has been shown to induce specifically the death of cancer stem-like cells (CSCs) [36]. EZH2 seems essential for glioblastoma cancer stem cell maintenance [42]. This is consistent with the key role of PRC in the commitment and differentiation of normal stem cells. A recent report described a greater efficacy of DZNep on MM CSCs having a CD138$^{low/-}$ compared to CD138$^{high/+}$ MM cells [32]. This constituted a supplemental argument for the epigenetic mode of action of the molecule. We have not directly assessed the

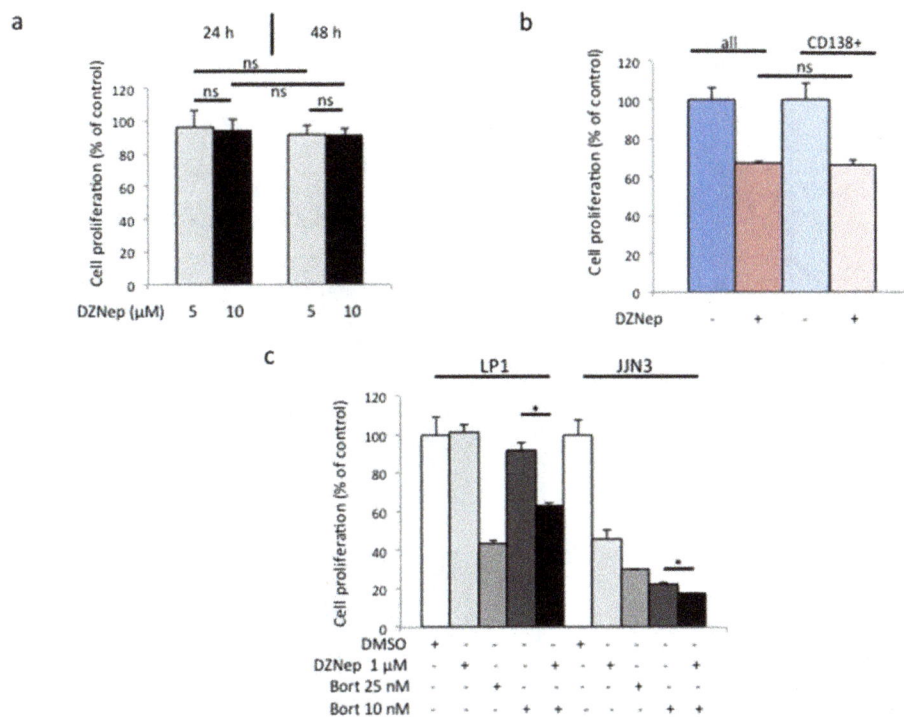

Figure 7. DZNep kills CD138⁺ MM cells and co-operates *in vitro* and *in vivo* with bortezomib. (a) Stromal HS-5 cells were seeded in 96-well plates at the density of 10^4 cells/well and cultured for three days. Vehicle or DZNep (1 µM) was further added in five wells per culture condition and plates incubated for 24 and 48 h. Cell viability was determined by a MTS assay. On the graph are the means and SD values. ns, not significant. (**b**) Exponentially growing 8226 cells were separated into CD138^{low} and CD138^{high} populations. The sensitivity of CD138^{high} population and global population to DZNep (1 µM for 72 h) was compared by the MTS assay as before. ns, not significant with the Student's *t*-test. (**c**) LP1 DZNep-resistant cells and JJN3 -sensitive cells were either treated with vehicle or DZNep 1 µM or bortezomib (Bort) 10–25 nM for 24 h or sequentially first with Bort then DZnep for 48 h. Cell proliferation was estimated by the MTS assay. Control samples referred to 100%. Here is shown a representative example from three independent experiments; each culture condition being in triplicate. Histograms show means ± SD, *$p<0.05$.

response of CD138$^{low/-}$ MM cells towards DZNep, but we showed here that MM cells expressing CD138 display similar sensitivity than the whole population. The precise phenotype of MM CSC or tumor-initiating cell is still debated. Recently, it was reported that exists a pool of CD19⁻CD138⁺ and CD19⁻CD138⁻ cells with an interconvertible phenotype that are functionally equivalent, having clonogenic properties and capable to propagate MM tumor *in vivo* [43]. From our data we can speculate that both cell types are sensitive towards DZNep.

Table 2. Additivity of DZNep and bortezomib proapoptotic effects on MM cells.

Cell line	Treatment	APO2.7+cells (%)
JJN3	Vehicle	4.3
	DZNep 1 µM	11.2
	Bortezomib 10 nM	43.7
	Bortezomib 25 nM	50.4
	DZNep 1+Bortezomib 10	54.9
	DZNep 1+Bortezomib 25	55.6
LP1	Vehicle	4.5
	DZNep 1 µM	1.9
	Bortezomib 10 nM	43.0
	Bortezomib 25 nM	54.9
	DZNep 1+Bortezomib 10	50.9
	DZNep 1+Bortezomib 25	55.4

JJN3 DZNep-sensitive cells and LP1 DZNep-resistant cells were either treated with vehicle or DZNep 1 µM or bortezomib (Bort) 10–25 nM for 48 h or sequentially first with bortezomib for 24 h then DZnep for 24 h. Apoptosis was estimated after anti-APO2.7 staining of cells and cytometry sorting. At least, 2×10^4 events were gated.

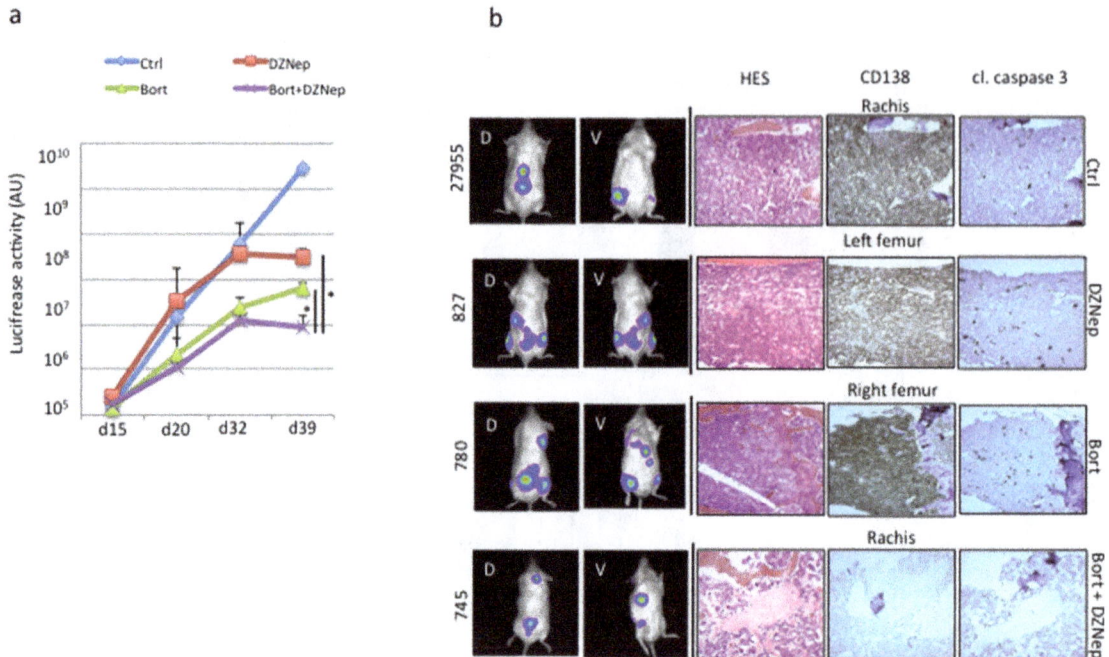

Figure 8. DZNep co-operates *in vivo* with bortezomib. (a) RPMI 8226-GFP-Luc cells were injected into the caudal vein of NSG mice (n = 20) at day 1 (5×10^6 cells were injected per animal). Ten days later, mice were separated into four groups (n = 5 in each group), one received vehicle for control, one was treated with 12.5 μg bortezomib i.p. twice a week, one was treated with 50 μg DZNep i.p. every two days, one was treated with bortezomib plus 50 μg DZNep i.p. every two days. Mice were imaged at days 15, 20, 32 and 39. At day 40, all mice (except three, see below) were euthanized. Two mice in the bortezomib-treated group and one in the bortezomib plus DZNep group died at day 32. BLI of the dorsal and the ventral sides of mice was taken at these time points and added. The luciferase activity (in arbitrary unit) representative of tumor growth in each series (mean ± SD) is represented in the graph; in blue the control group, in red the DZNep-treated group, in green the bortezomib-treated group and in purple the bortezomib/DZNep group. *$p<0.05$ with the Student's *t*-test. **(b)** Examples of histological analyses (HES, CD138 and cl. caspase 3 staining) from rachis (mouse #27955 from control group and mouse #745 from DZNep/borezomib group), left femur (mouse #827) from DZNep-treated group, and right femur (mouse #780) from bortezomib group. CD138-positive MM cells invaded bone tissues causing destruction and disorganization. In DZNep- or bortezomib-treated animals a high caspase 3 activity underlined therapeutic efficacy. Impressively, in mice #745 treated by both compounds, little CD138-positive cells were detected suggesting a possible cure.

This implies that contrary to most anti-myeloma drugs, DZNep will be able to eliminate all the cell types constituting the tumors.

DZNep is a promising tool for cancer therapy. It induces the apoptosis of cancer cells but not of their normal counterparts: epithelial cells and fibroblasts [14] or more importantly hematopoietic cells [44]. We show here that DZNep does not trigger the death of stromal cells surrounding tumor cells in the bone marrow. Importantly, DZNep and bortezomib co-operate to eliminate *in vitro* and *in vivo* MM cells. The response of MM cells to DZNep deserves further exploration however our data suggest that lower doses of bortezomib, which have adverse effects in patients, could be administered in association with DZNep in patients with bad prognosis or relapse.

Acknowledgments

The authors thank Anne Barbaras for help with cell cultures, Didier Bouscary (Institut Cochin, Paris, France) and Régis Bataille (IRS-UN, Nantes, France) for the gift of MMCLs, Didier Goux for transmission electronic microscopy analysis and Nicolas Elie for image analysis (CMaBio, Université de Caen, France), Arthur Vincent-Coves for reading the manuscript, the SFR 4206 (ICORE, Université de Caen, France) for flow cytometry facility, the Service Commun d'Expérimentation Animale (SCEA), the platform of Imagerie and Cytométrie (Valérie Rouffiac) and the service d'Anatomie pathologique (Paule Opolon and Olivia Bawa), IGR, Villejuif, France.

Author Contributions

Conceived and designed the experiments: JG JMR BS. Performed the experiments: JG FM JC LD JMR. Analyzed the data: JG FM JC JMR BS. Contributed reagents/materials/analysis tools: ACM. Contributed to the writing of the manuscript: JG JC JMR BS.

References

1. Palumbo A, Anderson KC (2011) Multiple myeloma. N Engl J Med 364: 1046–1060.
2. Smith EM, Boyd K, Davies FE (2010) The potential role of epigenetic therapy in multiple myeloma. Br J Haematol 148: 702–713.
3. Su IH, Dobenecker MW, Dickinson E, Oser M, Basavaraj A, et al. (2005) Polycomb group protein Ezh2 controls actin prolymerization and cell signaling. Cell 121: 425–436.
4. Chase A, Cross NCP (2011) Aberrations of EZH2 in cancer. Clin Cancer Res 17: 2613–2618.
5. Morin RD, Johnson NA, Severson TM, Mungall AJ, An J, et al. (2010) Somatic mutations altering EZH2 (Tyr641) in follicular and diffuse large B-cell lymphomas of germinal-center origin. Nat Genet 42: 181–185.
6. Velichutina I, Shaknovich R, Geng H, Johnson NA, Gascoyne RD, et al. (2010) EZH2-mediated epigenetic silencing in germinal center B cells contributes to proliferation and lymphomagenesis. Blood 116: 5247–5255.
7. Sneeringer CJ, Porter Scott M, Kuntz KW, Knutson SK, Pollock RM, et al. (2010) Coordinated activities of wild-type plus mutant EZH2 drive tumor-

associated hypermethylation of lysine 27 on histone H3 (H3K27) in human B-cell lymphomas. Proc Natl Acad Sci USA 107: 20980–20985.

8. Yap DB, Chu J, Berg T, Schapira M, Cheng SW, et al. (2011) Somatic mutations at EZH2 Y641 act dominantly through a mechanism of selectively altered PRC2 catalytic activity. Blood 117: 2451–2459.

9. Croonquist PA, Van Ness B (2005) The polycomb group protein enhancer of zest homolog 2 (EZH2) is an oncogene that influences myeloma cell growth and the mutant *ras* phenotype. Oncogene 24: 6269–6280.

10. Kalushkova A, Fryknäs M, Lemaire M, Fristedt C, Agarwal P, et al. (2010) Polycomb target genes are silenced in multiple myeloma. PLoS ONE 5: e11483.

11. van Haaften G, Dalgliesh GL, Davies H, Chen L, Bignell G, et al. (2009) Somatic mutations of the histone H3K27 demethylase gene UTX in human cancer. Nat Genet 41: 521–523.

12. Xie Z, Bi C, Cheong LL, Liu SC, Huang G, et al. (2011) Determinants of sensitivity to DZNep induced apoptosis in multiple myeloma cells. PLoS ONE 6: e21583.

13. Tan J, Yang X, Zhuang L, Jiang X, Chen W, et al. (2007) Pharmacological disruption of Polycomb-repressive complex 2-mediated gene repression selectively induces apoptosis in cancer cells. Genes Dev 21: 1050–1063.

14. Fiskus W, Rao R, Balusu R, Ganguly S, Tao J, et al. (2012) Superior efficacy of a combined epigenetic therapy against human mantle cell lymphoma cells. Clin Cancer Res 18: 6227–6238.

15. Pegoraro L, Malavasi F, Bellone G, Massaia M, et al. (1989) The human myeloma cell line LP-1: a versatile model in which to study early plasma-cell differentiation and c-myc activation. Blood 73: 1020–1027.

16. Gazdar AF, Oie HK, Kirsch IR, Hollis GF (1986) Establishment and characterization of a human plasma cell myeloma culture having a rearranged cellular myc proto-oncogene. Blood 67: 1542–1549.

17. Duperray C, Klein B, Durie BG, Zhang X, Jourdan M, et al. (1989) Phenotypic analysis of human myeloma cell lines. Blood 73: 566–572.

18. Katagiri S, Yonezawa T, Kuyama Y, Kanayama Y, Nishida K, et al. (1985) two distinct human myeloma cell lines originating from one patient with myeloma. Int J Cancer 36: 241–246.

19. Sola B, Poirot M, de Medina P, Bustany S, Marsaud V, et al. (2013) Antiestrogen-binding site ligands induce autophagy in myeloma cells that proceeds through alteration of cholesterol metabolism. Oncotarget 4: 911–922.

20. Cahu J, Bustany S, Sola B (2012) Senescence-associated secretory phenotype favors the emergence of cancer stem-like cells. Cell Death Dis 3: e446.

21. Ruifrok AC, Johnston DA (2001) Quantification of histochemical staining by color deconvolution. Anal Quant Cytol Histol 23: 291–299.

22. Roerdink J, Meijster A (2000) The Watershed Transform: Definitions, Algorithms and Parallelization Strategies. Fundamenta Informaticae 41: 187–228.

23. Rozemuller H, van der Spek E, Bogers-Boer LH, Zwart MC, Verweij V, et al. (2008) A bioluminescence imaging based *in vivo* model for preclinical testing of novel cellular immunotherapy strategies to improve the graft-versus-myeloma effect. Haematologica 93 : 1049–1057.

24. Urbinati G, Audisio D, Marsaud V, Plassat V, Arpicco S, et al. (2010) Therapeutic potential of new 4-hydroxy-tamoxifen-loaded pH-gradient liposomes in a multiple myeloma experimental model. Pharm Res 27: 327–339.

25. Hoang B, Benavides A, Shi Y, Frost P, Lichtenstein A (2009) Effect of autophagy on multiple myeloma cell viability. Mol Cancer Ther 8: 1974–1984.

26. Cirstea D, Hideshima T, Rodig S, Santo L, Pozzi S, et al. (2010) Dual inhibition of Akt/mammalian target of rapamycin pathway by nanoparticle albumin-bound-rapamycin and perifosine induces antitumor activity in multiple myeloma. Mol Cancer Ther 9: 963–975.

27. Kepp O, Galluzzi L, Lipinski M, Yuan J, Kroemer G (2011) Cell death assays for drug discovery. Nat Rev Discov 10: 221–237.

28. Zhou J, Bi C, Cheong LL, Mahara S, Liu SC, et al. (2011) The histone methyltransferase inhibitor, DZNep, up-regulates TXNIP, increases ROS production and targets leukemia cells in AML. Blood 118: 2830–2839.

29. Gannon OM, Merida de Long L, Endo-Munoz L, Hazar-Rethinam M, Saunders NA (2013) Dysregulation of the repressive H3K27 trimethylation mark in head and neck squamous cell carcinoma contributes to dysregulated squamous differentiation. Clin Cancer Res 19: 428–441.

30. Choudhury SR, Balasubramanian S, Chew YC, Han B, Marquez VE, et al. (2008) (-)-Epigallocatechin-3-gallate and DZNep reduce polycomb protein level via a proteasome-dependent mechanism in skin cancer cells. Carcinogenesis 32: 1525–1532.

31. Matsui W, Wang Q, Barber JP, Brennan S, Smith BD, et al. (2008) Clonogenic multiple myeloma progenitors, stem cell properties, and drug resistance. Cancer Res 68: 190–197.

32. Reghunathan R, Bi C, Liu SC, Loong KT, Chung T-H, et al. (2013) Clonogenic multiple myeloma cells have shared stemness signature associated with patient survival. Oncotarget 4: 1230–1240.

33. Rajkumar SV. (2012) Doublets, triplets, or quadruplets of novel agents in newly diagnosed myeloma? Hematology Am Soc Hematol Educ Program 2012: 354–361.

34. Blotta S, Jakubikova J, Calimeri T, Roccaro AM, Amodio N, et al. (2012) Canonical and noncanonical Hedgehog pathway in the pathogenesis of multiple myeloma. Blood 120: 5002–5013.

35. Schueler J, Wider D, Klingner K, Siegers GM, May AA, et al. (2013) Intratibial injection of human multiple myeloma cells in NOD/SCID IL-2R2γ(null) mice mimics human myeloma and serves as a valuable tool for the development of anticancer strategies. PLoS ONE 8: e79939.

36. Crea F, Hurt EM, Mathews LA, Cabarcas SM, Sun L, et al. (2011) Pharmacologic disruption of polycomb repressive complex 2 inhibits tumorigenicity and tumor progression in prostate cancer. Mol Cancer 10: 40.

37. Branscombe Miranda T, Cortez CC, Yoo CB, Liang G, Abe M, et al. (2009) DZNep is a global histone methylation inhibitor that reactivates developmental genes not silenced by DNA methylation. Mol Cancer Ther 8: 1579–1588.

38. Martinez-Garcia E, Popovic R, Min DJ, Sweet SMM, Thomas PM, et al. (2011) The MMSET histone methyltransferase switches global histone methylation and alters gene expression in t(4;14) multiple myeloma cells. Blood 117: 211–220.

39. Hurt EM, Wiestner A, Rosenwald A, Shaffer AL, Campo E, et al. (2004) Overexpression of c-Maf is a frequent oncogenic event in multiple myeloma that promotes proliferation and pathological interactions with bone marrow stroma. Cancer Cell 5: 191–199.

40. Herath NI, Rocques N, Garancher A, Eychène A, Pouponnot C (2014) GSK3 mediated MAF phosphorylation in multiple myeloma as a potential therapeutic target. Blood Cancer J, in press.

41. Cheng LL, Itahana Y, Lei ZD, Chia N-Y, Wu Y, et al. (2012) TP53 genomic status regulates sensitivity of gastric cancer cells to the histone methylation inhibitor 3-deazaneplanocin A (DZNep). Clin Cancer Res 18: 4201–4212.

42. Suvà ML, Riggi N, Janiszewska M, Radovanovic I, Provero P, et al. (2009) EZH2 is essential for glioblastoma cancer stem cell maintenance. Cancer Res 69: 9211–9218.

43. Chaidos A, Barnes CP, Cowan G, May PC, Melo V, et al. (2013) Clinical drug resistance linked to interconvertible phenotypic and functional states of tumor-propagating cells in multiple myeloma. Blood 121: 318–328.

44. Fiskus W, Wang Y, Sreekumar A, Buckley KM, Shi H, et al. (2009) Combined epigenetic therapy with the histone methyltransferase EZH2 inhibitor 3-deazaneplaocin A and the histone deacetylase inhibitor panobinostat against human AML cells. Blood 114: 2733–2743.

27

MDM4 Overexpressed in Acute Myeloid Leukemia Patients with Complex Karyotype and Wild-Type *TP53*

Li Li[1,2], Yanhong Tan[1], Xiuhua Chen[1], Zhifang Xu[1], Siyao Yang[1], Fanggang Ren[1], Haixiu Guo[2], Xiaojuan Wang[1], Yi Chen[1], Guoxia Li[1], Hongwei Wang[1]*

1 Department of Hematology, the Second Hospital of Shanxi Medical University, Taiyuan, Shanxi, P.R. China, 2 Department of biology, School of Basic Medicine, Shanxi Medical University, Taiyuan, Shanxi, P.R. China

Abstract

Acute myeloid leukemia patients with complex karyotype (CK-AML) account for approximately 10–15% of adult AML cases, and are often associated with a poor prognosis. Except for about 70% of CK-AML patients with biallelic inactivation of *TP53*, the leukemogenic mechanism in the nearly 30% of CK-AML patients with wild-type *TP53* has remained elusive. In this study, 15 cases with complex karyotype and wild-type *TP53* were screened out of 140 *de novo* AML patients and the expression levels of MDM4, a main negative regulator of p53-signaling pathway, were detected. We ruled out mutations in genes associated with a poor prognosis of CK-AML, including *RUNX1* or *FLT3-ITD*. The mRNA expression levels of the full-length of *MDM4* (*MDM4FL*) and short isoform *MDM4* (*MDM4S*) were elevated in CK-AML relative to normal karyotype AML (NK-AML) patients. We also explored the impact of MDM4 overexpression on the cell cycle, cell proliferation and the spindle checkpoint of HepG2 cells, which is a human cancer cell line with normal MDM4 and TP53 expression. The mitotic index and the expression of p21, BubR1 and Securin were all reduced following Nocodazole treatment. Moreover, karyotype analysis showed that MDM4 overexpression might lead to aneuploidy or polyploidy. These results suggest that MDM4 overexpression is related to CK-AML with wild-type *TP53* and might play a pathogenic role by inhibiting p53-signal pathway.

Editor: Ken Mills, Queen's University Belfast, United Kingdom

Funding: This study was supported by Natural Science Fund (81241014) of China, Natural Science Fund (2014011039-2) of Shanxi Province, University of Shanxi Science and Technology Development Project (20121004), Shanxi Medical Innovation Fund (C01201006), and Foundation for phD scientific research of Shanxi Medical University (03201309). The funders had no role in study design, data collection and analysis, decision to publish, or preparation of the manuscript.

Competing Interests: The authors have declared that no competing interests exist.

* Email: wanghw68@hotmail.com

Introduction

Acute myeloid leukemia patients with complex karyotype (CK-AML) account for approximately 10–15% of adult AML, and the incidence increases with age. CK-AML is characterized by chemoresistance, higher rates of refractory disease, and poor prognosis [1–3]. However, the molecular mechanisms mediating of leukemogenesis in CK-AML patients have remained elusive. A series of large sample studies show that nearly 70% of CK-AML cases carry *TP53* mutations and have biallelic inactivation of *TP53* [4,5]. p53 plays an important role in spindle damage induced mitotic arrest in proliferating T cells [6] and p53 lost myeloid progenitors exhibit aberrant self-renewal, thereby promoting AML[7]. Yet the question remains as to the leukemogenic mechanisms of the nearly 30% of CK-AML patients without *TP53* alterations.

MDM4 is a negative regulator of p53, and by binding p53, close the transcriptional activity domain and thereby inhibits p53 function [8]. The short isoform of MDM4 (MDM4S) is one of the MDM4 alternative splicing isoforms that results from the exclusion of exon 6 and termination of translation in exon 7. MDM4S is essentially a truncated protein that mainly consists of the p53-binding domain. MDM4S has been reported to bind and inhibit p53 more efficiently than full-length MDM4 (MDM4FL) [9].

Several recent studies suggest that an increased MDM4S/MDM4FL ratio may serve as both a more effective biomarker for p53 pathway attenuation in cancers than p53 gene mutation and as a poor prognostic indicator. [10,11]. The molecular mechanisms of myeloproliferative neoplasm (MPN) converting into AML were examined in 330 cases [12]. Among the 22 patients with transferred to AML, 10 (45.5%) cases had evidence of a p53-related defect mediated by gains (amplification) of chromosome 1q (which contains the potent p53 inhibitor MDM4) or *TP53* gene mutations. These reports suggest that overexpression MDM4 may be involved in the leukemogenic mechanisms of CK-AML patients without *TP53* alterations. This question has not been fully explored to date.

In this study, we detected the expression levels of *MDM4S* and *MDM4FL* in CK-AML patients with wild-type *TP53*. We also measured cell proliferation, cell cycle, proteins related to p53 pathway and spindle checkpoint expression levels, and analyzed karyotypes in MDM4-overexpressing tumor cell line with wild-type TP53. We used these approaches to investigate the possible pathogenesis of MDM4-overexpression in CK-AML patients lacking TP53 mutations.

Materials and Methods

Ethics Statement

This study complies with the Declaration of Helsinki, and has been approved by the Ethics Committee of Shanxi Medical University. The written informed consent was obtained from all patients and from the legal guardians in the case of minors.

Patients

Bone marrow samples were collected at the time of diagnosis of 140 non-M3 de novo AML patients. The fusion genes RUNX11/RUNX1T1, PML/RARα or CBFβ/MYH11 of the patients were identified to be negative at the time of enrollment.

Karyotype analysis

Conventional cytogenetics was performed at the time of diagnosis in 140 patients. Bone marrow cells were cultured in RPMI 1640 medium with 10% fetal bovine serum and penicillin-streptomycin for 24 hours, followed by treatment with 0.01 mg/ml colcemid for 60 min. Cells were harvested and placed in 0.075 M KCl for 15 min. After several changes in methanol-acetic acid fixative, slides were prepared by hot-plate drying. Metaphase chromosomes were banded by the trypsin-Giemsa or Phosphate R technique, and karyotyped according to the International System of Human Cytogenetic Nomenclature (ISCN 2005).

PCR and Gene sequencing

Exons 3–9 of the TP53 gene and exon 3–9 of RUNX1 were amplified by PCR from genomic DNA and sequenced directly in all cases with complex karyotype. TP53 deletions were detected by interphase FISH in complex karyotype cases. Fms-related tyrosine kinase 3 length mutation (FLT3-ITD) analysis was performed as published [13] in CK-AML with wild-type TP53 and NK-AML patients.

Real-time RT-PCR

For quantitative RT-PCR, cDNA was prepared using Prime-Script 1st Strand cDNA Synthesis Kit (TaKaRa, Shiga, Japan) and used in quantitative real-time PCR reactions with SYBR Premix Ex Taq (TaKaRa) and 0.5 μM of forward and reverse primers. For each gene analyzed, cDNA from 5×10^6 bone marrow cells of CK-AML or NK-AML patients were used for amplification. Primers used were as follows:

MDM4FL-F: 5'-CAGCAGGTGCGCAAGGTGAA-3'
MDM4FL-R: 5'-CTGTG CGAGA GCGAG AGTCTG-3'
MDM4S-F: 5'-CAGCAGGTGCGCAAGGTGAA-3'
MDM4S-R: 5'-GCACTTTGCTGTAGTAGCAGTG-3
ABL-F: 5'-GAGTTCATGACCTAC GGGAACCT-3'
ABL-R: 5'-GGTACTCCATGGCTGACGAGAT-3'

PCR conditions: initial denaturation at 95°C 10 s; denaturation 95°C 15 s, annealing 60°C 30 s, 40 cycles. The average Ct for MDM4FL, MDM4S, and ABL, as well as the ΔCt (CtMDM4FL-CtABL or CtMDM4S-CtABL) was determined. NK-AML patients were set to 1 and relative expression graphed for MDM4FL and MDM4S mRNA in CK-AML patients. $2^{-\Delta\Delta Ct}$ was used for calculating relative quantification.

Cell culture

HepG2 and 293T cell lines were obtained from the Institute of Cell Biology, Chinese Academy of Sciences, Shanghai, China. Cells were maintained in DMEM (Wuhan Boster, Biotechnology Ltd., Wuhan, China) supplemented with 10% fetal bovine serum (FBS; Gibco, Carlsbad, CA, USA), 100 U/ml penicillin, and

100 μg/ml streptomycin (Sigma, St. Louis, MO, USA). Nocodazole (Sigma) was dissolved in DMSO and used at either 0.1 μg/ml or 1 μg/ml.

Lentivector infection

For construction of the pCDH1-MDM4FL-EF1-copGFP and pCDH1-MDM4S-EF1-copGFP, MDM4FL or MDM4S fragments and pCDH1-MCS1-EF1-copGFP plasmid were digested by EcoR I and BamH I respectively, and then linked with T4 DNA ligase (TaKaRa). Plasmid sequences were confirmed by sequencing. Approximately 5×10^6 293T cells in 100 mm dishes was cotransfected with 10 μg pCDH1-MCS1-EF1-copGFP vector, pCDH1-MDM4FL-EF1-copGFP, or pCDH1-MDM4S-EF1-copGFP along with 10 μg packaging vector pPACKH1-GAG, pPACKH1-REV and pVSV-G using calcium phosphate precipitation. Media containing lentivirus were collected 48 and 72 hours after transfection and supernatant added to 5×10^5 HepG2 cells/well of a 6-well plate with 8 μg/ml polybrene (Sigma). For infection, cells were centrifuged at $1400 \times g$ for 2.5 hours at 32°C. GFP-positive cells were screened by limiting dilution, expanded in culture, and GFP-positive cells were pooled. To confirm that MDM4 was transfected into HepG2 cells, the expression levels of MDM4FL and MDM4S proteins were evaluated by western-blot analysis.

Cell cycle and cell proliferation assay

Cells stably expressing MDM4FL, MDM4S or vector control were cultured overnight and 0.1 μg/ml Nocodazole added the following day, and cells incubated for an additional 18 hours. Cells were stained by propidium iodine (PI) and cell cycle stage determined by flow cytometry (FCM). Cell proliferation was analyzed using the MTT assay. After 4 h incubation with MTT reagent, cells were lysed with DMSO for 10 min at 37°C and absorbance measured at 570 nm. The average percentage is shown for three independent HepG2 control, MDM4FL or MDM4S-expressing pools.

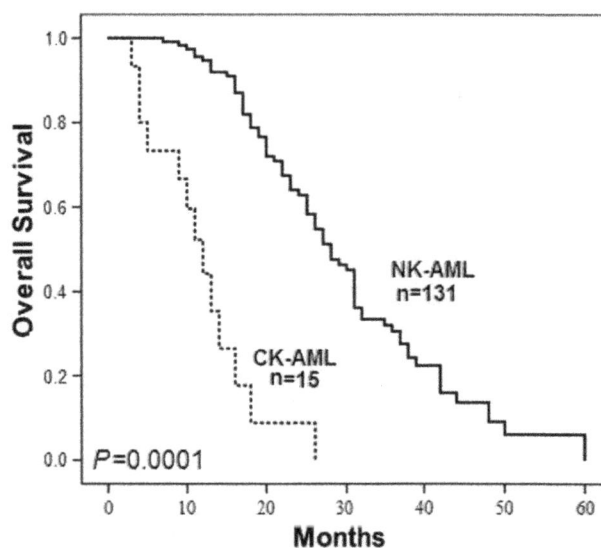

Figure 1. The overall survival of patients with NK-AML (solid line) and CK-AML (dotted line) analyzed by the Kaplan-Meier curve.

Table 1. General information, peripheral white blood cell count, outcome, karyotype, and survival time of 15 AML patients with complex karyotype.

patient	Age	Sex	FAB classification	WBC[1] (10^9/L)	outcome	karyotype	Overall survival (Mon[6])
1	59	F	M2	40.9	CR[2]	54, XXX,+8,+11,+15,+19,+20,+21,+22	3
2	76	M	M5	1.13	NT[3]	49, XY,+6, add(7)(p22),+8, add(11)(q25),+15	4
3	22	M	M2	18.9	CR	49, Y,+1,+5,−7,+8,−11, +13,+22,+t(11; 17) (q23; q21)	12
4	17	M	M5	106	PR[4]	51, XY,+13,+15,+16,+19,+22	17
5	44	M	M4	69.7	NR[5]	48, XXY,+1,−2,−5,+12, +18	9
6	62	F	M5	30	NR	50, XX,+1,−7,+8,+13,+15,+19	8
7	62	M	M5	0.77	NR	49, Y,+1,+5,−7,+8,+13, +21	11
8	64	F	M5	2.02	NR	50, XX, add(10)(p13),+16,+19,+21,+21	10
9	80	F	M4	83.7	NT	51, XX,−7,+13, +15,+21,+21,+21,+22	13
10	62	M	M4	26	PR	49, XY,+13,+19,+21	15
11	44	F	M4	79.9	NR	52, XXX,+10,+13,+16, −19,+21,+22,+der(19) t(11; 19)(q13; q21)	3
12	48	F	M0	4.17	NR	92, XXXX	2
13	55	M	M2	33.5	NR	47, XXY,+1,−2,−5,+19,+21,−22,+t(1; 17)(q31; q21)	25
14	67	M	M4	147	CR	56, XXXY,+1,−2,+10,+11,+12,+15,+20,+21,+21,+22	11
15	44	F	M2	2.48	CR	51, XXX,+8,+13,+15, +16	9

[1]WBC were detected at the time of diagnosis;
[2]CR: complete remission;
[3]NT: no treatment;
[4]PR: partial remission;
[5]NR: no remission;
[6]Mon: Month.

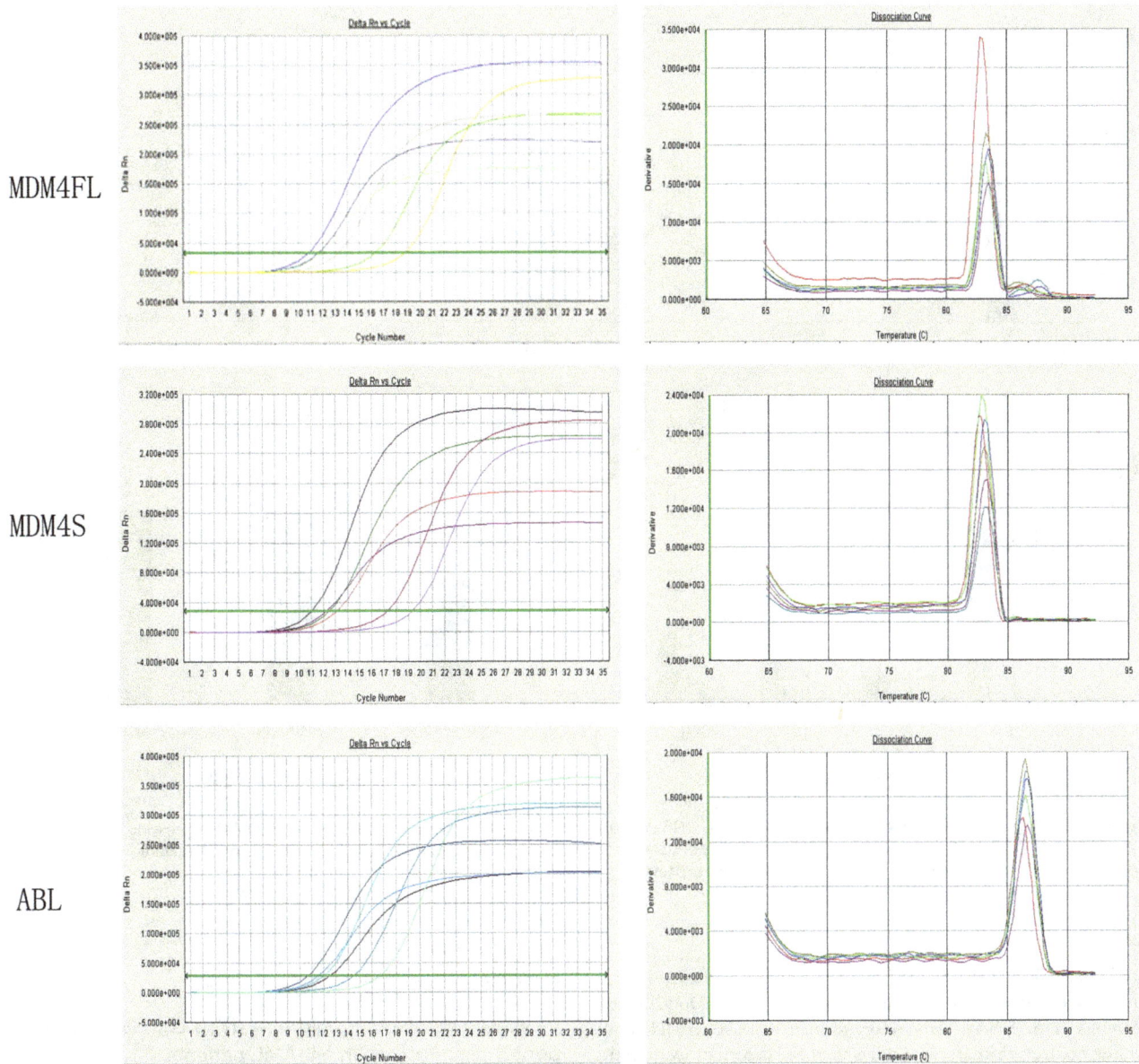

Figure 2. Amplification and melting curves of *MDM4FL*, *MDM4S* and *ABL*.

Western-blot analysis

After treatment with 1 µg/ml Nocodazole for 18 hours, total protein was extracted from approximately $5-10\times10^6$ control, MDM4FL or MDM4S-expressing cells, and stored at $-80°C$ before use. Lysates (30 µg) were resolved by 8–12% SDS-PAGE and gels transferred to nitrocellulose membrane. Membranes were blocked with 5% nonfat milk in PBST for 1 h followed by primary antibody and incubation overnight at 4°C with gentle rotation. Membranes were washed twice with PBS containing 0.2% Tween 20 and incubated with appropriate secondary antibodies for 1 h at room temperature with gentle rotation. Membranes were then washed twice with PBST and incubated with Super Signal West

Table 2. The relative expression levels of *MDM4FL* and *MDM4S* mRNA.

GENE	$\Delta Ct(\bar{x}\pm s)$ CK-AML	$\Delta Ct(\bar{x}\pm s)$ NK-AML	$\Delta\Delta Ct$	Normalized MDM4FL or MDM4S amount relative to NK-AML $2^{-\Delta\Delta Ct}$
MDM4FL	3.1300±2.5527	0.5882±1.2384	2.5418±1.8	5.82
MDM4S	6.1920±3.4192	1.7160±2.9743	4.4760±3.2	22.25

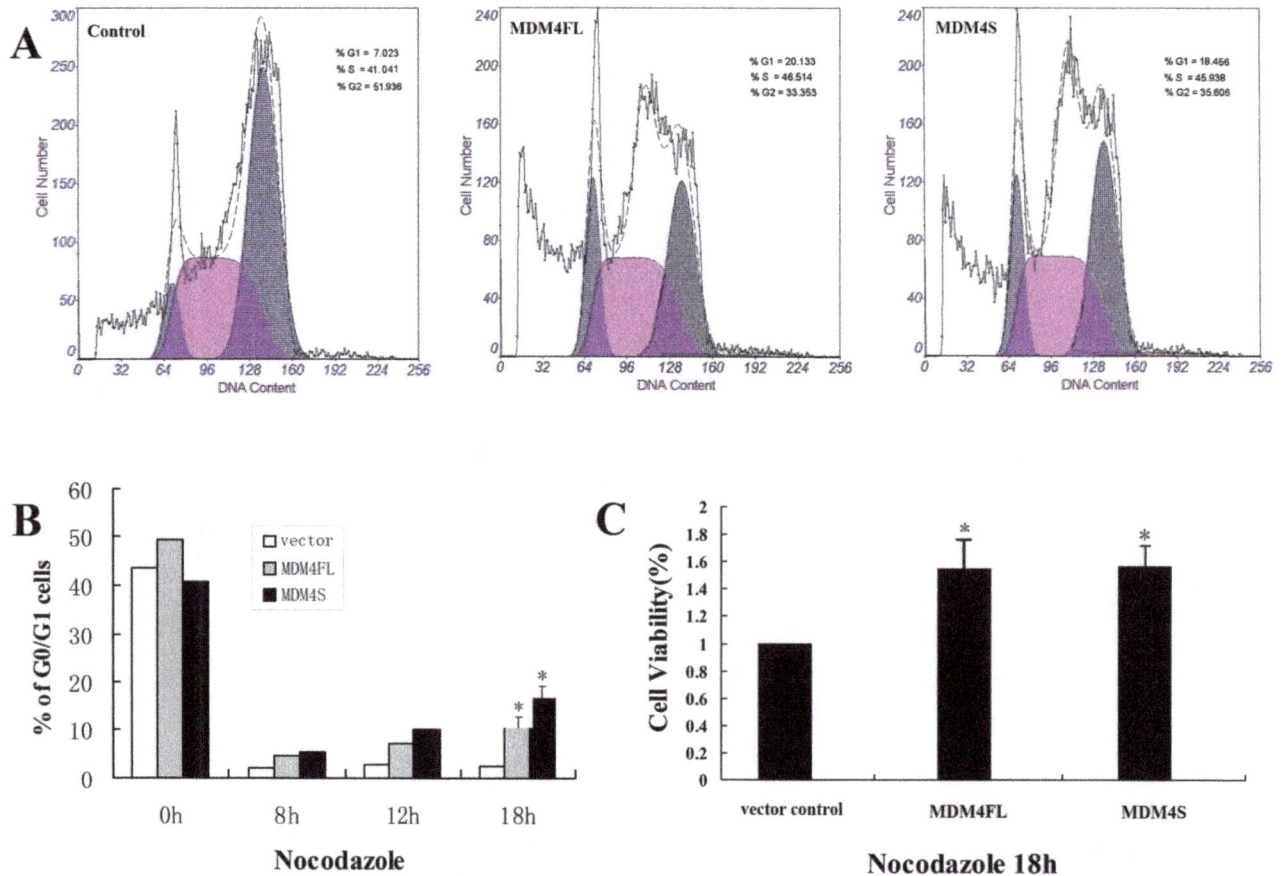

Figure 3. Cell cycle and cell proliferation analysis. A: DNA content detected by flow cytometry in MDM4FL, MDM4S-expressing or control cells. B: The proportion of G0/G1 phase cells at different time points after Nocodazole treatment. C: Cell proliferation assay. The average percentage of proliferating cells was increased in MDM4FL and MDM4S-expressing cells. *$P<0.05$.

pico (Pierce, Rockford, IL, U.S.A) for 1 minute and exposed to film. Images were captured using the Bio-Rad ChemiDoc Imager (Hercules, CA, USA). Data were normalized to GAPDH as a loading control. Primary antibodies used for detection were anti-P53 (1:400, Boster), anti-P21 (1:500, Bioworld Technology Inc, St. Louis, MO, USA), anti-BubR1 (1:500, Bioworld Technology), anti-Securin (1:500, Epitomics Burlingame, CA, USA), and anti-GAPDH (1:500, Santa Cruz Biotechnology, Dallas, TX, USA). Secondary antibodies conjugated to HRP were used at 1:2000 (Santa Cruz).

Mitotic chromosome and karyotype analysis

Chromosomes spreads were prepared from control, MDM4FL, MDM4S- expressing cells, and stained with Giemsa. Images were acquired with Motic high quality scientific grade CCD cameras (Hong Kong). Metaphase cells (75 per sample) from control, MDM4FL and MDM4S expressing pools were scored for chromosomes. Three independent chromosome counts were obtained for each data set, and the rank sum test used to compare chromosome number dispersion. Kruskal-Wallis was used to compare the medians of three ranked variables. All statistical analyses were performed using SPSS 16.0 (IBM, Chicago, IL, USA) and $P<0.05$ was considered significant.

Results

CK-AML patients with wild-type *TP53* correlated with poorer prognosis than NK-AML patients

This study cohort included 15 CK-AML patients with wild-type *TP53*, a male/female ratio of 1.14 (8:7) and median age of 59 years (range, 17–80 years), with seven patients (46.7%) ≥60 years. Two patients (13.3%) had WBC counts greater than 100×10^9/L. One patient was classified with M0, four with M2, five with M4 and five with M5 according to FAB classifications. Karyotype analysis showed monosomy 5 (−5) (n = 2), and monosomy 7 (−7) (n = 4). Of the 15 patients monitored for therapy response and survival, four achieved complete response (CR) and two achieved partial response (PR). The median survival time was 292 days (range, 66–738 days). The clinical characteristics of the 15 CK-AML karyotypes were provided in Table 1. The overall survival (OS) of NK-AML patients was significantly higher than that of CK-AML patients ($P = 0.001$) (Figure 1).

TP53 mutation and deletions were detected by genome PCR sequencing and interphase FISH in 24 CK-AML cases, and 15 CK-AML cases were wild-type *TP53*. In order to rule out other genes mutation associated with poor prognosis of CK-AML, we detected RUNX1 mutations in 15 CK-AML patients and *FLT3-ITD* mutation in 131 *de novo* AML cases (15 patients with wild-type *TP53* and 116 NK-AML patients.). Among the 15 CK-AML

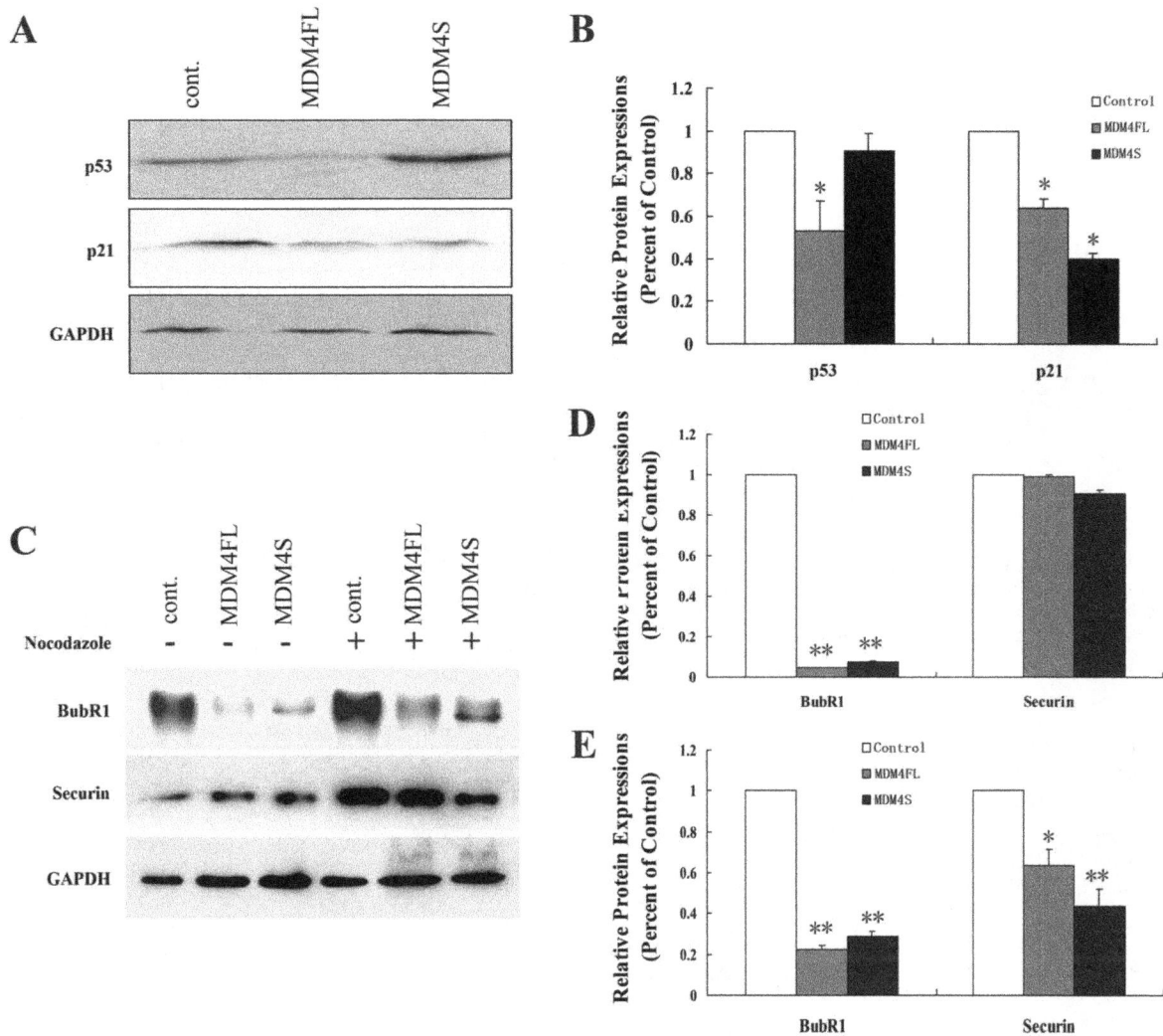

Figure 4. Dysregulation of p53 pathway and spindle checkpoint proteins are reduced in MDM4FL or MDM4S-expressing cells. A: Western blot analysis of p53 and p21 levels in control, MDM4FL, and MDM4S-expressing cells. B: Quantification of p53 and p21 expression levels in different cell groups. Levels were normalized against protein levels in control cells. * $P<0.05$. C: Western blot analysis of BubR1 and Securin in control, MDM4FL and MDM4S-expressing cells treated with 0.025% DMSO (−) or 1 μg/ml nocodazole (+) for 18 hours. D: BubR1 and Securin expression levels following treatment with 0.025% DMSO. E: BubR1 and Securin expression levels following treatment with 1 μg/ml Nocodazole. * $P<0.05$, ** $P<0.01$. Immunoblot for GAPDH confirms relative protein loading.

patients, no *RUNX1* mutations were detected. The positive rates of *FLT3-ITD* in CK-AML and NK-AML were 20% and 23.2%, there was no significant difference between the two groups. (*P>* 0.05).

The relative expression levels of *MDM4S* and *MDM4FL* were higher in CK-AML than in NK-AML

MDM4FL and *MDM4S* mRNA expression levels in CK-AML and NK-AML patients were assessed by real-time RT-PCR. The results indicated that normalized *MDM4FL* levels were 5.82 (1.67–20.28), while *MDM4S* levels were 22.25 (2.42–204.51). Both increased in CK-AML patients, with *MDM4S* showing a more notable increase (Table 2). The melting curve showed a single peak, suggesting a specific of amplified product (Fig. 2).

The metaphase arrest was reduced and cell proliferation activity increased in MDM4-expressing cells

HepG2 cells stably expressing MDM4FL, MDM4S or vector control were cultured overnight and 0.1 μg/ml Nocodazole added the following day and incubated for 18 hours. The percentage of M phase for control, MDM4FL and MDM4S-expressing cells were 51.94%, 33.35% and 35.61%, respectively. Compared with the control, there were fewer M phase cells in MDM4FL and MDM4S-expressing cells (*P<0.05*) (Fig.3A). We next examined the percentage of G0/G1 at different time points after Nocodazole treatment. Before Nocodazole treatment, the percentage of G0/G1 cells in all three lines was approximately 40–60%. Following Nocodazole treatment for 8 h, the percentage of G0/G1 cells in all three cell lines decreased sharply, and then gradually increased with prolonged treatment. At 18 h, the percentages of G0/G1 in MDM4FL and MDM4S-expressing cells were higher than that in control cells (*P<0.05*) (Fig. 3B). Finally, we examined cell

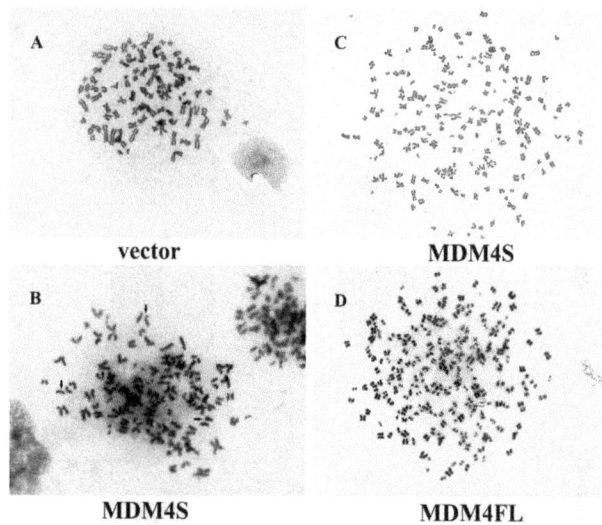

Figure 5. Prometaphase and mitotic of MDM4FL and MDM4S-expressing cells. A: Chromosome spread of a prometaphase vector control cell. B: Premature sister chromatid separation in an MDM4S prometaphase cell (indicated by arrows). C: Polyploidy in a MDM4S cell. D: Endoreduplication of a MDM4FL cell.

proliferation activity using MTT assay after 18 hours of Nocodazole treatment. The proliferation activities were 0.807 ± 0.071, 1.230 ± 0.082 and 1.253 ± 0.087 in control, MDM4FL, and MDM4S-expressing cells, respectively. Compared with the control, the average percentage of proliferating cells increased in MDM4FL and MDM4S-expressing cells ($P<0.05$) (Fig. 3C).

p21 expression levels decreased in MDM4-expressing cells

To explore whether MDM4 overexpression inhibited the activity of P53 pathway, p53 and p21 expression levels were

examined in the overexpressed MDM4 cell model. Our data showed that compared with control, p53 expression level decreased in MDM4FL-expressing cells ($P<0.05$), but it did not decline significantly in MDM4S-expressing cells ($P>0.05$). However, the p21 expression levels decreased in both MDM4FL and MDM4S-expressing cells compared with control ($P<0.01$) (Fig.4A–B).

BubR1 and Securin expression levels decreased in MDM4-expressing cells

The spindle checkpoint proteins, BubR1 and Securin, were assessed by western blot in control, MDM4FL or MDM4S-expressing cells. The results showed that the expression levels of BubR1 and Securin in MDM4FL and MDM4S-expressing cells decreased following Nocodazole treatment. However, control cells exhibited increased Securin levels, consistent with previous reports [14] that APC activity is required to destabilize Securin (Fig.4C–E).

Polyploidy and aneuploidy in MDM4FL and MDM4S-expressing cells

We then monitored chromosome number, premature sister chromatid separation and polyploidy or endoreduplication in control, MDM4FL and MDM4S-expressing cells. Karyotype analysis showed that prematurely dissociated sister chromatids prior to anaphase, polyploidy or endoreduplication were observed in MDM4FL or MDM4S-expressing cells, but not in control cells. (Fig. 5). Chromosome number data are expressed as medians (25th and 75th percentile). The median chromosome numbers were 81(52, 94) (range 45–120), 102 (86, 108) (range 45–284), and 100 (73, 102) (range 26–206) for control, MDM4FL and MDM4S-expressing cells, respectively (Kruskal-Wallis evaluation, $P<0.05$). Therefore, we conclude that at least one of these chromosome numbers had a different ranking distribution relative to the others. Boxplot analysis suggests that the MDM4S and MDM4FL cells most likely have different distributions from control cells. The chromosome numbers of each group reflects the range of chromosome numbers for MDM4S and MDM4FL, which were

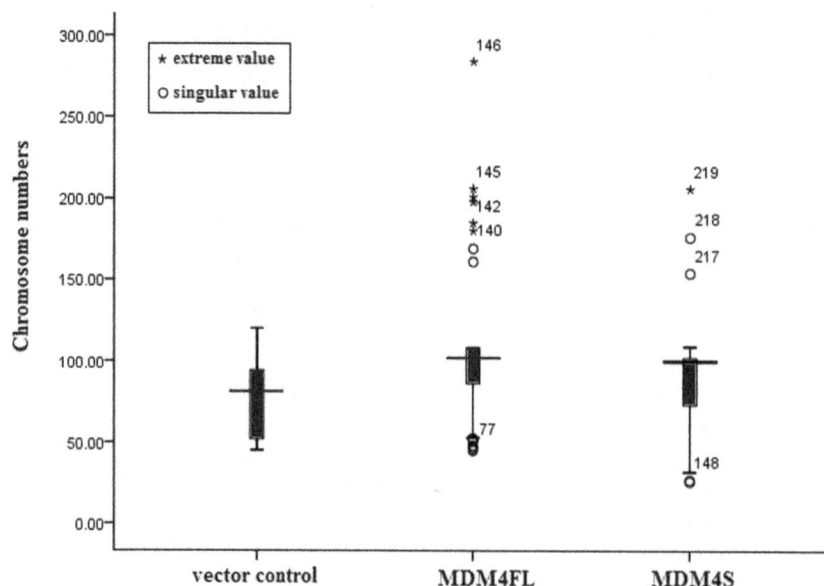

Figure 6. Boxplot reflecting the central tendency and dispersion tendency of the chromosome numbers of each group. * singular values, °extreme values.

much more diverse. There were several singular and outlier values in MDM4FL or MDM4S-expressing cells, however they were not found in control cells (Fig. 6).

Discussion

About 70% of CK-AML cases contain p53 mutations, and are often associated with poor prognosis [4,5]. Cell cycle regulation is closely related to the transcriptional activation of p53. Several studies have shown that Nocodazole, a spindle inhibitor, when applied to p53$-/-$ mouse fibroblasts, become polyploidy because of endoreduplication. This suggests an important role for p53 in regulating spindle checkpoint in mice [15–17]. p53 dysfunction leads to decreased p21 expression and a weakened spindle checkpoint. A cell with a chromosome aberration and with a weakened spindle checkpoint will continue to proliferate and exhibit aneuploidy or complex karyotype [18]. In this study, we ruled out mutations of some genes related to poor prognosis of CK-AML, including *RUNX1* [19], and *FLT3-ITD* in 15 CK-AML patients lacking *TP53* mutation. These results implied that there might be other important molecular events involved in the leukemogenic mechanisms that occur in CK-AML patients with wild-type *TP53*.

MDM4 is a negative regulation factor of p53, which exerts its effect by binding p53. *MDM4* has several transcript variants [20], with the *MDM4S* transcript obtained by exon 6 deletion, resulting in a truncated protein containing only the p53 binding domain. It has been reported that MDM4S affinity to p53 is approximately 10-fold higher than that of MDM4FL [21]. High levels of *MDM4S* mRNA expression are associated with short treatment free survival [11] and its overexpression was significantly correlated with an unfavorable prognosis in soft-tissue sarcoma patients [10,22]. Our results showed that *MDM4FL* and *MDM4S* expression levels were elevated in CK-AML patients relative to NK-AML patients. We thus speculate that *MDM4* overexpression may be involved in the leukemogenic mechanisms of CK-AML patients with wild-type *TP53*.

To prove the above speculation, we tried to find a leukemic cell line with wild-type p53 in the catalog of the American type culture collection (ATCC). However, all myeloid cell lines either contain mutant p53 or do not express p53 [23–26]. Taking into account the purpose of our experiments is just to investigate if MDM4 overexpression would influence p53 signal pathway in cancer cell with normal p53, we decided to choose other appropriate cancer cell to continue the study. The HepG2 cell line expresses wild-type p53, normal levels of MDM4, and low levels of MDM4S [27]. These characteristics were appropriate for our experiments. MDM4-expressing HepG2 cells displayed a reduced mitotic index following Nocodazole treatment, suggesting a failure in a subset of cells to undergo mitotic arrest through a functional spindle checkpoint. Additionally, MDM4-expressing cells had reduced levels of p21, an important effector molecule downstream of p53. This indicates that overexpression of MDM4FL or MDM4S inhibits p53 signaling pathway.

BubR1 is a critical component of the spindle checkpoint. BubR1 performs several roles during mitosis and ensures accurate chromosome separation [28]. Securin is one of the main substrates of APC/C [29]. The expression levels of BubR1 and Securin decreased in MDM4-expressing cells following Nocodazole treatment, suggesting that APC may be active in these cells because of a spindle checkpoint decline. However, following Nocodazole treatment, control cells had increased levels of Securin. These results indicate proper functioning of the spindle checkpoint and an inactive APC in control cells. Cells that continue to proliferate with an attenuated spindle checkpoint should missegregate chromosomes and become aneuploid. Previous reports indicate that Securin loss can lead to karyotype changes in cell lines [30]. Therefore, it is possible that the spindle checkpoint and APC activity, through BubR1 and Securin downregulation, contribute to the attenuation of cell cycle checkpoints.

Suppression BubR1 results in a dysfunction spindle checkpoint and leads to abnormal mitosis and aneuploidy [31]. CK-AML patients have been defined as the presence of at least five clonal aberrations or at least three abnormalities in the absence of t(8; 21), inv(16)/t(16; 16), and t(15; 17) [32]. Complex karyotype, like aneuploidy, may result from chromosome missegregation during mitosis. Our results suggest that MDM4 overexpression may cause aneuploid or polyploidy. We have not observed the association between specific chromosomal abnormalities and MDM4 overexpression because we only have 15 CK-AML patients with wild-type *TP53*. Although it is not well known if there is a causal relationship between MDM4 overexpression and aneuploidy, these date raise the possibility that MDM4 overexpression plays a role in CK-AML pathogenesis. It will be necessary to evaluate more patients and to further explore the molecular mechanisms of MDM4 overexpression and to develop targeted therapies for CK-AML patients. At least in theory, restoration of p53 function is a potential therapeutic approach in leukemia. Bista M et al [33] reported that SJ-172550, an inhibitor of the interaction between MDM4 and p53, may be a new option for the treatment of CK-AML. Their results suggest that the combination of a MDM4 inhibitor and traditional chemotherapy for refractory CK-AML may be worth evaluating.

MDM4 expression levels were elevated in CK-AML patients relative to NK-AML patients, MDM4-overexpressing HepG2 cell lines had a reduced mitotic index, reduced p21, BubR1 or Securin expression levels following Nocodazole treatment, and MDM4-overexpressing cells were aneuploidy or polyploidy. Based on data presented in this study, we speculate that the leukemogenic mechanism of CK-AML without *TP53* alternations is partly due to the p53 signaling pathway inhibited and the spindle checkpoint weakened by MDM4 overexpression. MDM4 may be a novel therapeutic target in the treatment of CK-AML patients with wild-type *TP53*.

Author Contributions

Conceived and designed the experiments: LL HWW. Performed the experiments: LL FGR HXG XJW SYY. Analyzed the data: YHT ZFX XHC. Contributed reagents/materials/analysis tools: YC GXL. Wrote the paper: LL HWW.

References

1. Bowen D, Groves MJ, Burnett AK, Patel Y, Allen C, et al. (2009) TP53 gene mutation is frequent in patients with acute myeloid leukemia and complex karyotype, and is associated with very poor prognosis. Leukemia 23: 203–206.
2. Perrot A, Luquet I, Pigneux A, Mugneret F, Delaunay J, et al. (2011) Dismal prognostic value of monosomal karyotype in elderly patients with acute myeloid leukemia: A GOELAMS study of 186 patients with unfavorable cytogenetic abnormalities. Blood 118: 679–685.
3. Yurlova L, Derks M, Buchfellner A, Hickson I, Janssen M, et al. (2014) The Fluorescent Two-Hybrid Assay to Screen for Protein-Protein Interaction Inhibitors in Live Cells: Targeting the Interaction of p53 with Mdm2 and Mdm4. J Biomol Screen 19: 516–525
4. Rücker FG, Schlenk RF, Bullinger L, Kayser S, Teleanu V, et al. (2012) TP53 alterations in acute myeloid leukemia with complex karyotype correlate with

specific copy number alterations, monosomal karyotype, and dismal outcome. Blood 119: 2114–2121.

5. Haferlach C, Dicker F, Herholz H, Schnittger S, Kern W, et al. (2008) Mutations of the TP53 gene in acute myeloid leukemia are strongly associated with a complex aberrant karyotype. Leukemia 22: 1539–1541.

6. Baek KH, Shin HJ, Yoo JK, Cho JH, Choi YH, et al. (2003) p53 deficiency and defective mitotic checkpoint in proliferating T lymphocytes increase chromosomal instability through aberrant exit from mitotic arrest. J Leukoc Biol 73: 850–861.

7. Zhao Z, Zuber J, Diaz-Flores E, Lintault L, Kogan SC, et al. (2010) p53 loss promotes acute myeloid leukemia by enabling aberrant self-renewal. Genes Dev 24: 1389–1402

8. Pei D, Zhang Y, Zheng J (2012) Regulation of p53: a collaboration between Mdm2 and MdmX. Oncotarget 3: 228–235.

9. Rallapalli R, Strachan G, Tuan RS, Hall DJ (2003) Identification of a domain within MDMX-S that is responsible for its high affinity interaction with p53 and high-level expression in mammalian cells. J Cell Biochem 89: 563–575.

10. Lenos K, Grawenda AM, Lodder K, Kuijjer ML, Teunisse AF, et al. (2012) Alternate splicing of the p53 inhibitor HDMX offers a superior pronistic biomarker than p53 mutation in human cancer. Cancer Res 72: 4074–4084.

11. Liu L, Fan L, Fang C, Zou ZJ, Yang S, et al. (2012) S-MDM4 mRNA overexpression indicates a poor prognosis and marks a potential therapeutic target in chronic lymphocytic leukemia. Cancer Sci 103: 2056–2063.

12. Harutyunyan A, Klampfl T, Cazzola M, Kralovics R (2011) p53 lesions in leukemic transformation. N Engl J Med 364: 488–490

13. Meshinchi S, Woods WG, Stirewalt DL, Sweetser DA, Buckley JD, et al. (2001) Prevalence and prognostic significance of Flt3 internal tandem duplication in pediatric acute myeloid leukemia. Blood 97: 89–94.

14. Jallepalli PV, Waizenegger IC, Bunz F, Langer S, Speicher MR, et al. (2001) Securin is required for chromosomal stability in human cells. Cell 105: 445–457.

15. Cross SM, Sanchez CA, Morgan CA, Schimke MK, Ramel S, et al. (1995) A p53-dependent mouse spindle checkpoint. Science 267: 1353–1356.

16. Taylor WR, Stark GR (2001) Regulation of the G2/M transition by p53. Oncogene 20: 1803–1815.

17. Zhi L, Zhang J, Jia Y, Shan S, Li Y, et al. (2011) Effect of G-rich oligonucleotides on the proliferation of leukemia cells and its relationship with p53 expression. Oligonucleotides 21: 21–27.

18. Gogolin S, Batra R, Harder N, Ehemann V, Paffhausen T, et al. (2013) MYCN-mediated over- expression of mitotic spindle regulatory genes and loss of p53–p21 function jointly support the survival of tetraploid neuroblastoma cells. Cancer Lett 331: 35–45.

19. Greif PA, Konstandin NP, Metzeler KH, Herold T, Pasalic Z, et al. (2012) RUNX1 mutations in cytogenetically normal acute myeloid leukemia are associated with a poor prognosis and up-regulation of lymphoid genes. Haematologica 97: 1909–1915.

20. Mancini F, Di Conza G, Moretti F (2009) MDM4 (MDMX) and its transcript variants. Curr Genomics 10: 42–50.

21. Rallapalli R, Strachan G, Cho B, Mercer WE, Hall DJ (1999) A novel MDMX transcript expressed in a variety of transformed cell lines encodes a truncated protein with potent p53 repressive activity. J Biol Chem 274: 8299–8308.

22. Bartel F, Schulz J, Böhnke A, Blümke K, Kappler M, et al. (2005) Significance of HDMX-S (or MDM4) mRNA splice variant overexpression and HDMX gene amplification on primary soft tissue sarcoma prognosis. Int J Cancer 117: 469–475.

23. Lübbert M, Miller CW, Crawford L, Koeffler HP (1988) p53 in chronic myelogenous leukemia. Study of mechanisms of differential expression. J Exp Med 167: 873–886.

24. Danova M, Giordano M, Mazzini G, Riccardi A (1990) Expression of p53 protein during the cell cycle measured by flow cytometry in human leukemia. Leuk Res 14: 417–422.

25. Sugimoto K, Toyoshima H, Sakai R, Miyagawa K, Hagiwara K, et al. (1992) Frequent mutations in the p53 gene in human myeloid leukemia cell lines. Blood 79: 2378–2383.

26. Berglind H, Pawitan Y, Kato S, Ishioka C, Soussi T (2008) Analysis of p53 mutation status in human cancer cell lines: a paradigm for cell line cross-contamination. Cancer Biol Ther 7: 699–708.

27. He M, Zhao M, Shen B, Prise KM, Shao C (2011) Radiation-induced intercellular signaling mediated by cytochrome-c via a p53-dependent pathway in hepatoma cells. Oncogene 30: 1947–1955.

28. Karess RE, Wassmann K, Rahmani Z (2013) New Insights into the Role of BubR1 in Mitosis and Beyond. Int Rev Cell Mol Biol 306: 223–273.

29. Kim S, Yu H (2011) Mutual regulation between the spindle checkpoint and APC/C. Semin Cell Dev Biol 22: 551–558.

30. Jallepalli PV, Waizenegger IC, Bunz F, Langer S, Speicher MR, et al. (2001) Securin is required for chromosomal stability in human cells. Cell 105: 445–457.

31. Ikawa-Yoshida A, Ando K, Oki E, Saeki H, Kumashiro R, et al. (2013) Contribution of BubR1 to oxidative stress-induced aneuploidy in p53-deficient cells. Cancer Med 2: 447–456.

32. Byrd JC, Mrózek K, Dodge RK, Carroll AJ, Edwards CG, et al. (2002) Pretreatment cytogenetic abnormalities are predictive of induction success cumulative incidence of relapse, and overall survival in adult patients with de novo acute myeloid leukemia: results from Cancer and Leukemia Group B (CALGB 8461). Blood 100: 4325–4336.

33. Bista M, Smithson D, Pecak A, Salinas G, Pustelny K, et al. (2012) On the mechanism of action of SJ-172550 in inhibiting the interaction of MDM4 and p53. PLoS One 7: e37518.

Permissions

List of Contributors

Jie Jin, Chao Hu, Mengxia Yu, Feifei Chen, Li Ye, Xiufeng Yin and Hongyan Tong
Department of Hematology, the First Affiliated Hospital of Zhejiang University, Hangzhou, People's Republic of China
Institute of Hematology, Zhejiang University School of Medicine, Hangzhou, People's Republic of China

Zhengping Zhuang
Surgical Neurology Branch, National Institute of Neurological Disorders and Stroke, National Institutes of Health, Bethesda, Maryland, United States of America

Jahangir Abdi, Johan Garssen and Frank A. Redegeld
Division of Pharmacology, Utrecht Institute for Pharmaceutical Sciences, Faculty of Science, Utrecht University, Utrecht, the Netherlands

Tuna Mutis
Department of Clinical Chemistry and Hematology, University Medical Center Utrecht, Utrecht, the Netherlands

Ruihua Mi, Jing Ding, Xianwei Wang, Jieying Hu, Ruihua Fan, Xudong Wei and Yongping Song
Henan Institute of Hematology, Affiliated Tumor Hospital of Zhengzhou University, Zhengzhou, Henan, China

Xiaodong Lyu
Henan Institute of Hematology, Affiliated Tumor Hospital of Zhengzhou University, Zhengzhou, Henan, China
Division of Molecular Pathology, Department of Pathology, University of Maryland School of Medicine, Baltimore, Maryland, United States of America

Yaping Xin
Department of Endocrinology and Metabolic Diseases, the Second Affiliated Hospital of Zhengzhou University, Zhengzhou, Henan, China

Richard Y. Zhao
Division of Molecular Pathology, Department of Pathology, University of Maryland School of Medicine, Baltimore, Maryland, United States of America

Hsiu-Hsia Lin, Shang-Ju Wu, Wen-Hui Chuang and Shang-Yi Huang
Department of Internal Medicine, National Taiwan University Hospital, Taipei, Taiwan

Shiaw-Min Hwang and Lee-Feng Hsu
Bioresource Collection and Research Center, Food Industry Research and Development Institute, Hsinchu, Taiwan

Yi-Hua Liao and Yi-Shuan Sheen
Department of Dermatology, National Taiwan University Hospital, Taipei, Taiwan

Heng Zhang, Yan Zhou, Yaoyao Rui, Yaping Wang, Liuchen Rong and Yongjun Fang
Department of Hematology and Oncology, Nanjing Children's Hospital Affiliated to Nanjing Medical University, Nanjing, China

Jie Li
Department of Hematology and Oncology, Soochow Children's Hospital Affiliated to Soochow University, Suzhou, China

Meilin Wang, Na Tong and Zhengdong Zhang
Department of Molecular and Genetic Toxicology, Cancer Center of Nanjing Medical University, Nanjing, China

Jing Chen
Department of Hematology and Oncology, Shanghai Children's Medical Center Affiliated to Shanghai, Jiao Tong University, Shanghai, China

Pamela Thompson
Paediatric and Familial Cancer Research Group, Institute of Cancer Sciences, University of Manchester, St Mary's Hospital, Manchester, United Kingdom

Patricia Buffler and Anand Chokkalingam
School of Public Health, University of California, Berkeley, Berkeley, California, United States of America

Kevin Urayama
School of Public Health, University of California, Berkeley, Berkeley, California, United States of America
Department of Human Genetics and Disease Diversity, Tokyo Medical and Dental University, Tokyo, Japan

Jie Zheng
School of Computer Engineering, Nanyang Technological University, Singapore
Genome Institute of Singapore, A STAR (Agency for Science, Technology, and Research), Biopolis, Singapore

Peng Yang
Data Analytics Department, Institute for Infocomm Research, A*STAR, Singapore

Matt Ford
Research Computing Services, Faculty of Medical and Human Sciences, University of Manchester, Manchester, United Kingdom

Tracy Lightfoot
University of York, Heslington, York, United Kingdom

Malcolm Taylor
Independent Researcher, Handforth, Cheshire, United Kingdom

Danjie Jiang, Qingxiao Hong, Yusheng Shen, Yan Xu, Huangkai Zhu, Yirun Li, Chunjing Xu and Shiwei Duan
Zhejiang Provincial Key Laboratory of Pathophysiology, School of Medicine, Ningbo University, Ningbo, Zhejiang, China

Guifang Ouyang
Department of Hematology, Ningbo First Hospital, Ningbo, Zhejiang, China

Nicole Bäumer, Annika Krause, Stephanie Lettermann, Georg Evers, Sebastian Bäumer and Wolfgang E. Berdel
Department of Medicine, Hematology/Oncology, University of Muenster, Muenster, Germany

Lara Tickenbrock
Department of Medicine, Hematology/Oncology, University of Muenster, Muenster, Germany
Hochschule Hamm-Lippstadt, University of Applied Science, Hamm, Germany

Carsten Müller-Tidow
Department of Medicine, Hematology/Oncology, University of Muenster, Muenster, Germany
Interdisciplinary Center for Clinical Research IZKF, University of Muenster, Muenster, Germany
Dept. of Medicine IV, Hematology and Oncology, University of Halle, Halle, Germany

Gabriele Köhler
Gerhard Domagk Institute for Pathology, University of Muenster, Muenster, Germany

Antje Hascher
Hochschule Hamm-Lippstadt, University of Applied Science, Hamm, Germany

Vít Procházka and Tomáš Papajík
Department of Hemato-Oncology, Faculty of Medicine and Dentistry, Palacky´ University, Olomouc, Czech Republic

Robert Pytlík and Marek Trněný
First Internal Department, Charles University General Hospital, Prague, Czech Republic,

Andrea Janíková and David Šálek
Department of Internal Medicine-Hematooncology, University Hospital Brno, and Faculty of Medicine, Masaryk University, Brno, Czech Republic

David Belada
Second Department of Medicine, Department of Hematology, University Hospital and Faculty of Medicine, Hradec Králové, Czech Republic

Vít Campr
Department of Pathology and Molecular Medicine, Charles University, and Second Medical School and Faculty Hospital in Motol, Prague, Czech Republic

Tomáš Fürst and Jana Furstova
Department of Mathematical Analysis and Applications of Mathematics, Faculty of Science, Palacký University, Olomouc, Czech Republic

King Yiu Lee, Kathy Yuen Yee Chan, Pak Cheung Ng, Chi Kong Li, Kam Tong Leung and Karen Li
Department of Paediatrics, The Chinese University of Hong Kong, Hong Kong

Kam Sze Tsang
Department of Anatomical and Cellular Pathology, The Chinese University of Hong Kong, Hong Kong

Yang Chao Chen and Hsiang-fu Kung
Centre for Emerging Infectious Diseases, Department of Medicine and Therapeutics, The Chinese University of Hong Kong, Hong Kong

Inés Gómez-Seguí, Esperanza Such, Irene Luna, María López-Pavía, Mariam Ibáñez, Eva Villamón, Carmen Alonso, Iván Martín, Pau Montesinos, Carolina Cañigral, Blanca Boluda and Claudia Salazar
Hematology Department, Hospital Universitari i Politècnic La Fe, Valencia, Spain

Jose Cervera
Hematology Department, Hospital Universitari i Politècnic La Fe, Valencia, Spain
Genetics Unit, Hospital Universitari i Politècnic La Fe, Valencia, Spain

Miguel A. Sanz
Hematology Department, Hospital Universitari i
Politècnic La Fe, Valencia, Spain
Department of Medicine, University of Valencia,
Valencia, Spain

Dolors Sánchez-Izquierdo
Array's Unit. Instituto Investigación Sanitaria
Fundación La Fe, Valencia, Spain

**Eva Barragán, Marta Llop, Sandra Dolz and Óscar
Fuster**
Laboratory of Molecular Biology, Department of
Clinical Chemistry, University Hospital La Fe,
Valencia, Spain

Pei-Ching Hsiao
School of Medicine, Chung Shan Medical University,
Taichung, Taiwan
Department of Internal Medicine, Chung Shan Medical
University Hospital, Taichung, Taiwan

Ying-Erh Chou and Hui-Yu Chen
Institute of Medicine, Chung Shan Medical University,
Taichung, Taiwan

Shun-Fa Yang
Institute of Medicine, Chung Shan Medical University,
Taichung, Taiwan
Department of Medical Research, Chung Shan Medical
University Hospital, Taichung, Taiwan

Peng Tan
Graduate Institute of Clinical Medicine, Taipei Medical
University, Taipei, Taiwan,

Ming-Hsien Chien
Graduate Institute of Clinical Medicine, Taipei Medical
University, Taipei, Taiwan,
Wan Fang Hospital, Taipei Medical University, Taipei,
Taiwan

Wei-Jiunn Lee and Liang-Ming Lee
Department of Urology, Wan Fang Hospital, Taipei
Medical University, Taipei, Taiwan

Jyh-Ming Chow
Department of Internal Medicine, Wan Fang Hospital,
Taipei Medical University, Taipei, Taiwan

Chien-Huang Lin
Graduate Institute of Medical Sciences, Taipei Medical
University, Taipei, Taiwan

**Jiaoyang Luo, Yichen Hu, Weijun Kong and Meihua
Yang**
Institute of Medicinal Plant Development, Chinese
Academy of Medical Sciences and Peking Union
Medical College, Beijing, P.R. China

**Justin Rendleman, Christina Adaniel, Yongzhao
Shao and Tomas Kirchhoff**
NYU School of Medicine, New York University, New
York, New York, United States of America

**Yevgeniy Antipin, Boris Reva, Jennifer A. Przybylo,
Ana Dutra-Clarke, Nichole Hansen, Adriana Heguy,
Kety Huberman, Laetitia Borsu, Chris Sander,
Andrew Zelenetz, Robert J. Klein, Mortimer Lacher,
Joseph Vijai and Kenneth Offit**
Memorial Sloan-Kettering Cancer Center, New York,
New York, United States of America

Ora Paltiel and Dina Ben-Yehuda
Hadassah-Hebrew University Medical Center,
Jerusalem, Israel

Jennifer R. Brown and Arnold S. Freedman
Dana Farber Cancer Center, Harvard University,
Boston, Massachusetts, United States of America

Xiaotong Hu
Biomedical Research Center, Sir Run Run Shaw
Hospital, Zhejiang University and Key Laboratory of
Biotherapy of Zhejiang Province, Hangzhou, China

**Han Xuan, Huaping Du, Hao Jiang and Jinwen
Huang**
Department of Hematology, Sir Run Run Shaw
Hospital, Zhejiang University, Hangzhou, China

**Ye Yao, Wei Wei, Xiaohui Deng, Linjun Chen, Liyuan
Ma and Siguo Hao**
Department of Hematology, Xinhua Hospital Affiliated
to Shanghai Jiaotong University School of Medicine,
Shanghai, China

Chun Wang and Chang Shen
Department of Hematology, The First People's
Hospital of Shanghai Affiliated to Shanghai Jiaotong
University, Shanghai, China

**Eahsan Rasul, Daniel Salamon, Noemi Nagy,
Benjamin Leveau, George Klein and Eva Klein**
Department of Microbiology, Tumor and Cell Biology
(MTC), Karolinska Instititet, Stockholm, Sweden

Ferenc Banati and Kalman Szenthe
RT-Europe Nonprofit Research Ltd, Mosonmagyaróvár,
Hungary

Anita Koroknai
Microbiological Research Group, National Center for
Epidemiology, Budapest, Hungary

Janos Minarovits
Microbiological Research Group, National Center for
Epidemiology, Budapest, Hungary

University of Szeged, Faculty of Dentistry, Department of Oral Biology and Experimental Dental Research, Szeged, Hungary

Elias Hallack Atta, Danielli Cristina Muniz de Oliveira, Luis Fernando Bouzas and Eliana Abdelhay
CEMO, Instituto Nacional de Câncer, Rio de Janeiro, Brazil

Márcio Nucci
University Hospital, Universidade Federal do Rio de Janeiro, Rio de Janeiro, Brazil

Ashish Narayan Masurekar and Catriona A. Parker
Children's Cancer Group, Centre for Paediatric, Teenage and Young Adult Cancer, Institute of Cancer, Manchester Academic Health Science Centre, Central Manchester University Hospitals Foundation Trust, The University of Manchester, Manchester, United Kingdom

Milensu Shanyinde and Sharon B. Love
Centre for Statistics in Medicine, University of Oxford, Oxford, United Kingdom

Anthony V. Moorman
Leukaemia Research Cytogenetics Group, Northern Institute for Cancer Research, Newcastle University, Newcastle upon Tyne, United Kingdom

Jeremy P. Hancock
Bristol Genetics Laboratory, Southmead Hospital, Bristol, United Kingdom

Rosemary Sutton
Children's Cancer Institute Australia, Lowy Cancer Research Centre, University of New South Wales, Sydney, Australia

Philip J. Ancliff and Nicholas J. Goulden
Great Ormond Street Hospital, London, United Kingdom

Mary Morgan
Child Oncology and Haematology Centre, Southampton General Hospital, Southampton, United Kingdom

Chris Fraser
Queensland Children's Cancer Centre, Brisbane, Australia

Peter M. Hoogerbrugge
Childrens Hospital, Radboud University Nijmegen Medical Centre, Nijmegen, The Netherlands Dutch Childhood Oncology Group, The Hague, The Netherlands

Tamas Revesz
Department of Haematology-Oncology, SA Pathology at Women's and Children's Hospital and University of Adelaide, Adelaide, Australia

Philip J. Darbyshire
Department of Haematology, Birmingham Children's Hospital, Birmingham, United Kingdom

Shekhar Krishnan and Vaskar Saha
Paediatric Oncology, Tata Translational Cancer Research Centre, Kolkata, India

Rie Nakamoto-Matsubara and Terukazu Enami
Department of Hematology, Graduate School of Comprehensive Human Sciences, University of Tsukuba, Tsukuba, Ibaraki, Japan

Mamiko Sakata-Yanagimoto, Hideharu Muto, Naoshi Obara, Naoki Kurita and Yasuhisa Yokoyama
Department of Hematology, Graduate School of Comprehensive Human Sciences, University of Tsukuba, Tsukuba, Ibaraki, Japan
Department of Hematology, Faculty of Medicine, University of Tsukuba, Tsukuba, Ibaraki, Japan
Department of Hematology, University of Tsukuba Hospital, Tsukuba, Ibaraki, Japan

Takayasu Kato and Shigeru Chiba
Department of Hematology, Graduate School of Comprehensive Human Sciences, University of Tsukuba, Tsukuba, Ibaraki, Japan
Department of Hematology, Faculty of Medicine, University of Tsukuba, Tsukuba, Ibaraki, Japan
Department of Hematology, University of Tsukuba Hospital, Tsukuba, Ibaraki, Japan
Life Science Center, Tsukuba Advanced Research Center, University of Tsukuba, Tsukuba, Ibaraki, Japan

Seiichi Shimizu
Department of Hematology, University of Tsukuba Hospital, Tsukuba, Ibaraki, Japan
Department of Hematology, Tsuchiura Kyodo General Hospital, Tsuchiura, Ibaraki, Japan

Takuya Komeno
Department of Hematology, University of Tsukuba Hospital, Tsukuba, Ibaraki, Japan
Department of Hematology, Mito Medical Center, National Hospital Organization, Ibaraki-machi, Ibaraki, Japan

Kenichi Yoshida, Yusuke Shiozawa, Masashi Sanada and Seishi Ogawa
Department of Pathology and Tumor Biology, Graduate School of Medicine, Kyoto University, Sakyo-ku, Kyoto, Japan

Shintaro Yanagimoto
Division for Health Service Promotion, The University of Tokyo, Bunkyo-ku, Tokyo, Japan

Tohru Nanmoku
Department of Clinical Laboratory, University of Tsukuba Hospital, Tsukuba, Ibaraki, Japan

Kaishi Satomi
Department of Pathology, University of Tsukuba Hospital, Tsukuba, Ibaraki, Japan

Koji Izutsu
Department of Hematology, Toranomon Hospital, Minato-ku, Tokyo, Japan
Okinaka Memorial Institute for Medical Research, Minato-ku, Tokyo, Japan

Yasunori Ota
Department of Pathology, Toranomon Hospital, Minato-ku, Tokyo, Japan

Yuji Sato
Department of Hematology, Tsukuba Memorial Hospital, Tsukuba, Ibaraki, Japan

Takayoshi Ito
Department of Hematology, JA Toride Medical Center, Toride, Ibaraki, Japan

Issay Kitabayashi
Division of Hematological Malignancy, National Cancer Center Research Institute, Chuo-ku, Tokyo, Japan

Kengo Takeuchi
Pathology Project for Molecular Targets, The Cancer Institute, Japanese Foundation for Cancer Research, Koto-ku, Tokyo, Japan

Naoya Nakamura
Department of Pathology, Tokai University School of Medicine, Isehara, Kanagawa, Japan

Hosadurga K. Keerthy and Basappa
Laboratory of Chemical Biology, Department of Chemistry, Bangalore University, Bangalore, India

Manoj Garg, Vikas Madan and Deepika Kanojia
Genomic Oncology Programme, Cancer Science Institute of Singapore, National University of Singapore, Singapore, Singapore

H. Phillip Koeffler
Genomic Oncology Programme, Cancer Science Institute of Singapore, National University of Singapore, Singapore, Singapore
Division of Hematology and Oncology, Cedar-Sinai Medical Centre, Los Angeles, California, United States of America

Chakrabhavi D. Mohan, Shivananju Nanjundaswamy and Kanchugarakoppal S. Rangappa
Department of Studies in Chemistry, University of Mysore, Manasagangotri, Mysore, India

Rangappa Shobith
Interdisciplinary Research Group of Infectious Diseases, Singapore-MIT Alliance for Research and Technology Centre (SMART), Singapore, Singapore

Daniel J. Mason and Andreas Bender
Unilever Centre for Molecular Science Informatics, Department of Chemistry, University of Cambridge, Cambridge, United Kingdom

Michaela Reagan, Yong Zhang, Yuji Mishima, Siobhan Glavey, Salomon Manier, Antonio Sacco, Aldo M. Roccaro and Irene M. Ghobrial
Department of Medical Oncology, Dana-Farber Cancer Institute, Harvard Medical School, Boston, Massachusetts, United States of America

Wenjing Zhang
Department of Medical Oncology, Dana-Farber Cancer Institute, Harvard Medical School, Boston, Massachusetts, United States of America
Nanfang Hospital, Southern Medical University, Guangzhou, China

Yu Zhang
Department of Medical Oncology, Dana-Farber Cancer Institute, Harvard Medical School, Boston, Massachusetts, United States of America
The First People's Hospital of Yunnan Province, Kunming University of Science and Technology, Kunming, China

Xavier Leleu
Department of Medical Oncology, Dana-Farber Cancer Institute, Harvard Medical School, Boston, Massachusetts, United States of America
Department of Hematology, Hopital Claude Huriez, Hospital of Lille (CHRU), Lille, France

Bo Jiang
Nanfang Hospital, Southern Medical University, Guangzhou, China

Yaoyu E. Wang
Center for Cancer Computational Biology, Dana-Farber Cancer Institute, Harvard Medical School, Boston, Massachusetts, United States of America

Michael C. R. Alavanja, Jonathan N. Hofmann, Kathryn H. Barry, Stella Koutros, Gabriella Andreotti, Jay H. Lubin, Aaron Blair and Laura E. Beane Freeman
Division of Cancer Epidemiology and Genetics, National Cancer Institute, Rockville, Maryland, United States of America

Charles F. Lynch
College of Public Health, University of Iowa, Iowa City, Iowa, United States of America

Cynthia J. Hines
National Institute for Occupational Safety and Health, Cincinnati, Ohio, United States of America

Joseph Barker and Dennis W. Buckman
IMS, Inc, Calverton, Maryland, United States of America

Kent Thomas
National Exposure Research Laboratory, U.S. Environmental Protection Agency, Research Triangle Park, North Carolina, United States of America

Dale P. Sandler and Jane A. Hoppin
Epidemiology Branch, National Institute for Environmental Health Sciences, Research Triangle Park, North Carolina, United States of America

Miho Sasaki, Misa Sumi, Sato Eida, Ikuo Katayama, Yuka Hotokezaka and Takashi Nakamura
Department of Radiology and Cancer Biology, Nagasaki University School of Dentistry, Nagasaki, Japan

Monique Terwijn, Wendelien Zeijlemaker, Angèle Kelder, Arjo P. Rutten, Alexander N. Snel, Willemijn J. Scholten, Sonja Zweegman, Gert J. Ossenkoppele and Gerrit J. Schuurhuis
Department of Hematology, VU University Medical Center, Amsterdam, The Netherlands

Thomas Pabst
Department of Medical Oncology, Inselspital, Bern University Hospital, University of Bern, Bern, Switzerland

Gregor Verhoef
Department of Hematology, University Hospital Leuven, Leuven, Belgium

Bob Löwenberg
Department of Hematology, Erasmus University Medical Center, Rotterdam, The Netherlands

Jérémie Gaudichon, Francesco Milano, Julie Cahu and Brigitte Sola
Equipe Associée 4652, Université de Caen, Normandie Univ, Caen, France

Lætitia DaCosta and Jack-Michel Renoir
Institut National de la Santé et de la Recherche Médicale U749, Institut Gustave Roussy, Villejuif, France

Anton C. Martens
Department of Immunology, University Medical Center Utrecht, Utrecht, The Netherlands

Yanhong Tan, Xiuhua Chen, Zhifang Xu, Siyao Yang, Fanggang Ren, Xiaojuan Wang, Yi Chen, Guoxia Li and Hongwei Wang
Department of Hematology, the Second Hospital of Shanxi Medical University, Taiyuan, Shanxi, P.R. China

Li Li
Department of Hematology, the Second Hospital of Shanxi Medical University, Taiyuan, Shanxi, P.R. China
Department of biology, School of Basic Medicine, Shanxi Medical University, Taiyuan, Shanxi, P.R. China

Haixiu Guo
Department of biology, School of Basic Medicine, Shanxi Medical University, Taiyuan, Shanxi, P.R. China

Index

www.ingramcontent.com/pod-product-compliance
Lightning Source LLC
Chambersburg PA
CBHW061331190326
41458CB00011B/3963